Educational Review Manual in General Surgery

8th Edition – 2009

Edited by

Samuel Eric Wilson, MD
Professor, Department of Surgery and Associate Dean
University of California, Irvine School of Medicine, Orange, CA

Editorial Assistant

Khushboo Kaushal, BS
University of California, San Diego School of Medicine

Ortho-McNeil® had no influence on the content of this publication which may include information about off-label uses for Ortho-McNeil® products. Please see full Prescribing Information for Ortho-McNeil® products.

CCGMP
Castle Connolly Graduate Medical Publishing

Castle Connolly Graduate Medical Publishing, Ltd.
17 Battery Place, Suite 643 • New York, NY 10004 • Tel: 212.644.9696 • Fax: 646.827.6443 • www.ccgmp.com • e-mail: info@ccgmp.com

Castle Connolly Graduate Medical Publishing, Ltd, publishes review manuals to assist residents and fellows in preparing for board certification exams.

NOTICE

This book is intended for use by licensed physicians only, and only for their use in preparing for the written examination for board certification in general surgery. It is not intended for use in the delivery of health care services, and cannot replace sound clinical judgment or individualized patient care for such purposes.

The authors, publishers, distributors, and sponsors of this book expressly disclaim all warranties, express or implied, with respect to this book and its contents, including any warranties as to the quality, accuracy, completeness or suitability of the information contained in this book for any particular purpose. Without limiting the foregoing, they caution the reader that use of this book does not guarantee passage of any board certification exams, written or otherwise.

The authors, publishers, distributors and sponsors of this book expressly disclaim any liability to any person or organization for any loss or damage caused by any errors or omissions in this book.

Our thanks to Copy Editor Sarah Herndon

Contents

Preface

8th Edition

Through the generous educational support of Ortho-McNeil™, we are very pleased to provide you with the revised 8th edition of the *Educational Review Manual in General Surgery.* This manual was developed by a distinguished group of clinician-educators to assist in preparation for the surgery board certification and in-service examinations. Our objective is to provide you with an up-to-date and comprehensive summary of core concepts that will facilitate critical self-review and independent preparation for test-taking.

I wish to thank the contributors whose considerable scholarship, creativity, and practical clinical insights are evident in each of the chapters. I am particularly indebted to the surgical faculty of UCI for their support of this project.

I would also like to acknowledge Michael D. Wolf, Ph.D., whose editorial expertise and counsel were truly invaluable. Finally, I thank Susan Nicholson, MD, Ortho-McNeil Janssen Scientific Affairs, LLC. who shared the vision for this book and Ortho McNeil for its continued commitment to educational excellence through sponsorship of this project.

Sincerely,

Samuel E. Wilson, MD
University of California, Irvine
Orange, CA
Editor

Castle Connolly Graduate Medical Publishing, Ltd., New York, NY.

ORTHO-McNEIL®
Division of
Ortho-McNeil-Janssen
Pharmaceuticals, Inc.

June 19, 2009

Dear Surgery Resident:

Ortho-McNeil® is proud to sponsor the *Educational Review Manual In General Surgery* 2009.

This manual is a tool to assist you through the completion of your residency training. It was prepared under the guidance of editor-in-chief Samuel Eric Wilson, M.D., Professor of Surgery and Associate Dean of the University of California, Irvine School of Medicine. Written by expert educators from medical centers around the US, this manual will be an invaluable tool for you in the months and years ahead.

As a leader in anti-infectives, Ortho-McNeil® is committed to developing new antimicrobials that will help healthcare professionals care for their patients.

Ortho-McNeil® is committed to the continued education of healthcare professionals and commends the authors and the esteemed editor for an outstanding effort in developing this review.

We hope that the wealth of information presented herein will enrich your understanding of General Surgery and help you during your training.

If you are licensed in any State or other jurisdiction, or an employee or contractor of any organization or governmental entity, that limits or prohibits any items of value from pharmaceutical companies, your name, the value, and purpose of this educational gift may be reported as required by state or federal law. Once reported, this information may be publicly accessible.

Regards,

Susan Nicholson MD

Susan Nicholson MD
Therapeutic Area Lead, Anti-Infective Franchise
Ortho-McNeil Janssen Scientific Affairs, LLC

Test Taking Strategies

Samuel E. Wilson, MD

1. Stress, anxiety and fear engendered through anticipation of testing are powerful factors adversely affecting an individual's performance on multiple choice examinations. Find a regular outlet for stress and anxiety reduction—running, working out in the gym or simply reading a novel at the end of the day—and stick to it as you prepare for the examination.

2. "Cramming" of factual information immediately before an examination has not been demonstrated to significantly improve performance. Additionally, fatigue from an "all- nighter" can impair cognitive processes and negatively affect performance. Controlled and methodical preparation for an examination is vastly preferable for the majority of test takers. Aim to peak the intensity and duration of self-study approximately one month before the examination date, and continue at a steady pace thereafter.

3. Identify and focus study efforts on areas of knowledge deficit. While it's usually less anxiety-provoking and more fun to study areas of interest and to add to one's fund of knowledge, the strategy of preparation aimed exclusively at one's strengths often increases depth of knowledge at the expense of breadth of information. On examinations designed to test both, this is usually not a wise choice.

4. Practice for the examination by taking and answering real multiple choice questions. Many books of questions have been published but the American College of Surgeons' SESAP is probably the best.

5. At the beginning of the examination, plan how you will use the time available. Estimate how many minutes will be required to complete each section and then pace yourself. Do not allow yourself to be distracted by the pace of others or to be thrown off pace by lingering over difficult questions. Move ahead and return to the difficult questions later.

6. Rely as much as possible on your own knowledge to answer questions. Attempting to discern patterns of responses during the test and then applying these patterns to answer subsequent questions is not prudent and is not recommended.

7. For multiple choice questions, read the "stem" of each question with the intention of answering it without the choices that follow. This should focus attention and increase concentration. Proceed by reading the choices, but be careful not to jump to conclusions by selecting the first choice that approximates your answer. Sometimes, two choices will be deliberately made to read quite similarly.

8. If you have to guess the answer to any multiple choice questions, several strategies may be useful. Eliminate answers that use specific grammatical determiners like "never" or "everyone" or "always;" choose answers that are more descriptive or detailed; apply a true-false test to each choice and eliminate the choices adjudged false; strongly consider the choice that is most convergent (includes the most elements in common with the other options).

9. When answering true-false questions, look for extreme modifiers that tend to make the response false such as invariably, never, always or absolutely. Also look for qualifiers that tend to make the response true such as usually, often, seldom, or frequently.

10. When reviewing completed questions, do not change an answer unless you are convinced that it is an error. Usually, the initial response to a question proves to be the correct one. However, anxiety engendered during the review process can raise doubts about selected answers and prompt ill-conceived changes in responses causing more harm than good.

11. It is always easier to read about a condition that you are currently treating or expect to operate upon, but read in depth – recent journal articles, published reviews, or specialized textbooks.

12. *Selected Readings in General Surgery*, from UT Southwestern in Dallas, is an invaluable source for recent articles and the reviews are expert.

13. Take a standard major textbook of surgery, divide it into weekly allotments, and systematically work through the text over the months before the exam. Making notes as you read helps you to remember.

14. Prepare seriously for the In-Service Exams and the board exam will be a breeze!

My thanks go to Robert M. Lembo, MD, New York University School of Medicine, for assistance in the preparation of the tips and strategies listed above.

Chapter 1: Preoperative and Anesthetic Management of the Surgical Patient

Debra E. Morrison, MD
Anna L. Harris, MD

Contents

1. The Anesthesiologist and the Surgical Team

Surgeons and anesthesiologists together constitute a team of physicians dedicated to the care of the surgical patient. The practice of anesthesiology emerged from the practice of surgery, out of a need to maintain patients in a safe, compliant, immobile and pain-free state during the course of an operation. Evolution of surgical technique has necessitated and inspired improved anesthesia techniques, which in turn have allowed surgical techniques both to evolve and to be tolerated by a wider range of patients.

The interest of the surgical patient is best served if members of the combined operative team assume their individual responsibilities yet understand and respect the skills and concerns of the team members working over the ether screen. Collaboration begins in the preoperative period and continues into the postoperative period. During the course of the operation itself, surgeons and anesthesiologists communicate succinctly regarding the status of the patient to ensure that all proceeds smoothly without either team disturbing the other's concentration. At the same time, there is often continuous idle chatter and music playing, which to an outsider might seem distracting, but is actually a means of relieving tension and aiding concentration.

While the surgeon is the star of the opera at center stage, the anesthesiologist is the impresario and the stage manager, or sometimes the conductor, often both of the operating room and the combined Operating Rooms, helping to keep things running smoothly. The surgeon is often unaware of the seemingly rapid passage of time from "skin to skin," from the cutting to the closing of the wound, but is painfully aware of the eternity from "skin to skin," between the closing of one wound and the opening of the wound on the next patient, and this is a constant source of friction. The surgeon comes to the operating room several times a week, balancing operating time with hours spent in clinic, lab, meetings, consultations and hospital rounds. Anesthesiologists reside there, hurrying from preop clinic to preop holding area, to the operating room "board," to see what cases can be squeezed into small open blocks of time, to meetings and postop rounds, to a sudden call for airway intervention in another part of the hospital and back to the recovery room to check on the previous patient, while the surgeon is waiting to proceed with the next operation. Time wasted through lack of communication affects everyone and extends the day in a painful manner, but time spent in preparation for safe anesthesia is no more wasted than time spent in careful suturing. Both the surgeon and the anesthesiologist care for the same patients, and they should attempt to understand each other's slightly different points of view and share an overlapping body of knowledge and experience.

2. Preoperative Evaluation and Assessment of Anesthetic Risk

The anesthesiologist's job is best performed when involvement begins in the preoperative period, days to weeks prior to the planned elective operation. The anesthesiologist can assist in or help to orchestrate identification of coexisting medical problems. Too often, parallel investigations of multiple "chief complaints" result in the discovery of an unresolved comorbidity as the day of surgery is approaching, and the anesthesiologist, with the input of other involved physicians, must help to address conflicting concerns. Once all appropriate data and medical opinion is compiled, the anesthesiologist can render an opinion regarding whether or not the patient's medical problems are managed optimally, and whether or not a reasonable anesthesiologist would proceed. Optimal management reduces anesthetic risk to that which is unavoidable, and allows the surgeon and the anesthesiologist to determine the ratio of risk to realistically obtainable benefit more accurately. Identification and management of problems in advance of the day of surgery can prevent surprises, delays, cancellations, and most importantly, complications that adversely affect patients, but affect surgeons and anesthesiologists as well.

Toward this effort, the patient's primary care physician or specialist should be consulted, either formally or informally. Even though the patient's physician may have referred the patient for a surgical consultation, optimal medical management for daily living may not be the same as optimal medical management for surgery and anesthesia. Given the opinion that the patient may benefit from surgery, the patient's physician should be offered the opportunity to participate in risk assessment and risk reduction. In the end, however, given all of the available information regarding the patient and the medical status, as well as the proposed surgery, the anesthesiologist is in a unique position in determining whether and how to proceed, assuming the worst and determining strategies to minimize patient risk in the operating room.

Cardiac complications are among the most ominous perioperative complications. In 2002, the American College of Cardiology (ACC) and the American Heart Association (AHA) coauthored a series of guidelines for perioperative cardiac evaluation and management of patients with cardiovascular disease. This risk assessment strategy represented an organized approach for physicians to follow during the perioperative workup. The guidelines were modified and updated in 2007 to provide evidence-based parameters for assessing patients with cardiac disease undergoing cardiac surgery. The ACC/AHA 2007 Guidelines were published online at **http://circ.ahajournals.org/cgi/content/full/116/17/1971** before appearing in print and contain tables and algorithms as quick references for decision making.

The purpose of evaluation is rarely to give "medical clearance," but is instead to assess the patient's current medical status, determine risk of perioperative cardiac problems, make recommendations for management, and allow informed decisions to be made regarding the plan of care during the perioperative period. Tests are not recommended unless they are likely to influence patient treatment. The goal is simply optimal care of the patient, whether the case is elective or whether it is an emergency in which worst must be assumed and anticipated.

The 2002 guidelines used major, intermediate and minor risk factor categories and, combined with the risk of the procedure and consideration of the patient's functional capacity, served to guide physicians in determining appropriate testing and/or treatment to improve outcomes. ***The 2007 Revised Cardiac Risk Index (RCRI)*** considers active cardiac conditions that when present indicate major risk, a group of clinical risk factors from the index initially excluding of the type of surgery, which is considered later in the algorithm in the approach to the patient.

2007 RCRI major risk factors include active conditions that are associated with major risk. These include unstable coronary conditions including unstable or severe angina or recent myocardial infarction (MI), decompensated heart failure (New York Heart Association ([NYHA]-Class IV), significant arrhythmias and severe valvular disease such as aortic stenosis or symptomatic mitral stenosis.

2007 RCRI clinical risk factors include history of heart disease (history of MI or Q waves by ECG), history of compensated or prior heart failure, history of cerebrovascular disease, diabetes mellitus and renal insufficiency (Cr level .2 mg/dL).

Using the stepwise approach to assessment using the RCRI:

Step 1 considers the urgency of noncardiac surgery. Emergent surgery may not allow for preoperative assessment or treatment but outcome may be improved by surveillance and perioperative medical management. If not emergent, proceed to Step 2.

Step 2 considers whether the patient has active cardiac conditions or clinical risk factors. If yes, patient should be evaluated and treated per ACC/AHA guidelines then proceed to the operating room. If not, proceed to Step 3.

Step 3 considers whether or not surgery is low risk. If so, proceed to the operating room. If not, proceed to Step 4.

Step 4 considers whether or not patient's functional capacity is greater than or equal to 4 METs without symptoms. If so, proceed to the operating room. If not, or functional capacity is unknown, proceed to Step 5.

Step 5 involves counting the patient's number of clinical risk factors, then determining whether surgery is high or intermediate risk. For vascular surgery with 3 or more clinical risk factors, testing should be considered if it will change management. For intermediate risk surgery with 1-3 or more clinical risk factors or vascular surgery with 1 or 2 clinical risk factors, consider noninvasive testing if it will change management or proceed with planned surgery with heart rate control (which will be discussed further). If no clinical risk factors, proceed with planned surgery.

The surgery-specific risk of noncardiac surgery is related to type of surgery as outlined below:

Cardiac[a] Risk Stratification for Noncardiac Surgical Procedures

Vascular (reported cardiac risk often more than 5%)

Aortic and other major vascular surgery, peripheral vascular surgery

Intermediate (reported cardiac risk generally 1%-5%)

Intraperitoneal and intrathoracic surgery

Carotid endarterectomy

Head and neck surgery

Orthopedic surgery

Prostate surgery

Low[b] (reported cardiac risk generally less than 1%)

Endoscopic procedures

Superficial procedure

Cataract surgery

Breast surgery

Ambulatory surgery

[a]Combined incidence of cardiac death and nonfatal myocardial infarction
[b]These procedures do not generally require further preoperative cardiac testing

End-organ effects of risk factors vary from patient to patient, and functional capacity may be discovered by history and patient-reported "exercise" capacity. Careful questioning may be required in order to determine just what a patient is able to do without symptoms. Questions about activities of daily living may be more useful than queries using the words "exercise" or "activity." It is useful to discover whether or not there has been a change in activity and whether or not this change is related to ominous symptoms, rather than pain or physical disability.

The use of beta blockers and Clonidine must be discussed here. The 2007 RCRI Guidelines stated that beta blockers should be continued in patients undergoing surgery who are already "receiving beta blockers to treat angina, symptomatic arrhythmias, hypertension, or other ACC/AHA Class I guideline indications." They further stated that "Beta blockers should be given to patients undergoing vascular surgery who are at high cardiac risk owing to the finding of ischemia on perioperative testing," are "probably recommended for patients undergoing vascular surgery in whom preoperative assessment identifies coronary heart disease," "...probably recommended for patients in whom preoperative assessment for vascular surgery identifies high cardiac risk, as defined by the presence of more than 1 clinical risk factor," and are "probably recommended for patients in whom preoperative assessment identifies coronary heart disease or high cardiac risk, as defined by the presence of more than 1 clinical risk factor, who are undergoing intermediate-risk or vascular surgery." However, "the usefulness of beta blockers is uncertain for patients who are undergoing either intermediate-risk procedures or vascular surgery, in whom preoperative assessment identifies a single clinical risk factor" and for "patients undergoing vascular surgery with no clinical risk factors who are not currently taking beta blockers." The Guidelines also stated that "Alpha-2 agonists for perioperative control of hypertension may be considered for patients with known CAD or at least 1 clinical risk factor who are undergoing surgery."

Patients who have contraindications to beta blockers or alpha-2 agonists should not be given these drugs. Patients who are on these drugs should not be taken off them. However, recent studies suggest that the rush to develop perioperative beta blocker protocols may have been premature or applied too widely. Publication of the landmark Perioperative Ischemic Evaluation (POISE) trial online May 12, 2008 in *Lancet* has resulted in debate on the pros and cons of using beta blockers perioperatively in noncardiac surgery. The study found that beta blockers do more harm than good, in particular when patients become hypotensive with resulting cerebral hypoperfusion, although the study's protocol was then criticized. At this time, the best course of action is to use beta blockers in certain patients, understanding that not everyone will benefit, and that some patients risk increased harm from the use of these drugs. One should consider the perioperative addition of Clonidine in the same light.

Patients with pulmonary disease should be queried about their exercise or activity tolerance, and whether they are at their baseline at the time of surgery. Smokers, whether or not they carry a diagnosis of chronic lung disease, can benefit from decreased wound infections from reduction or cessation of smoking in the weeks prior to surgery. Major risk factors for postoperative pneumonia include type of surgery (abdominal aortic aneurysm, thoracic, upper abdominal), age greater or equal to 60, poor functional status and poor nutritional status, most of which cannot be modified. Minor risk factors include history of COPD, general anesthesia, impaired mental status, history of stroke, poor renal function, transfusion greater than 4 units, emergency surgery, chronic steroid use, current or recent smoking, and significant alcohol intake. ***Risk stratification may be more likely to predict the hospital course rather than to improve it.***

The anesthesiologist helps to widen the focus of the patient and the surgeon. Both patient and surgeon may be primarily focused on the part of the body that requires surgical treatment, especially if that part causes pain, is malfunctioning or threatens the patient's life, and the patient may innocently withhold information about coexisting medical problems. Patients may defer mentioning other concerns to the surgeon because they assume these problems are not relevant or important, or because they may be embarrassing, thinking that they can more easily be dealt with after the operation. The patient may decide that if the surgeon wanted to know something, he or she would have asked specifically, and may not volunteer any apparently irrelevant information. The anesthesiologist plays the part of a neutral third party who must act as advocate for both the patient and the surgeon.

When the patient and the anesthesiologist confer by telephone or meet in person, the anesthesiologist's preoperative evaluation inspires confidence. It begins with the history of the surgical complaint, and expresses sympathy and concern for the patient's welfare, then advances subtly but relentlessly to a deliberate but apparently guileless highly detailed review of systems, in the manner of actor Peter Falk's "Columbo" detective character. The aim is really to secure evidence that the patient has the constitution to endure the operation and its sequelae, while attempting to discover any previously unknown organ system dysfunction that should be addressed to optimize the surgical outcome and anesthetic management. The astute surgeon will learn to preempt the anesthesiologist in this discovery process in order to compile an unassailable documentation of the patient's fitness for the planned operation.

Because the patient's surgical pathology may limit mobility, it is important to elicit a sense of the patient's premorbid exercise tolerance and learn of any related symptoms of cardiac or respiratory disease. It is reassuring to discover that the patient has endured some activity at least as stressful as the planned trip to the operating room without symptoms of organ failure. Ultimately, a review of the chart including background lab tests and studies, any appropriate communication with the patient's primary care physician, and, especially, an analysis of the patient's medications, will help to complete the picture of the patient's general health and how well coexisting problems are being managed. The anesthesiologist is also alert for signs and symptoms of an acute or very recent upper respiratory infection (URI), since the airway, particularly the pediatric airway, is far more irritable during and after a URI, and risk for bronchospasm and laryngospasm is increased.

Baseline vital signs are useful. Poorly controlled hypertension can be identified in advance, allowing time for medical management. Uncontrolled hypertension places the patient at risk for intraoperative hemodynamic lability. Waiting to treat hypertension until the patient is unconscious introduces the risk of cerebral hypoperfusion and is not safe practice.

Studies and laboratory tests are now used less frequently by anesthesiologists to screen for unsuspected coexisting disease. There is no convincing evidence that random screening decreases risk. History should alert the surgeon and anesthesiologist to potential problems, and studies and lab tests should be used to confirm and then quantify or qualify the existence of these problems. An active person is unlikely to have significant anemia or a clinically significant abnormality on a chest radiograph. A lab abnormality in a patient at low risk for a specific problem is more likely to be a lab error, which necessitates further workup with no ultimate benefit. More can be gained by discovering that a patient is able to walk 18 holes carrying a golf bag on a golf course than by obtaining tests. This approach is more economical, as well as more pleasing to the patient.

An atypical ECG on a healthy, asymptomatic athlete may actually be normal for that person. Baseline ECGs are obtained for patients at risk of cardiovascular problems (often men over 40 and women over 50, as well as patients with specific risk factors such as morbid obesity and diabetes and symptomatic or known heart disease) because the ECG is followed intraoperatively, and because cardiac ischemia carries a major risk of morbidity and mortality. All ECG abnormalities must still be evaluated in relation to clinical history. A change in an ECG may be more ominous than a stable abnormality.

Thus, lab tests and studies are useful to evaluate the current status of a sick or unstable patient, but not useful out of context to patient history. Existing labs in the medical record can be reviewed for a pattern of stability of a known problem, such as whether there is a pattern of good control of glucose in a diabetic. A glucose level is usually obtained in the morning before surgery if the patient is diabetic, but a level taken the week before is less useful than a normal glycosylated hemoglobin, which is evidence of good long-term control. Likewise, a potassium level just before surgery is more useful than the last post-dialysis potassium level. A random Dilantin or digoxin level may be too high or too low, depending on the time the sample is drawn. Instead of checking levels, it would be more useful to ask whether the patient's seizures are controlled or to check a pulse for evidence of rate control, and inquire about symptoms of toxicity. The physician who prescribes the Dilantin or digoxin probably monitors levels and clinical efficacy vs. toxicity as a matter of routine.

If a procedure is planned which is absolutely contraindicated in the presence of a particular problem, and the consequence of proceeding is grave, it is important to rule out that problem. Coagulopathy and pregnancy must be ruled out prior to proceeding with lithotripsy, for example.

Obtaining every conceivable lab test to "prevent anesthesia cancellation" due to a missing bit of irrelevant data is not productive, and may be more likely to lead to cancellation of surgery. It often seems that the likelihood of a false positive finding in a patient with low risk is greater than that of a true positive finding, especially if an operation is at risk for cancellation.

The anesthesiologist also elicits a past surgical history, with particular attention to details of past anesthetics and complications, especially complications that place the patient at particular risk for further complications. Past experiences may also predispose a patient to anxiety, and the patient's concerns should be addressed in appropriate detail. Often questions the patient has about past experiences can be answered as a bridge to proposing a plan for anesthesia that will prevent unpleasantness and minimize risk of complications. Of interest are postoperative nausea and vomiting, difficult intubation, intolerance or allergy to medication, intraoperative awareness, a family history of problems related to anesthesia or surgery, prolonged postoperative intubation, bleeding problems, nerve injury or anything the patient is concerned about. The anesthesiologist may also be able to reassure the patient that his or her choice of a surgeon is a wise one. The surgeon can help by notifying the anesthesiologist in advance that a patient may require special attention for any reason.

Although it is difficult to separate the risk of anesthesia from the risk specific to the individual patient and the risk of the operation itself, it is estimated that the chance of death totally attributable to anesthesia is rare, approximately 1 in every 100,000 to 250,000 anesthetics. The patient's disease(s), the type of surgery and possibly the location of surgery and postoperative care have a greater impact on the patient's overall outcome. Of the above, patient disease has the greatest impact on outcome. Specific diseases which are associated with increased risk for the patient include cardiovascular disease, pulmonary disease, renal failure and diabetes mellitus. Patients who are extremely old or extremely young or who require emergency surgery are at increased risk of perioperative complications.

Anesthetic causes of death or coma are equipment failure, intubation complications, and aspiration of gastric contents, postoperative respiratory depression, anaphylactoid shock and cardiac arrest. Potential complications can include allergic drug reactions, failure to intubate or provide adequate oxygenation and ventilation, nerve damage, eye damage, tooth damage and malignant hyperthermia (a potentially fatal hypermetabolic syndrome triggered by certain anesthetic drugs that occurs because of a genetic defect). Morbidity and mortality from general anesthesia does not really differ from that from spinal or epidural anesthesia. Morbid events associated with anesthesia include pneumonia, congestive heart failure, myocardial infarction, pulmonary embolism, respiratory failure and stroke.

ASA Classification

Patients are classified into American Society of Anesthesiologists (ASA) Class 1-6.

Class 1. Normal healthy patient: healthy with no systemic disease and the pathologic process for which surgery is to be performed is localized, without systemic effect. Example: a healthy athlete scheduled for knee surgery.

Class 2. Patient with mild systemic disease: mild to moderate systemic dysfunction caused by a coexisting systemic disease or by the pathologic process for which surgery is to be performed. Examples: controlled hypertension, controlled diabetes, upper respiratory infection, smoking and thyroid tumor that does not threaten the airway. Pregnancy and extremes of age are sometimes included in this category.

Class 3. Patient with severe systemic disease: multiple-system disease or controlled major system disease that affects activity. Examples: chronic obstructive pulmonary disease, chronic stable angina, obesity (which is a multisystem disease), lung tumor that decreases pulmonary function and pheochromocytoma after medical optimization.

Class 4. Patient with severe systemic disease that is a constant threat to life: may not be correctable by medical management or operation. Examples: congestive heart failure, unstable angina, severe pulmonary or hepatic dysfunction, major trauma, prematurity with respiratory distress and necrotizing enterocolitis, and pheochromocytoma prior to medical optimization.

Class 5. Moribund patient who is not expected to survive without the operation: little chance of survival with or without surgery, but no chance of survival without surgery. Examples: ruptured aortic aneurysm, major trauma and massive intracerebral injury.

Class 6. Declared brain-dead patient whose organs are being removed for donor purposes.

E is used as a modifier to denote emergency operation, with no time to optimize the medical condition. A healthy patient with an acute appendicitis would be classified 1E. E also implies increased risk.

Class 4 and 5 patients are at increased risk for morbidity and mortality, with mortality rates from 7%-50%.

Plan for Management

When the anesthesiologist is confident that the entire picture of the patient's physical health status is clear and optimal and the constraints of the operation are understood, an appropriate plan for management is discussed with the patient, with an outline of options and their risks and benefits. The operation planned, and the necessary positioning, individual aspects of the operation in relation to the patient or the surgeon, and the preferences of both surgeon and patient are considered. It is inappropriate for medical consultants to recommend a plan for anesthesia or monitoring requirements, just as it is inappropriate for medical consultants to prescribe the mode of surgical intervention. The medical consultant can affirm that the patient is in optimal condition from a medical standpoint, but cannot "clear" a patient for a particular operation or anesthetic. The anesthesiologist will perform an appropriate anesthetic and adapt the plan according to intraoperative events. Thus, a monitored anesthesia care (MAC) anesthetic, combining local anesthetics by the surgeon with sedation, may not be tolerated, or a spinal may wear off before the operation is over, so the anesthesiologist must proceed with general anesthesia. Any patient may become unstable and require escalation of monitoring and/or pharmacotherapy.

Increasingly, the preoperative visit with the anesthesiologist occurs on the morning of surgery, since most patients are not admitted in advance. The surgeon should learn to think like an anesthesiologist and provide the anesthesiologist with appropriate data in advance for evaluation, if there is concern that a problem will be considered cause for delay or cancellation if it is not addressed before the day of surgery. The anesthesiologist should be a willing consultant in the preoperative process.

3. Preparation of the Surgical Patient

NPO Orders

ASA Practice Guidelines for Preoperative Fasting are now focused on type of substance ingested, not age of patient. Recommended practice should be modified appropriately for patients with co-existing conditions or diseases that might affect gastric emptying or fluid volume (pregnancy, obesity, diabetes, hiatal hernia, gastroesophageal reflux, bowel obstruction, emergency care, enteral tube feeding, anticipated difficult intubation or already intubated), or patients who will not be given sedation or systemic analgesia.

Before a procedure requiring general or regional anesthesia or sedation/analgesia (monitored anesthesia care or moderate sedation/analgesia, deep sedation):

It is appropriate, regardless of patient age, for patients to fast from intake of clear liquids for 2 hours. There is no demonstrated benefit from abstention from clear liquids for more than 4 hours. Clear liquids include, but are not limited to, water, fruit juices without pulp, carbonated beverages, clear tea and black coffee. Alcohol is not included as an acceptable clear liquid. The type of liquid ingested is more important than the volume of liquid.

All neonates and infants, regardless of postconceptual age, should abstain from breast milk for 4 hours and infant formula for 6 hours.

All patients, regardless of age, should fast from intake of a light meal or non-human milk for 6 hours.

Fatty or fried foods, meat or a large amount of food may prolong emptying time and patients should fast for 8 hours prior to an elective procedure.

It is reasonable to require that patients fast for longer than the minimum recommended time in order to allow for flexibility in the operating room schedule.

NPO guidelines are based on reasonable interpretations of studies and vary between institutions. Guidelines should be applied appropriately after considering the individual patient. A trauma patient should be assumed to have a full stomach. Emergency surgery may necessitate proceeding before the stomach is likely to be empty, and the existence of intraabdominal pathology may prevent gastric emptying. A perfectly healthy young person who has been NPO for many hours and has been waiting nervously all day for surgery may also have increased production and delayed emptying of gastric fluids. Risks of aspiration should be considered while determining whether or not to proceed immediately. There is no solid evidence to suggest that pharmacologic intervention can reliably hasten gastric emptying or reduce the risk of pulmonary aspiration.

Medications

A complete list of medications and dosages should be obtained from each patient as part of the preoperative assessment. This allows insight into the patient's actual state of health and management of coexisting diseases, and helps in planning for surgery and in postoperative management. If the patient neglects to take necessary medications, time will be saved if the dose and the medication are already known.

Patients should continue necessary medications to retain a baseline steady state blood level of chronic medications. Necessary medications include antihypertensives, cardiac medications, epilepsy medications, hormone replacement, ulcer medications, antibiotics, narcotics and benzodiazepines. Other medications are also important.

Additional medication may be indicated during the perioperative period. Patients with pheochromocytoma should first be completely alpha-blocked and rehydrated, then, if appropriate, be beta-blocked, well in advance of surgery.

After appropriate consideration, some blood pressure medications should be discontinued preoperatively. If the antihypertensive regimen includes a diuretic, and the patient is to have a bowel prep, it may be better to forgo the diuretic. Anecdotal evidence, at least, suggests that ACE inhibitors and ACE receptor blockers can be associated, in some patients, with severe hypotension during anesthesia.

Increasingly, patients may be on ***nonprescribed vitamins, herbs and supplements***. These substances have the potential to interact with prescribed medications as well as anesthetic drugs. A complete list of vitamins, herbs and supplements should be obtained preoperatively from each patient. Substances with the potential for undesired side effects should be discontinued leaving adequate time, depending on the individual half-life, for clearance prior to surgery. Diet drugs should be discontinued at least 1 week prior to surgery, allowing time for clearance, in order to prevent labile blood pressure intraoperatively.

If it is appropriate to discontinue ***aspirin***, it should be stopped 10-14 days prior to surgery. ***NSAIDs*** should be stopped 1-3 days prior to surgery, depending on the half-life of the drug. Other ***anticoagulants and antiplatelet agents*** should be stopped, if appropriate, only after consultation with the prescribing physician, since they are prescribed for a variety of reasons, and some patients may be in danger of morbidity if the drugs are removed. Risks of increased bleeding and/or transfusion must be weighed against the benefits of the anti-inflammatory effects of the drugs, and the type of surgery must be considered in the decision. (Samama CM, Bastien O, Forestier F. Antiplatelet agents in the perioperative period. Expert Recommendations of the French Society of Anesthesiology and Intensive Care [SFAR]: Summary from SFAR National Congress; September 22, 2001.)

Particulate antacids can cause damage if aspirated, and should not be used for 8 hours prior to an anesthetic. Clear antacids are not a problem and can be continued.

Drugs like ***prednisone*** that cause nausea when taken on an empty stomach may not be tolerated on the morning of surgery and should be given intravenously.

Antirejection medication should be continued perioperatively.

The Patient with Diabetes Mellitus

Medical management of the patient with diabetes mellitus (DM) should be customized for the individual patient. In general, until sufficient evidence exists to support the routine use of tight glycemic control (blood glucose 80 to 110 mg/dL) and the technology exists to reliably detect and prevent hypoglycemia, the goal for glucose control during surgery should be to maintain the glucose level in a range between 110 to 150 mg/dL during surgery to protect against hypoglycemia. Patients, especially those with type 1, should be consulted on insulin management, since some patients practice very tight control during their daily lives and are experts in their own management, but the goal of tight control should be relaxed in the perioperative period. Intensive insulin therapy (IIT) has been shown in some studies to reduce morbidity and mortality among the critically ill, decrease infection rates and improve survival after cardiac surgery, and improve outcomes in acute neurologic injury and acute MI, but recent reports of adverse events associated with IIT and severe hypoglycemia raise questions about the safety and efficacy of IIT. Thus, while avoidance of hyperglycemia is beneficial it is uncertain which patients will benefit from IIT, what glucose targets are both safe and beneficial and whether present technology is adequate to prevent hypoglycemia. In considering the individual patient, the physician who manages the patient may also be consulted for insight and customized management strategy. The anesthesiologist will also be involved in the management plan and execution.

Scheduling procedures early in the day or "first case" is best for individuals with DM, especially those scheduled for outpatient surgery. Those who are more difficult to manage should be scheduled first. For early-morning procedures of short duration where the patient may still be expected to eat according to his or her usual meal plan, it is easiest to have the patient continue the usual medications the night before, hold morning medications, and give the morning oral medication or insulin and food after the procedure. Shortening the intervals between later meals may compensate for this delay and gradually realign the patient's mealtimes back to the usual schedule. This operative schedule is the easiest for patients and physicians because it has the least disrupting effect on the diabetes regimen and should be advocated by both patient and the physician responsible for managing the diabetes.

A detailed assessment of each individual with diabetes is recommended because multiple factors influence blood glucose management. Specific guidelines will not fit every patient's needs. Consider the following criteria when making decisions and recommendations about preoperative and pre-procedure diabetes medications:

1. **Type:** Determine whether patient has type 1 or type 2 DM. Many patients are wrongly categorized. Type 1 diabetics should never have all insulin withheld.

2. **Age of onset and duration:** Determine age of onset and duration of diagnosis of DM. Both types 1 and 2 can occur at any age. Long duration (over 10 years with type 2) usually means greater insulin deficiency and/or greater insulin resistance. Type 1 diabetics can become more resistant to insulin and type 2 diabetics can become insulin-deficient.

3. **Body habitus:** Overweight people (both types) have more insulin resistance and require larger amounts of insulin for control.

4. **Medical regimen:** Determine type/amount/frequency of medication(s) being taken.

5. **Insulin therapy:** Continuous insulin therapy started within 6 months of diagnosis usually means severe insulin therapy or type 1.

6. **Co-morbid conditions:** Document extent of complications to help avoid worsening during procedure, eg, neuropathic, insensate feet need protection to help prevent pressure ulcers; nephropathy means renal blood flow must be protected or patient may be on dialysis; infection may necessitate change in insulin management.

7. **Glucose control:** Check blood glucose control, not just random glucose levels. Assess recent hemoglobin A1c result and self-monitored glucose log, then check glucose in preoperative area.

8. **Awareness:** Does the patient have the ability to recognize symptoms of hypoglycemia and know treatment used for hypoglycemia? If patient complains of symptoms of hypoglycemia, and bedside glucometer does not confirm this, check a laboratory value. Glucometer readings can be incorrect.

9. **Hypoglycemia:** Guidelines include treating blood glucose 80 mg/dL or below with 15 grams glucose, retesting glucose in 15 minutes, and retreating/retesting every 15 minutes until glucose is at least 100 mg/dL.

In general, for patients with type 1 DM:

1. **Basal insulin:** Always continue basal insulin source (NPH, Lente, Ultralente, glargine [Lantus], insulin pump or intravenous insulin infusion) in order to prevent ketoacidosis. Morbidity and mortality is primarily due to lack of insulin in these patients.

2. **Non-peaking insulin:** Type 1 patients on glargine (Lantus) can be considered to be on a "poor man's pump" which should be continued without diminishing the dose. Glargine is usually taken every 24 hours at night as a basal dose, does not peak and is dosed unrelated to food intake. Type 1 patients should receive the usual dose of glargine every 24 hours whether it is taken at night or in the morning, including prior to surgery.

3. **Peaking basal insulins:** Dose may need to be adjusted for peaking insulins (NPH, Lente, Ultralente). Give/have patient take the usual dose of NPH insulin the night before procedure. Inpatients should have IV/have outpatients come to hospital and start IV then give 2/3 the usual dose of NPH insulin the morning of procedure; note that intravenous dextrose piggyback may be needed to decrease risk of hypoglycemia. After an outpatient procedure,

when patient is able to resume oral intake, test blood glucose and give remainder of usual morning dose of NPH insulin with extra rapid- or short-acting insulin as needed. Individuals who take long-acting peaking insulin (Ultralente) and short-acting insulin may be switched to an intermediate-acting type (NPH) a day or two before surgery.

4. **Short-acting insulin:** Omit fast- or rapid-acting (regular or Humalog) injected insulin the morning of procedure.

5. **Continuous insulin:** Patients treated with continuous insulin infusion therapy (insulin pumps) may be continued with their usual basal insulin rate.

6. **Complex patients:** Involve patient's endocrinologist or endocrinology consultant for complex or high risk patients.

7. **For a long procedure (over 4 hours):** Consider omitting all subcutaneous insulin and starting intravenous insulin infusion the morning of procedure, use ICU insulin infusion protocol when indicated. Intravenous regular insulin is indicated during the perioperative period for previously insulin-treated patients undergoing long, complex operative procedures, patients who require emergency surgery while in ketoacidosis and patients with unstable type 1 DM.

In general, for patients with type 2 DM:

1. **Short-acting insulin:** Omit fast- or rapid-acting injected insulin the morning of procedure.

2. **NPH insulin:** Follow guidelines for type 1 diabetes above.

3. **Glargine insulin (Lantus):** Type 2 diabetes patients may be prescribed glargine insulin as a basal dose OR may have a larger dose prescribed (sometimes in divided doses) to compensate in part for meals. Patients taking glargine at bedtime should take approximately 3/4 the usual dose the night before procedure. Patients taking glargine in the morning should take approximately 3/4 the usual dose the morning of procedure.

4. **For a long procedure (over 4 hours):** Consider omitting all subcutaneous insulin and starting intravenous insulin infusion the morning of procedure, use ICU insulin infusion protocol when indicated.

5. **Oral medications:** Omit glucophage XR the evening before procedure or earlier if the patient will be NPO longer or has decreased oral intake as part of the prep. Omit all glucophage the morning of procedure. Alterations in renal function arising intraoperatively may potentiate the risk for development of lactic acidosis. In type 2 diabetes, glucophage should not be resumed for 72 hours postoperatively after surgery where GI or renal function may be altered, when serum creatinine is measured to document the absence of any perfusion or contrast related renal toxic effects and the return of normal renal function. Hold sulfonylureas and nonsulfonylurea secretagogues (Glipizide, glyburide, Glimepride; Prandin, Starlix) the morning of procedure and restart when patient can resume diet. Hold chlorpropamide 24 hours prior to procedure. Thiazolidiones (avandia, actos) may be continued if used as monotherapy unless concern exists for fluid retention, but are usually held on the morning of surgery. Patients taking 2 or more oral agents should be placed on insulin (RISS) in the perioperative period. Hold alpha-glucosidase inhibitors (precose, glyset, Voglibose) until patient is eating usual meals. Other oral diabetes medications should be held until patient is eating usual meals.

6. **Other medications:** Omit GLP analogs (Byetta), amylin analogs (Symlin) and DPP VI inhibitors (Galvus, Januvia) on the morning of procedure and resume when patient is eating usual meals.

An NPO outpatient who is being driven to the hospital should not take a dose of NPH insulin at home. A traffic jam or other delay in reaching the preop holding room could result in hypoglycemia. NPH insulin should therefore be held until arrival at the hospital, and preferably until safe arrival in the preoperative area.

Surgical patients should have a stable, uninterrupted baseline of necessary medication as long as the medication does not increase perioperative risk.

Dialysis

Hemodialysis is best done 6-24 hours prior to surgery for optimal fluid status. Potassium can be checked just prior to the operation. The need for dialysis access usually does not require an emergency trip to the operating room and patients should be optimized before surgery and anesthesia, even MAC anesthesia, which sometimes proceeds to general anesthesia if there is a problem (eg, the patient cannot lie flat for a prolonged period of time without experiencing respiratory distress, or vascular injury from placing a dialysis catheter leads to the need for a thoracotomy or other operation).

Premedication

Patients are given premedication to decrease stomach acidity (liquid sodium citrate and citric acid), speed gastric emptying (metaclopromide) and block H2 receptors. There is no regimen that prevents aspiration. Patients are also given anxiolytics (midazolam) and pain medication if appropriate. Children are given midazolam orally or, in some cases, intranasally, when they do not already have an IV. Other medications may be administered for specific medical problems. These include antibiotics, hormones and clotting factors.

4. Intraoperative Monitoring and Intervention

Responsibility of the Anesthesiologist

One of the primary intraoperative responsibilities of the anesthesiologist is monitoring of the patient's physiological function. After a baseline is established, continuous acquisition of physiologic data and rapid interpretation of that data in terms of subjective knowledge allow the anesthesiologist and the surgeon to assess the patient's condition throughout the procedure, and to make therapeutic interventions necessary to maintain stability. The anesthesiologist keeps a record of data, events, impressions and interventions during the course of anesthetic management. The record may be a paper chart, but electronic records are becoming more widely used in the operating room.

Routine Intraoperative Monitoring

The ASA has established basic standards for routine intraoperative monitoring. Continuous monitoring of a patient's ventilation, circulation, oxygenation and temperature is standard. Each parameter is assessed by a combination of monitors. No individual monitor is without potential for artifact, and the array of data must be continuously surveyed and assessed by the anesthesiologist.

Ventilation
A precordial or esophageal stethoscope can be used to listen to breath sounds and to determine the rate and depth of respirations. Chest rise and fall and condensation of expired breath on a face mask can provide visual evidence of ventilation. The fingers holding the mask to the face can be used to palpate the vibration from the face and neck caused by air flowing through the airway, and fingers cupped near the mouth can feel warm expired air. A disposable device which changes color in the presence of carbon dioxide can be positioned near the airway to provide further evidence of ventilation. Use of capnometry and capnography, however, have become so prevalent as to be considered routine. The presence and amount of carbon dioxide in gases aspirated from or near the patient's airway provides clear evidence, both qualitative and quantitative, of ventilation. The capnometer provides a numerical measurement of the partial pressure or concentration of carbon dioxide in or at the airway during the ventilatory cycle, and capnography is the graphic

display of the waveform of carbon dioxide versus time. Capnography allows assessment of alveolar ventilation, airway integrity, function of the breathing circuit and ventilator, cardiac and pulmonary function, and detection of rebreathing and airway disconnection. In most settings today, the capnometer is part of the respiratory gas monitor measuring inspired and expired oxygen, carbon dioxide, nitrogen, nitrous oxide and volatile anesthetic gases.

Circulation

While palpation of the pulses and observation of color (as well as observation and inquiry regarding the status of organs in the surgical field) are means of assessing circulation and appropriate function of end organs (appropriate mentation in the awake patient or normal urine output) gives evidence of adequate perfusion, the circulation is usually assessed by intermittent blood pressure measurement and continuous electrocardiogram. The mercury sphygmomanometer, the standard of blood pressure measurement, is rarely used, and blood pressure is approximated oscillotomometrically by an automated noninvasive blood pressure cuff. The electrocardiogram can be monitored in 2 or more leads, usually II (most sensitive for cardiac dysrhythmias) and V5 (most sensitive for myocardial ischemia). Change in carbon dioxide waveform can signal a change in pulmonary artery perfusion and/or cardiac output. Pulse oximeters can also be used to detect changes in perfusion.

Oxygenation

Again, patient color allows some assessment of oxygenation, but routine use of pulse oximetry provides information on systemic oxygenation and heart rate with each heartbeat.

Temperature

Continuous monitoring of temperature using external (skin) or internal (rectal, urinary bladder, intravascular, esophageal or nasal) probes allows detection of changes in temperature and timely intervention to maintain normothermia and optimal physiologic performance. Temperature monitoring is critical for procedures that require cooling and rewarming, for early detection of malignant hyperthermia or other abnormal hypermetabolic states, and for detecting hypothermia.

Specialized Intraoperative Monitoring

When the surgical procedure is complex and/or the patient is at higher risk for intraoperative morbidity and mortality, or questions arise which cannot be satisfactorily answered with routine data, special monitors may be appropriate. Special or invasive monitoring can provide useful data which must be evaluated for artifact, but also carries the potential for complications.

Cardiovascular

Continuous intra-arterial pressure monitoring. Placement of an intra-arterial catheter allows access for blood sampling and constant measurement of the blood pressure, within constraints of artifact. Observation of the waveform in response to changes in intrathoracic pressure caused by positive pressure ventilation gives some information about volume status. Complications include infection, blood vessel perforation, and thrombogenesis. Noninvasive methods for continuous monitoring of arterial pressure are being developed.

Central venous catheter. Placement of a central venous catheter may allow more accurate assessment of volume status and access for rapid infusion of fluids (a catheter wider in caliber and shorter in length has the least resistance to flow). Complications include cardiac dysrhythmias, pneumothorax, hemothorax, nerve injury, hematoma, vessel injury, cardiac injury, infection and thrombogenesis.

Pulmonary artery catheter. A pulmonary artery catheter, or Swan-Ganz catheter, is a flow-directed catheter with the tip positioned in the pulmonary artery distally such that an inflated balloon at the tip can occlude flow. The catheter allows sampling of mixed-venous blood samples to help assess oxygen delivery and consumption, and allows approximate measurement of cardiac output and approximate assessment of left ventricular function. The catheter can carry a fiberoptic oximeter probe. Continuous monitoring of mixed-venous saturation aids in detecting and defining compromise from decreased oxygen carrying capacity, decreased cardiac output, decreased systemic vascular resistance, or abnormalities of ventilation and pulmonary perfusion. Multiple ports allow infusion of vasoactive drugs directly into the central circulation. The introduction of a pulmonary artery catheter through a central venous catheter (sheath) does compromise the flow characteristics of the central venous catheter. Complications include cardiac dysrhythmias, pneumothorax, hemothorax, nerve injury, hematoma, vessel injury (including pulmonary artery rupture), infection and thrombogenesis.

ST-segment analysis. Patterns of ST-segment change that fulfill criteria for myocardial ischemia have been extensively studied, and ST-segment analysis has been applied to anesthetized patients. Intraoperative ECG, however, is electronically filtered to remove artifact, which may distort waveforms and mimic ischemia. A standard 12-lead ECG may be necessary to confirm the significance of changes seen on the continuous intraoperative monitor.

Transesophageal echocardiography (TEE). With equipment in the hands of a trained operator/observer, TEE affords assessment of myocardial performance, valvular function, ventricular function and regional wall motion.

Pulmonary

Inspired and expired gas analysis. Gas analysis goes beyond the measurement of carbon dioxide at the airway to confirm ventilation. Inspired gases can be monitored for the presence of adequate oxygen to prevent delivery of a hypoxic gas mixture. Inspired and expired concentrations of anesthetic agents can be monitored, allowing accurate assessment of concentration of anesthetic gases in the brain, and taking much of the guesswork and calculation out of determining depth of anesthesia or time to awakening. End-tidal carbon dioxide waveforms can be analyzed to obtain information about the state of the patient's pulmonary disease, or to detect the presence of a pulmonary embolism. With both blood gas analysis and expired gas analysis, defects in ventilation and pulmonary perfusion can be detected. Expired carbon dioxide may be normal or low, with normal or increased ventilation, but if arterial carbon dioxide remains high, it should be obvious that pulmonary perfusion is being compromised, either by pulmonary embolism, pulmonary vasoconstriction, mechanical obstruction of the pulmonary arterial bed or by other causes of impaired pulmonary blood flow.

Pressure and volume measurement. Airway pressure and volume alarm and monitoring systems allow monitoring of peak airway pressure, tidal volume, inspiratory time and minute ventilation. Changes in pulmonary physiology can be detected as well as disconnections in the airway circuit, and kinking or obstruction of the endotracheal tube.

Renal

Bladder catheterization for accurate measurement of urine output is used routinely. Urine can easily be obtained for laboratory analysis or inspected for the presence of blood or injected dye.

Hematologic

The coagulation system can be assessed clinically as well as through the use of tests performed in the laboratory or operating room. Hemoglobin and hematocrit can be assessed clinically by estimating blood loss in the field, by observation of the consistency and color of intravascular blood, and by blood gas analysis and laboratory testing. Technology involving spectroscopy similar to that which is used in pulse oximetry is being developed to measure hemoglobin noninvasively.

Metabolic

Metabolic and electrolyte abnormalities can be assessed rapidly by blood gas analysis, and more extensively but not as rapidly by chemistry analysis.

Neurologic

Assessment is performed by electroencephalogram, bispectral index, intracranial pressure measurement, motor- and sensory-evoked potential monitoring, and intracranial pressure monitoring. Some neurological monitoring strategies require avoidance or minimal use of volatile anesthetic agents or neuromuscular blocking drugs.

Interventions

Airway

The anesthesiologist is responsible for and expert in airway management. In airway management, as in surgery, judgment must be exercised in conjunction with technical skill, and the ability to manage an airway problem strategically, considering all options and available tools, is critical.

The rigid laryngoscope, which consists of a handle, a blade and a light source, is the standard means of exposing the larynx for intubation. The laryngoscope is designed to be held in the left hand, while the endotracheal tube is placed with the right hand. Although there are dozens of blade styles, the 2 most commonly used blades are the Miller and the MacIntosh. The Miller, or straight blade, is usually used to pick up the epiglottis, while the MacIntosh, or curved blade, is placed in the vallecula, and upward traction is used to lift the epiglottis and expose the larynx.

There are 2 main airway considerations: whether or not the patient can be ventilated, and whether or not the patient can be intubated, because the larynx cannot either be visualized or reached. History (prior airway problems, sleep apnea) and airway examination (poor mouth opening with poor visibility of structures in the pharynx, small chin, overbite, neck extension is poor or contraindicated obesity) can help to anticipate potential problems with ventilation and intubation. Even if the patient can be ventilated, positive pressure ventilation of an unprotected airway (by mask) is unadvisable if the patient has or is suspected to have a full stomach because air introduced into the stomach can displace stomach contents upwards. If it is highly likely that the patient can be ventilated, and ventilation by mask is not contraindicated, it is reasonable to induce anesthesia and attempt to intubate.

If it is unlikely that the patient can be ventilated, and/or the patient is suspected to have a full stomach, but it is highly certain that the patient is intubatable, rapid-sequence induction (an induction agent and a rapid-onset muscle relaxant [both must be rapid, short-acting agents] given in quick succession while cricoid pressure is held to compress the esophagus and prevent passive [not active regurgitation or vomiting] regurgitation) and immediate intubation without attempt to mask is appropriate. In the event intubation is impossible at this point, attempt is made (likely to be unsuccessful) to perform mask ventilation with cricoid pressure until the anesthetic wears off. If the anesthetic does not wear off quickly enough, the anesthesiologist must resort quickly to advanced airway techniques for ventilation and/or intubation, or a surgical airway must be established.

If it appears that ventilation and intubation are both likely to be problematic, induction of anesthesia should occur after safe intubation of the awake patient. There are circumstances, such as when the patient has an unstable spine, when both intubation and positioning should occur while the patient is awake. Awake intubation is usually accomplished using a fiberoptic bronchoscope after topical or infiltration anesthesia of the lingual branch of the glossopharyngeal nerve, the superior laryngeal nerve, and the recurrent laryngeal nerve. After intubation, the awake patient should be able to tolerate the presence of the endotracheal tube, even while being positioned prone, until safe induction of anesthesia occurs. Awake intubation is not always an option in an emergency or with an uncooperative patient, and there are devices designed to facilitate difficult ventilation and/or intubation.

Oral airways and nasal trumpets may aid in maintaining an open airway during mask ventilation and various cuffed oropharyngeal airways can be connected to the anesthesia circuit.

Laryngeal mask airways (LMA) may allow mask ventilation by delivering the oxygen source to the glottis and creating a seal. Patients can be given positive pressure ventilation or may breathe spontaneously. However, the devices do not protect against aspiration of stomach contents or secretions. A small endotracheal tube can be introduced through an LMA using a fiberoptic bronchoscope.

Fastrach laryngeal mask airway is an LMA with a curved metal barrel through which an endotracheal tube can be introduced blindly, with or without carbon dioxide guidance, or with the help of a fiberoptic bronchoscope, with a high success rate. A variant of this device has a screen which displays a view of the larynx. Until the endotracheal tube is in place, the patient is not protected from aspiration.

Esophageal tracheal combitube is a tube that can be placed blindly and usually goes into the esophagus. A second lumen is ventilated after the esophageal lumen is sealed. If the device has gone into the airway, the first lumen is then ventilated. A similar device is designed always to be placed in the esophagus with a second lumen open to the airway and connected to the anesthesia circuit.

In addition to the fiberoptic bronchoscope, there are other indirect fiberoptic laryngoscopes, including the GlideScope©, the McGrath©, and the Storz© video laryngoscope. None requires neck extension and all display a view of the larynx. If the vocal cords can be seen but not reached, a fiberoptic bronchoscope can be used by a second operator to introduce the endotracheal tube to the vocal cords.

Jet ventilation can be used to force oxygen through a small airway placed through the cricothyroid membrane until a definitive airway is established.

Stylets, guides, tube changers, tracheal tube introducers or bougies, lighted stylets, and other devices are available to aid in intubation and/or in changing one endotracheal tube for another without losing control of the airway.

Many other devices exist or are in development. More important than the devices themselves are the skill and experience shown in using them and the thought process involved in predicting, preventing and solving strategic airway problems. The anesthesiologist develops a multitude of strategies using different combinations of these devices.

Often the combined efforts of the surgeon and the anesthesiologist are required for airway management such as in tracheostomy, bronchoscopy, surgery and anesthesia in the patient with an unstable cervical spine, and in the unstable trauma patient with trauma to or near the airway.

Maintaining the Internal Milieu

The skill of the anesthesiologist lies in manipulating vascular space and intravascular volume with fluids and vasoactive drugs that are rapidly titratable, anticipating changes in the surgical field to maintain constant perfusion pressure and oxygen delivery to vital organs, and anticipating and treating perturbations in the intravascular milieu to maintain normal electrolytes and temperature. Oxygenation and ventilation must be maintained, compensating for anticipated and unanticipated surgical effects on the lungs. Constant vigilance allows miniscule interventions to compensate for subtle changes as well as aggressive interventions to treat massive changes.

Patients may begin surgery with volume deficit due to fasting, sepsis, bleeding, recent dialysis and/or bowel prep. They may begin surgery with excess or abnormally distributed volume due to congestive heart failure, renal failure or hepatic failure. Volatile anesthetics cause vasodilation and exaggerate the effects of hypovolemia. Narcotics and other anesthetics blunt catecholamine response and compensatory mechanisms. Patients with hypotension and cardiovascular dysfunction have impaired compensatory mechanisms. The anesthesiologist must anticipate these problems and address them with infusion of appropriate fluids, as well as adjusting hemodynamic parameters with appropriate drugs. As the operation proceeds, blood loss ensues and trauma to tissue as well as exposure to the environment result in further fluid shifts, so the anesthesiologist must continue to compensate. With massive fluid shifts, electrolyte abnormalities eventually occur, and these must be anticipated and treated. Positioning requirements and special surgical techniques requiring insufflation of the pleural or peritoneal cavity such as thoroscopy and laparoscopy place demands on the patient's heart and lungs, requiring compensation. However, the development of the same techniques has allowed more medically fragile patients to recover more easily from operations that previously necessitated large incisions.

Hypothermia results in delayed metabolism of drugs as well as delays in coagulation, and is associated with increased risk of ischemia, even in the absence of shivering. The most effective means of preventing heat loss and of active warming is the warm air blanket. Warming intravenous fluids also prevents heat loss, but is less effective in active warming.

5. Anesthetic Drugs

The drugs used by the anesthesiologist include general anesthetics, either inhaled or intravenous, local anesthetics, neuromuscular blocking agents, analgesics, anxiolytics, vasoactive agents, antiemetics and other adjunct agents.

The ideal anesthetic should have a rapid onset of action with predictable and rapid recovery from its effects, and an absence of persistent effect on the brain or other organs after the time of anesthesia. It should be easy to administer, and administration should be guided by clear signs of the depth of anesthesia. It should have a wide safely margin in all patients. Drugs that act quickly and have a short half-life with inactive metabolites are ideal for use as and with anesthetics, because they can be quickly titrated to effect and their effect rapidly wanes after the drug is discontinued.

The goal of the anesthesiologist is to convince the body that nothing is happening to disturb homeostasis, while a series of noxious stimuli are delivered to it. Anxiety, fear, manipulation of the airway, surgical incision and manipulation with resultant tissue damage, disturbance in bowel function, changes in intravascular volume and ischemic pain from application of a tourniquet all threaten to disturb equilibrium. Their effects must be anticipated and pharmacologically blunted.

The intent of general anesthesia is to render the patient unconscious or unaware, to provide amnesia and analgesia, and to prevent the patient from moving, while maintaining perfusion, oxygenation and ventilation. No one drug does all of this. Thus, a patient can move while remaining unconscious and unaware or a patient can be aware and uncomfortable while unable to move and communicate.

General Anesthetics

Mechanism

General anesthetics most likely induce unconsciousness by causing hyperpolarization of thalamocortical neurons, thus changing their firing from a tonic to a burst pattern, according to current research.

Inhaled Anesthetics

(Volatile Anesthetics and Nitrous Oxide)

Anesthetic uptake and distribution. The route of entry and elimination of inhaled anesthetics is the respiratory tract. An adequate partial pressure of an inhaled anesthetic in the brain is required to induce anesthesia. The partial pressure of the anesthetic in the alveoli determines the partial pressure in all body tissues, including the brain. The route of delivery to the tissues is the arterial blood, the partial pressure in which is also determined by alveolar partial pressure.

The alveolar anesthetic partial pressure rises to equilibrate with the concentration of inspired anesthetic following an asymptotic curve. There is a steep initial increase in concentration, then a long slow progression towards equilibrium. Increasing the inspired concentration to greater than the desired partial pressure (overpressure) will shorten the time needed to reach the desired alveolar partial pressure. An increase in the minute ventilation will also promote more rapid alveolar uptake of the drug, as will increasing the volume of the breathing circuit.

Again, alveolar anesthetic partial pressure determines partial pressure in the brain, and despite the fact that the anesthetic is delivered by the blood, decreased removal from the alveolus by the blood promotes a greater anesthetic effect. Thus, ***decreased cardiac output favors more rapid induction*** of inhaled anesthetic. Decreased alveolar-venous anesthetic gradient and decreased solubility of the anesthetic in blood also favor more rapid induction of inhaled anesthetic. Conversely, delayed induction results from increased cardiac output, increased alveolar-venous anesthetic gradient and increased solubility of the anesthetic in blood.

Emergence from volatile anesthetic follows an asymptotic curve as well, with a rapid decrease in concentration, followed by a long slow progression towards equilibrium. The expired concentration cannot be reduced to less than zero, thus the differential gradient is between the brain, the blood, the alveoli and zero. Increasing minute ventilation and the volume of the breathing circuit promote elimination of anesthetic from the body and speeds recovery.

Inhaled anesthetics are categorized by their physical and physiological characteristics.

MAC is defined as the minimum alveolar concentration (partial pressure) of an inhaled anesthetic at 1 atmosphere, which prevents skeletal muscle movement in response to a noxious stimulus (surgical skin incision) in 50% of patients. Thus, MAC represents 1 point on the dose response curve of effects produced by inhaled anesthetics, and is the most important index of potency of inhaled anesthetics.

Comparing the volatile anesthetics in current (or recent) use, 1 MAC of inhaled anesthetic at equilibrium equals 0.75 volume percent halothane, 1.15 volume percent isoflurane, 1.68 volume percent enflurane, 2.0 volume percent sevoflurane or 7.0 volume percent desflurane. By comparison, another inhaled anesthetic, the inert gas nitrous oxide at 105.0-110.0 volume percent equals 1 MAC, thus nitrous oxide cannot be used alone as an anesthetic at 1 atmosphere pressure. ***MAC values for combinations of inhaled anesthetics are probably additive,*** however, thus nitrous oxide can be used in combination with a volatile anesthetic (and oxygen) to reduce the volume percent of the volatile required to produce anesthesia. Volatile anesthetics are not used in combination with each other.

MAC is unchanged by duration of the anesthetic, serum potassium levels, degree of metabolism of inhaled anesthetic, thyroid function, gender, blood pressure (above a mean of 40 mm Hg), arterial partial pressure of carbon dioxide (within the range of 15-95 mm Hg) and arterial partial pressure of oxygen (above 38 mm Hg).

MAC is increased by hyperthermia, hypernatremia, chronic ethanol abuse and by drugs that increase central nervous system catecholamine levels (monoamine oxidase inhibitors [MAOIs], tricyclic antidepressants [TCAs], acute cocaine intoxication, acute amphetamine ingestion).

MAC is decreased by hypothermia, hyponatremia, pregnancy, lithium, magnesium, lidocaine, pancuronium, physostigmine, arterial partial pressure of oxygen below 38 mm Hg, increased age, preoperative medication (sedatives, narcotics), acute ethanol ingestion and by drugs that decrease central nervous system catecholamine levels (alpha-methyldopa, clonidine, chronic amphetamine ingestion).

When comparing inhaled anesthetics by MAC, one might conclude that halothane, the most potent, would be the anesthetic of choice. However, other characteristics do not correlate with MAC.

Solubility is expressed in terms of blood:gas or tissue:blood ***partition coefficients***. At equilibrium, the partial pressure of anesthetic is the same in blood and gas (alveolus) and in tissue (brain is usually the tissue of interest) and blood. Although the partial pressures are the same in both phases at equilibrium, concentrations in one phase can be greater than in the other. If an agent has a blood:gas partition coefficient of 2, that agent will reach twice the concentration (in volume percent) in the blood phase as in the gas phase at equal partial pressures. If an agent has a tissue:blood coefficient of 2, that agent will reach twice the concentration (in volume percent) in the tissue phase as in the blood phase at equal partial pressures.

Insolubility in blood (lower blood:gas partition coefficient) ***favors rapid uptake*** of anesthetic. From most soluble to least soluble volatile agents (with blood:gas partition coefficients at 37°C), are halothane (2.4), enflurane (1.7), isoflurane (1.4), sevoflurane (0.64) and desflurane (0.42). By comparison, nitrous oxide is 0.47.

The time necessary for equilibration of the tissue with the blood is determined by the tissue:blood partition coefficient. This time can be predicted by calculating a time constant (amount of inhaled anesthetic that can be dissolved in the tissue divided by tissue blood flow) for each tissue. Complete equilibrium of inhaled anesthetic in any tissue, including the brain, with inhaled agent in the blood, requires at least 3 time constants. The time constant for volatile anesthetics is approximately 5 minutes, and the time constant for nitrous oxide is approximately 6 minutes because it is less soluble in brain tissue.

Tissue (particularly lipid-rich tissue like the brain) solubility and high blood flow to a given tissue favor rapid equilibrium at induction of anesthesia, thus well-perfused tissues equilibrate rapidly and poorly perfused tissues equilibrate very slowly.

Recovery is more rapid with decreased solubility and increased blood flow to tissues and is slower after an anesthetic of long duration (due to the presence of more anesthetic dissolved in tissues over time). Note that partition coefficients given are for 37°C. Hypothermia speeds induction and delays emergence.

Pungency of inhaled anesthetics varies. Very pungent anesthetics are not only unpleasant to smell, they are irritating to the upper airway and may induce coughing and laryngospasm, and are therefore not suitable for delivery through a mask until a patient is deeply anesthetized. The 2 least pungent volatile anesthetics are halothane and sevoflurane. Both are used for mask induction of anesthesia, although halothane, the more soluble of the 2, is associated with a longer induction time and a more prolonged recovery. Sevoflurane is widely in use, while halothane now used less frequently. Nitrous oxide is nonpungent. Enflurane was the most pungent of the volatile agents and is no longer in use.

Nitrous oxide is unique in that high partial pressures are achieved in blood because of its low solubility and low potency. Nitrous oxide is slightly more soluble than nitrogen (the major component of air) in blood, thus it ***diffuses into body cavities containing air*** faster than nitrogen diffuses out, until equilibrium is reached, increasing the volume of the air-filled cavities. If a cavity is nondistensible, the pressure in the cavity increases. During prolonged anesthesia at high inspired concentrations, there can be considerable distention of the bowel, an effect which ranges from inconvenient to dangerous, depending on the condition of the patient. Intrapleural gas volume also increases, thus nitrous oxide is inappropriate for use in a patient with a pneumothorax. Lung cysts and bullae will also increase in volume. The middle ear is also an air-filled cavity; nitrous oxide can be used to advantage to "tent" the tympanic membrane to facilitate tympanostomy, but is contraindicated for tympanoplasty because it will displace the graft. A pneumoencephalocele will expand, thus causing an increase in intracranial pressure. A patient who has just undergone a craniotomy or pneumoencephalogram should not be given nitrous oxide. The volume of air emboli will also expand, thus suspicion of air embolus also contraindicates use of nitrous oxide. Nitrous oxide is used during induction of anesthesia because of its rapid uptake, which reduces the volume of gas in the alveolus, allowing a mass movement of inspired gas at increased concentration into the alveolus from the tracheobronchial tree and into the tracheobronchial tree from the circuit, thus increasing alveolar delivery of the volatile anesthetic used: this is called the second gas effect. Nitrous oxide is also used during mask induction to moderate the awareness of the more pungent volatile anesthetic. It also diffuses rapidly out of the body, thus its inconvenient effect on the bowel is reversible. Unfortunately, it also diffuses rapidly into the alveolus, reducing the partial pressure of carbon dioxide and oxygen, and may cause ***diffusion hypoxia***, the effects of which can be prevented by increasing the fraction of inspired oxygen for 2 or 3 minutes after the termination of nitrous oxide. Both nitrous oxide and nitrogen, in equilibrium, serve as inert expanders of alveoli, allowing free diffusion of oxygen and carbon dioxide into and out of open alveoli, and preventing ***diffusion atelectasis.***

Inhaled anesthetics produce dose-dependent and agent-specific effects on physiology, thus potency and rapidity of uptake are not the only considerations for choosing a volatile anesthetic agent. Comparison of these agents was performed on healthy volunteers in the absence of extraneous influences such as other drugs, surgical stimulation, extremes of age, coexisting diseases or abnormal intravascular volume status.

Respiratory physiology. The spontaneous respiratory pattern during inhalation of anesthetic concentrations of volatile agents becomes regular, unlike the awake pattern in which breaths vary in length. The respiratory rate increases but tidal volume decreases, resulting in a decrease in alveolar ventilation. The central chemosensory apparatus in the brainstem presumably becomes less responsive to hydrogen ions, thus the ventilatory response to decreased pH is decreased, allowing an increase in the partial pressure of arterial carbon dioxide. Intercostal muscle function is impaired, particularly by halothane, and although the diaphragm is relatively spared, the chest is allowed to collapse inward, thus reducing lung volumes, particularly functional residual capacity (FRC). Mucociliary function is impaired, in particular by halothane, enflurane or the addition of nitrous oxide, leading to retention of secretions and potential atelectasis or pneumonia. This effect can persist for hours after discontinuation of halothane. Volatile agents attenuate bron chospasm in bronchoconstricted patients, but do not really affect airway resistance in normal patients. Volatile agents attenuate hypoxic pulmonary vasoconstriction (HPV), the reflex constriction of pulmonary arterioles in areas of atelectasis in an attempt to prevent perfusion of nonventilated alveoli. Nitrous oxide probably does not affect HPV.

Cardiovascular physiology. Parameters of interest are stroke volume, heart rate, cardiac output, systemic vascular resistance, blood pressure, rhythm, pulmonary vascular resistance and coronary perfusion. ***Stroke volume (SV):*** all volatile agents decrease SV. Enflurane and sevoflurane decrease SV the most (-40%), followed by halothane and desflurane (-20%), then isoflurane (-10%). Nitrous oxide does not change SV. ***Heart rate (HR):*** sevoflurane causes the greatest increase in HR (+30%), followed by isoflurane and enflurane (+20%, although isoflurane's effect is not dose-dependent), then desflurane (+10%), and nitrous oxide (minimal increase). Halothane does not increase HR. ***Cardiac output (CO):*** enflurane and sevoflurane cause the greatest decrease in CO (-25%), followed by halothane (-20%). Isoflurane and desflurane do not decrease CO. Nitrous oxide causes a mild increase in CO, probably because it is a mild sympathomimetic. ***Systemic vascular resistance (SVR):*** isoflurane and desflurane cause the greatest decrease in SVR (-25%), followed by enflurane and halothane (-10%). Sevoflurane causes little decrease in SVR (-5%). Nitrous oxide causes no significant change in SVR. ***Blood pressure (BP):*** enflurane and desflurane decrease BP most (-35%), followed by sevoflurane (-34%), then halothane and isoflurane (-25%). Nitrous oxide causes no change in BP. ***Cardiac rhythm:*** halothane sensitizes the myocardium to the effects of epinephrine by slowing transmission through the His-Purkinje system, predisposing the patient to dysrhythmias and suppressing sinus node activity. Halothane, enflurane and isoflurane slow transmission through the atrioventricular node. Pulmonary vascular resistance can be increased by nitrous oxide in patients with pulmonary hypertension. Halothane and isoflurane reduce coronary perfusion and myocardial oxygen consumption, apparently as a result of a decrease in myocardial oxygen demand. Sympathetic response to surgical stimulation both attenuates the effect of anesthetic agents on cardiac physiology, and is opposed by volatile agents.

Cerebral circulation. All inhalation anesthetics are direct cerebral vasodilators and depress cerebral autoregulation and cerebral metabolism. Increased arterial carbon dioxide also contributes indirectly to cerebral vasodilation, but this effect is mitigated by controlling the respiratory rate.

Splanchnic circulation. Volatile anesthetics reduce splanchnic perfusion pressure. Nitrous oxide does not.

Renal circulation. Inhaled anesthetics, including nitrous oxide, increase renal vascular resistance and decrease renal blood flow, decreasing glomerular filtration rate (GFR) by 19%-55% and renal plasma flow (RPF) by 36%-67%.

Skin and muscle circulation. Inhaled anesthetics, including nitrous oxide, all dilate cutaneous vessels, possibly by interfering with thalamic temperature regulating mechanisms, resulting in heat loss. Inhaled anesthetics do not have a direct effect on skeletal muscle blood flow.

Muscle relaxation. Volatile anesthetics all provide some degree of muscle relaxation while nitrous oxide does not. Airway muscle tone is also reduced by volatile anesthetics.

Metabolism and toxicity. Inhaled anesthetics can undergo varying degrees of metabolism in the liver and to a lesser extent in the lungs, kidneys, and gastrointestinal tract. ***Metabolism, because the amount metabolized is relatively insignificant, does not influence induction, maintenance, or emergence from inhaled anesthetics***.The degree of metabolism is dependent on the induced activity of hepatic enzymes, as well as genetic factors and the chemical structure of the individual anesthetic agent.

Halothane undergoes significant metabolism, but metabolites are not likely to be toxic. Halothane-associated hepatic dysfunction, which is rare, is associated with eosinophilia and repeat exposure, thus allergic reaction is the suspected cause of liver damage. Hepatic dysfunction after an anesthetic is statistically more likely to be the result of underlying liver disease and/or hypoperfusion. Nevertheless, halothane is not the agent of choice in the patient with liver disease. Enflurane undergoes minimal metabolism, which can result in elevated serum fluoride concentrations in obese patients. Fluoride-induced nephrotoxicity, in which there is a transient decrease in urine concentrating ability, is remotely possible after prolonged exposure to enflurane. Enflurane is not the agent of choice in the patient with renal disease. Sevoflurane also has potential for nephrotoxicity after prolonged exposure, but this effect is mitigated by avoiding low air and oxygen flows. Isoflurane and desflurane undergo insignificant metabolism. Nitrous oxide produces inhibition of the mobilization of polymorphonuclear leukocytes, potentially suppressing inflammatory response in a dose-dependent manner. Synthesis of chromosomal protein may be inhibited by inactivation of methionine synthetase by nitrous oxide, thus nitrous oxide is usually avoided in the pregnant patient. Volatile anesthetics are triggering agents in patients with genetic susceptibility for malignant hyperthermia and should not be used in these patients.

Intravenous Anesthetics

Intravenous agents are routinely used for the induction of anesthesia, and some of these agents can also be used for maintenance of anesthesia. With the exception of ketamine, these agents are not analgesics; in fact, barbiturates are antalgesic.

Sodium thiopental is a thiobarbiturate with rapid onset and rapid awakening after an induction dose of 3-5 mg/kg. Awakening after a single dose is due to redistribution of the drug to inactive tissue sites, but elimination half-life is at least 9 hours. Unconsciousness is prolonged after doses sufficiently saturate inactive sites. Administration of thiopental reduces BP, increases HR, depresses the myocardium, decreases SVR and venous return to the heart, and reduces sympathetic tone. These effects are exaggerated in the hypovolemic patient. Thiopental depresses ventilation and produces transient apnea and unconsciousness, but does not suppress laryngeal reflexes or attenuate bronchospasm. The drug is a potent cerebral vasoconstrictor that also decreases cerebral metabolism and oxygen utilization, and suppresses the electroencephalogram, making it ideal for patients undergoing neurosurgical procedures. Thiopental is highly alkaline, and extravascular injection can result in local irritation and tissue necrosis. Intra-arterial injection can cause profound arterial vasoconstriction, distal cyanosis, and gangrene, and the artery should immediately be injected with lidocaine or procaine (to promote vasodilatation) and heparin (to minimize thrombosis). Sympathetic nervous system innervation to the limb may be blocked to minimize pain. Finally, thiopental and other barbiturates are contraindicated in patients with porphyria.

Methohexital is an oxybarbiturate with rapid onset and rapid awakening after an induction dose of 1-2 mg/kg. Elimination half-life is only 1.5 hours. Methohexital can be used for induction or infused for sedation. Effects on hemodynamics and ventilation are similar to the effects of thiopental. Methohexital evokes electroencephalographic evidence of epileptic foci, and is preferred for electroconvulsive therapy.

Ketamine, a phencyclidine, produces dissociative anesthesia, in which the patient is in a cataleptic state with open eyes, nystagmatic gaze, increased skeletal muscle tone and profound analgesia. HR, BP, CO and pulmonary artery pressure are increased in the patient with an intact and nondepressed central nervous system. Ketamine use may be undesirable in patients with cardiac ischemia, mitral valve lesions or some congenital heart lesions. Ketamine is useful for induction of anesthesia in a moderately hypovolemic patient, but can cause hypotension in a severely hypovolemic patient who is depleted of catecholamines. Upper airway patency is facilitated by increased skeletal muscle tone. Laryngeal reflexes are only slightly depressed, and ventilatory response to carbon dioxide is maintained unless large doses are given. Ketamine acts as a bronchodilator in bronchoconstricted patients. Ketamine increases salivary secretion, thus patients are often pretreated with an anticholinergic such as glycopyrrolate, with a quaternary structure that does not, unlike atropine, cross the blood-brain barrier. Ketamine is associated with unpleasant emergence dreams and hallucinations, the memory of which can be attenuated by concomitant use of a benzodiazepine such as midazolam. Ketamine 1-2 mg/kg IV has an onset within 1 minute and 4-6 mg/kg IM has an onset within 2-4 minutes. Redistribution is responsible for much of the recovery from the drug within 15-30 minutes. Elimination half-life is 2-3 hours. The drug is used extensively for burn dressing changes and debridements, and for suturing wounds. Because ketamine is also an analgesic, it can be used for reducing fractures and dislocations without risk of respiratory depression which can be caused by residual narcotic. Doses for moderate sedation are .25-.50 mg/kg IV. Ketamine is contraindicated in patients with intracranial pathology because it increases cerebral blood flow and cerebral metabolic oxygen requirements as well as intracranial pressure.

Etomidate is a carboxylated imidazole that produces unconsciousness in less than 1 minute with recovery in 4-10 minutes. Most of the drug is metabolized by the liver and eliminated in the urine. Induction dose is 0.4 mg/kg, although a smaller dose should be used in unstable patients. Etomidate is used in patients who are hemodynamically unstable because it produces minimal changes in HR and BP, and minimal alteration in ventilation. Etomidate causes a decrease in cerebral blood flow through cerebral vasoconstriction. Pain occurs on injection and myoclonic movements not associated with epileptiform activity occur frequently, and etomidate also causes transient suppression of adrenocortical function.

Propofol is an alkylphenol in a milky white soy lecithin emulsion, which causes discomfort, but not vascular damage, on injection. Propofol is used as an induction agent as well as for anesthetic maintenance. It is also used for short periods of sedation as well as for more prolonged sedation of adult patients in intensive care units. In small doses, propofol behaves like a mild sedative, and in larger doses, it behaves like a profound general anesthetic. An induction dose of 2.5 mg/kg produces unconsciousness within 1 minute. Recovery occurs within 3 minutes. The drug is rapidly metabolized in the liver by conjugation to inactive water soluble compounds which are excreted by the kidneys. Clearance is actually out of proportion to hepatic blood flow, thus it is proposed that an additional route of metabolism and elimination exists, possibly the lungs. Propofol affects the respiratory system in a manner similar to barbiturates, with an induction dose causing apnea, which may be prolonged. A maintenance infusion allows spontaneous ventilation much in the manner of a volatile anesthetic. Induction with propofol produces a decrease in BP, CO, SV and SVR, due to both vasodilation and myocardial depression, without increasing HR. Propofol does not affect hepatic, hematologic, fibrinolytic or immunologic function, and is not a triggering agent for malignant hyperthermia. Propofol infusion has become the agent of choice for induction and maintenance of general anesthesia in the patient at risk for malignant hyperthermia. Because no anesthesia machine is required, propofol infusion, which can be administered via a small syringe pump, is often the agent of choice for procedures done away from the operating room when an anesthesia machine is not available. Propofol infused rapidly or over a long period of time places the patient at risk for irreversible acidosis and complications as a result of an overdose of soy lecithin emulsion.

Local Anesthetics

Local anesthetics are used by the surgeon on the field for infiltration anesthesia, both preemptively and at the end of an operation, and for nerve blocks. They are used by the anesthesiologist for nerve blocks and neuraxial (spinal and epidural) anesthesia. In addition, intravenous lidocaine is used for intravenous regional anesthesia (Bier block), and to moderate response to airway manipulation and painful injection. Lidocaine can be sprayed directly into the airway as a topical anesthetic.

The toxicity of local anesthetics first excites, then depresses, the central nervous system. Lidocaine typically causes tingling and numbness of the lips and tongue, light-headedness, ringing in the ears and some visual changes at low serum concentrations (up to 10 mg/mL), followed by muscular twitching, convulsions and coma (at 18 mg/mL), and finally respiratory and cardiac arrest at 25 mg/mL. The effect is exacerbated by arterial hypoxemia. Lidocaine is relatively short-acting, and initial benign symptoms manifest themselves at much lower serum concentrations than the concentration at which ominous symptoms appear. Conversely, bupivacaine is longer acting, and cardiac arrest may occur, without warning, as a result of the same dose which causes seizures. Cardiac arrest from bupivacaine is extremely difficult to reverse due to prolonged blockade of sodium channels. Bupivacaine should never be given intravascularly.

Local anesthetics injected into different sites diffuse into blood at different rates, depending on blood flow to the site. Serum concentrations become elevated to toxic levels when diffusion into the blood is more rapid than metabolism. Typically, the nerve block associated with the most rapid diffusion into blood is the intercostal block, followed by caudal, epidural, brachial plexus and femoral sciatic. A local anesthetic should be chosen for use in a given site with potential toxicity in mind, and used in the smallest doses possible to accomplish the clinical goal.

Maximum doses for infiltration for local anesthetics are:

Amides
Lidocaine 7 mg/kg (moderate duration)
Mepivacaine 7 mg/kg (moderate duration)
Bupivacaine 2.5-3 mg/kg (long duration)
Ropivacaine 4 mg/kg (long duration)

Esters
Tetracaine 1.5 mg/kg (long duration)
Procaine 14 mg/kg (short duration)
2-Chlorprocaine 20 mg/kg (short duration)

Bupivacaine is used quite frequently for infiltration to minimize postoperative pain, because it has long duration. It usually comes in .25% and .5% strengths. By moving the decimal point one place to the right, mg/mL can be determined, thus quarter percent contains 2.5 mg/mL. The safe dose of quarter percent is therefore 1 mL/kg and the safe dose of half percent is .5 mL/kg.

Bupivacaine is not the local anesthetic of choice for a Bier block, since it will be administered intravenously, and tourniquet release will result in intravascular spread of the drug. Lidocaine would be a more appropriate choice, since duration of action of a Bier block is determined by how long the tourniquet is tolerated (1-1.5 hours), not by the duration of the local anesthetic. (Bupivacaine can be used in caudal, epidural, and spinal anesthesia, and in brachial plexus, cervical plexus and intercostal blocks.)

Epinephrine slows uptake of some local anesthetics into the blood, leading to a decrease in the potential for systemic toxicity for a given dose, thus larger doses of the local anesthetic are permitted. Lidocaine can be given in greater doses when combined with epinephrine. Epinephrine also acts as a marker for intravascular lidocaine by causing tachycardia, but it can cause dysrhythmia.

Neuromuscular Blocking Agents

Depolarizing Agent

Succinylcholine is the sole agent of this class of drug. It is simply a double molecule of acetylcholine (ACh) and acts by activating all skeletal muscle neuromuscular junctions, causing massive fasciculation, thus blocking the receptor slightly longer than ACh does, since its breakdown is slowed by its bulk. It is inactivated by circulating plasma cholinesterase.

The action of succinylcholine is prolonged by monoamine oxidase inhibitors, herbicide toxicity, nitrogen mustard and cyclophosphamide, and in malnutrition, severe liver disease, pregnancy, patients with congenital atypical pseudocholinesterase and in myasthenia gravis patients on pyridostigmine.

Succinylcholine is contraindicated or relatively contraindicated in patients with upper or lower motor neuron disease or spinal cord injury more than 24 hours old, patients who have been on prolonged bed rest, have myotonic disease or burns more than 5 days old and, even if well healed, less than 60 days old, with crush injuries, sepsis, intraabdominal infection, an open globe, elevated intracranial pressure from closed head injury, pheochromocytoma, malignant hyperthermia and hyperkalemia. This is because succinylcholine causes potassium efflux from normal muscle cells (0.5 mEq/L). If potassium is already high, muscle cells are injured, or central nervous system injury causes up regulation of active sites at the neuromuscular junction (the latter two conditions resulting in increased potassium efflux [1-6 mEq/L]), or the patient is susceptible to malignant hyperthermia triggered by succinylcholine, the serum potassium level could rise to levels sufficient to cause dysrhythmias and cardiac arrest. The concern with open globe injury is related to the rise in intraocular pressure from fasciculation, not to potassium efflux. The concern with malignant hyperthermia not limited to potassium efflux is the triggering of the entire syndrome. Pretreatment with a nondepolarizing muscle relaxant will not prevent potassium efflux, elevated intraocular pressure or malignant hyperthermia. In patients with pheochromocytoma, succinylcholine may trigger release of catecholamines. Succinylcholine may also cause bradycardia, and is used as little as possible in infants and children.

The use of cricoid pressure during rapid sequence induction has nothing to do with attenuating the effects of succinylcholine. Succinylcholine is indicated for rapid sequence induction and cricoid pressure is used, with less than 100% success, to prevent insufflation of air into the stomach and passive regurgitation during rapid sequence induction in the patient who may have a full stomach.

Nondepolarizing Agents

Nondepolarizing agents combine with the cholinergic receptors but do not activate them. If a sufficient number of receptors are occupied by a nondepolarizing muscle relaxant, they are not available to ACh. Thus blockade is postsynaptic and competitive.

Reversal of nondepolarizing muscle relaxants is traditionally achieved by blocking acetylcholinesterase (after giving an anticholinergic to prevent bradycardia and/or asystole) and making more ACh available to compete with the neuromuscular blocker for the receptors. Sugammadex, a new drug, reverses relaxation by encapsulating the rocuronium molecule, rendering it inactive.

Nondepolarizing agents include pancuronium, vecuronium, rocuronium, atracurium and cis-atracurium. Actions of concern are onset, duration, side effects, metabolism, excretion and/or elimination. Pancuronium lasts the longest, requires renal excretion and causes tachycardia. Vecuronium and rocuronium have no cardiovascular side effects. Rocuronium is faster and shorter acting than vecuronium. The action of pancuronium, vecuronium and rocuronium can be prolonged by other drugs and all require some metabolism or renal excretion. Atracurium causes histamine release, and cis-atracurium, the cis-enantiomer, does not. Both are relatively rapid in onset, and atracurium is shorter in duration than cis-atracurium. Both are degraded by Hoffman elimination which is not dependent on renal or hepatic function.

Another agent, rapacuronium, had the quickest onset and the shortest duration, and was potentially the best replacement for succinylcholine for rapid sequence induction when succinylcholine is contraindicated. It could not be redosed and did not require reversal. It was taken off the market because of its association with severe bronchospasm.

Narcotics (Opioids)

Opioid receptors are found throughout the brain and in the spinal cord around the C-fiber terminal zone and substantia gelatinosa. Opioids are classified by strength (weak vs. strong), derivation (natural vs. synthetic), and as agonists, partial agonists, agonist/antagonists or antagonists.

Full agonists include the alkaloids, some of which are semisynthetic (morphine, codeine, hydromorphone, oxycodone, oxymorphone, heroin, hydrocodone and dihydrocodone) and synthetic opioids (levorphanol, fentanyl, sufentanil, alfentanil, remifentanil, meperidine, methadone and propoxyphene).

Partial agonists include buprenorphine (semisynthetic alkaloid), dezocine (synthetic opioid) and tramadol.

Mixed agonists include nalbuphine (semisynthetic alkaloid), pentazocine and butorphanol (synthetic opioids).

Antagonists include naloxone, naltrexone, and nalmefene. Endogenous opioids are beta-endorphin, dynorphin and enkephalin.

Opioid Systemic Effects

- Central nervous system depression, nausea and vomiting, pupillary constriction, depressed cough reflex, analgesia, central nervous system excitation and seizures (meperidine in high doses), and hyperactive spinal reflexes.

- Bradycardia due to vagal stimulation, tachycardia (meperidine only), arteriolar and venous dilation leading to orthostatic hypotension, cardiac depression (meperidine) and histamine release (morphine and meperidine).

- Increased arterial carbon dioxide tension, decreased respiratory rate, increased depth of breathing, decreased minute ventilation, brainstem depression and chest wall rigidity.

- Urinary retention, slow gastric emptying and spasm of sphincter of Oddi (less with meperidine).

- Cutaneous localized histamine release (not allergic reaction).

- Tolerance and physical dependence. There is increasing evidence that opioids may enhance sensitivity to pain.

- Drug interaction with monoamine oxidase inhibitors: respiratory depression and hyperthermia (meperidine).

Neuraxial Opioids

Opioids with higher lipid solubility (fentanyl) have faster onset of action, bind to a smaller area of distribution along the spinal cord resulting in a more limited area of analgesia and have faster clearance from the neuraxis, shorter duration of action and higher blood concentrations with more systemic side effects. Opioids with lower lipid solubility (morphine) are slower in onset, bind to a wider area along the spinal cord and have slower clearance, with side effects resulting from direct effects on the central nervous system.

Comparative Potency of Opioids

Comparing intramuscular (IM) doses, 10 mg morphine is equivalent to 75 mg meperidine, 10 mg methadone, or 1.5 mg hydromorphone. Comparing oral (PO) doses, 30 mg morphine is equivalent to 300 mg meperidine, 12.5 mg methadone, 7.5 mg hydromorphone or 30 mg oxycodone. Comparing intravenous doses, .01 mg sufentanil is equivalent to .1 mg fentanyl, 1 mg alfentanil, 1 mg hydromorphone, 10 mg morphine and 100 mg meperidine.

Intravenous opioids differ in rapidity of onset, distribution and elimination. Remifentanil has rapid onset and elimination without residual effects. Fentanyl has rapid onset and redistributes into inactive sites until they are saturated, but has a relatively long elimination half-time (185-219 minutes). Morphine has a slower onset than fentanyl, does not redistribute, and has a shorter elimination half-time than fentanyl (102-132 minutes). Thus remifentanil might be used for a prolonged procedure that is extremely stimulating but does not cause residual tissue damage (diagnostic bronchoscopy), and fentanyl might be used for a shorter, highly stimulating procedure, or a longer, less stimulating procedure that results in some tissue damage. Morphine might be used for a long, painful procedure expected to result in significant postoperative pain. Used preemptively, a baseline stable blood level can be achieved with narcotics before the patient becomes aware of pain, and patient-controlled analgesia (PCA) can be used effectively.

Commonly Used Opioids

Morphine relieves constant dull pain better than sharp intermittent pain. It should be used preemptively. Morphine is well-absorbed IM, onset takes 15-30 minutes, peak action occurs at 45-90 minutes and duration of action is about 4 hours. Morphine has low lipid solubility, and thus poor central nervous system penetration, after IV administration. Metabolism is by the liver (may be impaired by monoamine oxidase inhibitors) and kidneys, and elimination may be impaired in patients with renal failure. Plasma concentration is increased in the elderly, during the first 4 days of life and in patients with renal failure. Morphine may cause more sedation than analgesia in many patients, thus patients may appear to be comfortable, but may in reality be uncomfortable but too sedated to complain.

Meperidine, unlike morphine, is well absorbed from the gastrointestinal tract. It is structurally similar to atropine, and confers an antispasmodic effect. It is the opioid least likely to cause spasm of the sphincter of Oddi. It can cause tachycardia, mydriasis, and decreased myocardial contractility. 90% of the drug is metabolized to normeperidine, the effects of which are not antagonized by naloxone, and which may cause seizures. It is effective in small doses for treating postoperative shivering.

Fentanyl is more rapid in onset and has shorter duration than morphine due to increased lipid solubility, although elimination half-life is longer than that of morphine. A low dose (1-3 mg/kg) is used to blunt circulatory response to sudden stimuli. A higher dose (50-150 mg/kg) can be used to provide surgical anesthesia in critically ill patients who cannot tolerate volatile agents, but will not prevent patient awareness. Fentanyl does not cause histamine release, but can cause bradycardia, and can cause transiently increased intracranial pressure in patients with severe head injury.

Remifentanil is related to fentanyl. Rapid hydrolysis of the drug to inactive metabolites makes it the first ultra short-acting opioid.

Opioid Antagonists

Naloxone and naltrexone are pure opioid antagonists, and naltrexone is effective orally. Naloxone is available in multiple or single dose vials or ampules. For treatment of postoperative respiratory depression in adults, naloxone incremental doses of 0.005-0.04 mg IV can be titrated at 2-3 minute intervals, which promptly reverses both analgesia and respiratory depression. Duration of action is about 30-40 minutes, so repeated doses or an IV infusion are needed for opioid overdose. Smaller doses can be used to reverse mild ventilatory depression without causing severe pain and sympathetic response. Continuous infusion can be used to treat side effects without reversing analgesia.

Sedatives (Benzodiazepines)

Benzodiazepines are GABA receptor agonists with minimal cardiovascular effects, although midazolam may cause a decrease in peripheral vascular resistance with a resultant drop in blood pressure. This effect is enhanced by coadministration of fentanyl. Benzodiazepines do cause respiratory depression. Central nervous system effects include decreased cerebral oxygen consumption, intracranial pressure and cerebral blood flow. Benzodiazepines are used to prevent and control grand mal seizures. They also cause mild muscle relaxation at the spinal cord level. Benzodiazepines reduce minimum alveolar concentration of inhaled anesthetics by 30% and act as amnestics and anxiolytics.

Midazolam is the most commonly used benzodiazepine for premedication and sedation. Unlike diazepam, it does not cause pain on injection. Onset is quicker than with diazepam, and half-life (1-4 hours) is much shorter than diazepam (21-37 hours) or lorazepam (10-20 hours).

Benzodiazepines can be antagonized by flumazenil, which is a competitive inhibitor of GABA. The dose is 0.2-1.0 mg IV every 20 minutes for a 70-kg person. A dose of 3-5 mg IV used to reverse overdose may induce seizures, acute withdrawal, nausea, dizziness and agitation.

Dexmedetomidine

Dexmedetomidine is a relatively selective alpha2-agonist approved for continuous IV sedation in the intensive care setting of initially intubated and mechanically ventilated patients in the ICU setting for up to 24 hours. It enhances or decreases the need for sedation and analgesia without causing significant respiratory depression. It is also used in the operating room to prevent anxiety and pain without respiratory depression by minimizing the need for benzodiazepines and opioids.

6. Anesthetic Techniques

Anesthesiologists use a large armamentarium of techniques in the care of the surgical patient. General anesthesia, and regional or local techniques with sedation (MAC) can be used alone or in combination, or in association with other techniques, to provide appropriate care for an individual patient for a specific operation.

General Anesthesia

General anesthesia can be defined as a state of induced unconsciousness, in which the patient is pain-free, unaware or without the capability of forming memory, and immobile.

Regional Anesthesia

Regional anesthesia includes neuraxial anesthesia and specific nerve blocks, as well as intravenous (Bier) block. ***Neuraxial anesthetics include caudal, epidural, and spinal anesthesia.*** Only preservative-free anesthetics are used for neuraxial techniques. All neuraxial techniques can cause sympathectomy and vasodilation, with resultant decreases in blood pressure, and all can be used for surgical anesthesia. Vasodilation can be an advantage during and after vascular surgery. Narcotics placed neuraxially can cause nausea and vomiting, pruritus, sedation and respiratory depression, and urinary retention, as can intravenous narcotics.

The spinal anesthetic involves local and/or narcotic being placed directly into the spinal fluid, while both epidural and caudal involve local and/or narcotic being placed into the epidural space. The spinal requires a very small volume of local anesthetic, usually about one-tenth the volume required to achieve a similar level of anesthesia with an epidural, therefore local anesthetic toxicity is less likely with a spinal anesthetic. The narcotic dose for spinal anesthesia is usually less than one-tenth the epidural dose. Both techniques involve a needle, but the spinal needle is much thinner. While the spinal approach necessitates deliberate puncture of the dura, the resulting tear from a 27g, 25g or 22g needle is much smaller than an accidental tear resulting from a 17g Tuohy needle used to place an epidural catheter. The spinal anesthetic is limited in duration, since a catheter is usually not placed to allow redosing.

Local anesthetic placed into the spinal fluid can be directed. Mixed with 10% dextrose, or hyperbaric, the solution descends with gravity, and can be directed caudally if the patient is seated, or to one side if the patient is placed in the lateral position. Undiluted, or isobaric, the solution diffuses evenly. Mixed with preservative-free water, or hypobaric, the solution rises with gravity, and can be directed rostrally if the patient is seated, or caudally if the patient is in jackknife position. ***The caudal approach*** is used in infants and small children. Access is through the sacral hiatus into the caudal epidural space, which is below the cauda equina. The maximum safe dose of bupivacaine can be introduced into the space (2.5 mg/kg or 1 mL/kg of 0.25%) for surgical anesthesia or postoperative analgesia. An epidural catheter is sometimes used, allowing for redosing or continuous infusion.

The epidural approach is usually lumbar for abdominal surgery and postoperative analgesia. However, epidural catheters can be placed at any spinal level for analgesia. The technique for placement (loss-of-resistance technique) involves repeated attempts to inject air or preservative-free saline into the interspinous ligament. After each attempt, the styletted Tuohy needle is advanced a minute distance. After the needle pierces the interspinous ligament, it is possible to inject the air or saline without resistance. This is evidence that the needle is in the epidural space. A test dose is given before injecting any large volume of local anesthetic into the space to ensure that the needle or catheter is not puncturing an epidural vein, which would result in intravascular (systemic) spread of the local anesthetic. Eventually local anesthetics and narcotics diffuse into the vasculature, but the rate at which they diffuse does not usually result in toxic effects. An epidural anesthetic can be redosed or infused continuously, and the catheter can be left in place for postoperative analgesia.

Specific nerve blocks include blocks such as femoral sciatic block, cervical plexus (deep and superficial) blocks, brachial plexus (supraclavicular, interscalene, and axillary) blocks, and intercostal blocks as well extremity blocks (ankle, wrist, finger, etc).

Catheters and devices can also be placed intrapleurally, into joints, and near nerve plexuses for continuous analgesia. Devices which can utilized to deliver local anesthetics subcutaneously can be placed by the surgeon.

MAC

Monitored anesthesia care (MAC) consists of monitoring with or without appropriate pharmacologic intervention to ensure that an awake patient with or without local infiltration by the surgeon is comfortable, calm, safe and cooperative.

7. Subspecialty Anesthesia

Anesthesiologists with specialized training, knowledge, and experience, who are familiar with the routines and idiosyncrasies of specialized surgeons and the operations they perform, are a critical element in operations where timing is crucial and the potential for complications is great. The surgeon and the anesthesiologist grow accustomed to each other, and anticipate each other's needs and concerns, ensuring greater safety for the patient. While immediate communication is important, it is impossible for a surgeon to inform an anesthesiologist unfamiliar with a given procedure on a moment-by-moment basis and still achieve an operation with the best possible result. The informed anesthesiologist can anticipate events and interpret the nuances of a familiar operation performed by a familiar surgeon, and can detect flaws in the normal routine that may presage a problem, allowing rapid intervention to prevent it.

Cardiac Anesthesia

The cardiac anesthesiologist has usually completed a post residency fellowship, although at present no board examination exists.

Evaluation and Plan

The anesthesiologist shares a body of knowledge and experience with the cardiac surgeon and the cardiologist, which informs interpretation of preoperative data including ECG, echocardiogram, nuclear medicine scans and angiography. The anesthesiologist appreciates the anatomical and physiological pathology, the implications for the planned operation, as well as coexisting disease processes and their implications, and outlines an anesthetic plan, including monitors, drugs and postoperative management appropriate for the individual patient and the planned operation.

Monitors

Standard monitors, plus continuous arterial pressure monitoring are standard, with many patients also needing central venous pressure and pulmonary artery pressure, cardiac output, mixed venous saturation and transesophageal echocardiographic (TEE) monitoring. A means of determining coagulation status is also necessary.

Anesthetic Management

The cardiac patient is potentially most unstable preoperatively, during induction of anesthesia, and until safely on cardiopulmonary bypass (CPB), and the anesthesiologist, the pump technician and the surgeon must all be prepared to accelerate the process of anesthetizing the patient and placing him or her on CPB should the patient become irreversibly unstable. Both intravenous and inhaled anesthetics can be used for cardiac surgery. Ideally, the anesthetic should not cause myocardial depression, and should not contribute to prolongation of postoperative intubation.

Cardiopulmonary Bypass

The cardiac anesthesiologist has extensive knowledge of CPB, although a pump technician actually operates the pump, and the anesthesiologist anticipates potential malfunctions and complications related to CPB as well as to the operation. Knowledge of the CPB circuit, the oxygenators and priming solutions used, and position and order of cannula placement is essential. Intravascular anticoagulation and reversal, and measurement of degree of anticoagulation, are performed by the anesthesiologist, who must be familiar with timing and aware of cues on the field. Hemodynamic changes are anticipated and pharmacologic and fluid interventions are instituted. Pump flow and mean arterial pressure (usually 40-70 mm Hg) must be monitored to ensure organ perfusion. Normal blood gas values and a hematocrit (usually at least 20%) are maintained. The anesthesiologist participates in and must understand myocardial preservation and cardioplegia (antegrade and retrograde), cooling and rewarming, and the process of going on and coming off of CPB.

Depth of Anesthesia

The anesthesiologist continuously evaluates depth of anesthesia, sometimes with the use of EEG or bispectral index (BIS) monitoring, and administers drugs as needed to prevent awareness and ensure amnesia. Adequate depth of anesthesia is critical during rewarming. Drugs and fluids can be given via the CPB circuit during CPB.

Rewarming

During rewarming, the anesthesiologist also evaluates hematocrit, serum potassium and calcium, arterial blood gas, anticoagulation status and hemodynamics. By the time CPB is discontinued, the patient should be warmed to 36°C or greater, and must have a cardiac rhythm which supports an adequate cardiac output. Dysrhythmias must be evaluated to determine if the cause is reversible or ominous. If a pacemaker is necessary, the anesthesiologist manages the nonsterile equipment. Ventilation of the lungs is reinstituted and evaluated for adequacy. The surgeon vents arterial air from the great vessels. Emboli may be detectable in the pulmonary arterial bed by noting an abrupt decrease in end tidal carbon dioxide, but cannot be detected instantaneously in the brain. Vasoactive agents are used to adjust preload, afterload, rate, rhythm and contractility for optimal performance. After decannulation, anticoagulation is reversed with protamine slowly titrated to effect to avoid hypotension.

Recovery

Patients are transported to the ICU, usually still intubated, with oxygen and ventilatory support, and monitoring of ECG, pulse oximetry and arterial blood pressure, with drugs and equipment necessary to maintain stability on transport and until the intensive care team is prepared to assume full responsibility. After a full report is given to the ICU team, including history, intraoperative course, medications given and most recent laboratory data, if the patient is stable the ICU team assumes care. At no time is monitoring interrupted. The trend is to "fast track" cardiac surgery patients, with a brief period of ventilatory support, full recovery, then extubation once patient is awake and alert, hemodynamically stable and warm, has appropriate oxygenation and ventilation not requiring assistance, and has normal blood gas values. At this time anesthetic drug effects should be minimal, with the only active anesthetic drugs being those given for relief of pain.

Anesthesia for Thoracic Surgery

Most anesthesiologists routinely perform anesthetics for thoracic surgery, although there are some specialized fellowships.

Evaluation and Plan

While cardiac surgery is expected to improve cardiac function acutely, thoracic surgery and anesthesia rarely improve pulmonary function acutely. Thus, preoperative evaluation of the patient is crucial, especially if there is clinical evidence of pulmonary dysfunction or if pulmonary tissue is to be resected to a degree sufficient to cause pulmonary dysfunction.

Preoperatively, coexisting disease and the extrathoracic effects of the intrathoracic disease must be assessed. Important elements of history include the patient's exercise tolerance, history of exposure to tobacco or other substances toxic to the lungs such as asbestos or bleomycin, and symptoms of respiratory distress. It is important to try to differentiate pulmonary from cardiac causes of poor exercise tolerance. Cardiac problems may well be masked by a pulmonary patient's inactivity because pulmonary limitations limit exercise to a level insufficient to stress the heart and cause symptoms.

A thorough physical examination of the chest is appropriate, looking for evidence of wheezing, obstruction, pulmonary edema, pleural effusion or other abnormalities, and lips and extremities should be examined for cyanosis, clubbing or edema. Airway evaluation is important, since intubation for thoracic surgery is made more difficult by the specialized endotracheal tubes used.

History and physical examination determine selection of lab tests and studies. A test should be ordered to confirm or measure an abnormality that is strongly suspected to exist, and to assess the patient's ability to tolerate lung resection. Chest radiograph, arterial blood gas analysis, ECG, spirometry and flow-volume loops, and split-lung function tests are frequently ordered in association with thoracic surgery. If a patient's lungs are likely to be colonized or infected preoperatively, it may be appropriate to identify and treat (or be prepared to treat) the infection. Chronic hypoxemia may result in elevated hemoglobin and hematocrit, while other disease processes may result in low hemoglobin and hematocrit. A suspected problem should be confirmed. Other labs are appropriate based on coexisting problems. Certainly, if endocrine problems, related or unrelated to the intrathoracic process, are suspected, their existence should be confirmed. However, checking labs without specific indications is not helpful.

Optimization

When the extent of the patient's problems is clear, every effort is made to ensure that the patient's physical status is optimized in order to decrease the potential for perioperative complications. Smoking cessation (at least 3 days), pulmonary toilet and bronchodilator therapy, and antibiotic therapy may be recommended. The patient with myasthenia gravis scheduled for thymectomy will require continued attention from a neurologist. A patient with pleural effusion scheduled for mediastinotomy may require pleurocentesis prior to induction of anesthesia. A patient with a thyroid tumor may require medication to regulate thyroid function prior to proceeding with surgery. Suspected metastatic disease that would change indications for surgery, change management, or increase risk of complications of surgery and/or anesthesia should be evaluated prior to surgery. The patient with an anterior mediastinal mass should be evaluated functionally as well as by CT scan to determine whether the airway or great vessels are threatened with obstruction, and may need radiation or chemotherapy to shrink the mass before proceeding with general anesthesia or even sedation safely. After induction, the patient with an anterior mediastinal mass may have obstruction of the trachea that is distal to the end of the endotracheal tube inserted by the anesthesiologist. The patient must be turned quickly into lateral position or prone, or have an experienced rigid bronchoscopist available to stent open the airway once patency is lost. Diagnosis may be necessary via lymph node biopsy under local anesthesia prior to radiation or chemotherapy. The patient scheduled for rigid bronchoscopy and stenting for tracheal stenosis may have severe coexisting disease, but threatened loss of airway patency overrides any other concerns.

Anesthetic Management

Anesthetic technique is planned after considering whether the airway is to be shared (as in a bronchoscopy), whether or not there is a practical means of delivering inhaled anesthesia, or whether the only reliable route is intravenous (as in a bronchoscopy), whether the patient will require lung isolation (when one lung is infected) or bronchial intubation and one lung ventilation (for lung resection), and the desired position and whether the patient will tolerate it. The type of operation and the pathophysiology determine choice of anesthetic (usually general anesthesia) and extent of special monitoring techniques.

Monitors

Standard monitoring with continuous arterial pressure monitoring is appropriate, although central intravascular pressure monitoring may be necessary for safe anesthesia in a sicker patient. More than 1 pulse oximeter may be helpful, if compression of any large vessel is likely (as in thoracoscopy or mediastinoscopy, in a patient with anterior mediastinal mass or for repair of a tracheo-innominate artery fistula), with one oximeter probe used for continuous monitoring placed on an unthreatened limb, and the other for comparison and detection of poor flow placed on the threatened limb (right upper extremity). The arterial catheter is placed on an unthreatened limb.

Airway Management

The special device for thoracic surgery is the double-lumen endotracheal tube. Absolute indications for use of a double-lumen endotracheal tube are: to protect one lung from the other; to allow ventilation of one lung when the other lung has a bronchopleural fistula; a massive hemorrhage or a unilateral infection such as a lung abscess; to allow resection of a pulmonary cyst; or to perform unilateral bronchopulmonary lavage. Relative indications are to allow surgical exposure for pneumonectomy, upper lobectomy and thoracic aneurysm repair. Each lung can theoretically be ventilated with a different mode of ventilation or different peak inspiratory pressures by using a double-lumen endotracheal tube and 2 ventilators. Lung isolation can also be achieved by inflating an Arndt endobronchial blocker or a Fogarty vascular catheter in one mainstem bronchus, or by using a UniVent®(by Fuji) endotracheal tube, which incorporates a retractable bronchial blocker. Other devices are in development.

The double-lumen endotracheal tube is usually placed in the left mainstem bronchus (tubes come left- or right-sided) because the distance between the carina and the left upper lobe bronchus is usually greater than the distance between the carina and the right upper lobe bronchus. In fact, in some cases the right upper lobe bronchus is at the level of the carina. The device consists of an endotracheal tube with a cuff, and at the side (left side for left-sided placement) there is an endobronchial tube, also with a cuff that is smaller and rounder than the tracheal cuff. The tracheal cuff is clear and the bronchial cuff is blue. When the appropriate-sized device is placed properly, the tracheal cuff can be inflated between the larynx and the carina, and the bronchial cuff can be inflated between the carina and the takeoff of the upper lobe. Either lumen can be clamped (with a rubber-shod clamp) and either lumen can be connected to a ventilator or oxygen source, or neither lumen can be clamped and both lumens can be connected to a ventilator or oxygen source. Position is confirmed after placement or patient positioning by alternately clamping each side and confirming no breath sounds on the clamped side and normal breath sounds on the unclamped side, and by deploying a fiber optic bronchoscope down the tracheal lumen and confirming that just enough of the inflated bronchial cuff is visible such that it appears as a blue crescent-moon shape.

Physiology of One-Lung Ventilation

In the lateral position, the dependent lung is better perfused than the nondependent lung due to the effect of gravity. When the right lung is dependent, it receives 65% of the total pulmonary blood flow, as compared to 55% in the upright position. When the left lung is dependent, it receives 55% of the total pulmonary blood flow, as compared to 45% in the upright position. When both lungs are participating in gas exchange in the lateral position, the nondependent lung is better ventilated than the dependent lung due to the pleural pressure gradient that allows greater volume in the nondependent alveoli. Thus, there is ventilation-perfusion mismatch even before anesthesia or one-lung ventilation. When the nondependent lung is collapsed and ceases to participate in gas exchange in the absence of volatile anesthetics, hypoxic pulmonary vasoconstriction (HPV) occurs, resulting in a further decrease in blood flow to the nondependent, now nonventilated lung, decreasing ventilation-perfusion mismatch. Volatile anesthetics inhibit HPV however, and increase the intrapulmonary shunt, thus contributing to hypoxemia. Volatile anesthetics do have some more desirable effects in thoracic surgery, such as inhibiting bronchoconstriction and allowing rapid recovery from anesthesia, and are used in combination with narcotics to achieve a balanced anesthetic.

The solution to this problem is to first increase delivery of oxygen to the collapsed and still perfused nondependent lung by subtle insufflation, with low flow (1-2 L) continuous positive airway pressure (CPAP), at about 5 cm, which should not interfere with exposure. Next, after this has been instituted, ventilation of the well-perfused dependent lung is optimized with positive end expiratory pressure (PEEP) at 5-10 cm. This measure also decreases perfusion to the dependent lung to some degree, thus ventilation-perfusion matching is improved. Additional maneuvers include adjusting ventilator parameters and pulmonary artery pressures, and ultimately, particularly during pneumonectomy, the surgeon may need to clamp the ipsilateral pulmonary artery to control the shunt. Other intraoperative concerns include undesired changes in endotracheal tube position, acid-base disturbances, dysrhythmias, ischemia and hemodynamic instability.

Recovery
If the patient is awake, stable and has adequate pulmonary function, and pain is well controlled enough to allow coughing to clear secretions, immediate extubation is reasonable. Pain is controllable with thoracic epidural analgesia or intercostal nerve blocks as well as with patient-controlled intravenous analgesia. Pain control without sedation is desirable in patients with marginal pulmonary function if the patient is to remain extubated. Patients with poor pulmonary function may require prolonged ventilation postoperatively, and should understand this in advance.

Anesthesia for Vascular Surgery

Disease of the vasculature presents as diseases caused by poor perfusion of organs or limbs. Since vascular disease is usually widespread, it should be assumed that other organs or limbs are also threatened. Anesthesia for vascular surgery is the ultimate test of the anesthesiologist's skill in manipulating vascular space and intravascular volume with titratable vasoactive drugs and appropriate fluids, since the major physiological system the anesthesiologist manipulates is often horribly damaged. Vascular access for monitoring may be difficult, hemostasis may be difficult to achieve, and the vasculature is unpredictable. The perfusion pressure of organs such as the brain, the heart and the kidneys must be kept constant, within 10%-20% of baseline, while cross-clamping and unclamping abruptly alters afterload on the heart, bleeding alters preload, and reperfusion alters contractility by redistribution of unoxygenated and acidic blood.

Pediatric Anesthesia
Anesthesia for pediatric patients is part of the scope of practice of all anesthesiologists. Fellowship training exists for pediatric anesthesia, although there is currently no board certification in this subspecialty. Pediatric anesthesiologists gain more experience with extremely young (less than 1 year of age), extremely high-risk pediatric patients or patients for complex and high-risk operations.

The pediatric patient differs anatomically and physiologically, as well as emotionally and medicolegally, from the adult patient. Disease states that necessitate surgery are often embryological or congenital, rather than acquired. The pediatric patient also requires that every procedure be accomplished in miniature. The normal pediatric patient has more physiological reserve than the elderly patient.

The pediatric patient is not a consenting patient, and should not be assumed to be cooperative. The anesthesiologist should not imply to the child that there is a choice unless the anesthesiologist is willing to allow the child to refuse. Rapport must be established with the parents as well as the child. Preoperative evaluation unique to the child is the attention paid to gestational age and intrauterine development, and to the child's relationship with his or her parents. Children old enough to be anxious about separation from parents are premedicated, usually orally, to cause amnesia and decrease anxiety to the point of sedation. Oral midazolam is the preferred anxiolytic, although a smaller dose of intranasal midazolam may be used for patients who cannot tolerate oral medication.

The usual method of induction of anesthesia in a child without a preexisting IV is by mask, first with oxygen/nitrous oxide, then with a volatile agent (previously halothane, now usually sevoflurane) or by mask with oxygen/nitrous oxide/high percent sevoflurane. An IV is then placed, usually prior to intubation, although there are many variations.

Nitrous oxide used only for induction has no effect on distension of a closed space.

The pediatric airway is different from the adult airway. The narrowest part of the airway is the subglottis, and to prevent damage to the airway, the endotracheal tube should be smaller than the subglottis, as demonstrated by a small leak around the endotracheal tube. Cuffed tubes are traditionally not used on children under 8-10 years of age, although this practice is being examined. Fluids and drugs are all administered based on weight, and management is meticulous.

Small children cannot follow commands to demonstrate readiness for extubation. Readiness must be based on other clinical criteria, such as the ability to spontaneously lift the knees to the chest, the reestablishment of a normal breathing pattern and purposeful attempts to remove the endotracheal tube. If no muscle relaxant has been used, or a laryngeal mask airway (LMA) has been used, the child may be extubated "deep" and allowed to wake up slowly, if there is no risk of airway obstruction or aspiration.

Postoperative pain control strategies include rectal acetaminophen, intravenous ketorolac, carefully titrated narcotics and local anesthetic, either by caudal or by infiltration. PCA has been used successfully on younger patients beginning from ages 5 or 6.

Geriatric Anesthesia

While it is accepted that the elderly patient is physiologically different from a younger patient, it is difficult to establish just when a patient fits the definition of being elderly, since physiological age may not correlate with chronological age. A physiologically young patient who presents with correctable disease in a single organ might safely be assumed to have an ill matched set of organs, one of which has a shorter life span than the rest of the body, thus the failure of one organ early in life may not predict imminent failure of other organs. Failure of a single organ in a physiologically aged patient may be seen as a potential "herald event," which sets off a chain of organ failures.

Resilience and reserve decline with senescence in almost all physiologic parameters: myocardial function, vascular integrity, autonomic nervous system function, neuroimmunoendocrine response to stress, respiratory function and central nervous system function. Hepatic and renal dysfunction causes delays in protein synthesis, metabolism, clearance and elimination. Volume of distribution as well as elimination half-life of drugs will be altered. In addition, patients may require (and tolerate) less anesthetic and analgesic.

Operations may be emergent or involve major organ systems, both of which increase risk. In addition, drugs which may be more potent may have delayed onset due to poor cardiac output, and may last longer due to impaired metabolism and elimination. It is easy to become impatient after giving a drug and seeing no immediate effect, then to give more, only to discover that once all of the drug has taken effect, the drug has an exaggerated effect which is prolonged. Apparently well-compensated physiology can become remarkably decompensated. Thus, exquisite attention to detail and careful, deliberate, patient titration of drugs is important. Maintaining homeostasis as much as possible includes maintenance of normothermia, preservation of cerebral perfusion pressure, optimizing myocardial supply and demand, and maintaining fluid and electrolyte normality. Older and sicker patients are undergoing surgery with good outcomes due to careful management.

The elderly patient is at increased risk for ***postoperative cognitive dysfunction*** (POCD), and, although no single risk factor has been identified, can benefit from avoidance, as much as possible, of drugs that alter the central nervous system.

Outpatient Anesthesia

More and increasingly complex operations are performed on an outpatient basis, with patients arriving from home just prior to surgery and leaving within an hour after surgery. Their expectation is not to be "sick" or in pain. Appropriate anesthetics are short-acting, and prevention of pain and nausea is paramount.

Outpost Anesthesia

Anesthetics are not confined to the operating rooms and the labor and delivery area. Anesthetics are given for surgical procedures in remote locations such as MRI, brain scan, and CT, in gastroenterology endoscopic procedures labs, cardiac cath labs, angiography suites, urodynamics laboratories and radiation oncology, as well as intensive care units from the NICU and PICU to the SICU, when a patient who is too unstable to be moved needs an operation. Anesthesiologists are called on to give anesthesia for elective cardioversions and electroconvulsive therapy. In addition, anesthesiologists are consulted to perform blood patches to treat spinal headaches, most often the results of diagnostic lumbar punctures, although some are from spinal and epidural anesthetics. There are also consultations to request lumbar punctures and IV access.

8. Postanesthesia Care Unit

The postanesthesia care unit, or PACU, is the anesthesiologist's acute critical care unit. Because the period of emergence from anesthesia is a time of rapid physiologic and pharmacologic change, immediate identification and aggressive management of problems rather than noting and following trends is necessary. There is a very low patient-to-nurse care ratio, often 2:1, 1:1, or 1:2, and nurses are usually experienced critical care RNs. Anesthesiologists and surgeons are nearby. The PACU team receives a detailed report from the anesthesiologist regarding history, intraoperative events, drugs, fluid status and plan for management. The anesthesiologist and the surgeon continue to care for the patient through the PACU team even while continuing with the next scheduled case, receiving information about vital signs, hemodynamics, any labs or studies ordered, airway and ventilatory status, complications, pain management, nausea and vomiting, bleeding and other issues. The PACU can and does function as an extension of the surgical intensive care unit (SICU) for patients who are too unstable for transport or who may need to return to the operating room, or when the SICU is full. Patients recovering from interventional cardiology or interventional radiology procedures may also receive care in the PACU. Because of the presence of the anesthesiologists, emergency drugs can be obtained more quickly than an order can be written. Anesthesiology is one of the 3 pathways to critical care board certification (surgery, anesthesiology, pulmonary medicine), and the PACU is often managed by a team of anesthesiologists board-certified in critical care.

9. Acute Pain Management

Traditionally, pain after surgical incision was managed with intramuscular narcotics on an as-needed (PRN) basis. A patient had to wait until his or her allotted time limit was up, then call to the nurse, then wait further for his or her "shot," then wait for the injection to work. The waiting, the anxiety and the anticipation exacerbated the pain, and underscored the punishment and reward aspect of finally receiving the injection, placing the patient at greater risk for addictive behavior. Blood levels and pain relief oscillated from extremely low to extremely high. Attention is currently paid to at least the concept of ***preemptive analgesia***, in which neither pain nor unwanted sedation as a side effect of swings in blood level of pain medication is allowed to reach extremes. Ongoing and future research promises to reveal more about the mechanisms and appropriate treatment strategies for acute as well as chronic pain. It is recognized that pain is associated with sympathetic nervous system outflow, stress, and morbidity and mortality. In addition, other modes of delivering pain relief have evolved.

Intravenous Patient-Controlled

Analgesia (PCA)

PCA involves a pump that can be programmed for the individual patient, allowing continuous infusion as well as small patient-controlled doses. This eliminates waiting, assessment by a third party, and the unpredictability of intramuscular delivery. The patient is initially given a loading dose, preferably before emergence from anesthesia, and started on a combination of continuous infusion and patient-controlled doses. The pump can be interrogated to evaluate the patient's diminishing use of medication, allowing elimination of the continuous dose, followed by the patient-controlled doses, once usage is minimal and the patient is able to tolerate oral pain medication. Using PCA, patients usually require less pain medication and have less sedation and other side effects of narcotics such as inactivity and ileus. It seems to take more pain medication to relieve pain than to prevent it in the first place, partly because pain is both a physical and an emotional experience.

The loading dose is ideally given before the patient wakes up to the awareness of pain, or it can be programmed to be delivered by the PCA pump. The maintenance dose is manipulated by the patient pushing a button. Dose can initially be determined by patient weight, although it can be adjusted to the individual patient's tolerance after the patient begins to use the pump, by interrogating the pump and examining patterns of use, then adjusting the dose upward for repeated attempts and downward for excessive sedation. Computer order entry systems can help eliminate accidental overdosing due to misplaced decimals and illegible handwriting.

Lockout Interval

The PCA pump is set to be refractory to demands by the patient for a period after a dose is given. Redosing before the previous dose takes effect would result in over sedation. Drugs with faster onset can have shorter lockout intervals than drugs with slower onset, but should be given in smaller doses. Conversely, drugs with slower onset should have longer lockout intervals so that the patient is able to assess whether or not the dose was effective before initiating another dose.

Continuous Infusion

A constant rate infusion can be administered and adjusted in addition to or instead of the maintenance dose. When an infusion is started, the plasma level of the opioid rises until the rate of infusion matches the rate of elimination. When infusion is used alone, the patient has no control. PCA plus an infusion allows patient control and requires less narcotic.

Choice of Narcotics

Morphine, meperidine, fentanyl and hydromorphone are used in PCA pumps. Fentanyl has the most rapid onset, and thus the shortest lockout interval. Morphine and meperidine have slower onset, and thus longer lockout intervals. Loading doses are proportional to potency, as are individual PCA doses. Morphine is used most commonly in PCA. While meperidine is also used, its use is complicated by the possible accumulation of normeperidine, which can cause seizures in a dose-dependent manner.

Monitoring

Patients on PCA should be monitored for level of pain and sedation and respiratory rate.

Complications

The most dangerous complication of PCA is respiratory depression, detected by following respiratory rate and level of sedation. Respiratory depression may lead to accumulation of carbon dioxide and carbon dioxide narcosis. Oxygen therapy and reversal with naloxone (carefully titrated in increments of no more than .04 mg for an adult, rather than by the ampule) are necessary. The opioid should be discontinued and, if later restarted, the dosage should be decreased. Opioids also contribute to nausea and vomiting, which can be treated by changing the opioid or by administering an antiemetic. Other complaints are pruritus and urinary retention, which can be treated by changing the drug or with a low-dose naloxone infusion.

Epidural Analgesia

Epidural anesthesia using opioids and/or local anesthetics is used extensively to manage postoperative pain acutely. Opioids diffuse from the epidural space to the spinal cord, and after some delay, into the blood. Local anesthetics work on nerves or on spinal roots. While opiates decrease pain, local anesthetics affect pain, sensation and motor function. Epidural anesthesia allows excellent pain relief with much less sedation, and can be achieved in a segmental manner, at or near the level of catheter placement.

Common side effects of epidural opioids are nausea, pruritus and urinary retention, all of which can be treated with low-dose naloxone infusion. Sedation and delayed respiratory depression are more serious side effects, and are thought to be caused by rostral spread of the narcotic to the brainstem in addition to systemic absorption. Epidural local anesthetics may cause hypotension, motor block or sensory loss. Agitation and seizures may result from systemic absorption of local anesthetic.

Spinal Analgesia

Local anesthetics are not routinely infused into the CSF for postoperative pain relief. However, preservative-free narcotics, in particular morphine, can be injected in a single low dose into the CSF and will last for 18-24 hours. All of the side effects of central nervous system narcotics can occur. The spinal dose of morphine is less than one-tenth the epidural dose.

Intrapleural Analgesia

Intrapleural catheters may be placed to decrease pain from open cholecystectomy or rib fractures.

Ketorolac

Ketorolac is an IV or IM form of NSAID (oral preparation also available). It is an effective analgesic with few side effects when used short-term. The usual dose is 30 mg IV or IM every 6-8 hours. In patients weighing less than 30 kg, the dose is .5-1.0 mg/kg. Smaller doses should be used in elderly or very young patients or those with severe systemic disease, or patients in whom bleeding would be too great a risk. (There is a risk of enhanced surgical or GI bleeding, renal dysfunction or platelet dysfunction.) Ketorolac should not be used for more than 5 days. It is useful as a nonsedative pain medication for a patient who is not yet able to take PO medication.

Acetaminophen

Acetaminophen is used routinely orally and rectally as a benign pain medication. It is manufactured in combination with narcotics, in increasing narcotic potencies. If a patient gets inadequate pain relief from the prescribed dose and takes a larger dose of the acetaminophen-containing product, he or she runs the risk of hepatic toxicity from the acetaminophen, which may potentially be fatal. The antidote, if given on time, is n-acetyl cysteine. A preparation of acetaminophen-containing narcotic with adequate narcotic potency should be chosen in order to avoid the risk of acetaminophen toxicity.

10. Sedation

Not all procedures require the care of an anesthesiologist, and sedatives and analgesics are given for sedation and analgesia under the supervision of, but not by, the surgeon performing the procedure. A state of moderate sedation/analgesia may be produced by the use of intravenous, oral, transmucosal or intramuscular narcotics, sedatives, hypnotics or anxiolytics. Moderate sedation/analgesia is defined by the purpose for and degree of sedation, not the specific agent used or the route by which it is administered. The safe sedation of patients for diagnostic and therapeutic procedures requires a combination of skilled personnel, appropriate selection of patients and drugs, appropriate physical facilities, minimum standards of monitoring and proper recovery of patients.

Practical Definition of Levels of Consciousness

Analgesia or Anxiolysis

This level of consciousness occurs when anxiolytic or analgesic drugs are used for the specific purpose of achieving a state of consciousness in which the patient is without anxiety or pain, but is fully awake and responsive to his or her surroundings. This definition is not associated with a procedure being performed. This usually implies the use of 1 appropriate agent (not combinations of narcotics and sedatives), although there may be situations in which both pain and anxiety must be treated. The dosages of drugs used to achieve these goals would fall within the lower recommended range specified by the ***Physicians' Desk Reference*** guidelines for these purposes. Patients vary in response to drugs, thus a patient may become overly sedated despite staying within dosing guidelines. The elderly patient, in particular, may require reduced and less frequent dosing. Other patients may exhibit significant tolerance to sedatives or analgesics, and may require larger doses to achieve analgesia or anxiolysis. Examples include administering narcotics to treat pain and administering small doses of benzodiazepines to reduce anxiety or to promote sleep at night. The patient receiving analgesia or anxiolysis does not require constant monitoring other than routine nursing floor monitoring.

Moderate Sedation/Analgesia

This is a medically controlled state of depressed consciousness that allows protective reflexes to be maintained, retains the patient's ability to maintain a patent airway independently and continuously, and permits appropriate response by the patient to physical stimulation or verbal command. Examples include administering sedatives and/or narcotics to facilitate invasive procedures that are only moderately uncomfortable or are supplemented with local anesthesia, leaving the patient mildly drowsy but awake and easily arousable to voice. When sedative drugs are given to achieve this level of consciousness, adherence to a moderate sedation/analgesia protocol is appropriate. Moderate sedation/analgesia implies that the sedation is time-limited and reversible, and that the patient is fully monitored by a qualified person other than the person performing the procedure. Monitoring the patient and administering medications for moderate sedation/analgesia can be done by a registered nurse or another qualified person, either of whom should be trained and certified to administer moderate sedation and analgesia. A clinician administering moderate sedation/analgesia must be prepared at all times to manage a patient who becomes sedated beyond intentions and expectations.

Deep Sedation

Deep sedation is a medically controlled state of depressed consciousness or unconsciousness from which the patient is not easily aroused, or may be aroused only by vigorous stimulation. Partial loss of protective reflexes may occur, as well as the inability of the patient to maintain a patent airway independently and respond purposefully to physical stimulation or verbal command. Examples include administering anxiolytics and narcotics for procedures that are very stimulating, such as endoscopy or emergency fasciotomy. When sedative drugs are given to achieve this level of consciousness, adherence to a deep sedation protocol is appropriate. Patients in intensive care may be deeply sedated to allow them to tolerate prolonged tracheal intubation and ventilation, and may indeed undergo procedures while in this state, but this falls outside the realm of deep sedation for procedures. Deep sedation for procedures implies that the sedation is time-limited and reversible, and that the intent is for the patient to recover his or her baseline level of consciousness after the procedure is over. Monitoring the patient and administering deep sedation should only be done by a physician, such as a critical care physician, an emergency medicine physician, or an oral surgeon, whose training and privileges include this treatment, and who is not the person performing the procedure.

General Anesthesia

General anesthesia is a medically controlled state of unconsciousness accompanied by deliberate ablation of protective reflexes, in which the airway is controlled, and the patient is unable to respond purposefully to physical stimulation or verbal command. Only an anesthesiologist or a certified registered nurse anesthetist (CRNA) under the direction of a qualified physician should administer general anesthesia. (Anesthesiologists and anesthetists routinely move patients through various levels of consciousness, including those defined above as deep and conscious sedation, and may even simply monitor patients without altering consciousness in any way. Thus, care by an anesthesiologist or anesthetist is not defined as sedation, but is part of a range of monitored care by specifically trained physicians and nurses that potentially encompasses any baseline or induced state of consciousness or unconsciousness.)

The Practice of Moderate Sedation/Analgesia

Identification

Patients undergoing moderate sedation/analgesia should have an identification armband in place prior to the start of the sedation or procedure.

Preprocedure Assessment

A focused history is taken that includes history of adverse reactions to sedation in the past, allergies, current medications, cardiac and pulmonary history, airway history (sleep apnea, snoring, surgery, difficult intubation), and pathology potentially affecting distribution, metabolism or excretion of drugs, in addition to anything relevant to the planned procedure.

An examination of the airway is performed focusing on potential airway difficulties such as morbid obesity, small submental space (signified by large overbite, retrognathia, mental-thyroid distance less than 3 of the patient's fingerbreadths), evidence of prior airway surgery, trauma or congenital anomalies, large tongue, high arched palate, narrow jaw, and decreased mobility of jaw or neck such as that seen in patients with rheumatoid arthritis or other cervical spine pathology.

Auscultation of heart and lungs is performed, with attention to signs of heart failure, dysrhythmias and pulmonary pathology.

Baseline level of consciousness is determined, which will be altered, then returned to baseline state. The ability to move extremities voluntarily or on command and response to auditory and tactile stimuli should be assessed and documented.

Preprocedure vital signs are taken, including blood pressure, heart rate, respiratory rate, temperature, and oxygen saturation (with fraction of inspired oxygen if patient is not on room air). An ECG rhythm strip may be appropriate.

Vital statistics are recorded, including age, weight in kilograms, and height, if weight and height appear disproportionate.

Any appropriate labs or studies are done. Again, patient history drives the necessity for labs or studies. It is inappropriate to obtain labs or studies just to check for unsuspected problems.

Patient's ASA classification is determined. Moderate sedation/analgesia is best used with patients who are ASA I, II or III. Patients who are ASA IV and above, or who require a prolonged or complicated procedure, may not be appropriate for moderate sedation/analgesia and may benefit from an anesthesia consultation.

NPO status should be documented (time and nature of last oral intake). NPO guidelines for sedation should mirror those for anesthesia. Necessary medications should be continued as scheduled. NPO guidelines are based on reasonable interpretations of studies, and vary between institutions. Instructions should be altered with consideration for coexisting medical problems such as pregnancy, obesity, trauma, uremia or diabetes which may slow gastric emptying.

Informed consent should be obtained for sedation and procedure.

Procedure Area Requirements

Moderate sedation/analgesia should be performed in designated procedure areas or intensive care units. Adequate lighting should be available for observation of the patient, the monitors and the procedure taking place, with a back-up source of light in case of power failure.

Sufficient space for operative personnel, monitoring equipment, and emergency equipment should exist. Adequate power and emergency power outlets should be at hand for necessary equipment, as should a reliable means of summoning help should it become necessary. A reliable means of changing patient position is needed, including to the Trendelenburg position. Monitoring equipment should be visible at all times to the person monitoring the patient as well to as the person performing the procedure. The person monitoring the patient should be able to see and interact with the patient. Resuscitation equipment should be available immediately.

An oxygen source adequate to provide the patient with at least 10 L/min flow for a minimum of 2 hours is needed, as well as devices needed for the appropriate delivery of oxygen (oxygen regulators, nasal cannula or oxygen mask) and a full back-up source (E cylinder) and regulator. A functional self-inflating bag and mask system appropriate for the patient is needed. A functional system for suctioning the patient, with suction catheters sized appropriately for the patient should be at hand. Reversal agents (flumazenil and naloxone) should be immediately available and recognizable, and the appropriate dose for the patient should be calculated in advance.

Monitoring

The patient should be ***monitored continuously*** from the time of drug administration until recovery is judged adequate, usually at least 30 minutes after the procedure is over or discharge criteria are met, whichever occurs later. The person monitoring the patient must have the patient in his or her sight at all times, although other minor tasks can be performed as long as they are not distracting and attention to the patient can be maintained. The following parameters should be monitored: pulse oximetry with heart rate should be continuous and level of consciousness, respiratory rate and blood pressures should be determined repeatedly. An electrocardiogram may be appropriate for patients with preexisting cardiac disease. Parameters should be documented before administration of each dose of medication, after medication, and at least every 15 minutes thereafter throughout the recovery period. Baseline oxygen saturation prior to adding supplemental oxygen may provide a benchmark for comparison at the end of the procedure. Temperature monitoring may be appropriate in patients at risk of becoming hypothermic or hyperthermic. Because drugs given intramuscularly or transmucosally have unpredictable onset, patients receiving sedation by this route should be monitored for at least 90 minutes after the last dose has been given. The record should be designed to allow easy analysis of cause and effect in order to quickly spot trends, and identify the probable cause of undesirable changes in hemodynamics or level of consciousness.

Personnel

The surgeon performing the procedure has primary responsibility for the patient, and orders the medications to be administered based on the type of procedure, the projected length of the procedure, the degree of discomfort likely and the individual patient. The surgeon in charge and the appropriate person monitoring the patient should be trained and certified in giving moderate sedation. Basic life support skills are necessary for all involved, and one available person should be trained in advanced cardiac life support (or pediatric advanced life support if the patient is a child). Availability of backup personnel should be assessed.

If the patient progresses to deep sedation or unconsciousness, or cannot tolerate the procedure, options such as terminating the procedure and/or calling for anesthesia consultation should be considered in a timely manner.

Selection of Patients and Drugs

Assessment of the patient allows selection of patients who are fairly healthy (ASA I-III) and have a low risk of airway obstruction or difficult intubation. Drugs should be selected based on the type and length of the procedure, and how stimulating, painful, or distressing the procedure will be. The usefulness of "verbal Valium" should not be underestimated. Both patient and drug should be considered in terms of initial dose and how quickly doses are titrated. Drugs with slow onset and patients with low cardiac output require more patience. Redosing before the first dose has had time to take effect can result in overdose and over sedation or hypotension. Drugs with long half-lives and patients with impaired metabolism or elimination can tie up personnel long after the procedure is over. It is a good idea to consult with an anesthesiologist before designing a moderate sedation/analgesia regimen for a given procedure, especially if the procedure is one that will be done on a series of patients. Choosing the best drugs for the task at hand, and learning to use them will make both the procedure and the sedation easier.

Recovery and Transportation

The recovery period begins after the procedure is finished, not as the last drug dose is given. Patient status should be assessed and documented on arrival to the recovery site, and documented at least every 15 minutes until discharge criteria are met and at least 30 minutes beyond that point. The surgeon should be available and made aware of any changes in the patient's condition. The patient should be considered recovered if activity, respiration, airway reflexes, circulation, level of consciousness and oxygen saturation have returned to baseline levels. Recovery is often based on objective data, plus a scoring system such as the Johns Hopkins Hospital Level of Consciousness Scale. The Hopkins scale gives 5 points for Aware, alert, oriented; 4 points for Drowsy, easily aroused to voice; 3 points for Drowsy, responds to repeated commands; 2 points for Drowsy, arouses to tactile stimuli; 1 point for Response to pain only; and 0 points for No responses. The patient should be discharged when the Hopkins score reaches 5 or the patient's baseline score; when cardiovascular function and airway patency are satisfactory and stable; respiratory pattern and rate are normal; and oxygen saturation is not less than 95% on room air for 30 minutes or has been stable at the patient's baseline. Pain should be controlled and score 4 or less by the patient's subjective rating on a scale of 1-10, and the patient should be mobile consistent with baseline and procedure. If appropriate, the patient should be able to retain oral fluid.

Finally, following the administration of naloxone or flumazenil, the patient should not be discharged for a minimum of 90 minutes. This is because the half-life of naloxone and flumazenil are shorter than the half-life of the drugs (narcotics and benzodiazepines) they reverse, and the patient must be monitored until the danger of resedation is past. The use of naloxone or flumazenil is considered a failure of technique, not a clever way to bring sedation to a screeching halt the moment the procedure is over, and use of these drugs indicates the need to investigate the quality of care being delivered.

Most hospital policies require patients who have just undergone moderate sedation/analgesia to travel to bed or car via wheelchair, on a gurney or in an age-appropriate mode of transportation such as a crib, rather than being allowed to walk away from the procedure area. Practice should be tailored to the procedure performed and the drugs used. Discharge instructions for outpatients should be given to a designated responsible adult, and that adult must be available to drive the patient home. Patients should not drive home or go home unaccompanied in a bus or taxi. Patients who are to be transported to a hospital bed, particularly if recovery has been prolonged and they may need a monitored bed, should be accompanied by someone capable of assessment and intervention if there is any likelihood of problems.

Administering moderate sedation/analgesia safely and effectively is difficult, and requires planning, practice and care. A drug regimen should be chosen for the particular patient as well as for the particular procedure involved, and skills developed using that regimen. The ability to intervene should over sedation occur is a fundamental prerequisite for the surgeon who administers moderate sedation/analgesia.

11. References

1. Allen JN, Blenko JW. Moderate Sedation Best Practice Recommendations. University Health-System Consortium.

2. Alkire MT, Haier RJ, Fallon JH. Toward a unified theory of narcosis: brain imaging evidence for a thalamocortical switch as the neurophysiologic basis of anesthetic-induced unconsciousness. *Consciousness Cognition*. 1999;7:1-17.

3. American Society of Anesthesiologists. ASA Physical Status Classification System. 2005. Available at www.asahq.org.

4. Barash PG, Cullen BF, Stoelting RK, eds. *Clinical Anesthesia*. 5th ed. Philadelphia, PA: Lippincott; 2006.

5. Cohn SL, Goldman L. Preoperative risk evaluation and perioperative management of patients with coronary artery disease. *Medical Clinics of North America*. 2003;87:111-136.

6. Eagle KA , Berger PB, Calkins H, . ACC/AHA Guideline update for perioperative cardiovascular evaluation for noncardiac surgery. *J Am College Card*. Feb 2002;39 (3):542-553.

7. Lee TH et al. Derivation and prospective validation of a simple index for prediction of cardiac risk of major noncardiac surgery. *Circulation*. 1999;100:1043-1049.

8. Mangano DT et al. Effect of atenolol on mortality and cardiovascular morbidity after noncardiac surgery. *NEJM*. 1996;335:1713-1720.

9. Marks JB. Perioperative management of diabetes. *Am Fam Physician*.2003;67:93-100.

10. McAnulty GR et al. Anaesthetic management of patients with diabetes mellitus. *Br J Anaes*. 2000;85(1):80-90.

11. Miller RD, ed. *Anesthesia*. 6th ed. New York, NY: Churchill Livingstone; 2004.

12. Pasternak LR, chair. American Society of Anesthesiologists Task Force on Preanesthesia Evaluation. Practice Advisory for Preanesthesia Evaluation. Park Ridge, IL: American Society of Anesthesiologists.

13. Pietropaolo M. An 18-year-old patient with Type 1 diabetes undergoing surgery. *PLoS Med*. 2005;2(5):e140.

14. Smetana GW, Cohn SL, Lawrence VA. Update in perioperative medicine. *Ann Int Med*. 2004;140:452-461.

15. Lipshitz AKM, Gropper MA. Perioperative glycemic control: an evidence-based review. *Anesthesiology* 2009;110:408-421.

16. Fleischer LA, Beckman JA, Brown KA, ACC/AHA guidelines on perioperative cardiovascular evaluation and care for noncardiac surgery: executive summary. *Circulation* 2007;116:1971-1996.

17. London MJ. Quo vadis, perioperative beta blockade? Are you "POISE'd" on the brink? *Anesth. Analg*. 2008;106:1025-1030.

12. Questions

1. Because of specific side effects, succinylcholine can be harmful to which of the following patients?

A. A patient with an open eye injury

B. A patient with papilledema, confusion, and a space-occupying intracranial lesion

C. A patient whose legs have just sustained a severe crush injury

D. A patient with a history of malignant hyperthermia

2. 15 minutes after administration of an uncomplicated hyperbaric bupivacaine spinal placed with patient in the seated position, the patient in jackknife position becomes bradycardic and hypotensive, then apneic and unresponsive. What is the mechanism?

A. The patient has a high spinal due to position

B. The spinal has blocked cardiac accelerator fibers in the spinal cord

C. The spinal has caused sympathectomy and vasodilation

D. The bupivacaine has gone intravascular and caused cardiac toxicity

3. Which of the following statements is true regarding malignant hyperthermia?

A. Patients with a suspicious history should be tested for the disease

B. Patients with Duchenne's muscular dystrophy may be at risk

C. Nondepolarizing muscle relaxants are permissible in patients with MH and may in fact cause muscle relaxation and treat the disease

D. Succinylcholine and volatile agents can trigger MH

4. Comparing spinal anesthesia with epidural anesthesia, which statements are true?

A. Epidural anesthesia requires higher volumes of local anesthetics

B. Spinal anesthesia alone places patients at risk for dural puncture headaches because the epidural is placed superficial to the dura

C. Both spinal and epidural anesthesia can produce sympathectomy

D. A single-shot epidural anesthetic lasts longer than a single-shot spinal and provides superior analgesia

5. Which of the following statements are true regarding propofol?

A. Propofol is suspended in a soy emulsion

B. Propofol can be administered in small boluses, induction dose amounts, or by continuous infusion for sedation or for general anesthesia

C. Propofol does not cause nausea and vomiting

D. Propofol has a very short distribution and elimination half-life

E. All of the above are true

6. When using a MacIntosh blade for laryngoscopy:

A. The epiglottis is lifted directly

B. The laryngoscope is held in the left hand

C. The laryngoscope enters the mouth on the left and pushes the tongue to the right

D. The tip of the blade is advanced into the vallecula

7. Pulse oximeters:

A. Are based on Beer's law

B. Use a single wavelength of red light

C. Can differentiate carboxyhemoglobin from oxyhemoglobin

D. Can differentiate methemoglobin from oxyhemoglobin

8. The laryngeal mask airway (LMA):

A. Protects against aspiration as well as an endotracheal tube

B. May prevent airway obstruction during monitored anesthesia care

C. Requires a laryngoscope for insertion

D. Prevents laryngospasm

E. Permits positive pressure ventilation

9. Factors which increase the difference between arterial and measured end-tidal carbon dioxide include:

A. Ventilation and perfusion mismatch

B. Pulmonary embolism

C. Pulmonary artery vasospasm

D. High cardiac output

E. Anemia

10. Hypoxic vasoconstriction is prominent in the:

A. Lungs

B. Brain

C. Heart

D. Skin

E. Liver

Answers

1. A., B., C., D.

Succinylcholine is a depolarizing muscle relaxant that acts rapidly by mimicking the action of acetylcholine on neuromuscular junctions in a global manner, causing skeletal muscle fasciculation and contraction. Duration of action is longer than acetylcholine due to delayed breakdown of the molecule because it is a double ACh molecule. Succinylcholine is used when rapid onset and quick reversal are required, classically in the patient with a presumed full stomach who may aspirate if ventilated by mask with positive pressure, or in the patient who is likely to be difficult or impossible to mask and rapid ease of intubation is desirable. Fasciculation of the extrinsic muscles of the eye increases intraocular pressure, which is undesirable in patients with glaucoma or open globe. Succinylcholine also increases intracranial pressure, and may lead to herniation in a patient at risk. However, laryngoscopy can also increase intraocular and intracranial pressure, so risks of aspiration must be weighed against risks of injury to the eye or herniation, and laryngoscopy must be atraumatic and the airway reflexes blunted pharmacologically. Depolarization also results in efflux of potassium from skeletal muscle cells, raising serum potassium. Significant hyperkalemia may occur in patients with burns, crush injuries or conditions associated with denervation of skeletal muscle and upregulation of receptor sites, such as in spinal cord injury and upper motor neuron disease. The patient who is already hyperkalemic, such as the patient in renal failure, may also experience efflux of enough potassium to cause cardiac arrest. Succinylcholine is a known triggering agent of malignant hyperthermia (MH), and should not be given to patients with known or suspected MH. Use of cricoid pressure to occlude the esophagus during rapid sequence induction with succinylcholine has no effect on fasciculation.

2. A., B., C.
Hyperbaric spinal anesthetic solution, or local anesthetic mixed with dextrose, is heavier, or has higher baricity than CSF, and falls with gravity to the lowest part of the CSF. Isobaric spinal anesthetic solution, or undiluted local anesthetic, is distributed without regard to position. Hypobaric spinal anesthetic solution, or local anesthetic mixed with preservative-free water, rises to the highest part of the CSF. Spinal for jackknife position is often placed in that position, and a hypobaric solution is used. Hyperbaric bupivacaine can be used, but sufficient time is needed for the bupivacaine to bind before positioning should take place. Hyperbaric lidocaine can be expected to bind more quickly, especially if it contains epinephrine. The patient probably has a high spinal due to movement up the spinal cord after positioning. In addition, a high spinal can block cardiac accelerator fibers. A spinal does cause sympathectomy and vasodilation. In addition, a high enough spinal can block the cervical spine and the phrenic nerve and cause apnea and paralysis, prior to unconsciousness, which is a result of hypoperfusion and hypoxia. Less than 2 mL of local anesthetic is unlikely to cause cardiac toxicity, and local anesthetic placed correctly into CSF has a fairly certain location. Epidural bupivacaine is given in 10 times the volume, and is more likely to become intravascular, which can result in cardiac toxicity. A test dose of lidocaine with epinephrine is given epidurally before injecting bupivacaine, to test for intravascular (epidural vein) placement of the epidural needle or catheter.

3. B., D.
Because of the risk of a false negative or false positive test, muscle biopsy testing is not completely reliable. Patients with a suspicious history should be treated as if they may have the disease, and anesthesia with nontriggering agents can proceed. Patients with a family history may be at risk, as may patients with Duchenne's. Succinylcholine and volatile agents should be avoided in patients at risk. The defect in MH occurs distal to the neuromuscular junction, therefore nondepolarizing muscle relaxants have no effect on MH. If muscle relaxation does occur as a result of administration of a nondepolarizer, the problem is occurring proximal to the neuromuscular junction in the central nervous system, and is therefore not MH.

4. A., C.
Epidural anesthesia requires about 10 times the volume of local anesthetic, which may produce systemic effects. Both methods can produce sympathectomy, although the epidural can be activated slowly, thus mitigating the effect of a sudden sympathectomy. Although the spinal needle is used to cause deliberate dural puncture, this thin needle does not always result in a headache. The epidural needle, if it causes an unintended dural puncture, causes a much larger tear, thus creating a headache. A single-shot epidural does not last any longer than a single-shot spinal, and may actually provide a less "dense" analgesia.

5. E.
All are true.

6. B., D.
The tip of the MacIntosh blade is held in the left hand, enters the mouth on the right and pushes the tongue to the left, then is placed into the vallecula in order to lift the epiglottis indirectly.

7. A.
Pulse oximeters are based on Beer's law, and use two wavelengths of light, red and infrared. They can distinguish oxyhemoglobin from deoxyhemoglobin, but cannot distinguish it from carboxyhemoglobin or methemoglobin.

8. E.
The LMA does not protect against aspiration or prevent laryngospasm. It is not tolerated without general anesthesia, therefore is not used for monitored anesthesia care. It is inserted by hand, not by laryngoscopy, although sometimes a laryngoscope is used as a tongue blade. It does permit positive pressure ventilation and prevents airway obstruction during general anesthesia.

9. A., B., C.

The first 3 are correct, since PE and low pulmonary perfusion from any cause increases dead space, thus increasing the difference.

10. A.

Only the pulmonary bed vasoconstricts in response to hypoxemia, in order to reduce shunt and mismatch. All the other tissue beds above dilate. Volatile anesthetics inhibit hypoxic pulmonary vasoconstriction.

Chapter 2: Preoperative Cardiac Risk Assessment

Christian de Virgilio, MD
Phillip Ge, BA

Contents

1. Introduction

Adverse cardiac events are a major source of morbidity and mortality following noncardiac surgery. Up to 50% of all perioperative deaths are cardiac related. This is likely the result of the high prevalence of coronary artery disease (CAD) in the aging US population. Over the next 30 years, the number of noncardiac procedures will increase by 50% (to 38 million) and the percentage of surgical patients over the age of 65 will increase 25% to 35%. It then follows that the number of older noncardiac surgical patients with possible CAD will double from 6 million to 12 million.[1]

Cardiac risk assessment is used to identify patients at greatest risk for adverse cardiac events and to prevent a negative outcome. It begins with a thorough history and physical examination. Following the history and physical exam, one of various cardiac risk scoring systems can be used to further identify which patients are at greatest risk. 4 major indices that are used to stratify patients are DrippsASA, Goldman, Detsky and Lee. Each index has its own advantages and shortcomings. In some instances, additional preoperative tests are administered to further stratify patients. In this chapter we will define the problem, discuss the rationale for cardiac risk assessment, describe the various noninvasive tests available and their limitations, and outline an algorithm for the individual patient. In creating an algorithm, one must keep in mind that the entire field of cardiac intervention is in a constant state of flux. As such, there is no consensus as to which noninvasive cardiac test is ideal, nor is there uniform agreement as to optimal preoperative management.

2. Scope of the Problem

Prevalence of CVD

Cardiovascular disease (CVD) is the leading cause of death in the United States, Canada, Europe and Japan.[2] It affects 25% of the US population and about 1 million people die each year from its complications.[1,3] The mortality rate for CVD exceeds that of all other diseases combined and accounts for 1 of every 2 deaths in the United States.[1,3] Each year, 7-8 million noncardiac surgical patients are at risk for cardiac morbidity or mortality. Of this number, about 1 million have diagnosed CAD (classical angina or Q waves on ECG), 2-3 million have 2 or more major risk factors for CAD, and 4 million are over 65 years of age.[1] The annual incidence of cardiac morbidity exceeds 1.9 million. This includes 1.5 million myocardial infarctions (MI) and 400,000 cases of congestive heart failure (CHF). About 10% of the US population is over 65 years of age, and with the continued growth of this age group coupled with advancements in medical technology, it is expected that by the middle of the next century the over-65 population will increase to 66 million, many of whom will have CVD.

Currently, the largest number of operations and the most days in hospital occur in the over-65 age group.[1] Nearly 8 million of the 25 million operations performed a year in the United States are on patients over age 65. 1 of every 4 major operations (ie, intraabdominal, thoracic, vascular, neurologic and orthopedic) are performed in patients considered at high risk for postoperative complications, and 50% of all postoperative complications are cardiovascular.[3] It is predicted that over the next few decades, more than 37 million patients will undergo surgery each year and 40% will have, or be at risk for, coronary artery disease.[2] Current statistics underestimate the number of people with CAD, since an estimated 2-5 million others have silent myocardial ischemia.

Perioperative Cardiac Mortality

Perioperative cardiac morbidity is the leading cause of death following anesthesia and surgery.[1] Adverse postoperative cardiac events are defined as myocardial ischemia/unstable angina, myocardial infarction, dysrhythmias, congestive heart failure and cardiac death.

Myocardial Ischemia/Unstable Angina

Perioperative myocardial ischemia can be detected in 18%-74% of noncardiac surgical patients with CAD through the use of a combination of ECG and transesophageal echocardiography (TEE). Such transient ischemic events are most commonly noted by ST changes in the lateral leads or by segmental wall motion abnormalities. Though the routine use of intraoperative TEE is impractical, it is important to note that several factors can precipitate ischemic changes.[1] These factors include tachycardia, hypertension, anemia, stress, sympathomimetic drugs or the discontinuation of beta-blockers, all of which increase the demand on myocardial oxygen consumption.

Myocardial Infarction

The rate of postoperative MI in the general population is fairly low, ranging from 0% to 0.7%. This rate increases to 1.8% in patients over age 40. Infarction rates in patients with prior MI are even higher. Classic dogma states that the rate of reinfarction is over 30% if the previous MI was less than 3 months prior, 15% if the MI was 3 to 6 months prior, and 6% if greater than 6 months prior.[4] However, most of these data are derived from studies done in the 1960s and 1970s. More recently, Rao and colleagues found an overall MI rate of 1.9% in patients with prior infarction and only a 5.7% MI rate in patients with recent (within 3 months) MI.[5] This lower rate of MI may be a reflection of improved anesthetic and surgical techniques, coupled with improvements in perioperative monitoring.

Many MIs occur silently (non-Q wave) during the postoperative period, and therefore are detected only by serial measurement of cardiac enzymes. Such events typically occur on postoperative days 3-5, but may occur as late as 7 days postoperatively or beyond. Recently, the significance of a non-Q wave MI in the postoperative period has come into question. Taylor and colleagues noted that patients suffering a non-Q wave MI postoperatively have a similar long-term prognosis as patients who did not suffer a cardiac event.[6] They further noted that patients with a non-Q wave MI did not have any appreciable change in left ventricular ejection fraction. The results of this study therefore question the need for routine use of serial cardiac enzymes after surgery in the absence of cardiac symptoms.

The etiology of postoperative MI is still unclear. The effects of surgery and anesthesia may lead to increased coronary artery shear stress as a result of changes in contractility, blood pressure, coronary blood flow and coronary tone. This in turn may disrupt a preexisting atherosclerotic lesion. Platelet aggregation may be enhanced as a result of catecholamine surges, blood viscosity and coronary blood flow changes, and alterations in hemostasis. Finally, coronary vasospasm may be induced by various stress mediators.[1]

Ellis et al[7] analyzed the coronary angiograms of 63 patients undergoing major nonthoracic vascular surgery. They found that coronary occlusion proximal to viable myocardium was associated with an increased rate of perioperative MI and death. The findings suggested that revascularization of coronary occlusions might reduce the frequency of adverse events. However, in the same study, a significant number of milder, nonobstructive lesions were also associated with MI and death. These findings are consistent with other studies that show that severe coronary artery stenosis may not always be the source of a perioperative MI, and that coronary thrombosis frequently occurs at sites of subcritical stenosis, due to inflammation and plaque destabilization. Thus, preoperative revascularization of severe stenoses may not reduce perioperative ischemic complications.

Congestive Heart Failure

Congestive heart failure (CHF) is increasingly a significant source of postoperative morbidity and mortality. Rao and associates noted a 4.8% rate of postoperative CHF in patients with a prior MI,[5] whereas Mangano and Goldman reported a 3.6% rate of CHF in patients over 40 years of age.[2] Postoperative CHF develops as a result of impaired diastolic relaxation or systolic contraction, which may be precipitated by local or global ischemia or infarction. Preexisting cardiomyopathy and/or valvular heart disease may also exacerbate CHF.

Dysrhythmias

The risk of suffering from a perioperative dysrhythmia has been documented to range from 13%-84%, and ventricular dysrhythmias occur in 3%-60% of patients.[1] A serious dysrhythmia (defined as persistent multifocal premature ventricular contractions, ventricular tachycardia or ventricular fibrillation) occurs in 0.9%-6.0% of patients.[1]

Cardiac Death

Foster and associates found patients with CAD to have a 2.4% risk of cardiac mortality, compared to a 0.5% risk in patients without CAD.[8] Patients over age 40 also proved to have higher cardiac mortality (1.9%) with or without CAD.[1] Although cardiac death may be precipitated by many confounding factors, perioperative MI has been found to be the precipitating factor in 36%-70% of cases.[1]

3. Goals of Preoperative Evaluation

There are 2 primary goals of preoperative cardiac risk assessment. The first goal is to identify whether a patient is at increased risk for an adverse perioperative cardiac event. An increased cardiac risk may be a reflection of the operative procedure (eg, aortic surgery) or patient risk factors (eg, recent MI). Identifying a patient at increased cardiac risk may be accomplished by applying 1 of numerous clinical indices (eg, Goldman, Detsky, Lee) and/or by performing a noninvasive cardiac test (eg, dobutamine echocardiography), both of which will be described in detail later. Once a patient has been recognized to be at higher cardiac risk, the second goal is to prevent or reduce the risk of perioperative complications such as cardiac death, MI, transient myocardial ischemia, arrhythmia and CHF. In theory, this may be accomplished in several ways: 1.) medical management (ie, adding a beta-blocker perioperatively); 2.) invasive cardiac testing (coronary angiography) followed by coronary revascularization; 3.) alteration of the operative procedure to a less stressful one (ie, axillofemoral bypass instead of aortobifemoral bypass); or 4.) cancellation of the operation.

4. Risk Associated with the Type of Operation

The type of operation has been strongly associated with the risk of perioperative cardiac complications as seen in Table 1. Low-risk operations, with a reported cardiac risk of <1%, include endoscopic, superficial, cataract and breast operations.[9] Intermediate-risk procedures have a reported cardiac risk of >1% but <5%. These operations include carotid endarterectomy, head and neck operations, intraperitoneal, intrathoracic, orthopedic and prostate operations. High-risk procedures are associated with a cardiac risk >5%. These include emergent major operations (particularly in elderly patients), aortic and other major peripheral vascular operations, and procedures with an anticipated prolonged duration and associated with large fluid shifts or blood loss.

5. Cardiac Risk Assessment

Every patient undergoing major surgery should have an assessment of their cardiac risk. Even a low-risk operation can be associated with major cardiac morbidity and mortality in a patient with significant cardiac symptoms. Thus a detailed cardiac history and review of systems, as well as a careful physical examination, should be performed in all patients. Particular attention should be paid to identifying patients at highest cardiac risk: unstable angina, decompensated CHF, serious ventricular arrhythmias, symptomatic aortic stenosis or myocardial infarction within the last month. Patients should be asked about other evidence of coronary artery disease (remote history of MI or angina), congestive heart failure, symptomatic arrhythmias and valvular disease. Based on these findings, the patient can be classified into 1 of 3 general risk classes (Table 2), as defined by the American College of Cardiology/American Heart Association Task Force. Patients can be further stratified into different levels of cardiac risk by applying 1 of 4 commonly used cardiac risk assessment indices to assess an individual patient's cardiac risk.

Dripps-ASA Index

Dripps and colleagues derived a classification system by modifying the American Society of Anesthesiologists (ASA) index of physical status (Table 3). The Dripps-ASA index is used to predict cardiac death within 48 hours of surgery. Patients are categorized into 5 different types of physical status according to cardiac history. A patient classified as ASA 1 is a normal, healthy patient undergoing an elective operation. An ASA 2 patient has mild systemic disease. An ASA 3 patient has severe systemic disease that limits activity but is not incapacitating. An ASA 4 patient has incapacitating systemic disease that is a constant threat to life. Finally, ASA 5 status is reserved for moribund patients that are not expected to survive 24 hours with or without an operation.[10] Correlation between mortality rates for elective and emergent procedures and ASA classification status is listed in Table 4. The mortality rates after elective surgery range from 0.07% for class 1 to 8.1% for class 5 (note that figures in Table 3 combine data from elective and emergency procedures).[10] With specific regard to cardiac morbidity and mortality, Goldman and colleagues[11] noted life-

Table 1

Cardiac Risk Stratification for Noncardiac Surgical Procedures

High	
(Reported cardiac risk often greater than 5%)	
	Emergency and major operations, especially in the elderly
	Aortic and major vascular surgery
	Peripheral vascular surgery
	Anticipated prolonged surgical procedures associated with large fluid shifts and poor blood loss
	Examples include Whipple procedure, abdominal perineal resection
Intermediate	
(Reported cardiac risk generally less than 5%)	
	Carotid endarectomy
	Head and neck surgery
	Intraperitoneal and intrathoracic surgery
	Orthopedic surgery
	Urologic surgery, including prostate surgery
Low	
(Reported cardiac risk generally less than 1%)	
	Endoscopic procedures, including bronchoscopy, hysteroscopy or cystoscopy
	Superficial procedures
	Ophthalmologic procedures, including cataract surgery
	Breast surgery

Table 2

Clinical Predictors of Increased Perioperative Cardiac Risk

Major	
Unstable coronary syndromes Recent MI with evidence of important ischemia Unstable or severe angina (Canadian Class 3 or 4)	
Decompensated CHF	
Significant arrhythmias High-grade atrioventricular block Symptomatic ventricular arrhythmias with underlying heart disease Supraventricular arrhythmias with uncontrolled ventricular rate	
Severe valvular disease	
Intermediate	
Mild angina pectoris (Canadian Class 1 or 2)	
Prior myocardial infarction (by history or by Q waves)	
Compensated or prior CHF	
Diabetes mellitus	
Minor	
Advanced age	
Abnormal ECG findings (LV hypertrophy, left bundle branch block, ST-T wave changes)	
Rhythm other than sinus	
Low functional capacity	
History of stroke	
Uncontrolled systemic hypertension	

Eagle KA, Brundage BH, Chaitman BR, et al. Guidelines for perioperative cardiovascular evaluation for noncardiac surgery. Report of the American College of Cardiology/American Heart Association Task Force on Practice Guidelines (Committee on Perioperative Cardiovascular Evaluation for Noncardiac Surgery). Circulation. *1996;93:1278-1317.*

Table 3

The Dripps-ASA Classification of Physical Status

Physical Status	Description
1	A normal healthy patient
2	A patient with mild systemic disease
3	A patient with a severe systemic disease that limits activity, but is not incapacitating
4	A patient with an incapacitating systemic disease that is a constant threat to life
5	A moribund patient not expected to survive 24 hours with or without operation

Note: In the event of an emergency procedure, an "E" is placed before the number.

Table 4

Mortality Rates for Each ASA Physical Status

Physical Status	Anesthetic Procedures	Deaths	Mortality rate, percent*[a]
1	50,703	43	0.08
2	12,601	34	0.27
3	3626	66	1.8
4	850	66	7.8
5	608	57	9.4
Total	**68,388**	**266**	**0.39**

*[a] *Includes the combined totals of emergency and elective procedures.*

Vacanti CJ, Van Houten RJ, Hill RC. A statistical analysis of the relationship of physical status to postoperative mortality in 68,388 cases. Anesth Analg. *1970;49:564-566.*

Table 5

Correlation Between Preoperative Dripps-ASA Classification and Cardiac Complications

Classification	No or only minor complications	Life-threatening complications	Cardiac death
1 (N = 129)	129 (100%)	0	0
2 (N = 408)	398 (97%)	7 (2%)	3 (1%)
3 (N = 323)	302 (93%)	13 (4%)	8 (2%)
4 (N = 112)	87 (78%)	19 (17%)	6 (5%)

Class V was not assigned to any patient in this study.
Goldman L, Caldera DL, Nussbaum SR, et al. Multifactorial index of cardiac risk in noncardiac surgical procedures.
N Engl J Med. *1977;297(16):835-850.*

Table 6

The Goldman Multifactorial Cardiac Risk Index

Criterion	Points
1. History	
Age ≥70 years	5
MI in previous 6 months	10
2. Physical examination	
S_3 gallop or JVD	11
Important valvular aortic stenosis	3
3. Electrocardiographic findings	
Rhythm other than sinus or premature atrial contractions on last preoperative ECG	7
>5 Premature ventricular contractions/min documented at any time before operation	7
4. General status	
Po_2,60 mm Hg or Pco_2 >50 mm Hg	
K<3 mEq/L or HCO_3 <20 mEq/L	
BUN >50 mg/dL or Cr >3 mg/dL	
Abnormal SGOT, signs of chronic liver disease or patient bedridden from noncardiac causes	3
5. Operation	
Intraperitoneal, intrathoracic, or aortic	3
Emergency	4
Total	**53**

threatening complication rates of 0%, 2%, 4% and 17%, respectively, for ASA classes 1 through 4, and a cardiac death rate of 0%, 1%, 2% and 5%, respectively, for the same classes (Table 5). Critics of the ASA classification system feel the index is subjective and poorly reproducible, particularly in the elderly, the obese, in patients with a history of prior MI and those with mild systemic disease.[4]

Goldman Multivariate Risk Assessment

Goldman and colleagues[11] devised a multifactorial approach for risk assessment after recognizing the shortcomings of the Dripps-ASA index. In a landmark study, 1001 patients over age 40 years undergoing major noncardiac operations were prospectively evaluated to determine which preoperative factors might affect the development of postoperative cardiac complications. The multifactorial index was then derived retrospectively. A multivariate analysis of 39 variables was performed to determine which factors predicted perioperative cardiac complications. From the history, physical examination, ECG, laboratory data and operation, 9 variables were found to have statistically significant independent correlations with cardiac outcome. Each of these factors was assigned a discriminant function coefficient reflecting its relative weight in statistical analysis. The coefficients were used to assign a point value for each variable, and the point scores were used to define the 4 classes (Class I = 0-5 points, Class II = 6-12 points, Class III = 13-25 points and Class IV = ≥26 points) of the preoperative cardiac risk index.

The 9 factors, in order of decreasing significance, are: S3 gallop or jugular vein distention (JVD) on preoperative examination; MI in the preceding 6 months; rhythm other than sinus or premature atrial contractions on preoperative ECG; > 5 premature ventricular contractions/min documented at any time before operation; intraperitoneal, intrathoracic, or aortic operation; age > 70 years; important valvular aortic stenosis; emergency operation; and poor general medical condition. Poor general status was defined as $PO_2 < 60$ mmHg or $P_{CO2} > 50$ mm Hg, K < 3.0 mEq/L or $HCO_3 < 20$ mEq/L, BUN > 50 mg/dL or Cr > 3.0 mg/dL, abnormal AST (SGOT), signs of chronic liver disease or patient bedridden from noncardiac causes (Table 6).[11]

The progression from risk Class I to Class IV showed a stepwise increase in the proportion of patients who had life-threatening cardiac complications or cardiac death. Class I patients have a 0.7% risk of life-threatening complications (ie, MI, pulmonary edema or ventricular tachycardia), and a 0.2% risk of cardiac death. Class II patients have a 5% risk of life-threatening complications, and a 2% risk of cardiac death. Class III patients have an 11% risk of life-threatening complications, and a 2% risk of cardiac death. Finally, Class IV patients have a 22% risk of life-threatening complications, and a 56% risk of cardiac death.[4]

Surprisingly, many important variables (ie, diabetes, pulmonary vascular disease [PVD], stable angina, old MI by history or ECG, ST segment and T wave changes on ECG, bundle branch blocks or CHF without an S3 gallop or JVD) were not found to be significant in the Goldman index. The Dripps-ASA index was also evaluated in the study and was not found to be an independent predictor of complications. Numerous subsequent studies have confirmed the Goldman index to be objective, reliable and valid.

In recent years, the utility of the Goldman index has come into question. Jeffrey and associates[12] showed that the index is not helpful in predicting cardiac risk in patients undergoing elective aortic surgery. Others have verified that the index is less reliable for risk stratification for patients undergoing major vascular surgery. The index has a low sensitivity in vascular patients, and may overlook important CAD, especially in the elderly.[4,13] This is of critical importance because vascular patients are precisely the ones that have the highest operative risk, and would therefore theoretically benefit most from a reliable index. Another limitation of the Goldman index is that it is based on data from the mid-1970s, and it therefore may not properly reflect the recent advances in anesthesia, medicine and surgery.

Modified Goldman Index (Detsky)

Detsky and associates[14,15] modified the Goldman multivariate index to add more objectivity and to correct its other perceived inadequacies. Angina and alveolar pulmonary edema were added as risk factors. Under the category of angina, Canadian

Table 7

The Modified Multifactorial Cardiac Risk Index (Detsky)

Variables	Points
CAD	
MI within 6 months previously	10
MI more than 6 months previously	5
Canadian Cardiovascular Society angina	
Class 3	10
Class 4	20
Unstable angina within 3 months previously	10
Alveolar pulmonary edema	
Within 1 week previously	10
Ever	5
Valvular disease	
Suspected critical aortic stenosis	20
Arrhythmias	
Sinus plus atrial premature beats or rhythm other than sinus on last preoperative ECG	5
>5 Ventricular premature beats at any time before surgery	5
Poor general medical status	5
Age >70 years	5
Emergency operation	10

According to the CCS, Class 3 angina is defined as having a marked limitation of ordinary activity, such as angina when walking 1-2 blocks on level terrain or climbing up 1 flight of stairs in normal conditions and at a normal pace. Class 4 angina is defined as the inability to carry on any physical activity without discomfort; anginal syndrome ***may be*** *present at rest.*

Goldman L, Hashimoto B, Cook EF, Loscalzo A. Comparative reproducibility and validity of systems for assessing cardiovascular functional class: Advantages of a new specific activity scale. Circulation. *1981;64(6):1227-1234.*

Table 8

Lee's Revised Cardiac Risk Index – Predictors for Major Cardiac Complications

1. High-risk type of surgery
   Includes any intraperitoneal, intrathoracic or suprainguinal vascular procedures
2. History of ischemic heart disease
   History of myocardial infarction
   History of positive exercise test
   Current complaint of chest pain secondary to myocardial ischemia
   Use of nitrate therapy
   ECG with pathological Q waves
3. History of heart failure
   History of congestive heart failure, pulmonary edema or paroxysmal nocturnal dyspnea
   Physical examination showing bilateral rales of S3 gallop
   Chest radiograph showing pulmonary vascular redistribution
4. History of cerebrovascular disease
   History of transient ischemic attack or stroke
5. Diabetes mellitus requiring treatment with insulin
6. Preoperative serum creatinine >2.0 mg/dL (177 μmol/L)

Lee TH, Marcantonio ER, Mangione CM, et al. Derivation and prospective validation of a simple index for prediction of cardiac risk of major noncardiac surgery. Circulation. *1999;100(10):1043-1049.*

Table 9

Estimated Rate of Major Perioperative Cardiac Event According to Number of Risk Factors in Lee's Revised Cardiac Risk Index

Number of Risk Factors	Risk of Major Perioperative Cardiac Event, % (95% CI)
0	0.4 (0.1 – 0.8)
1	1.0 (0.5 – 1.4)
2	2.4 (1.3 – 3.5)
3 or greater	5.4 (2.8 – 7.9)

Major perioperative cardiac events described in this table include cardiac death, nonfatal myocardial infarction and nonfatal cardiac arrest. Postoperative cardiogenic pulmonary edema and complete heart block were also included as outcomes in the Lee index but are not included in this table.

Devereaux PJ, Goldman L, Cook DJ, et al. Perioperative cardiac events in patients undergoing noncardiac surgery: a review of the magnitude of the problem, the pathophysiology of the events and methods to estimate and communicate risk. CMAJ. *2005;173(6):627-634.*

Table 10

A Summary of Studies Investigating Myocardial Perfusion Imaging for Preoperative Assessment of Cardiac Risk

Total number of studies, 1985-1997	Total number of patients enrolled	Positive Predictive Value	Negative Predictive Value
27	3718	13% (180/1307)	99% (1549/1571)

Table 11

A Summary of Studies Examining the Value of Dobutamine Stress Echocardiography for Preoperative Risk Assessment

Total number of studies, 1985-1997	Total number of patients enrolled	Positive Predictive Value	Negative Predictive Value
12	1699	15% (74/484)	99% (1203/1213)

Cardiovascular Society (CCS) Class 3 and Class 4 angina were added, as was unstable angina within the previous 3 months. CCS Class 3 angina is defined as angina that occurs when walking 1-2 blocks on level terrain or up 1 flight of stairs at a normal pace. CCS Class 4 angina is defined as occurring during any type of physical activity or occurring at rest.[16] Alveolar pulmonary edema was further categorized into recent (within 1 week) and remote. Myocardial infarction was also temporally defined as recent (within the previous 6 months) or remote (>6 months previously). The scoring system was also simplified by assigning either 5, 10, 15 or 20 points to each cardiac risk factor (Table 7).

Based on these changes, patients were stratified into 3 risk classes: Class 1 (0-15 points), Class 2 (15-30 points) and Class 3 (>30 points). The maximum point score a patient could receive was 105, but patients rarely had a total over 40. Another change Detsky made was to factor in the type of surgical procedure outside of the scoring system. The type of operation was weighed and calculated as a separate risk value (or pretest probability). The pre-test probability reflected the overall complication rate for all patients undergoing a specific type of operation. This value was then converted into a post-test probability, which was the patient's cardiac risk within a specific risk group (ie, Class 1 [0-15 points]). The post-test value was calculated using a likelihood ratio and was derived from a nomogram.

Though Detsky and coworkers made important modifications to the Goldman index, applying the Detsky scoring system is somewhat cumbersome. To apply the index requires that one know the overall rate of cardiac complications for each type of operation at one's own institution. Second, it requires having a nomogram in order to apply the likelihood ratios.

The Detsky modification, as well as the other cardiac risk indices, have other shortcomings. These classification schemes place patients into broad categories, thus limiting the usefulness of the system. Also, these indices do not take into consideration unpredictable stresses that may occur during major vascular or thoracic operations.

Lee's Revised Cardiac Risk Index

The most recent and now most widely utilized risk stratification system is the Lee Revised Cardiac Risk Index. Lee and colleagues[17] further revised the original Goldman cardiac risk index in an attempt to simplify the prediction of risk. Their study monitored 2893 patients with a mean age of 66 years who were undergoing elective major noncardiac procedures, and identified 6 independent predictors of major cardiac complications, each of them of approximately equal prognostic importance. Major cardiac complications were defined as having myocardial infarction, pulmonary edema, ventricular fibrillation or primary cardiac arrest, or complete heart block.

The 6 independent predictors of major cardiac complications are listed in Table 8 and include: 1.) high-risk type of surgery including any intraperitoneal, intrathoracic or suprainguinal vascular procedures; 2.) history of ischemic heart disease as defined by a history of a previous myocardial infarction, positive exercise test, current complaint of chest pain considered to be secondary to myocardial ischemia, use of nitrate therapy or ECG with pathological Q waves; 3.) history of congestive heart failure including either pulmonary edema, paroxysmal nocturnal dyspnea, physical examination showing bilateral rales or S3 gallop or chest radiograph showing pulmonary vascular redistribution; 4.) history of cerebrovascular disease as defined by a history of either a transient ischemic attack or stroke; 5.) diabetes mellitus requiring treatment with insulin; and 6.) preoperative serum creatinine > 2.0 mg/dL (177 μmol/L).[17] Patients who had prior coronary revascularization procedures were considered as having ischemic heart disease only if they also had the listed criteria for ischemic heart disease.[17] The 6 predictors were validated in a cohort of 1422 patients, and the predictive value was shown to be statistically significant in all types of major elective noncardiac surgery (including thoracic, abdominal, orthopedic and vascular) except for abdominal aortic aneurysm (AAA) surgery.[17]

Current literature suggests the Lee index to be the most accurate estimation of perioperative cardiac risk for generic and practical use. Devereaux and colleagues[18] determined that the rate of cardiac death, nonfatal myocardial infarction and nonfatal cardiac arrest are 0.4% (95% CI 0.1%-0.8%) in patients with zero risk factors, 1.0% (95% CI 0.5%-1.4%) in patients with 1 risk factor, 2.4% (95% CI 1.3%-3.5%) in patients with 2 risk factors and 5.4% (95% CI 2.8%-7.9%) in patients with 3 or more risk factors (Table 9). Auerbach and Goldman[19] studied the rate of major cardiac complications according to both the number of risk factors and the use or nonuse of beta-blockers. They found the rate to be 0.4%-1.0% without beta-blockade vs. < 1% with beta-blockade in patients with zero risk factors, 2.2%-6.6% without beta-blockade vs. 0.8%-1.6% with beta-blockade in patients with 1 or 2 risk factors and >9% without beta-blockade vs. > 3% with beta-blockade in patients with 3 or more risk factors.[19]

However, the Lee index is not without its own shortcomings. In particular, this model has shortcomings for vascular surgery—only 21% of the patients used in deriving the index underwent vascular surgery, and many vascular procedures were by definition considered as high-risk. Furthermore, the index does not account for age, which itself is oftentimes regarded as an independent risk factor for postoperative mortality. To address these issues, Welton and colleagues[20] studied the influence of aging on the prognostic value of Lee's revised cardiac index in a study involving 2642 patients over a 13-year period who underwent open vascular surgery including carotid endarterectomy, elective infrarenal abdominal aortic surgery, acute infrarenal AAA surgery and lower limb arterial reconstruction procedures. They found that the predictive value of Lee's index is highest among patients under 55 years of age and lowest among patients over 75 years of age.[20] However, they found that adjustment of Lee's index for age, presence of hypertension, and risk of surgical procedure improved the prognostic value of the index in the population of patients over 75 years of age.[20]

6. Preoperative Tests

Twelve-Lead Electrocardiogram (ECG)

A routine ECG is not necessary in every patient prior to surgery, however it is useful in men over age 40 years and women over age 55 years. It is also useful in patients with positive cardiac findings on history or physical examination. 40%-70% of patients with CAD have abnormalities on preoperative ECG. ST-T wave changes are most common, followed by signs of left ventricular hypertrophy, and Q waves.[1] Although some authors have found a correlation between ST-T wave changes, left ventricular hypertrophy and adverse cardiac events, most authors would agree that the Q wave is the most significant predictor. In patients undergoing open and endovascular aortic aneurysm repair, de Virgilio and associates[21] noted a 25% cardiac event rate in patients with a Q wave on ECG vs. a 1.6% event rate without a Q wave.

Chest Radiography (X-Ray)

Routine chest x-ray is not necessary in every patient prior to surgery. It is most helpful in patients with evidence of prior pulmonary and cardiac disease and those with abnormal findings on cardiac and pulmonary examination. In the elderly, the chest x-ray is used routinely, because this population has a high prevalence of coexisting pulmonary disease. A preoperative chest radiograph is particularly useful if it demonstrates evidence of ventricular function abnormalities. In patients with CAD, the finding of cardiomegaly is associated with a low ejection fraction in 70% of cases.[1] Whether a low ejection fraction is predictive of adverse cardiac events is debatable.[1]

Functional Capacity

A measure of functional capacity can be determined by metabolic equivalent of the task (MET) levels. One MET is the equivalent of the oxygen consumption of a 40-year-old man (weight, 70 kg) at a resting state (3.5 mL/kg/min). The inability to achieve over 4 METs has been associated with a higher likelihood of adverse perioperative cardiac events. Examples of activities that require more than 4 METs are climbing hills, moderate cycling, singles tennis and jogging, whereas activities requiring less than 4 METs are baking, golfing with a cart and walking at a speed of approximately 2-3 mph.[9]

In addition to the preoperative ECG, chest x-ray and an assessment of the patient's functional capacity by calculation of maximum METs, some authors recommend further noninvasive cardiac stress testing in select patients who are found to be at moderate risk for adverse cardiac events. These additional tests may identify significant CAD or dysrhythmias that may place the patient at high risk for an adverse cardiac event. Whether further cardiac testing and subsequent preoperative cardiac intervention actually reduces the rate of adverse cardiac events is the subject of intense debate that will be discussed later in the chapter.

It should be noted that *patients with very high cardiac risk (ie, unstable angina, decompensated CHF, serious ventricular arrythmias, recent MI) should not undergo stress testing because the stress test itself may precipitate myocardial ischemia.* Rather, such patients should proceed directly to coronary angiography prior to surgery. Conversely, patients at low risk for an adverse cardiac event are not likely to benefit from additional stress testing and therefore can proceed to surgery without additional tests.

Exercise ECG

Exercise electrocardiography (ECG) is one of the most commonly used noninvasive cardiac stress tests for determining the degree of CAD. The test provides an estimate of functional capacity, hemodynamic response to exercise, potential for catecholamine-induced cardiac arrhythmias and exercise myocardial ischemia threshold.[22] Gianrossi and associates performed a meta-analysis of 147 consecutive series with 24,074 patients who underwent both coronary angiography and exercise testing.[22] The mean sensitivity of exercise electrocardiography for multivessel CAD was 81% (range, 40%-100%) with a mean specificity of 66% (range, 17% - 100%). However, the sensitivity of exercise ECG is reduced in patients who cannot reach maximum levels of exercise, and in those with extensive Q wave anterior MI on resting ECG.[22] An important limitation of exercise electrocardiography in vascular patients is that 30%-50% of patients referred to a cardiologist are unable to reach maximum levels of exercise.[22]

Other investigators have suggested that low exercise capacity itself is an indicator of cardiac risk. Cutler and associates studied 130 patients who underwent exercise electrocardiography before vascular surgery.[23] Of the patients who were able to achieve greater than 75% of predicted maximum heart rate, none suffered a postoperative cardiac complication. Patients who had inducible ischemia at low workloads (<75% of predicted maximum heart rate) were found to have the greatest risk of cardiac complications (38% cardiac event rate). Thus, low exercise tolerance does not necessarily preclude use of this test, because some valuable information can still be obtained.[23] The most important findings are the ability to achieve >75% of age-predicted maximum heart rate without chest pain, arrhythmia or ST-segment depression greater than or equal to 1 mm. The treadmill is most commonly used, but the bicycle is another option. For patients with claudication, arm ergometry is sometimes used. Stress imaging conducted with either echocardiography or nuclear perfusion increases the accuracy of the test results.[23]

There are 2 advantages of standard exercise ECG testing: its wide availability and its low cost. However, exercise testing with ECG monitoring has its limitations. First of all, its sensitivity (65%-70%)[24] is reportedly lower than nuclear imaging techniques. Second, its specificity is poor in the presence of ST-T abnormalities on a resting ECG or in patients on digoxin. It also does not accurately illustrate the extent of ischemia nor provide any information on left ventricular function.[24] Its greatest liability is that it is not useful if the patient is unable to exercise because of a disability or incapacity, a frequent occurrence in vascular patients. Unfortunately, these are precisely the patients that may most benefit from stress testing. In such patients, a pharmacologic stress test should be considered.

Pharmacologic Stress Testing (Dipyridamole/Sestamibi-Thallium)

Pharmacologic stress testing involves the administration of agents (dipyridamole, adenosine) that mimic the coronary vasodilator response associated with exercise. Upon administration, dipyridamole and adenosine cause coronary vasodilatation and increase coronary blood flow to levels 3-4 times those of normal vessels.[24] Dipyridamole, a known antiplatelet agent, is a potent vasodilator if administered at 5-10 times its antiplatelet dose. The difference in augmentation of resting coronary blood flow in normal vs. diseased coronary arteries allows demonstration of regional differences in myocardial perfusion by thallium or sestamibi scintigraphy. Coronary arteries with severe stenosis have an abnormal flow reserve, which shows up as perfusion defects on nuclear images. If a perfusion defect is present at both stress and at rest, this is thought to represent an old infarct (fixed defect), whereas if the defect disappears at rest, the area of myocardium is thought to be ischemic (reversible defect). Patients with large reversible defects or reversible defects in 2 or more areas of myocardium are considered at greatest risk for an adverse cardiac event.

Dipyridamole-thallium (DTHAL) and sestamibi (DIMIB) are commonly used in patients with physical limitations (ie, claudication, orthopedic or neurologic disease, amputation and advanced age) that prevent exercise ECG testing.[2] Contraindications for both dipyridamole and adenosine are obstructive lung disease, pronounced bronchiospastic airway disease, patients at risk for severe complications from prolonged hypotension and patients on xanthine derivatives.[24]

DTHAL scintigraphy has been shown to have a high degree of sensitivity and specificity for the detection of hemodynamically significant CAD when compared to angiography in human studies. However, controversy exists as to whether an abnormal DTHAL is useful in predicting which vascular patients are at increased risk for perioperative adverse cardiac events. In a review of 254 vascular patients referred to a nuclear cardiology laboratory, Eagle and colleagues noted that the DTHAL results were best used when combined with clinical risk factors.[25] In patients with 1 or 2 clinical risk factors, they noted a 29.6% cardiac event rate with reversible ischemia on DTHAL vs. only a 3.2% event rate without reversible ischemia. In a report by Vanzetto et al,[26] 517 consecutive patients were evaluated before abdominal aortic surgery. If no major or fewer than 2 intermediate clinical cardiac risk factors were present, patients went directly to elective surgery. The authors noted a 5.6% incidence of cardiac events in those patients with 1 risk factor and a rate of 2.4 % in those with no cardiac risk actors. All high-risk patients underwent dipry-mamode thallium SPECT imaging, and those with a normal scan had a cardiac event rate of 2% in contrast to a rate of 23% in 43 patients (36%) demonstrating reversible thallium defects. In several publications by Hendel et al,[27] Lette et al[28], and Brown et al,[29] the scoring or quantification of scan abnormalities had a significant impact on improving risk assessment and positive predictive value. The data suggest that as the size of the defect increases to a moderate degree, the cardiac risk significantly increases.

More recently, the utility of DTHAL/DMIBI as a preoperative cardiac screening tool has come into question.[30-35] In 2 retrospective studies, de Virgilio and associates found that DTHAL and DMIBI redistribution were not predictive of adverse cardiac events in patients without severe cardiac symptoms (recent MI, unstable angina, decompensated CHF).[30,31] The positive predictive value of DTHAL and DMIBI for adverse cardiac events was 6% and 10%, respectively. In a prospective study of 457 consecutive patients undergoing abdominal aortic surgery, Baron and colleagues also found that DTHAL results did not accurately predict adverse cardiac outcomes.[32] Stratmann and coworkers noted a 3% cardiac event rate in 87 patients with a normal DMIBI and a 5% event rate in 110 patients with an abnormal DMIBI (P = NS).[33] Mangano and colleagues found no association between DTHAL redistribution and perioperative cardiac ischemia in 60 consecutive patients undergoing vascular surgery.[34] In a more recent prospective, blinded study, de Virgilio and associates again found no association between a reversible defect on DTHAL/DMIBI and adverse cardiac events in 82 patients undergoing elective vascular surgery.[36] The adverse event rate was 13.8% for patients with a reversible defect and 9.8% for patients without (P= 0.7).[36] For patients with 2 or more reversible defects, the cardiac event rate was 12.5% vs. 11.1% for less than 2 reversible defects.

The use of DTHAL in preoperative risk assessment was evaluated in 27 studies, all published since 1985 as seen in Table 10. This revealed an overall 13% positive predictive value and a 99% negative predictive value. Thus, though DTHAL is useful in identifying CAD in ambulatory patients, it has a very low positive predictive value perioperatively and thus is losing favor as a preoperative tool.

Exercise/Dobutamine Echocardiography (ECHO)

Stress ECHO can be performed with treadmill exercise. It has the advantage over DTHAL in that it assesses ventricular and valvular function while simultaneously detecting regional wall motion at rest and at stress. A drop in ejection fraction, an increase in end-systolic volume or multiple regional wall motion abnormalities during exercise or after dobutamine infusion suggest an increased likelihood of left main or 3-vessel disease. Stress ECHO is less expensive than nuclear imaging. The disadvantages are that unsatisfactory images are produced in about 5% of patients and expertise is required to obtain and analyze the images.

Dobutamine is administered in patients with exercise intolerance. Dobutamine is a synthetic sympathomimetic agent that causes an increase in myocardial contractility and heart rate that leads to an increased myocardial oxygen demand. One of the main disadvantages of dobutamine infusion is that several side effects may occur, including chest pain, arrhythmia, headache, tremor, palpitations, and either hyper- or hypotension.[24]

Several reports have documented the accuracy of dobutamine stress echo to identify patients at risk for perioperative cardiac events. The use of dobutamine stress echo in preoperative risk assessment was evaluated in 12 studies, all published since 1991 as seen in Table 11. The data indicates that dobutamine stress echo can be performed safely and with acceptable patient tolerance. In the series by Poldermans et al,[37] the presence of a new wall motion abnormality was a powerful determinant of an increased risk of perioperative events after multivariate adjustment for different clinical and echocardiographic variables. Several studies suggest that the extent of the wall motion abnormality and/or wall motion changes at low ischemic thresholds are especially important. These findings have been shown to be predictors of long-term and short-term outcome.[38-41] Although hypotension during dobutamine testing is generally not well correlated with degree of underlying CAD, in 1 recent report, hypotension was an independent predictor of perioperative complications.[41] Eichelberger and colleagues studied 75 consecutive patients who had dobutamine ECHO prior to major vascular surgery.[42] This was the only prospective blinded study of consecutive patients who underwent dobutamine ECHO. 16 patients (21%) had significant adverse effects from the dobutamine infusion, including hypotension (11%) and severe hypertension (>240 mm systolic, 4%). The postoperative ischemic cardiac event rate was 7%. All 5 patients with cardiac events had positive dobutamine stress tests (sensitivity, 100%). The negative predictive value was also 100%. However, 22 patients with a positive stress test did not have an event, thus the positive predictive value was only 19%.[42] Therefore, it appears that dobutamine stress echocardiography may be most useful when results are negative.

Coronary Angiography

The ultimate gold standard for preoperative cardiac assessment is coronary angiography. In a landmark study, Hertzer and colleagues[43] reported a series of 1000 consecutive patients who underwent coronary angiography prior to peripheral vascular surgery. They identified surgically correctable CAD in 25%. In current practice, most institutions recommend coronary angiography for patients with severe cardiac symptoms (severe or unstable angina, recent MI, decompensated CHF). Another indication for coronary angiography, though controversial, is its use in patients who have a positive noninvasive stress test. If operable CAD is detected, it can be corrected via percutaneous transluminal coronary angioplasty (PTCA) or coronary artery bypass grafting (CABG).

7. Risks/Benefits of Coronary Revascularization

In determining whether preoperative coronary revascularization is justified prior to surgery, it is important to be aware of the risks of intervention. Coronary arteriography carries a 0.15% risk of MI, and a 0.3% risk of mortality.[44] Percutaneous transluminal coronary angioplasty has a 6% risk of MI and a 1.8% risk of mortality.[44] Patients with peripheral vascular disease, and those with diabetes in particular, have higher mortality following CABG than those without peripheral vascular disease. Hertzer and associates reported an operative mortality rate of 5% for CABG in patients with peripheral vascular disease compared to a 1.2% mortality rate for those without.[43] In a study from the Mayo Clinic, the mortality rate of CABG for patients 80 years of age and older increased from 4% without peripheral vascular disease to 16% when peripheral vascular disease was present.[45]

Several studies suggest that prophylactic coronary revascularization lowers the risk of subsequent adverse cardiac events during vascular surgery. In a series of 1000 consecutive patients who underwent coronary angiography prior to elective vascular surgery at the Cleveland Clinic Foundation, 216 patients underwent CABG with an operative mortality of 5.5%. Of the 130 patients who subsequently underwent vascular surgery, there was only 1 death (0.8% mortality).[43] In the Coronary Artery Surgery Study, patients who underwent CABG before noncardiac surgery had a lower mortality (0.9%) when compared with patients with significant CAD who were randomized to medical therapy before noncardiac surgery (2.4%).[8] Mahar and associates noted a 5% MI rate following noncardiac surgery in 49 patients with angiographically demonstrated CAD who did not undergo preoperative CABG, as compared to a 0% MI rate in 99 patients with preoperative CABG who underwent 168 subsequent procedures.[46]

Fewer data are available regarding the role of preoperative PTCA prior to noncardiac surgery. Huber and colleagues studied 55 consecutive patients with significant CAD referred for preoperative PTCA prior to noncardiac surgery.[47] During PTCA, 1 patient had abrupt closure of the coronary artery leading to hemodynamic instability and emergent CABG. Another patient had a coronary artery dissection requiring CABG. In 3 others, the coronary lesions could not be traversed, requiring CABG, thus PTCA was unsuccessful in 9%. Of the 50 patients with successful PTCA, 1 patient had a non-Q wave MI following PTCA. Another patient had a fatal MI following thoracoabdominal aneurysm repair despite the PTCA. 2 other patients had non-Q wave MIs. The overall perioperative MI rate was 5.6% and the postoperative mortality rate was 1.9%.[47] In a cohort of 2452 patients undergoing AAA repair over a 10-year period at the Mayo Clinic, Elmore and associates noted that preoperative coronary revascularization was necessary in only 100 patients (4.1%).[48] 95 of these patients had symptomatic CAD (history of MI, angina, or CHF). The perioperative MI rate in these 100 patients was 5% with no postoperative mortality vs. an overall mortality of 2.9% for the entire series. The authors noted the late cardiac event rate was significantly higher in patients undergoing PTCA (56.5%) vs. those who had undergone CABG (27%).[48]

More recently, several authors have questioned the role of preoperative coronary revascularization. Using a decision model to compare treatment alternatives for patients at higher risk of perioperative cardiac complications after vascular surgery, Mason and colleagues concluded that proceeding directly to vascular surgery without preoperative coronary arteriography led to lower morbidity and less cost.[44] Subjecting a patient to preoperative invasive cardiac evaluation would expose them to risks of at least 3 procedures: coronary arteriography, coronary revascularization (PTCA and/or CABG) and the vascular operation. They stated that *preoperative coronary revascularization would only be beneficial if the estimated operative mortality of the vascular operation was substantially higher than 5% and if the estimated operative mortality of the CABG was in the 2%-3% range*.[44] Massie and colleagues compared 70 consecutive patients that underwent coronary arteriography because of 2 or more segments of redistribution on DTHAL with 70 matched patients with similar DTHAL findings who did not undergo additional evaluation.[49] They found that any possible benefit from invasive cardiac evaluation was offset by 3 deaths and 2 MIs that complicated the cardiac evaluation. There was no significant difference between the coronary angiography group and the matched control group with regard to perioperative nonfatal MI (13% vs. 9%), fatal MI (4% vs. 3%), late nonfatal MI (16% vs. 19%) or late cardiac death (10% vs. 13%).[49] In a prospective study over a 1-year period, Taylor and coworkers noted no fatal MIs and no operative deaths among 285 elective major vascular procedures.[6] The study is noteworthy in that only patients with severe symptomatic CAD (unstable angina, uncontrolled arrhythmia, severe CHF) underwent invasive cardiac testing, and only 3 patients had a prophylactic CABG. The authors concluded that invasive cardiac testing should be limited to patients with severe symptomatic CAD. In a prospective study, Seeger and associates compared 146 consecutive patients undergoing aortic reconstruction, DTHAL, and selective coronary revascularization with 172 historical controls who did not undergo extensive cardiac testing.[35] The authors noted no difference in cardiac mortality, serious cardiac complications or long-term cardiac mortality between the groups, in spite of the fact that 41% of the DTHAL group had undergone coronary arteriography and 11.4% had undergone coronary revascularization.[35] Our institutional results mirror those of Seeger and colleagues.[31] We limited coronary revascularization to patients with severe cardiac symptoms or recent cardiac events. Of the 8 patients that underwent preoperative coronary revascularization, 1 patient (12.5%) suffered a massive MI following preoperative PTCA.[31] The adverse cardiac event rate was no different when patients who underwent DTHAL testing with selective coronary revascularization were compared with those that did not undergo DTHAL testing.[50]

Due to the limited data, prophylactic preoperative PTCA cannot be advocated in trying to reduce perioperative cardiac complications in patients undergoing major vascular surgery. Until data is established proving the contrary, the indications of PTCA in the preoperative vascular patients is the same as those developed by the joint AHA outlining the indication for PTCA in the general patient population.

Coronary Artery Revascularization Prophylaxis (CARP) Trial

This study enrolled 510 patients from 18 US VA centers from 1997-2003 in order to assess the long-term benefit of preoperative coronary artery revascularization among patients with stable CAD scheduled for elective vascular surgery.[51] Subjects were scheduled for elective vascular surgery. To receive cardiac catheterization, patients were deemed by a cardiologist to be at increased risk of perioperative cardiac complications. Those who had angiographic evidence of stenosis greater than 70% in at least 1 coronary artery, were randomly assigned to coronary artery revascularization (CAR) or no revascularization before the vascular procedure. Percutaneous intervention was performed on 59% of the patients and CABG on 41%. The primary end was long-term mortality with a minimum follow-up of 1 year and a medical follow-up of about 2.5 years. Before vascular surgery, there were 10 deaths in the CAR group and 1 death in the no CAR group. However, 30-day mortality was similar in both groups (3.1% and 3.4%). Mortality was 22% and 23% at a median of 2.7 years after randomization for the CAR and no CAR groups, respectively. There were no differences in 30-day postoperative myocardial infarction rates between the 2 groups. Importantly, patients assigned to the CAR group had a significant delay of 54 days before receiving their vascular surgery procedure, in contrast to a delay of 18 days in the no CAR group. This is the first prospective randomized study that demonstrated no benefit in preoperative coronary artery revascularization prior to elective vascular surgery. This has led to a major change in preoperative recommendations as there is much less justification for performing preoperative coronary intervention in patients who have no coronary symptoms prior to a noncardiac operation.

8. Perioperative Medical Therapy

Beta Blockade

Studies Showing Benefit to Beta-Blockade

Beta-blockers form a class of agents with cardioprotective potential. Beta-blockers decrease myocardial oxygen demand by reduction of heart rate and myocardial contractility. Furthermore, beta-blockers reduce adrenergic activity, which results in reduced levels of free fatty acids, thus causing a shift in the myocardial metabolism towards glucose uptake.

Several studies have addressed the relationship between beta-blockers and perioperative myocardial ischemia. Stone et al[52] studied the effect of low dose beta-blockers, specifically labetolol, atenolol or oxprenolol, in 128 hypertensive patients undergoing noncardiac surgery. Patients who received beta-blocker had a lower incidence of myocardial ischemia, as determined by continuous 12 lead ECG monitoring, than patients without beta-blocker treatment. Mangano et al[53] conducted the first randomized controlled study evaluating the cardioprotective effect of beta-blockers in patients undergoing noncardiac surgery. 200 patients undergoing vascular surgery were randomized to atenolol treatment or placebo. No difference was observed in perioperative mortality between the 2 treatment arms. However, atenolol was associated with a significant lower mortality during the 2-year follow up.

The DECREASE study[54] clearly demonstrated a cardioprotective effect of bisoprolol, a selective beta-blocker, in high-risk patients undergoing major vascular surgery. Bisoprolol was associated with a significant reduction in cardiovascular death and myocardial infarction during the 30-day perioperative phase (3.3% vs. 34% events; *P*-value <0.01). Boersma et al[55] showed beta-blockers reduced the cardiac event rate even in patients with multiple cardiac risk factors and an abnormal ECHO. However, there was no difference in the incidence of cardiac events among patients with more extensive ischemia on dobutamine stress ECHO. Therefore, beta-blockers were beneficial in all but the subset of patients with more extensive ischemia.

McGory et al[56] performed a meta-analysis of 6 articles on preoperative beta-blockade published between 1966-2004. As part of their study, they performed a sensitivity analysis on outcomes of postoperative myocardial infarction and ischemia in patients undergoing lower risk surgery, such as general or orthopedic surgery, who had received beta-blockade. They demonstrated a significantly reduced benefit of preoperative beta-blockade in diminishing risk of myocardial infarction and ischemia in comparison to patients undergoing vascular surgery. They speculated that their results might have reflected the risk of the procedure type due to the decreased rate of cardiac events following abdominal or orthopedic surgery in contrast to patients undergoing vascular surgery.

The above findings are supported by a study by Lin et al.[57] In a retrospective study of 333 patients undergoing major abdominal surgery for gastrointestinal cancer, the authors reported very low adverse cardiac event rate (3.9%) and cardiac mortality (0.6%). Of note, only 20% received beta-blockers, supporting the fact that low or intermediate risk surgeries may not necessitate preoperative beta-blockade.

Studies Against the Routine Use of Beta-Blockade in All Noncardiac Surgeries

The POISE trial[58] is the largest trial to date that examined the effects of preoperative beta-blockade. This randomized controlled trial conducted in 190 hospitals in 23 countries consisted of 8351 patients with or at risk of atherosclerotic disease undergoing noncardiac surgery. Most of the patients had a revised cardiac risk index (see section above on Lee's revised cardiac index) of 1 or 2, and 42% were undergoing some form of vascular surgery. The patients were randomly assigned to either a fixed dose of metoprolol (100 mg extended release metoprolol succinate) or placebo given 2-4 hours before surgery, and repeated 0-6 hours after surgery. This was followed by either 200 mg metoprolol or placebo daily for 30 days. At 30 days, the study found a significant decrease in cardiovascular death, nonfatal myocardial infarction, or nonfatal cardiac arrest in the metoprolol group as compared to placebo (5.8% vs. 6.9%, HR 0.84, 95% CI 0.70-0.99).[58] Fewer patients in the metoprolol group had a myocardial infarction compared to placebo (4.2% vs. 5.7%, HR 0.73, 95% CI 0.60-0.89).[58] However, the study also found a higher mortality rate in the metoprolol group than in the placebo group (3.1% vs. 2.3%, HR 1.33, 95% CI 1.03-1.74), and also a higher incidence of stroke in the metoprolol group than in the placebo group (1.0% vs. 0.5%, HR 2.17, 95% CI 1.26-3.74).[58]

The results of the POISE study suggests that for every 1000 patients undergoing noncardiac surgery, extended-release metoprolol would prevent 15 patients from having a myocardial infarction, 3 from cardiac revascularization and 7 from developing clinically significant atrial fibrillation.[58] However, for every 1000 patients treated, there would also be an excess of 8 deaths, 5 patients with stroke, 53 with clinically significant hypotension and 42 with clinically significant bradycardia.[58]

Bangalore and colleagues[59] performed a meta-analysis of 33 trials that included 12,306 patients, of which the POISE study constituted the largest portion of their analysis. Their analysis showed no clear benefit of perioperative beta-blockade for the prevention of cardiovascular outcomes; every 1000 patients treated with beta-blockers resulted in 16 fewer non-fatal myocardial infarctions at the expense of 3 disabling strokes, 45 patients with clinically significant bradycardia, 59 patients with clinically significant hypotension and potentially increased mortality.[59] They furthermore found that the apparent benefit of beta-blockade is largely driven by high bias risk trials, whereas analysis of the more reliable trials with low bias risk affirms the findings of the POISE study of increased risk of mortality and non-fatal strokes.

Given the results of the POISE study, the evidence does not seem to suggest initiating prophylactic beta-blocker therapy in most patients undergoing noncardiac surgery. Although beta-blockers appear to decrease the risk of a perioperative myocardial infarction, the increase in the risk of stroke and mortality makes this benefit seem much less appealing, especially given that most myocardial infarctions are asymptomatic whereas most strokes are seriously disabling or incapacitating.

However, the POISE study is not without its limitations. The major limitation of the POISE study is that it uses a high and fixed dose of metoprolol that is not adjusted for heart rate, and that the therapy is initiated only 2-4 hours prior to surgery as compared to up to 30 days before surgery in some of the other trials.[58] The 100 mg starting dose of metroprolol succinate in the POISE study was 2-8 times the commonly prescribed dose, and up to 200 mg of metroprolol succinate administered on the first day of surgery represents 50% of the maximum daily therapeutic dose.[60] Furthermore, the findings of the POISE study[58] does not exclude potential benefits of beta-blockade in high risk patients with a revised cardiac risk index of 3 or higher, even though such patients only comprised about 2% of the population in a large retrospective observational study of 663,665 patients who underwent major noncardiac surgery between 2000-2001.[61] Similarly, the POISE study does not exclude the possible benefit of beta-blockers in patients with evidence of significant ischemia as demonstrated by stress tests and who do not undergo preoperative coronary revascularization.

Studies Using Targeted Beta-Blockade

There have also been a number of studies comparing the value of targeted beta-blockade especially in the setting of achieving tight individualized heart rate control prior to major surgeries. In one such study, Poldermans and colleagues[62] examined the value of preoperative cardiac stress testing in intermediate-risk patients undergoing major vascular surgery. In their study, 770 intermediate risk (1-2 risk factors using Lee's revised cardiac risk index) patients were randomized to receive either cardiac stress testing (via dobutamine echocardiography, dobutamine or dipyridamole perfusion scintigraphy) or no testing. At the same time, targeted beta-blockade bisoprolol was installed in all patients and tightly adjusted to achieve a resting heart rate of 60-65 beats/minute prior to surgery, after surgery and after discharge. The results of the study revealed that at 30 days after major vascular surgery, no difference in intermediate-risk patients was observed in the incidence of cardiac death and nonfatal myocardial infarction between the testing and no testing groups.[62] Furthermore, the incidence of perioperative cardiac death or myocardial infarction was significantly correlated with heart rate control; patients with heart rate of less than 65 beats/minute prior to surgery had a lower incidence of perioperative cardiac death or myocardial infarction than the remaining patients (1.3% vs. 5.2%, OR 0.24, 95% CI 0.09-0.66).[62] Thus, tight heart rate control using targeted beta-blockade was clearly associated with improved outcome.

In another recent study, de Virgilio and colleagues[63] demonstrated that targeted beta-blockade alone is more effective than selective cardiac stress testing and nontargeted beta-blockade in the prevention of cardiac morbidity in patients undergoing major lower extremity revascularization, carotid endarterectomy, or major lower extremity amputation. Their study compared 100 prospective patients receiving preoperative targeted beta-blockade and no cardiac stress testing, with 80 retrospective control patients of which 14% had underwent preoperative cardiac stress testing and 61% had received nontargeted beta-blockers preoperatively. Patients receiving preoperative targeted beta-blockade were given metoprolol at incrementally higher doses (starting from a mean of 4 days preoperatively) with the goal of achieving a targeted heart rate of 50-60 beats/minute; at time of surgery, median heart rate was 66 beats/minute compared to 77 beats/minute in the retrospective group receiving cardiac stress testing and/or nontargeted beta-blockade. After adjusting for the Lee's revised cardiac risk index score, the study demonstrated at 30 days after major vascular surgery a significantly lower cardiac complications rate among patients receiving targeted beta-blockade (OR 2.46, 95% CI 1.3-4.5) compared to patients receiving cardiac stress testing and/or nontargeted beta-blockade.[63] Again, tight heart rate control using targeted beta-blockade appears to be clearly associated with improved outcomes, and the results of this study further supports the notion that targeted beta-blockade started days in advance of surgery may serve an important role in improving outcomes in major noncardiac surgeries.

Current Recommendations on Beta-Blockade

Beta-blockers are the cornerstone in the medical treatment of coronary artery disease, with proven long term benefits.[64] A number of early studies showed significant benefits in the use of perioperative beta-blockade in reducing perioperative ischemia and the risk of myocardial infarction and death in high-risk patients undergoing moderate- to high-risk surgery. They recommended that when possible, beta-blockers should be started days or weeks before elective surgery, with the dose titrated to achieve a resting heart rate between 50-60 beats per minute. A subsequent meta-analysis by McGory et al[56] indicated that beta-blockade was not necessary in low-moderate risk patients undergoing low-risk surgery.

The findings of the POISE study group[58] and the Bangalore et al[59] meta-analysis of the various major clinical trials supports the notion that indiscriminate use of beta-blockade is not recommended. In particular, beta-blocker therapy that is initiated just before surgery without targeting the heart rate actually increases the risk of stroke and mortality. Given the increased risk of stroke, bradycardia and hypotension, the current literature suggests that beta-blockade should not be routinely used as perioperative prophylaxis of all patients undergoing noncardiac surgery. However, in patients who are already taking beta-blockers for clinically indicated reasons such as heart failure, coronary artery disease or a previous myocardial infarction, the beta-blockade should be continued. On the other hand, if a patient is undergoing a high risk procedure such as a major vascular operation, or if the patient has 3 or more clinical risk factors as determined by Lee's revised cardiac risk index, strong consideration should be given to instituting beta-blockade, provided it is done at least several days in advance and is appropriately titrated.

If beta-blockers are used in the preoperative setting, one is faced with a number of issues, including the choice of agent, the dose and timing of therapy, and possible adverse effects. Studies that reported cardiovascular benefit in perioperative beta-blockade used agents that are either moderately (atenolol and metoprolol) or highly (bisoprolol) beta-1 cardioselective.[59] However, there are no comparative trials of the different beta-1 cardioselective agents. In terms of dosing, the 2007 ACC/AHA guidelines on perioperative cardiovascular evaluation[65] recommend maintaining a heart rate of 60-65 beats per minute. In terms of timing, starting beta-blockers days to weeks before surgery should decrease the risk of hypotension in the perioperative period. In patients who do not require long-term beta-blockade, however, the drug must be carefully tapered after surgery to avoid potential adverse effects of rapid beta-blocker withdrawal such as accelerated angina, myocardial infarction, or cardiovascular mortality.[66] Targeted beta-blockade, when started well in advance of surgery and used for high risk surgical cases such as major vascular surgery, may also obviate the need to perform cardiac stress testing.

Statins

Coronary plaque rupture and erosions are recognized as precipitants of MIs, unstable angina and sudden death in the operative and nonoperative setting.[67-75] A number of perturbations induced by the perioperative status may precipitate plaque instability and thrombosis. These include increased sympathetic tone, anemia, pain, temperature fluctuation, activation of the coagulation system and abrupt changes in metabolic, hemodynamic and electrolytic parameters.[75] HMG-CoA reductase inhibitors or statins are considered a keystone in the primary and secondary prevention of cardiovascular disease. In addition to inhibiting development of atherosclerotic plaques through reduction of serum cholesterol as a long-term benefit, statins are anti-inflammatory, can improve endothelial function and coagulation, and produce a stabilizing effect on vulnerable plaques, even with short-term usage.[76] These properties may be especially beneficial in the perioperative period because the disruption of unstable plaques is believed to be responsible for most cases of perioperative myocardial infarction.[77]

Perioperative use of statins has been shown to reduce all causes of mortality in patients undergoing major vascular surgery. In a case control study, Poldermans et al[67] demonstrated that statin use among patients undergoing major vascular surgery was associated with a 4-fold risk reduction in perioperative all cause mortality. Atorvastatin was recently shown to reduce the incidence of cardiovascular events after vascular surgery by 68%, as compared with placebo in 570 patients who underwent AAA repair between 1991-2001.[78] Lindenauer et al[79] confirmed these results in a study of patients undergoing major noncardiac surgery. Statin therapy was associated with a 40% reduction of risk for postoperative death.

The Statins for Risk Reduction in Surgery (StaRRS) Study[80], a retrospective study of 1163 hospitalizations on 997 patients from 1999-2000, found that cardiovascular complications after noncardiac surgery were significantly decreased in patients receiving statins (9.9%) as compared to patients not receiving statins (16.5%). Even after adjusting for other significant predictors of perioperative complications such as age, gender, type of surgery, emergent surgery, left ventricular dysfunction and diabetes mellitus, the study found that statins still conferred a statistically significant protective effect (odds ratio 0.52).[80]

Durazzo and colleagues[81] conducted the first randomized controlled trial investigating the influence of statins on perioperative cardiovascular complications. In their trial, 100 patients were randomly to either receive 20 mg atorvastatin or placebo for 45 days, with vascular surgery performed on average 30 days after randomization. Within 6 months after surgery, they noted an 8.0% incidence of cardiovascular events (such as cardiac death, myocardial infarction, unstable angina or stroke) in those treated with atorvastatin compared to a 26.0% incidence in the placebo group, suggesting that even a short-term treatment with a statin can reduce the incidence of major cardiovascular complications after vascular surgery.[81] A meta-analysis by Hindler and colleagues[82] found that the use of preoperative statin therapy was associated with a 59% reduction in the risk of mortality after vascular surgery.

Thus far, long-term statin use is associated with reduced all cause and cardiovascular mortality, irrespective of clinical risk factors and beta-blocker use. While the optimal time of initiation and duration of statin therapy is still unclear, a small but growing number of studies are showing benefit in the use of statins in the perioperative setting for the reduction of major cardiovascular complications.[83] However, since there has only been 1 randomized controlled trial thus far investigating the influence of statins on perioperative complications, more studies are clearly needed to definitively demonstrate whether statin therapy truly has a benefit, and if so, to determine the magnitude of that benefit. Given the current level of evidence, patients undergoing major vascular surgery or those with known coronary disease should continue statin therapy if they are already being treated, and statin therapy should be initiated in previously untreated patients undergoing elective vascular surgery. Finally, it is critical that statins be continued postoperatively in patients who are on chronic statin therapy, because of the risk of postoperative myonecrosis and an increased risk of perioperative adverse cardiac events with postoperative statin withdrawal.[84]

Alpha^2-Adrenergic Agonists

The surgical stress response plays a key role in the pathogenesis of cardiovascular complications.[85,86] The alpha^2-adrenergic agonists attenuate the stress response and therefore potentially reduce cardiovascular complications. Unlike alpha^1-antagonists, which act on peripheral adrenergic receptors to inhibit vasoconstriction directly, alpha^2-agonists act on central and presynaptic receptors to inhibit central sympathetic outflow[87] and reduce peripheral norepinephrine release.[88] Alpha^2-agonists dilate poststenotic coronary vessels[89] and decrease the severity of perioperative hemodynamic abnormalities,[90,91] and consequently were classified as a grade IIb recommendation in the 2002 American College of Cardiology/American Heart Association Guideline Update on Perioperative Cardiovascular Evaluation for Noncardiac Surgery.[92]

Several recent studies examined the role of alpha agonists (clonidine and mivazerol) in perioperative cardiac protection. Oliver et al[93] reported a large randomized, placebo-controlled, multicenter trial of the alpha^2-agonist mivazerol in perioperative use. They randomized 2854 patients with known CAD or significant risk factors that were undergoing noncardiac surgery to 1.5 mcg per kg per hour infusion of mivazerol or placebo. Among patients with history of CAD who were undergoing general surgical procedures, the rate of MI was no different between the mivazerol and placebo groups, but the cardiac death rates were significantly reduced. Among patients undergoing vascular procedures, both cardiac death rate and the combined end point, eg, death or MI, were significantly reduced. The Multicenter Study of Perioperative Ischemia Research Group also reported the results of a placebo-controlled, randomized, double-blind study of perioperative mivazerol.[94] 300 patients with known CAD undergoing noncardiac surgery were randomized to high- or low-dose mivazerol or placebo. No differences in perioperative death or MI were observed,

Figure 1

Our proposed algorithm for preoperative cardiac risk assessment (Modified from Auerbach et al.[19])

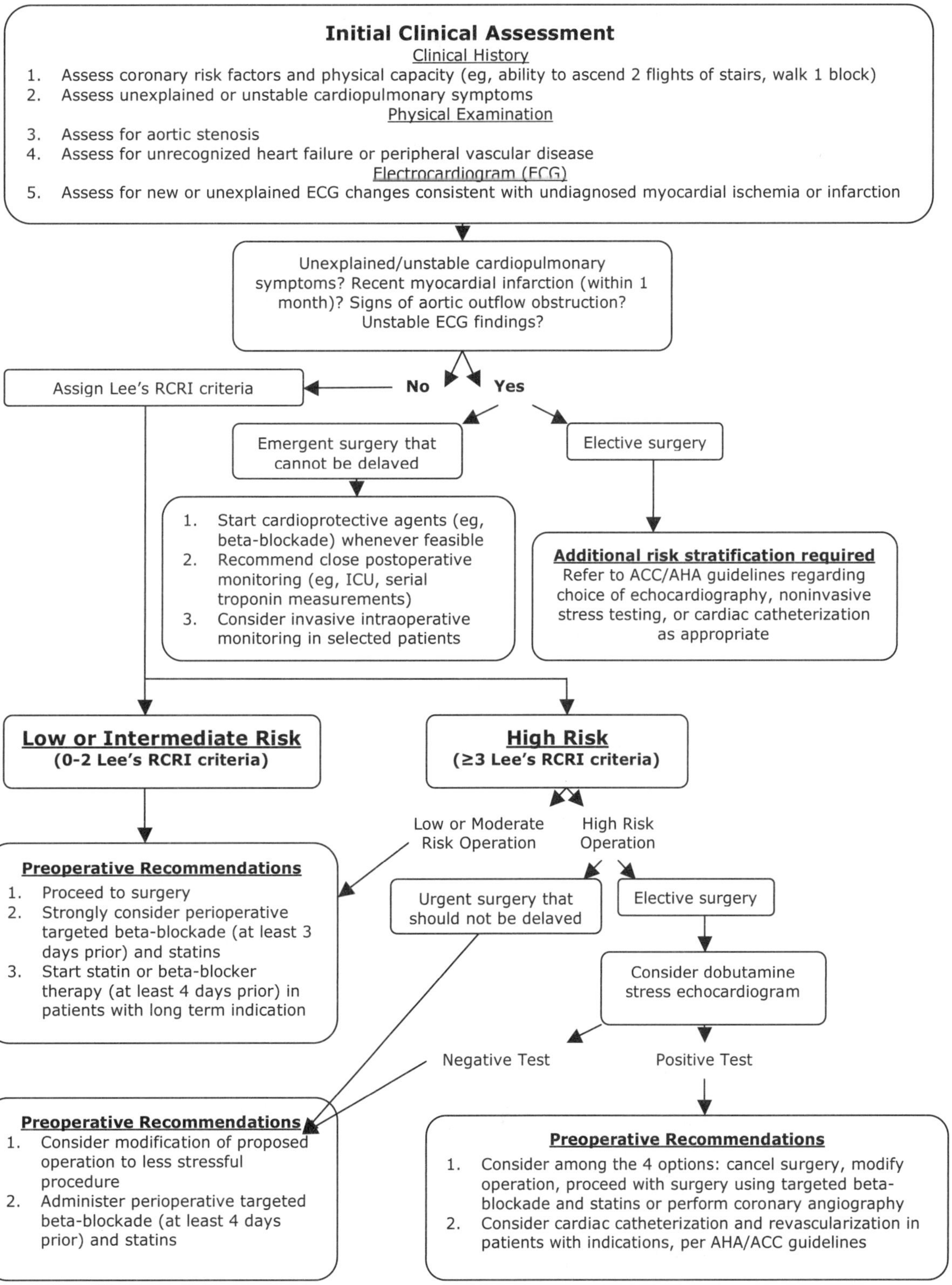

Figure 2

AHA guidelines for preoperative cardiac risk assessment

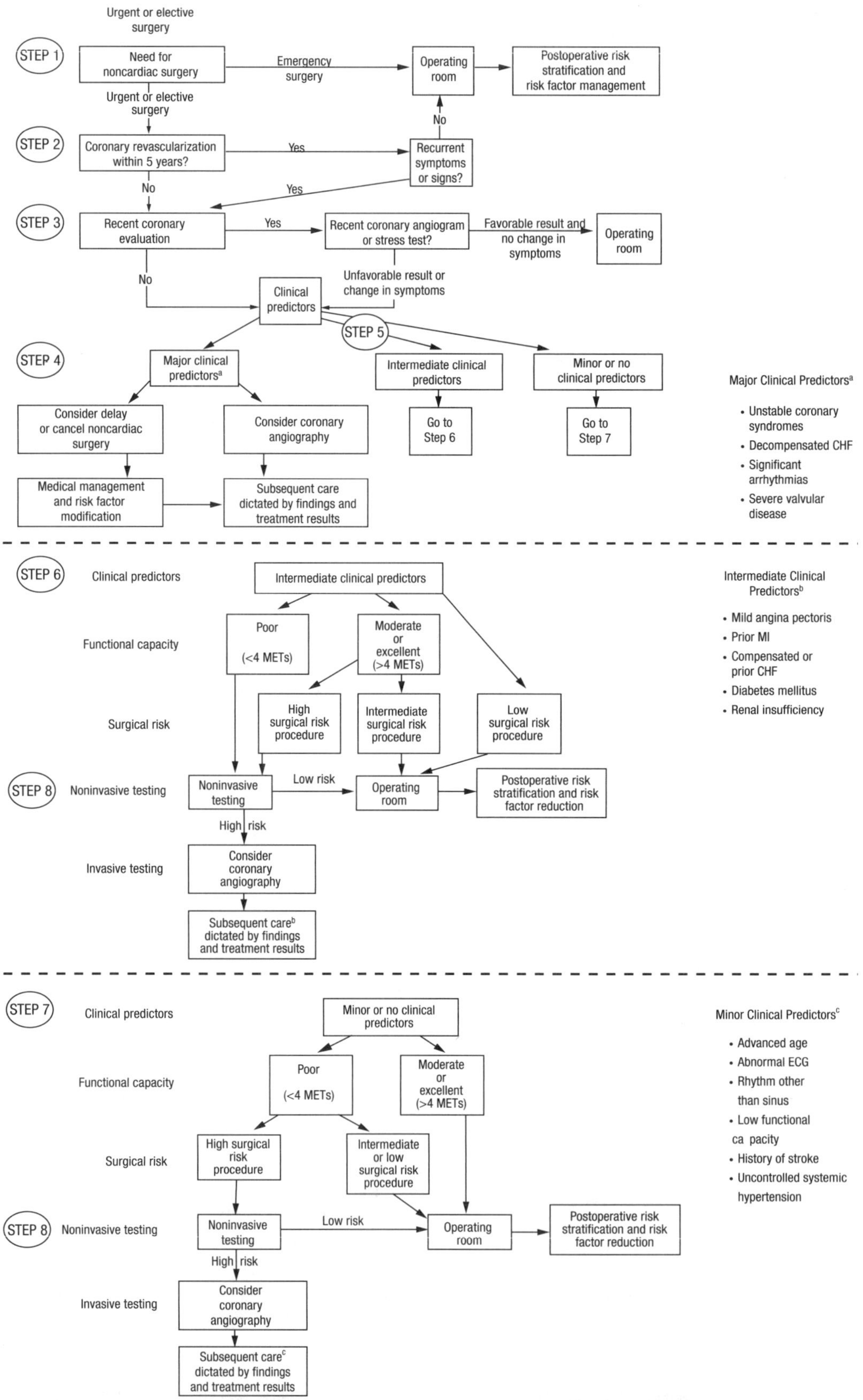

but the high dose had significantly less myocardial ischemia than the placebo group. 2 randomized placebo-controlled studies of clonidine for perioperative myocardial protection were performed in 297 patients undergoing vascular surgery[95] and 61 patients undergoing general surgery.[88] Both studies demonstrated a significant decrease in the incidence of myocardial ischemia.

Although these results support the use of alpha2-agonists for prevention of perioperative cardiovascular complications following vascular or cardiac surgery, their potential in improving perioperative outcomes should be clarified in large, randomized, controlled trials.

9. Costs of Preoperative Cardiac Testing

Cost must be recognized when considering whether to recommend further noninvasive or invasive testing. Although physicians should be concerned with improving the clinical outcome for their patients, cost is an appropriate consideration when different evaluation and treatment strategies are available.

Bry and colleagues estimated the cost of cardiac testing (including costs of DTHAL, selective coronary arteriography, and selective PTCA and CABG) to be $392,000 per life saved and $181,000 per MI prevented.[96] They further noted that the positive predictive value of DTHAL was only 19%.[96] In our own study, time from evaluation to surgery significantly increased from 12 days to 18 days ($P = .0003$) in patients undergoing DTHAL, without improving outcome.[31]

10. Clinical Significance of Postoperative Cardiac Events

Bry and associates noted a 5.9% MI rate and a 1.3% cardiac mortality rate following 237 major vascular procedures.[96] The authors noted that the majority of MIs were clinically insignificant. Pre- and post-infarction ECHO data were available in 11 of the 14 patients who suffered an MI. 8 of these 11 patients had no change in ejection fraction.[97] Yeager and colleagues reported that patients with a perioperative non-Q wave or "chemical" MI had a similar long-term cardiac prognosis as controls, suggesting that such an MI may not be a significant event.[97] Patients with a Q wave MI had a higher incidence of subsequent adverse cardiac events and coronary revascularization than patients without postoperative MI, but survival rates at 1 and 4 years were similar.[97]

11. Surgery in the High Cardiac Risk Patient

One would anticipate an unacceptably high cardiac event rate in patients with high surgical risk (ie, uncorrectable severe cardiac disease) who undergo aortic surgery. Thus, the tendency would be to deny such a patient a surgical option. However, McCann and Wolfe reported no difference in operative mortality between patients with low ejection fraction (35%, 5% mortality) and higher ejection fraction (>35%, 2% mortality).[98] There was also no difference in cumulative life-table survival. In a study of 106 high-risk patients from the Mayo Clinic, Hollier and associates reported only a 5.7% mortality rate.[99] Thus they argued that high-risk patients with large aortic aneurysms should not be denied surgical repair, because it can be performed with an acceptable morbidity and mortality.

12. Long-Term Benefits of Cardiac Revascularization

Johnston and associates noted that the late survival rate of patients with abdominal aortic aneurysm (AAA) was significantly lower than the age- and sex-matched normal population (60.2% vs. 79.2%), and that heart-related causes of late death were more frequent (44.4% vs. 34.1 %).[100] In a study of 680 patients following AAA repair, Hertzer and colleagues found that the cumulative 5-year survival rate (75%) and cardiac mortality rate (5%) after CABG were nearly identical to survival figures calculated for patients having normal coronary arteries.[101] In comparison, the cumulative survival and cardiac mortality rates for a small subset of patients with severe, uncorrected CAD were 29% and 34%, respectively.[101] However, these observations may be biased in favor of the CABG group because these patients had the most favorable coronary anatomy and were thus selected for revascularization. In contradiction, Massie and associates found that patients who underwent extended cardiac evaluation and treatment had a longer interval before their first MI, but did not demonstrate an improvement in the number of fatal and nonfatal cardiac events or in survival rate over the control group.[49]

13. Management Algorithm

In light of recently published studies, and most importantly the CARP trial, it is evident that very few surgical patients require an extensive preoperative cardiac work-up. We propose an algorithm as demonstrated in Figure 1, which we modified from the management algorithm proposed by Auerbach and Goldman.[19] Our algorithm slightly differs from the AHA guidelines as our algorithm also reflects the data from Poldermans and colleagues indicating that patients with 1-2 risk factors do not need stress testing but can be effectively managed with targeted perioperative beta-blockade.[62]

Every patient undergoing non-emergent surgery should undergo cardiac risk assessment. This assessment may be limited to a careful history and physical examination. The first goal is to identify the patient with high cardiac risk. Patients considered high risk include those with unstable angina, acute MI, symptomatic aortic stenosis or decompensated CHF. Major surgery poses an inordinate cardiac risk in these patients and should be postponed if the surgical condition is not immediately life-threatening. In this small subgroup of patients, a careful cardiac work-up should be performed and may include coronary angiography and echocardiography, where appropriate.

If high cardiac risk factors are not present, the next step is to compute the number of cardiac risk factors using Lee's Revised Cardiac Risk Index.[17] A score of 0-6 should be assigned. If the cardiac history is positive, it is important to establish whether the cardiac disease is active, the severity and whether coronary revascularization has been recently performed. If a patient has a cardiac history but has undergone coronary revascularization within the last 5 years and is now symptom free, such a patient has a low cardiac risk and can proceed to surgery. If the patient has a Revised Cardiac Risk Index of <3, the operation will carry a low predicted cardiac risk and can be performed without cardiac stress testing. Routine use of perioperative beta-blockade and statins is not necessary, but should be strongly considered in high risk surgery, provided the beta-blockade is targeted and instituted several days in advance. If the patient has a Revised Cardiac Risk Index of ≥ 3, one should consider the type of operation performed. If the proposed operation is low or moderate risk, the patient can proceed to surgery without additional testing. In these patients, again, strong consideration should be given for beta-blockade and statins. If the patient with a Revised Cardiac Risk Index of ≥3 is about to undergo a high-risk operation, the urgency of the operation must be considered (keeping in mind that this represents a very small subgroup of patients). If the patient has limb-threatening ischemia or very large or symptomatic nonruptured AAA, further cardiac testing should be omitted. For these patients, one can change the proposed operation to a less stressful procedure (ie, endovascular AAA repair instead of open repair, axillofemoral bypass instead of aortobifemoral bypass) or simply administer targeted perioperative beta-blockade and statins. In the patient with a Revised Cardiac Risk Index of ≥3 who is to undergo a purely elective case, dobutamine stress echocardiogram should be considered. If the results of the stress echocardiogram are normal, one can proceed with surgery. If the echocardiogram shows new wall motion abnormalities, the number of segments should be determined. If there are extensive areas of new wall motion abnormalities, there are 4 options: cancel surgery, modify the operation, proceed with surgery using targeted beta-blockade and statins, or perform coronary angiography. The decision of which option to choose must be individualized based on the indications for surgery, age, expected life span and the estimated risk of coronary intervention. Given the conflicting studies on the benefit of preoperative beta-blockade, indiscriminate use of these agents for all noncardiac patients is not recommended.

14. References

1. Mangano DT. Perioperative cardiac morbidity. *Anesthesiology*. 1990;72:153-184.

2. Mangano DT, Goldman L. Preoperative assessment of patients with known or suspected coronary disease. *N Engl J Med*. 1995;333(26):1750-1756.

3. Thompson ME. Assessing cardiac risk before noncardiac surgery: Basic principles. *Hosp Med*. August 1996;31-38.

4. Abraham SA, Coles NA, Coley CM, et al. Coronary risk of noncardiac surgery. *Prog Cardiovasc Dis*. 1991;34(3):205-234.

5. Rao TK, Jacobs KH, El-Etr AA. Reinfarction following anesthesia in patients with myocardial infarction. *Anesthesiology*. 1983;59: 499-505.

6. Taylor LM, Yeager RA, Moneta G, et al. The incidence of perioperative myocardial infarction in general vascular surgery. *J Vasc Surg*. 1992;15:52-59.

7. Ellis SG, Hertzer NR, Young JR, et al. Angiographic correlates of cardiac death and myocardial infarction complicating major non-thoracic vascular surgery. *Am J Cardiol*. 1996;77: 1126-1128.

8. Foster E, Davis K, Carpenter J, et al. Risk of noncardiac operation in patients with defined coronary disease: The Coronary Artery Surgery Study (CASS) registry experience. *Ann Thorac Surg*. 1986 Jan;41(1):42-50.

9. Eagle KA, Brundage BH, Chaitman BR, et al. Guidelines for perioperative cardiovascular evaluation for noncardiac surgery. Report of the American College of Cardiology/American Heart Association Task Force on Practice Guidelines. Committeee on Perioperative Cardiovascular Evaluation for Noncardiac Surgery. *Circulation*. 1996;93(6):1278-1317.

10. Vacanti CJ, Van Houten RJ, Hill RC. A statistical analysis of the relationship of physical status to postoperative mortality in 68,388 cases. *Anesth Analg*. 1970;49:564-566.

11. Goldman L, Caldera DL, Nussbaum SR, et al. Multifactorial index of cardiac risk in noncardiac surgical procedures. *N Engl J Med*. 1977;297(16):835-850.

12. Jeffrey CC, Kunsman J, Cullen DJ, et al. A prospective evaluation of cardiac risk index. *Anesthesiology*. 1983;58:462-464.

13. Bronson DL, Halperin AK, Marwick TH. Evaluating cardiac risk in noncardiac surgical patients. *Cleve Clin J Med*. 1995;62:391-400.

14. Detsky AS, Abrams HB, Forbath N, Scott JG, Hilliard JR. Cardiac assessment for patients undergoing noncardiac surgery: A multifactorial clinical risk index. *Arch Intern Med*. 1986;146:2131-2134.

15. Detsky AS, Abrams HB, McLaughlin JR, et al. Predicting cardiac complications in patients undergoing non-cardiac surgery. *J Gen Intern Med*. 1986;1:211-219.

16. Goldman L, Hashimoto B, Cook EF, Loscalzo A. Comparative reproducibility and validity of systems for assessing cardiovascular functional class: Advantages of a new specific activity scale. *Circulation*. 1981;64(6):1227-1234.

17. Lee TH, Marcantonio ER, Mangione CM, et al. Derivation and prospective validation of a simple index for prediction of cardiac risk of major noncardiac surgery. *Circulation*. 1999 Sep 7;100(10):1043-1049.

18. Devereaux PJ, Goldman L, Cook DJ, et al. Perioperative cardiac events in patients undergoing noncardiac surgery: a review of the magnitude of the problem, the pathophysiology of the events and methods to estimate and communicate risk. *CMAJ*. 2005;173(6):627-634.

19. Auerbach A, Goldman L. Assessing and reducing the cardiac risk of noncardiac surgery. *Circulation*. 2006;113(10):1361-1376.

20. Welten GM, Schouten O, van Domburg RT, et al. The influence of aging on the prognostic value of the revised cardiac risk index for postoperative cardiac complications in vascular surgery patients. *Eur J Vasc Endovasc Surg*. 2007;34(6):632-638.

21. de Virgilio C, Bui H, Donayre C, et al. Endovascular vs open abdominal aortic repair: a comparison of cardiac morbidity and mortality. *Arch Surg*. 1999;134(9):947-951.

22. Gianrossi R, Detrano R, Mulvihill D, et al. Exercise induced ST depression in the diagnosis of coronary artery disease: A meta-analysis. *Circulation*. 1989;80:87-98.

23. Cutler BS, Wheeler HB. Applicability and interpretation of electrocardiographic stress testing in patients with peripheral vascular disease. *Am J Surg*. 1981;141:501-506.

24. Mayo Clinic Cardiovascular Working Group on Stress Testing. Cardiovascular Stress Testing: A description of the vascular types of stress tests and indications for their use. *Mayo Clin Proc*. 1996;71:43-52.

25. Eagle KA, Coley CM, Newell JB, et al. Combining clinical and thallium data optimizes preoperative assessment of cardiac risk before major vascular surgery. *Ann Int Med*. 1989;110:859-866.

26. Vanzetto G, Machecourt J, Blendea D, et al. Additive value of thallium single-photon emission CT myocardial imaging for prediction of perioperative events in clinically selected high cardiac risk patients having abdominal aortic surgery. *Am Cardiol*. 1996; 77:143-148.

27. Hendel RC, Whitfield SS, Villegas BJ, et al. Prediction of late cardiac events by dipyridamole thallium imaging in patients undergoing elective vascular surgery. *Am Cardiol*. 1992; 70: 1243-1249.

28. Lette J, Waters D, Cerino M, Picard M, Champagne P, Lapinte J. Preoperative coronary artery disease risk stratification based on dipyridamole imaging and a simple three step, three segment model for patients undergoing noncardiac vascular surgery or major general surgery. *Am J Cardiol*. 1992; 69: 1553-1558.

29. Brown KA, Rowen M. Extent of jeopardized viable myocardium determined by myocardial perfusion imaging best predicts perioperative cardiac events in patients undergoing noncardiac surgery. *J Am Coll Cardiol*. 1993;21: 325-330.

30. de Virgilio C, Pak S, Arnell T, et al. Cardiac assessment prior to vascular surgery: Is dipyridamole-sestamibi necessary? *Ann Vasc Surg*. 1996 Jul;10(4):325-329.

31. de Virgilio C, Kirby L, Lewis RJ, et al. Limited utility of dipyridamole-thallium for predicting adverse cardiac events after vascular surgery. *Vasc Endovascular Surg*. 1998;32(3):275-279.

32. Baron JF, Munder O, Bertrand M, et al. Dipyridamole-thallium scintigraphy and gated radionuclide angiography to assess cardiac risk before abdominal aortic surgery. *N Engl J Med*. 1994;330:663-669.

33. Stratmann H, Younis L, Wittry M, et al. Dipyridamole technetium-99m sestamibi myocardial tomography in patients evaluated for elective vascular surgery: Prognostic value for perioperative and late cardiac events. *Am Heart J*. 1995;131:923-929.

34. Mangano D, London M, Tubau J, et al. Dipyridamole thallium-201 scintigraphy as a preoperative screening test: A reexamination of its predictive potential. *Circulation*. 1991;84:493-502.

35. Seeger J, Rosenthal G, Self S, et al. Does routine stress-thallium cardiac scanning reduce postoperative cardiac complications? *Ann Surg*. 1994;219:654-663.

36. de Virgilio C, Toosie K, Elbassir M, et al. Dipyridamole-thallium/sestamibi before vascular surgery: A prospective blinded study in moderate risk patients. *J Vasc Surg*. 2000 Jul;32(1):77-89.

37. Poldermans D, Fioretti PM, Forster T, et al. Dobutamine stress echocardiography for assessment of perioperative cardiac risk in patients undergoing major vascular surgery. *Circulation*. 1993;87:1506-1512.

38. Davila-Roman VG, Waggoner AD, Sicard GA, et al. Dobutamine stress echocardiography predicts surgical outcome in patients with an aortic aneurysm and peripheral vascular disease. *J Am Coll Cardiol*. 1993;21:957-963.

39. Poldermans D, Arnese M, Fioretti PM, et al. Improved cardiac risk stratification in major vascular surgery with dobutamine-atropine stress echocardiography. *J Am Coll Cardiol*. 1995;26: 648-653.

40. Day SM, Younger JG, Karavite D, et al. Usefulness of hypotension during dobutamine echocardiography in predicting perioperative cardiac events. *J Am Coll Cardiol*. 2000; 85:478-483.

41. Bigatel DA, Franklin DP, Elmore JR, et al. Dobutamine stress echocardiography prior to aortic surgery: long-term cardiac outcome. *Ann Vasc Surg*. 1999; 13:17-22.

42. Eichelberger J, Schwarz K, Black E, et al. Predictive value of dobutamine echocardiography just before noncardiac vascular surgery. *Am J Cardiol*. 1993;72:602-607.

43. Hertzer N, Beven E, Young J, et al. Coronary artery disease in peripheral vascular patients: a classification of 1000 coronary angiograms and results of surgical management. *Ann Surg*. 1984;199:223-233.

44. Mason J, Owens D, Harris R, et al. The role of coronary angiography and coronary revascularization before noncardiac vascular surgery. *JAMA*. 1995;273:1919-1925.

45. Mullaney C, Darling G, Pluth J, et al. Early and late results after isolated coronary artery bypass surgery in 159 patients age 80 years and older. *Circulation*. 1990;82(suppl IV):229-236.

46. Mahar L, Steen P, Tinker J, et al. Perioperative myocardial infarction in patients with coronary artery disease with and without aorta-coronary artery bypass grafts. *J Thorac Cardiovasc Surg*. 1978;76:533-537.

47. Huber K, Evans M, Bresnahan J, et al. Outcome of noncardiac operations in patients with severe coronary artery disease successfully treated preoperatively with coronary angioplasty. *Mayo Clin Proc*. 1992;67:15-21.

48. Elmore JR, Hallet J, Gibbons R, et al. Myocardial revascularization before abdominal aortic aneurysmorrhaphy: Effect of coronary angioplasty. *Mayo Clin Proc*. 1993;68:637.

49. Massie MT, Rohrer M, Leppo J, Cutler B. Is coronary angiography necessary for vascular surgery patients who have positive results of dipyridamole thallium scans? *J Vasc Surg*. 1997;25:975-983.

50. Bui H, de Virgilio C. Preoperative cardiac evaluation and interventions before aortic surgery: are they justified? *Perspect Vasc Surg Endovasc Ther*. 2000;12(2):25-41.

51. McFalls, EO, Ward HB, Moritz TE, et al. Coronary artery revascularization before elective major vascular surgery. *N Engl J Med*. 2004; 351:2795-2804.

52. Stone JG, Foex P, Sear JW, et al. Myocardial ischemia in untreated hypertensive patients: effect of a single small oral dose of a betaadrenergic blocking agent. *Anesthesiology*. 1988; 68:495-500.

53. Mangano T, Layug EL, Wallace A, et al. Effect of atenolol on mortality and cardiovascular morbidity after noncardiac surgery. Multicenter Study of Perioperative Ischemia Research Group. *N Engl J Med*. 1996;335:1713-1720.

54. Poldermans D, Boersma E, Bax JJ, et al. The effect of bisoprolol on perioperative mortality and myocardial infarction in high-risk patients undergoing vascular surgery. Dutch Echocardiography Cardiac Risk Evaluation Applying Stress Echocardiography Study Group. *N Engl J Med*. 1999;341: 1789-1794.

55. Boersma E, Poldermans D, Bax JJ, et al. Predictors of cardiac events after major vascular surgery: the role of clinical characteristics, dobutamine echocardiography, and beta blocker therapy. *JAMA*. 2001; 285:1865-1873.

56. McGory ML, Maggard MA, Ko CY. A meta-analysis of perioperative beta blockade: what is the actual risk reaction? *Surgery*. 2005 Aug;138(2):171-9.

57. Lin M, Haukoos J, Tahernia A, de Virgilio C. Cardiac morbidity and mortality after surgery for gastrointestinal carcinomas. *Am Surg*. 2005 Oct;71(10):833-6.

58. POISE Study Group, Devereaux PJ, Yang H, et al. Effects of extended-release metoprolol succinate in patients undergoing non-cardiac surgery (POISE trial): a randomised controlled trial. *Lancet*. 2008 May 31;371(9627):1839-47.

59. Bangalore S, Wetterslev J, Pranesh S, et al. Perioperative beta blockers in patients having non-cardiac surgery: a meta analysis. *Lancet*. 2008 Dec 6;372(9654):1962-76.

60. Fleisher LA, Poldermans D. Perioperative beta blockade: where do we go from here? *Lancet*. 2008 May 31;371(9627):1813-14.

61. Lindenauer PK, Pekow P, Wang K, et al. Perioperative beta-blocker therapy and mortality after major noncardiac surgery. *N Engl J Med*. 2005 Jul 28;353(4):349-61.

62. Poldermans D, Bax JJ, Schouten O, et al. Should major vascular surgery be delayed because of preoperative cardiac testing in intermediate-risk patients receiving beta-blocker therapy with tight heart rate control? *J Am Coll Cardiol*. 2006 Sep 5;48(5):964-9.

63. de Virgilio C, Yaghoubian A, Nguyen A, et al. Peripheral vascular surgery using targeted beta blockade reduces perioperative cardiac event rate. *J Am Coll Surg*. 2009; 208: 14-20.

64. Cruickshank JM. Beta-blockers continue to surprise us. *Eur Heart J*. 2000 Mar;21(5):354-64.

65. Fleisher LA, Beckman JA, Brown KA, et al. ACC/AHA 2007 guidelines on perioperative cardiovascular evaluation and care for noncardiac surgery: a report of the American College of Cardiology/American Heart Association Task Force on Practice Guidelines (Writing Committee to Revise the 2002 Guidelines on Perioperative Cardiovascular Evaluation for Noncardiac Surgery) developed in collaboration with the American Society of Echocardiography, American Society of Nuclear Cardiology, Heart Rhythm Society, Society of Cardiovascular Anesthesiologists, Society for Cardiovascular Angiography and Interventions, Society for Vascular Medicine and Biology, and Society for Vascular Surgery. *J Am Coll Cardiol*. 2007 Oct 23;50(17):1707-32.

66. Shammash JB, Trost JC, Gold JM, et al. Perioperative beta-blocker withdrawal and mortality in vascular surgical patients. *Am Heart J*. 2001 Jan;141(1):148-53.

67. Poldermans D, Bax JJ, Kertai MD, et al. Statins are associated with a reduced incidence of perioperative mortality in patients undergoing major noncardiac vascular surgery. *Circulation*. 2003; 107: 1848-1851.

68. Rosenson RS, Tangney CC. Antiatherothrombotic properties of statins: Implications for cardiovascular event reduction. *JAMA*. 1998; 279: 1643-1650.

69. Sacks FM, Pfeffer MA, Moyre LA, et al. The effect of pravastatin on coronary events after myocardial infarction in patients with average cholesterol levels. *N Engl J Med*. 1996;335:1001-1009.

70. Shepherd J, Cobbe SM, Ford I, Isles CG, et al. Prevention of coronary heart disease with pravastatin in men with hypercholesterolemia. *N Eng J Med*.1995; 333:1304-1407.

71. Scandinavian Simvastatin Survival Study Group. Randomized trial of cholesterol lowering in 4444 patients with coronary artery disease (4S). *Lancet*. 1994;344:1383-1389.

72. Downs JR, Clearfield M, Weis S, et al. Primary prevention of acute coronary events with lovastatin in men and women with average cholesterol levels. *JAMA*. 1998;279: 1615-1622.

73. Prevention of cardiovascular events and death with pravastatin in patients with coronary heart disease and a broad range of initial cholesterol levels. The long term Intervention with Pravastatin in Ischemic Disease (LIPID) Study Group. *N Engl J Med*. 1998. 339:1349-1357.

74. Schwartz GG, Oliver M, Exekowitz MD, et al. Rationale and design of the Myocardial Ischemia Reduction with Aggressive Cholesterol Lowering (MIRACL) study that evaluates atorvastatin in unstable angina pectoris and in non-Q-wave acute myocardial infarction. *Am J Cardiol*. 1998;81:578-581.

75. Schwartz GG, Olsson AG, Ezekowtiz MD, et al. Myocardial Ischemia Reduction with Aggressive Cholesterol Lowering (MIRACL) Study Investigators. Effects of atorvastatin on early recurrent ischemic events in coronary syndromes: a randomized controlled trial. *JAMA*. 2001;285:1758-1760.

76. Farmer JA. Pleiotropic effect of statins. *Curr Atheroscler Rep*. 2000;2:208 217.

77. Dawood MM, Gupta DK, Southern J, et al. Pathology of fatal perioperative myocardial infarction: implications regarding pathophysiology and prevention. *Int J Cardio*l. 1996;57:37-44.

78. Kertai MD, Boersma E, Westerhout CM, et al. Association between long term statin use and mortality after successful abdominal aortic aneurysm surgery. *Am J Med*. 2004116:96-103. Anesthesiology. 1995;82:620-633.

79. Lindenauer PK, Pekow P, Wang K, et al. Lipid lowering therapy and in hospital mortality following major noncardiac surgery. *JAMA*. 2004; 291: 2092-2099.

80. O'Neil-Callahan K, Katsimaglis G, Tepper MR, et al. Statins decrease perioperative cardiac complications in patients undergoing noncardiac vascular surgery: the Statins for Risk Reduction in Surgery (StaRRS) study. *J Am Coll Cardiol*. 2005 Feb 1;45(3):336-42.

81. Durazzo AE, Machado FS, Ikeoka DT, et al. Reduction in cardiovascular events after vascular surgery with atorvastatin: a randomized trial. *J Vasc Surg*. 2004 May;39(5):967-75.

82. Hindler K, Shaw AD, Samuels J, et al. Improved postoperative outcomes associated with preoperative statin therapy. *Anesthesiology*. 2006 Dec;105(6):1260-72.

83. Kapoor AS, Kanji H, Buckingham J. Strength of evidence for perioperative use of statins to reduce cardiovascular risk: systematic review of controlled studies. *BMJ*. 2006 Dec 2;333(7579):1149.

84. Daumerie G, Fleisher LA. Perioperative beta-blocker and statin therapy. *Curr Opin Anaesthesiol*. 2008 Feb;21(1):60-5.

85. Halter JB, Pflug AE, Porte D Jr. Mechanism of plasma catecholamine increases during surgical stress in man. *J Clin Endocrinol Metab*. 1977;45:936-944.

86. Roizen MF. Should we all have a sympathectomy at birth? Or at least preoperatively? *Anesthesiology*. 1988;68:482-484.

87. Muzi M, Goff DR, Kampine JP, et al. Clonidine reduced sympathetic activity but maintains baroreflex responses in normotensive humans. *Anesthesiology*. 1992;77:864-871.

88. Ellis JE, Drijvers G, Pedlow S, et al. Premedication with oral an transdermal clonidine provides safe and efficacious postoperative sympatholysis. *Anes Analg*. 1994; 79: 1133-1140.

89. Heusch G, Schipke J, Thamer V. Clonidine prevents the sympathetic initiation and aggravation of poststenotic myocardial ischemia. *J Cardiovasc Pharmacol*. 1985;7:1176-1182.

90. McSCPI-EUROPE Research Group. Perioperative sympatholysis: beneficial effects of the alpha 2 adrenoreceptor agonist mivazerol on hemodynamic stability and myocardial ischemia. *Anesthesiology*. 1997;86:346-363.

91. Talke P, Li J, Jain U, et al. Effects of perioperative dexmedetomidine infusion in patients undergoing vascular surgery. The Study of Perioperaive Ischemia Research Group. *Anesthesiology*. 1995 Mar;82(3):620-33.

92. Eagle Ka, Berger PB, Calkins H, et al. ACC/AHA guideline update on perioperative cardiovascular evaluation for noncardiac surgery. *Circulation*. 2002; 105:1257-1267.

93. Oliver MF, Goldman L, Julian DG, et al. Effect of mivazerol on perioperative cardiac complications during non cardiac surgery in patients with coronary heart disease: the European Mivazerol Trial (EMIT). *Anesthesiology*. 1999;91:951-961.

94. McSPI-Europe Research Group. Perioperative sympatholysis. Beneficial effects of the alpha-2 adrenoreceptor agonist mivazerol on hemodynamic stability and myocardial ischemia. *Anesthesiology*. 1997; 86: 346-363.

95. Stuhmeier KD, Mainzer B, Cierpka J, et al. Small, oral dose of clonidine reduced the incidence of intraoperative myocardial ischemia in patients having vascular surgery. *Anesthesiology*. 1996; 85: 706-712.

96. Bry J, Belkin M, O'Donnell T, et al. An assessment of the positive predictive value and costeffectiveness of dipyridamole myocardial scintigraphy in patients undergoing vascular surgery. *J Vasc Surg*. 1994;19:112-124.

97. Yeager R, Moneta G, Edwards J, et al. Late survival after perioperative myocardial infarction complicating vascular surgery. *J Vasc Surg*. 1994;20:598-606.

98. McCann R, Wolfe W. Resection of abdominal aortic aneurysm in patients with low ejection fractions. *J Vasc Surg*. 1989;10:240-244.

99. Hollier L, Reigel M, Kazmier F, et al. Conventional repair of abdominal aortic aneurysm in the high-risk patient: A plea for abandonment of nonresective treatment. *J Vasc Surg*. 1986;3:712-717.

100. Johnston KW and the Canadian Society for Vascular Surgery Study Group. Nonruptured abdominal aortic aneurysm: Six-year followup results from the multicenter prospective Canadian aneurysm study. *J Vasc Surg*. 1990;12:163-170.

101. Hertzer N, Young J, Beven E, et al. Late results of coronary bypass in patients with infrarenal aortic aneurysms: The Cleveland Clinic Study. *Ann Surg*. 1987;205:360-367.

15. Questions

1. According to the Dripps-ASA Classification, a patient with an ASA physical status 4 would:

A. Have an incapacitating systemic disease that is a constant threat to life and have a 7.8% operative mortality rate

B. Be moribund and have a 9.4% operative mortality rate

C. Have a severe systemic disease that is not incapacitating and have a 1.8% operative mortality rate

D. Have a severe systemic disease that is not incapacitating and have a 7.8% operative mortality rate

E. Have an incapacitating systemic disease that is a constant threat to life and have a 1.8% operative mortality rate

2. Under the Goldman Multifactorial Cardiac Risk Index, the highest operative risk (based on point assignment) would be given to a patient with:

A. A Po_2 <60 mm Hg

B. Age >70 years

C. S_3 gallop or JVD

D. Rhythm other than sinus

E. BUN >50 mg/dL

3. According to the American College of Cardiology/American Heart Association task force, clinical predictors of *major* cardiac risk include all of the following *except:*

A. Canadian Class III angina

B. Atrial fibrillation with uncontrolled ventricular rate

C. Decompensated CHF

D. Uncontrolled systemic hypertension

E. Severe aortic stenosis

4. According to the Eagle risk factors for patients undergoing vascular surgery, all of the following are considered criteria for increased cardiac risk except:

A. History of CHF

B. Q wave on ECG

C. Age >70 years

D. Smoking

E. Angina

5. Which of the following patients would have the *highest* predicted cardiac risk?

A. A 60-year-old diabetic undergoing an emergency cholecystectomy

B. A 75-year-old smoker undergoing carotid endarterectomy

C. A 60-year-old diabetic with controlled atrial fibrillation undergoing a femoral popliteal bypass

D. A 60-year-old with a history of CHF and a Q wave on ECG undergoing an aortobifemoral bypass

E. A 60-year-old hypertensive smoker who gets angina after walking 5 blocks undergoing aortic aneurysm repair

6. A 65-year-old female is being evaluated for repair of a 5.5 cm aortic aneurysm. On history, she reports angina on walking across her bedroom. What would be the *best* recommendation for this patient?

A. Postpone surgery and perform a dipyridamole thallium test

B. Postpone surgery and perform a dobutamine ECHO

C. Postpone surgery and perform a coronary angiogram

D. Postpone surgery and perform an exercise ECG

E. Proceed with surgery after medical optimization

7. A 55-year-old male is being evaluated for an elective total hip replacement. The patient reports a history of syncope. He denies angina or prior cardiac history. On physical examination you detect a loud systolic murmur over the aortic region radiating to the neck. The *best* recommendation for this patient would be:

A. Postpone surgery and perform a dobutamine ECHO

B. Postpone surgery and perform an exercise ECG

C. Postpone surgery and perform a carotid duplex scan

D. Postpone surgery and perform a transthoracic ECHO

E. Proceed with surgery after medical optimization

8. Detsky made important modifications to the Goldman Index. The *highest* cardiac risk (based on number of points) in this modified index is/are:

A. CCS Class 4 angina

B. Recent alveolar pulmonary edema

C. Suspected critical aortic stenosis

D. A. and C.

E. B. and C.

9. A 60-year-old female is being evaluated for symptomatic cholelithiasis. She has a remote history of MI but denies any active cardiac symptoms. The best recommendation for this patient would be:

A. Postpone surgery and perform a dipyridamole-thallium test

B. Postpone surgery and perform a dobutamine ECHO

C. Postpone surgery and perform a coronary angiogram

D. Postpone surgery and perform an exercise ECG

E. Proceed with surgery after medical optimization

10. A 60-year-old male is being evaluated for an elective aortobifemoral bypass for claudication. He reports having suffered an MI 1 month earlier. He denies any current cardiac symptoms. The *best* recommendation for this patient would be:

A. Postpone surgery and perform a dipyridamole-thallium test

B. Postpone surgery and perform a dobutamine ECHO

C. Postpone surgery and perform a coronary angiogram

D. Cancel the operation

E. Proceed with surgery after medical optimization

11. All of the following are proposed mechanisms of action by statins that support their use in the perioperative period *except:*

A. Anti-inflammatory

B. Improvement in endothelial function and coagulation

C. Stabilizing effect on vulnerable plaques

D. Dilate poststenotic coronary vessels

E. They reduce all cause mortality in patient undergoing major vascular surgery

Answers

1. A.

A patient classified as ASA 1 is a normal, healthy patient undergoing an elective operation. An ASA 2 patient has mild systemic disease. An ASA 3 patient has severe systemic disease that limits activity but is not incapacitating (answer C). An ASA 4 patient has **incapacitating systemic disease** (answer A) that is a constant threat to life. Finally, ASA 5 status is reserved for moribund patients (answer B) that are not expected to survive 24 hours with or without an operation. Mortality rates for the different ASA classes are 0.08%, 0.27%, 1.8% (answer C), 7.8% (answer A), and 9.4% (answer B), respectively, for classes 1 to 5. Answer D is not a correct match between ASA classification and mortality and is therefore incorrect.

2. C.

According to the Goldman Multifactorial Cardiac Risk Index, the factor with the highest point assignment is the finding of S3 or JVD (answer C), which is given 11 points. An MI in the previous 6 months is next highest with 10 points. Critics of the Goldman index point to the failure of the index to take into account the different classes of angina or a history of CHF. Rhythm other than sinus (answer D), age > 70 years (answer B), and poor general medical status such as PO2 < 60mmHg (answer A) and BUN >

50mg/dL (answer E) are also factors in the Goldman index, but are given lesser weight.

3. D.
The American College of Cardiology/American Heart Association has divided patients into 3 levels of cardiac risk based on clinical predictors. Predictors of major cardiac risk include unstable coronary syndromes such as recent MI with evidence of significant ischemia and unstable or severe angina (Canadian Class III or IV) (answer A), decompensated CHF (answer C), significant arrhythmias such as high-grade atrioventricular block, symptomatic ventricular arrhythmias with underlying heart disease, supraventricular arrhythmias with uncontrolled ventricular rate (answer B), and severe valvular disease (answer E). Uncontrolled systemic hypertension is not a predictor of cardiac risk according to this classification scheme (answer D).

4. D.
Lee and associates devised a Revised Cardiac Risk Index designed specifically for all patients undergoing major surgery. Its risk factors include 1) high-risk type of surgery, 2) history of ischemic heart disease (answer B), 3) history of congestive heart failure (answer A), 4) history of cerebrovascular disease (answer D), 5) diabetes mellitus requiring insulin, and 6) preoperative serum creatinine >2.0 mg/dL (answer E). The Revised Cardiac Risk Index does not account for age (answer C).

5. D.
In general, patients undergoing major aortic surgery have the highest cardiac risk. According to the Revised Cardiac Risk Index, patient A has a score of 0, patient B has a score of 0 (carotid endarterectomy is not considered a high risk procedure; see Table 1), patient C has a score of 1 (insulin-dependent diabetic), patient D has a score of 3 (1 point each for history of CHF, Q wave on ECG, and high risk procedure), and patient E has a score of 1 (high risk procedure). Although patient E has angina, it is mild angina. Smoking, hypertension, and atrial fibrillation are not part of the Revised Cardiac Risk Index. According to the American College of Cardiology/American Heart Association, controlled atrial fibrillation is a minor clinical predictor.

6. C.
The patient described above has severe angina (CCS Class 4) that occurs during any type of activity. Such a patient is at extremely high risk for an adverse cardiac event, and surgery should be postponed. In addition, a 5.5 cm AAA is not imminently life threatening as the annual rupture risk is only about 5%. Patients with severe overt cardiac symptoms should not undergo stress testing because this may precipitate worsening ischemia. As such, one should proceed directly to coronary angiography.

7. D.
According to both the Detsky index and the American College of Cardiology/American Heart Association, severe valvular disease (in particular severe aortic stenosis) places a patient at extremely high risk for an adverse cardiac event. Patients with severe aortic stenosis may manifest symptoms of angina, congestive heart failure, syncope, and are at risk for sudden death. Such a patient should not undergo stress testing, but rather should have a standard ECHO to assess valvular function.

8. D.
Critics of the Goldman index noted the failure to include angina and to characterize how recently the patient had CHF. Detsky added angina and more specifically categorized the type of angina. Additionally, the index identified whether the patient had ever had an episode of CHF. The highest point assignment (20 points) was given to CCS Class 4 angina and to suspected critical aortic stenosis (answer D).

9. E.
This patient has a history of MI, but no other cardiac risk factors, so her Revised Cardiac Index score is 1. Since cholecystectomy is not a high-risk procedure, and since the patient does not have any active severe cardiac symptoms, a detailed cardiac workup is not warranted. There would be no indication to place this patient on a beta blocker.

10. D.

Patients with a recent MI are at particularly high risk for an adverse cardiac event postoperatively. When assessing cardiac risk one must also consider the type of operation and its urgency. An aortobifemoral bypass is one of the higher operative risk procedures. Furthermore, the indication for the operation in this patient is claudication, which is not limb threatening. Claudication can be managed medically with smoking cessation and ambulation. Thus the most prudent thing to do would be to cancel the operation. Since he is not having postinfarction ischemia, there is no immediate indication for cardiac evaluation.

11. D.

HMG-CoA reductase inhibitors or statins inhibit development of atherosclerotic plaques through reduction of serum cholesterol as a long-term benefit. They are also anti-inflammatory (answer A), can improve endothelial function and coagulation (answer B), and produce a stabilizing effect on vulnerable plaques (answer C) even with short-term usage. Perioperative use of statins has been shown to reduce all cause mortality in patients undergoing major vascular surgery (answer E). Statins have not been shown to dilate poststenotic coronary vessels (answer D).

Chapter 3: Pathophysiology of Multiple-Organ Dysfunction Syndrome

Donald E. Fry, MD

Contents

1. History and Background

The failure of individual organ systems in critically injured and critically ill patients has been recognized as a complication in military casualties over the last century. The soldiers with severe injuries were initially identified as dying from cardiovascular failure, when in reality they died of shock due to hypovolemia. The development of intravenous fluid administration and the transfusion of red cells and plasma led to effective management of patients with shock. In the wake of effective management of shock by restoring injured patients to an acceptable blood pressure, renal failure emerged during World War II as the major organ failure complex in battlefield casualties that had survived their acute injuries. With better definition of volume resuscitation, renal failure became less of a problem, but in the Vietnam War, pulmonary failure became the new problematic clinical entity. The development of better support technology for managing pulmonary failure was the result of this experience.

In the 1960s and 1970s, as intensive care units and critical care medicine evolved, a single organ failure (eg, pulmonary or renal failure) in the critically ill surgical patient was not the most frequent cause of patient death; most often it was failure of multiple organ systems. For the last 30 years, the pursuit of a better understanding and development of a unifying concept to explain the failure of anatomically distinct organ systems has been a major focus in improving the outcome in injured and critically ill patients.

The origin of the concept of multiple organ failure (MOF) can be traced to any one of several different articles. Skillman and colleagues[1] identified a clinical association between sepsis, stress mucosal gastric ulceration, and pulmonary failure in the critically ill surgical patient in 1969, but did not use the term "multiple organ failure" in their report. In 1973, Tilney and coworkers[2] were the first to describe the failure of multiple organ systems in a group of patients who survived the initial surgical intervention for ruptured aneurysm. They identified a wide constellation of different organ systems that appeared to fail in sequence or in synchrony in this group of patients. They may have been the first to use the terminology of multiple, or sequential, organ failure. Eiseman and associates[3] identified multiple organ failure complexes in patients with uncontrolled intraabdominal infection. In 1975, Baue[4] put forth in an editorial the numerous clinical variables that were associated with the syndrome of multiple or sequential organ failure. He described many of the potential organ systems at risk and suggested mechanisms that might be responsible for triggering the failure of these diverse organ systems.

In the early 1980s,[5,6,7,8] our group produced a series of clinical reports which emphasized the strong relationship between the emergence of organ failure (pulmonary, hepatic, gastrointestinal [stress mucosal bleeding], and kidney failure) and severe infection in the surgical patient. In these studies, we used criteria of sepsis that commonly prevailed at the time. Those criteria were: 1.) fever and leukocytosis for 5 consecutive days; 2.) deep-seated suppurative infection (eg, abscess or empyema); 3.) positive blood cultures; 4.) positive cultures from a site presumed to be responsible for severe infection; and 5.) shock interpreted to be due to infection. Patients were identified as having sites of infection that were responsible for the development of these systemic signs of sepsis, and it was clearly evident in the data that the evolution of the sepsis syndrome was associated with the progressive cascade of organ failure. These studies defined a clinical sequence with which organ failure occurred and concluded that mortality rates increased as the number of failed organs increased.

However, Goris and colleagues[9] subsequently studied a large number of patients who seemingly had this same evidence of a systemic "septic" response, but the researchers were unable to determine from clinical criteria or postmortem examination that the majority of these patients actually had infection. A careful temporal analysis of the sequence of infectious complications in these patients raised the issue of whether infection, when present, was a consequence of organ failure or the cause of organ failure. They concluded that the nonspecific systemic activation of inflammation by any of a number of clinical variables set into motion a syndrome that had all of the hallmarks of what was commonly referred to as "sepsis," but was not consistently identified with uncontrolled infection. Experimental studies using nonspecific activators of the inflammatory cascade identified the experimental indicators of "septic" hemodynamic profiles, but no infection was present in the experimental animals.[10,11] Thus the concept evolved that the systemic activation of the inflammatory cascade was the important variable responsible for organ failure, not infection itself.

From the results of numerous clinical studies in the 1980's it became apparent that the terms "sepsis," "sepsis syndrome," "septicemia," and similar terms were being used without the existence of a consistent definition among the different investigators using them. Accordingly, in 1992 a consensus conference was convened and a standardized nomenclature was adopted.[12] The concept of the Systemic Inflammatory Response Syndrome (SIRS) was developed (Table 1). SIRS was defined as the nonspecific systemic activation of the human inflammatory response. ***Sepsis*** was defined as the activation of SIRS by invasive or severe infection. ***Septic shock*** was defined as hemodynamic instability that is the consequence of SIRS activated by infection. Furthermore, the phrase "multiple organ failure" was replaced with the concept of "multiple-organ dysfunction syndrome," or MODS, to reflect that this clinical syndrome has graduated levels of severity. While the concept of SIRS is still undergoing evolution, the presently-accepted hypothesis posits that those biological processes activated by the normal salutary events of the human inflammatory response become destructive when the domain of activation is systemic. Thus, the following discussion will focus on the normal human inflammatory response as it occurs in a wound or localized infectious process, and how activation of that beneficial local process can affect the patient on a systemic level and lead to SIRS and the development of the multiple-organ dysfunction syndrome (MODS) (Figure 1).

Table 1

Current Definition of the Systemic Inflammatory Response Syndrome (SIRS) and Related Terminology

Systemic Inflammatory Response Syndrome
The systemic inflammatory response to a variety of severe clinical insults. The syndrome is manifested by 2 or more of the following clinical conditions:

1. Core body temperature >38°C or <36°C
2. Heart rate >90 beats/minute
3. Respiratory rate >20 breaths/minute; or $Paco_2$ <32 mm Hg
4. White blood cell count >12,000 cells/mm^3, or <4000 cells/mm^3, or >10% immature (band) forms

Sepsis
The systemic inflammatory response syndrome secondary to infection.

Severe Sepsis
Sepsis associated with organ dysfunction, hypoperfusion, or hypotension. Hypoperfusion and perfusion abnormalities may include, but are not limited to lactic acidosis, oliguria and an acute alteration in mental status.

Septic Shock
Sepsis with hypotension despite adequate fluid resuscitation, along with the presence of perfusion abnormalities that may include but are not limited to lactic acidosis, oliguria, and an acute alteration in mental status. Patients who are taking inotropic or vasopressor agents may not be hypotensive when perfusion abnormalities are documented.

Hypotension
Systolic blood pressure <90 mm Hg or a reduction of >40 mm Hg from baseline in the absence of other causes of hypotension.

Multiple-Organ Dysfunction Syndrome
Presence of altered organ function in an acutely ill patient such that homeostasis cannot be maintained without intervention.

2. Biology of Inflammation

The biological processes involved in a soft tissue wound provide an organizational framework for the understanding of SIRS and the mechanisms of inflammation that are responsible for the development of MODS. The wound itself may stem from a mechanical injury due to penetrating or blunt trauma, or may be the result of a surgical incision. The wound may be thermal, caustic, cold injury or even ischemia reperfusion. The wounding process is associated with disruption of host cells and the introduction of microbes into the environment of injury. Ischemia of tissue and microbial proliferation make continued tissue injury a dynamic and ongoing process.

The host must recognized intrinsic or extrinsic signals to marshall the innate and adaptive host responses for the eradication of potential or established infection, removal of dead or effete host cells, and promotion of wound healing. All of these intrinsic and extrinsic signals can be collectively grouped as Damage-associated Molecular Patterns (DAMPs). These chemical signals are released into the injured tissue, bind to specific cell receptors or ubiquitous proteins, and in turn activate the subsequent initiator events described below. DAMPs can be subdivided into those signals which arise from bacterial cells and those that arise from acutely injured, disrupted or necrotic cells. Pathogen-associated Molecular Patterns (PAMPs) are structural or secreted products of bacterial cells.[13] Endotoxins and exotoxins are PAMPs. Distressed or damaged cells release endogenous signals that similarly promote the initiator events. Signals released from damaged or injured cells, or secreted by cells secondary to ischemia or other biological stresses, can by collectively referred to as alarmins. Alarmins are an area of very active research and it is certain that the list of potential cell products arising intrinsically from endogenous cellular sources will increase. At present, these alarmin signals include high mobility group box 1 (HMGB1) protein,[14] the S100 proteins,[15] heat shock proteins,[16] interleukin 1α,[17] and others.[18]

All of the different wounding processes DAMPs may activate the human inflammatory response through different receptor sites on the cell surface, but all seem to share a common intracellular mechanism that results in activation of innate and adaptive immune responses. PAMPs from multiple microbial sources

Figure 1

Diagram illustrating the severe clinical events that activate the human systemic inflammatory response, which leads to the Multiple-Organ Dysfunction Syndrome (MODS)

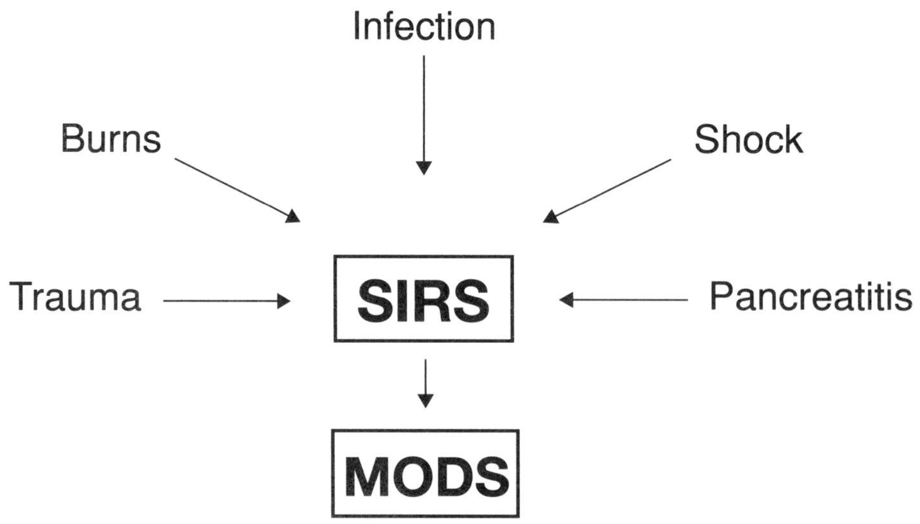

bind to the toll-like receptors.[19] IL-1 activates the cell via IL-1 receptors. Alarmins bind to receptors for advanced glycation end products, or RAGEs,[20] and likely other receptor groups yet to be identified. Binding to all surface receptors appear to share the common intracellular signaling pathway through NF-κB with a resultant commonality of proinflammatory effector responses.

The duplication and redundancy of these activators of inflammation and immunity are similarly shared by the initiators that represent effector signals of host response.[21,22] The net effect of DAMPs is to stimulate five separate but interactive initiator events. These initiator events are responsible for the subsequent physiologic changes that occur during the inflammatory process.

The first initiator of significance is the coagulation cascade.[23,24] Most surgeons are not accustomed to thinking of coagulation as being an initiating event in inflammation but rather consider it fundamental to hemostasis. The injury disrupts vascular structures and initiates the complex coagulation cascade. The activation of coagulation proteins produces several important and biologically-active protein products. Among these, activated factor XII is most significant, because it interacts with other initiator events to promote major microcirculatory and other changes that herald human inflammation.

The second initiator is the platelet.[27,28] Activation of coagulation also activates the platelets, a phenomenon which again is normally viewed as having hemostatic purposes. However, when the enzymes within the granules of the cytoplasm of the platelet are injected into experimental animals, they stimulate an extraordinarily robust inflammatory response. Degranulation of platelets *in vivo* undoubtedly serves an important role in the initiation of human inflammation.

The third major initiator of human inflammation is the mast cell.[19,20] The mast cell, when stimulated by activated factor XII or by products from platelet degranulation, releases histamine, neutral proteases, and other presynthesized components of the mast cell granule. Some recent researchers have even identified presynthesized tumor necrosis factor (TNF) within the granules of the mast cell.[29] In addition, stimulated mast cells will produce de novo, after stimulation, other vasoactive and proinflammatory cytokine signals.[30-32]

The fourth initiator event is the contact activating system.[33,34] Prekallikrein is a gamma globulin which is converted to kallikrein by the action of activated factor XII. Kallikrein then catalyzes the conversion of high molecular weight kininogen into bradykinin. Kallikrein also catalyzes the fibrinolytic process by the transformation of plasminogen into plasmin. Bradykinin becomes an important agonist signal, by binding to receptors on endothelial cells and stimulating the synthesis of nitric oxide synthase.[35] Nitric oxide is then produced, resulting in relaxation of vascular smooth muscle.

The fifth initiator pathway of inflammation is the complement cascade.[36,37] Complement is a complex series of serum proteins which can be activated by both the classical and alternative pathways. Tissue injury, endotoxin and activated factor XII, among other stimuli, activate complement through the alternative pathway. Antigen-antibody complex activates complement through the classical pathway. The cleavage products of complement serve important vasoactive opsonic and chemoattractant functions in the acute inflammatory process.

While the complex relationship among all five of these initiator events has yet to be defined, it is apparent that there is enormous redundancy and duplication in biological function among the products that spring from these specific initiators. It appears that activation of one initiator event results in the activation of all five. The redundancy of the mechanisms of the inflammatory cascade is clearly seen throughout its many steps of initiation. This redundancy makes apparent the therapeutic difficulties likely to be encountered when one attempts to use the strategy of blocking only one specific step.

Following activation of the initiators, phase I of inflammatory effects is seen. These changes consist of microcirculatory vasodilatation, increased microcirculatory permeability and tissue edema. The benefit to the host of these vasoactive changes consists of increased bulk flow from the circulation to the area of injury. Increased flow provides opsonic and other proteins to the injured area that are beneficial to the host as inflammation evolves, as well as facilitating the

Table 2

The New Chemokines[a]

Chemokine Group	Specific Leukocyte Group
Subgroup C-C (no amino acids between the cysteine residues) • Monocyte Inflammatory Proteins (MIP-1alpha; MIP-1beta) • Monocyte Chemoattractant Protein (MCP-1; MCP-2; MCP-3; MCP-4; MCP-5) • Regulated or Activated, Normal T Expressed and Secreted (RANTES) • I-309 • Eotaxin	Monocytes
Subgroup C-X-C (one amino acid between the cysteine residues) • Interleukin-8 (IL-8) • Growth-Related Oncogene (GRO-alpha; GRO-beta; GRO-gamma) • Granulocyte Chemotactic Protein-2 (GCP-2) • Epithelial Neutrophil Activating Protein-78 (ENA-78) • Platelet Basic Proteins (PBP) • Cleavage products of PBPs which include: Connective Tissue Activating Proteins-III (CTAP-III); Beta-Thromboglobulin (Beta-TG); and Neutrophil Activating Protein-2 (NAP-2) • Platelet Factor-4 (PF-4) • Interferon-gamma-inducible protein (IP-10) • Monokine induced by INF-gamma (MIG)	Neutrophils
Chemokine Subgroup C • Lymphotactin	unknown
Chemokine Subgroup C-XXX-C (three amino acids between the cysteine residues) • Fractalkine	unknown

[a] *The new chemokines are a chemically analogous group of chemoattractant cytokines that have specificity for selected leukocyte groups. The number of chemokines exceed 40 in number and the list above is not complete.*

delivery of large numbers of phagocytic cells to the area of injury. Dilatation results in reduced flow velocity through the microcirculation in the area of the injury. Reduced flow velocity is the initial biological process permitting margination of phagocytic cells to the surface of the vascular endothelium. Increased vascular permeability provides exit routes, allowing phagocytic cells to leave the microcirculation, and also results in edema formation in the soft tissues. Edema likewise facilitates opsonic protein delivery to the injured area. Perhaps the most important physiologic role for edema is providing aqueous conduits that facilitate phagocytic cell entry into the injured area.

A second important consequence of phase I of inflammation is the production of a vast array of chemoattractant compounds.[38-41] Cleavage products from the complement cascade and bradykinin also serve as chemoattractants. Significantly, mast cells and perhaps other populations of cells within the inflammatory milieu produce a wide variety of chemoattractant cytokines that are collectively referred to as chemokines. There are many chemokines and the list is constantly growing, with an incomplete listing of the early identified proteins in Table 2. They share an interesting chemical homology. The suble differences in the number of amino acids that are substituted between the cross-linking cysteine residues may create specificity of each chemokine for a specific phagocytic cell. One class of chemokines may be specific for attracting neutrophils, while another class may be specific for attracting monocytes, and still other classes of chemokines may be specific for basophils or eosinophils. Thus the appearance of specific phagocytic cells at different phases in the evolution of the inflammatory process is likely orchestrated by this complex array of chemokines that are produced within the wound itself. The density of chemokines produced within the wound dictates the speed at which the phagocytic phase of inflammation is initiated. As the number of chemokines increases, additional functions for these proteins are similarly being identified.[42]

At the start of phase II, the phagocytic cells have been identified within the inflammatory environment. The diffusion of chemokines from the area of injury results in transformation in the endothelial cell expression of adhesion proteins. This transformation results in the "rolling" of neutrophils on the surface of the vascular endothelium because this process dramatically slows the neutrophils on the surface of the endothelium in preparation for complete margination of these cells. This rolling is mediated through the selectin adhesion proteins present on both the surface of the neutrophil and on the surface of the endothelial cell.[43,44] Following the rolling process with selectins, the margination process is completed by the transformation of the constitutively expressed CD 11/18 complex, which forms a tight bond to the ICAM receptor on the endothelial surface.[45,46] Completion of the margination process of the neutrophil on the surface of the endothelium is then followed by the directional diapedesis process between endothelial cells and into the interstitium of the soft tissue. The chemoattractant and chemokine gradient direct the phagocytic cell to move toward the focus of injury and contamination in an orderly fashion. By similar mechanisms, monocytes are attracted to the same epicenter. The monocyte is a somewhat larger cell with a much larger nucleus, and it is thought that the delay in monocyte arrival at the acute inflammatory site relates in part to the greater mechanical difficulty involved in transport of the cell from the intravascular compartment to the site of injury. As was discussed above, differences in migration rates may be related to different specific chemokine signals.

Once the monocyte arrives in the inflammatory milieu, the intensity of the chemokine signal dictates the cytokine response of the monocyte cell. The monocyte activation from intense chemokine stimulation from the environment results in the production of tumor necrosis factor (TNF), interleukin 1, and other proinflammatory signals. The principal function of TNF in this phase of inflammation is to upregulate the phagocytic activity of neutrophils already present in the local environment.[47,48] The release of interleukin 1 presumably mediates the febrile response, the upregulation of acute phase reactants from the liver, and systemic neutrophilia, by direct stimulation of the bone marrow and mobilization of marginated neutrophils stored in reservoirs elsewhere in the host.[49]

When density of bacteria is very high within the injured area, or when a significant amount of necrotic tissue is present, the intense proinflammatory cytokine response results in frenzied phagocytic behavior by neutrophils. This results in the extracel

Figure 2A

Graph depicting the changes in cardiac output that occur in the patient with the 4 different stages of SIRS

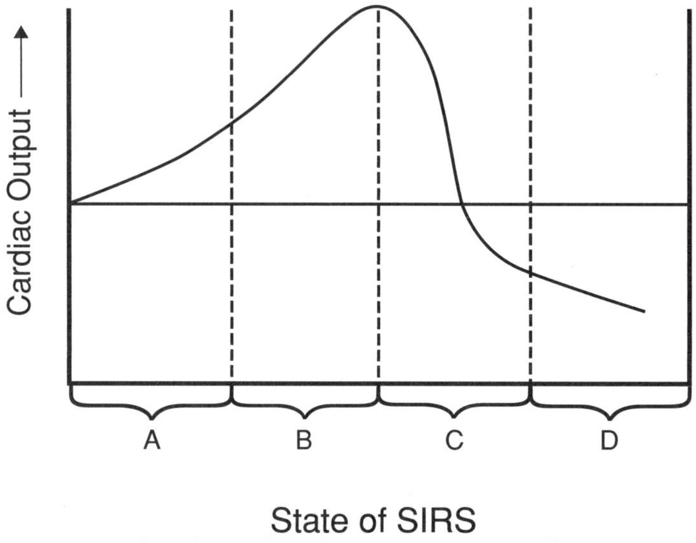

Figure 2B

Graph depicting the changes in systemic vascular resistance that occur in the patient with the 4 different stages of SIRS

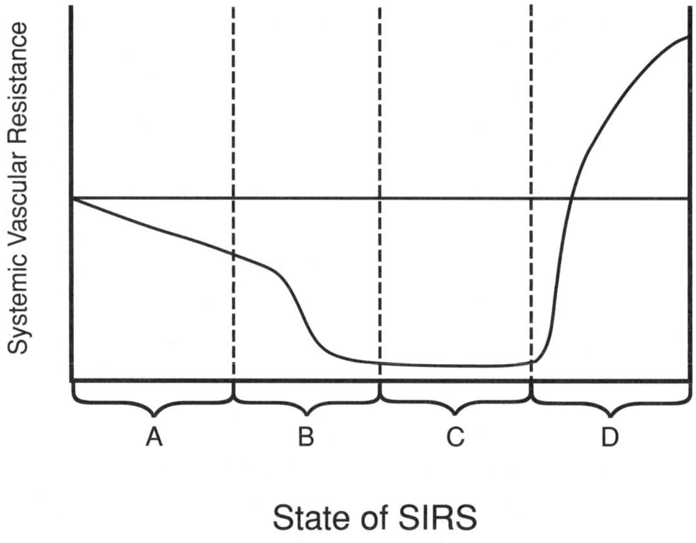

lular production by neutrophils of acid hydrolases and reactive oxygen intermediates.[50,51] This vigorous phagocytic activity and extracellular production of phagocytic enzymatic components result in lipid peroxidation, degradation of dead tissue, and ultimately the formation of pus at the area of injury or infection. Of course, the magnitude of contamination and the quantity of dead tissue at the site are directly responsible for the level of chemoattractant and chemokine production within the wound, and these are major fac tors in determining the intensity of the overall response of the phagocytic cell invasion of the site of injury.

The Stages of SIRS

The basic principle behind SIRS is that the normal inflammatory processes, when activated at a systemic level, result in destructive systemic consequences of inflammation.[52] Can these systemic consequences of inflammation be broken down into a clinical staging system? While not initially intended to define the stages of SIRS, a classic study by Siegel and colleagues[53] described a 4-stage classification system for sepsis. In examining the physiologic and metabolic patterns of patients with severe clinical infection, it is apparent that these authors did in fact identify the stages of SIRS, and also described how the specific normal physiologic events of inflammation become pathophysiologic events at the systemic level. It is important to note the characteristic changes in cardiac output and systemic vascular resistance and their relationship to each other during each of the physiologic stages of SIRS (Figures 2A, 2B).

Stage A was defined by these authors as the normal physiologic response to injury, operation or illness. Stage A is characterized by the patient experiencing a modest elevation in cardiac output and a modest reduction in systemic vascular resistance. Arterial venous oxygen differences remain constant, indicating that increased systemic perfusion due to the increase in cardiac output is associated with a systemic increase in oxygen consumption. This hypermetabolic response would appear to be an appropriate and proper response to injury and severe illness. Patients do not demonstrate an accumulation of lactate, indicating that systemic oxygenation and oxygen utilization are appropriate. Stage A occurs in virtually every surgical or trauma patient, and in the absence of complicating secondary events (eg, reoperation or infection) it spontaneously resolves during convalescence.

Stage B represents the exaggerated stress response and is actually the prototype state of patients with clinical SIRS. In Stage B, the patients have a steep reduction in systemic vascular resistance (to less than 800 dyne/sec/cm^{-5}). This loss of systemic vascular resistance, when managed with an appropriate amount of volume, support results in hyperdynamic cardiac output. Cardiac output may be dramatically increased, exceeding twice the normal values. Failure to provide adequate preload under these circumstances can cause arterial hypotension, which is actually a hypovolemic event, as opposed to a true septic shock event.

An interesting feature often seen with Stage B is the narrowing of the gap in the arterial-venous oxygen content. This emphasizes the apparent peripheral defect in oxygen utilization of the septic patient. The patient is truly hypermetabolic, but the increase in cardiac output is not associated with a linear increase in oxygen consumption. This peripheral defect is variously ascribed to either a direct transformation in the intermediate metabolism of the visceral and other cell populations of the body,[43] or related to microcirculatory changes.[54]

Stage B has particular significance because of the accumulation of lactate species seen in the patient. Lactate concentrations are increased, but compensatory mechanisms act to maintain normal systemic pH values. Increased lactate concentrations are associated with an equimolar increase in pyruvate concentrations. When an excess of lactate species are measured in the patient, one witnesses the emergence of the organ failure complexes. Adult respiratory distress syndrome emerges, and the patient begins to show evidence of chemical hyperbilirubinemia. If Stage B continues, an organ failure dysfunction syndrome results, with the patient ultimately experiencing renal failure. An important point to emphasize is that the emergence of multiple-organ dysfunction syndrome occurs at a point when overall systemic oxygen delivery appears to be adequate and the patient has normal arterial blood gases and arterial blood pressure. This dramatic vasodilatation and loss of vascular tone, as well as the diffuse edema resulting from changes in microcirculatory permeability, appear to represent systemic consequences of phase I of the inflammation, which were discussed earlier.

In Stage C, patients experience decompensation of systemic hemodynamics from the exaggerated stress response described in Stage B. The profound loss of systemic vascular resistance cannot be overcome by cardiac output. Cardiac output may appear to be normal or increased in comparison to the patient's unstressed level, but under circumstances of profound loss of systemic vascular resistance, the patient actually has arterial hypotension. This state of hypotension, accompanied by normal or even slightly increased cardiac output, commonly gives the patient in Stage C the appearance of "hot shock." This shock state with profound vasodilatation again underscores the extreme effects of the phase I vasodilatory influences on systemic activation of inflammation.

Stage D can be viewed as the preterminal phase of SIRS unless prompt and dramatic therapeutic interventions are undertaken. Stage D represents the frank imposition of cardiac failure on the fundamental disease process of SIRS. Cardiac output is extremely low and patients actually have a vasoconstrictive response, mediated by the autonomic nervous system which overrides the peripheral vasodilatation of Stages A, B, and C that was likely mediated by local metabolic events. Patients in Stage D have severe problems with both oxygen delivery and utilization. Cardiac output is inadequate, in addition to the systemic metabolic defects brought on by SIRS itself. Lactate concentrations are greatly elevated, out of proportion to pyruvate concentrations. This is commonly the preterminal event in the natural history of systemic inflammation.

Inflammation-Mediated MODS

SIRS is considered to be the clinical event that heralds the multiple organ failure cascade, more commonly referred to now as multiple-organ dysfunction syndrome (MODS). The basic tenet of this hypothesis is that the inflammatory mechanisms identified in the simple wound which normally serve a salutary autocrine and paracrine role become destructive to the host when they are activated at a systemic level and spread to the endocrine domain. Disseminated and unregulated systemic inflammation becomes the basis for microcirculatory and parenchymal injury of the target organs identified as failing in MODS. For the purpose of identifying the mechanisms and potential treatment strategies, this inflammatory self-destruction can be broken down into a 10-step process (Figure 3).

Step I: The Activators of Human Inflammation
Activation of systemic inflammation occurs via mechanisms similar to those seen in activation of local inflammation. Infection has been the most thoroughly explored mechanism for the activation of systemic inflammation. Invasive infection becomes an activator of systemic inflammation by several means. Obviously, microbial blood-borne infection in the form of bacteremia or fungemia results in activation of inflammatory events. Clinicians who have regularly performed blood cultures in severely septic patients have readily identified, however, that bacteremia is an inconsistently documented event even in patients with the most severe of clinical infections and clinical SIRS. This has led to considerable interest in the study of activation of systemic inflammation by endotoxins, as well as by other synthesized or structural products from pathogens. As with bacteremia, the documentation of endotoxemia in obviously infected patients has also been difficult to consistently document. It is likely that an intensely invasive infection such as severe acute bacterial peritonitis or burn wound sepsis could potentiate the excessive production of tissue-based, proinflammatory mediator signals, which are then distributed on a systemic level. It is the dissemination of the mediator signal rather than the microbe itself or microbial cell products that may actually be the seminal event precipitating systemic inflammation.

In recent years there has been considerable interest in the concept of microbial gastrointestinal translocation as a means of activation of the human inflammatory response.[55,56,57,58] Translocation suggests that the gut barrier has been compromised and that either microbes or microbial cell products escape from the lumen of the gut, thereby activating systemic inflammation. While it is commonly considered just another form of infection, microbial gastrointestinal

Figure 3

Flowchart illustrating the relationship of the 10 steps in the activation of SIRS which lead to MODS

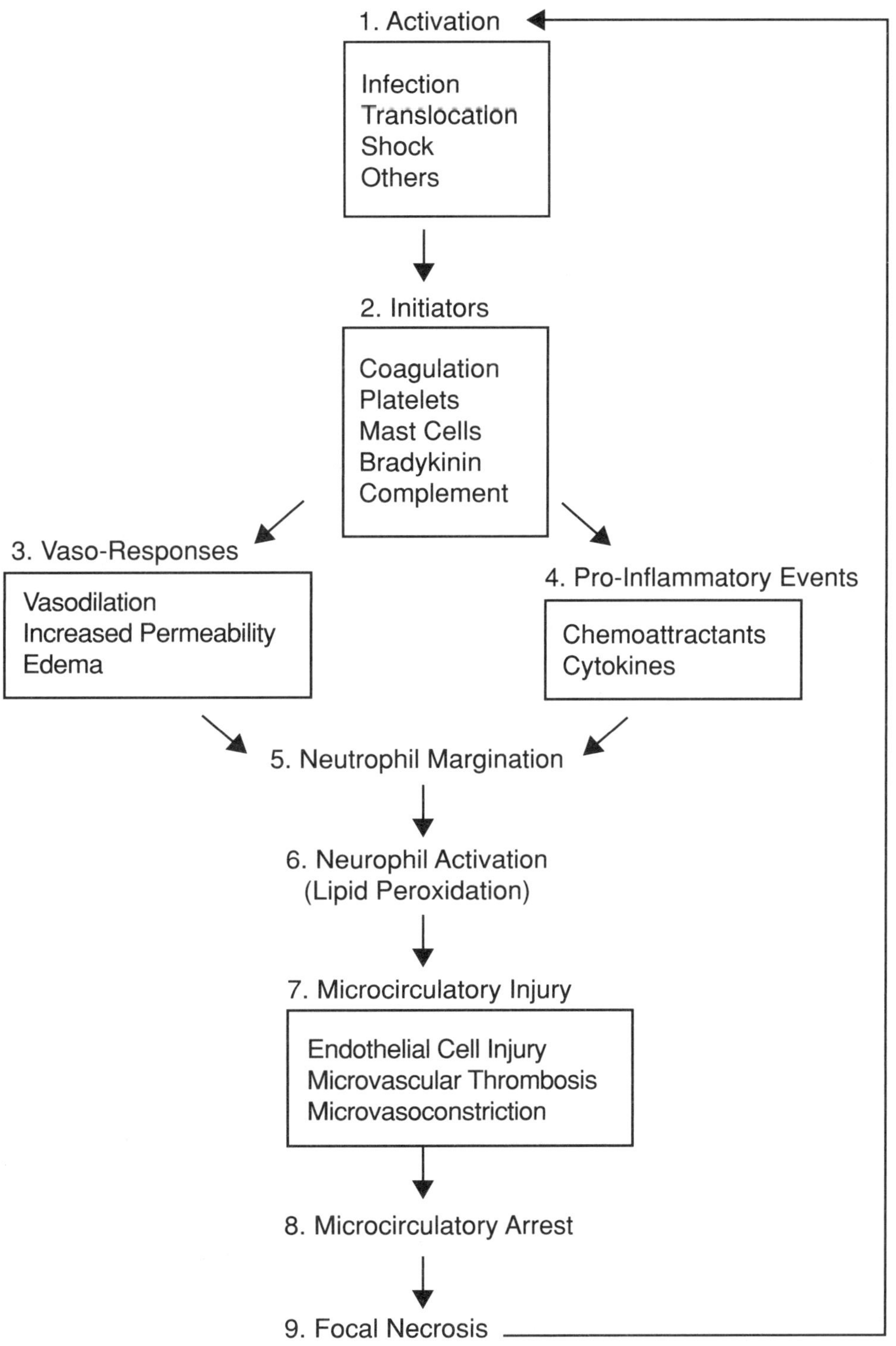

translocation represents failure of the host defenses, as well as a means of activation of systemic inflammation unlikely to respond to antimicrobial therapy. Thus, translocation must be viewed as a separate and distinct mechanism for the activation of inflammation. Similar to the model of peritonitis or severe burn wound sepsis discussed above, some evidence indicates that translocation of microbes and their byproducts from the gastrointestinal tract into the regional mesenteric lymph nodes may actually instigate a local inflammatory response within the lymph nodes. Inflammation within the lymph node results in the dissemination of proinflammatory signals. Thus microbial gastrointestinal translocation could potentially be an activator of widespread inflammation even though the microbe or endotoxin does not gain systemic access to the host.

Considerable attention has focused on noninfectious and nonmicrobial stimuli that may activate systemic inflammation. Multiple soft tissue trauma in selected patients may systemically activate inflammation in the same way that striking one's thumb with a hammer provokes a local inflammatory response. Systemic shock due to hemorrhage or other causes and sustained systemic hypoxemia may similarly act as signals that activate inflammation. Ischemia/reperfusion injury then becomes another potential mechanism of activation. Other sterile foci of inflammation (eg, acute fulminant pancreatitis[59]) may create a sufficiently intense local inflammatory response to cause dissemination of proinflammatory mediator signals that may then trigger a systemic inflammatory response. It is likely that the presence of necrotic tissue stimulates inflammation, and this may serve as a synergistic factor in fulminant pancreatitis, severe soft tissue trauma, and certain invasive infections, which then further potentiate the activation of inflammation. For many patients, it is the combination of several activator signals working in concert that precipitates the systemic inflammatory cascade. Yet other clinical events, such as cardiopulmonary bypass[60] or the generalized production of antigen-antibody complex, may occur with certain drug reactions and could similarly act to trigger one or more of the initiators of inflammation, resulting in systemic inflammation.

In recent years, attention has focused on the concept of the "two-hit" hypothesis of organ failure.[61,62] The two-hit hypothesis proposes that tandem proinflammatory activation events can work together to induce systemic inflammation. Central to this hypothesis is the idea that an initial activation event such as shock from hemorrhage or multiple soft tissue trauma results in a "priming" of the human inflammatory cascade. After this priming event, a second "hit" then results in an exuberant, excessive, and unregulated systemic inflammatory response. Severe infection, reoperation, or other post-injury or postoperative complications could act as the second hit. The idea of these dual biological events provoking systemic inflammation may in part explain the ongoing confusion about whether infection is the cause or a consequence of MODS. In complex clinical scenarios, what acts as the priming event and what acts as the second hit can be very difficult to determine. Obviously, severe primary events may precipitate the entire inflammatory process without the assistance of the second event. Furthermore, as will be discussed below, severe injury or infection and SIRS itself clearly are immunosuppressive to the host and may lead to infectious events secondary to the primary activating events. These infectious events secondary to immunosuppression may be the sustaining activating stimuli that provoke the sustained inflammatory response.

Step II: Activation of the Initiators of Inflammation

As was described in the discussion of the biology of the human wound, activation of systemic inflammation likely occurs through the common initiator pathways seen in tissue injury. The coagulation cascade is activated systemically and can clearly be associated with disseminated intravascular coagulation in the SIRS patient. Platelet activation is demonstrated by thrombocytopenia in patients with SIRS. Systemic activation of mast cells likely results in the systemic spread of histamine, neutral proteases and other mast cell signals. An important consequence of a generalized mast-cell response is the generalized elaboration of chemokine signals. Disseminated intravascular coagulation unquestionably activates the contact activating system and produces bradykinin in the host. Finally, considerable scrutiny has been given to systemic activation of the coagulation cascade in both clinical[63] and experimental infections.[64] The systemic liberation of complement cleavage products would clearly provoke systemic inflammatory events.

Step III: Systemic Consequences of Phase I of Inflammation

The systemic hemodynamic observations seen in SIRS patients are likely to be the consequence of vasoactive products of the initiator events seen in Step II. Systemic vasodilatation is likely to be an effect of histamine and bradykinin. Bradykinin and histamine both appear to have nitric oxide synthase-dependent pathways for initiating vasodilatation and the subsequent loss of systemic vascular resistance. This systemic vasodilatation results in an increase in vascular capacitance, hence the requirement for increased volume support in the SIRS patient. The systemic liberation of initiator products similarly results in an increase in microcirculatory permeability and the resultant systemic edema of the SIRS patient. Given adequate preload administration to the SIRS patient experiencing this systemic vasoactive assault, the result is increased cardiac output. The cardiac output is clearly driven by the afterload reduction that is the consequence of the loss of systemic vascular resistance.

Step IV: Systemic Distribution of Chemoattractant/Proinflammatory Signals

The generalized activation of the initiator events results in a systemic liberation of chemoattractants and chemokine signals. This generalized chemoattractant stimulation results in changes in endothelial adhesion receptors and initiates the process of neutrophil rolling, but without the gradient and direction that orchestrates the process in a localized soft tissue injury. Similarly, the systemic distribution of the potent chemoattractant signals results in a systemic monocyte activation that results in the production of proinflammatory cytokines in a generalized fashion within the SIRS patient.

Step V: Generalized Margination of Neutrophils

The generalized changes within the endothelial cell and the resultant rolling of neutrophils on the endothelial surface results in neutrophil margination in the same fashion that would occur at a local site of injury. The CD-11/18 complex of the neutrophil results in interaction with the ICAM on the endothelial surface, but unlike the case of a localized injury, the diffuse chemoattractant signal provides no direction for neuteophil migration and diapedesis. The marginated neutrophils on the surface of endothelial cells and in the perivascular spaces around the microcirculatory vessels are then subjected to the extreme proinflammatory stimulation of TNF, interleukin 1 and other monocyte-derived proinflammatory signals.

Step VI: Full Activation of Marginated Neutrophils

The orchestration and stimulation of neutrophil phagocytic activity by TNF and other proinflammatory cytokines is a prerequisite to the eradication of large concentrations of microbes in soft tissue as part of the normal inflammatory response to contamination. However, the stimulation of marginated neutrophils and neutrophils within the perivascular space caused by systemic activation of inflammation now results in autodestructive behavior by the neutrophils. The release of reactive oxygen intermediates results in lipid peroxidation, which is further enhanced by acid hydrolases and other lysosomal enzymes that are released. This can be clinically demonstrated by the identification of markers reflecting lipid peroxidation in patients and in experimental models of infection.

Step VII: Microcirculatory Injury and Vasoconstriction

The release of toxic products from the stimulated neutrophils results in severe endothelial injury. This chemical injury becomes an additional means of activation for the inflammatory cascade. Local injury provokes the coagulation cascade and platelet aggregation, resulting in the local release of thromboxane A_2, which then has a local vasoconstrictive effect.[65,66] The consequence of neutrophil-mediated microcirculatory injury is the creation of local thrombus and vasoconstriction.

Step VIII: Microcirculatory Arrest

One consequence of injury of the endothelial cells may be local thrombus and this, combined with vasoconstriction, may produce reduced microcirculatory flow through the affected vascular unit. This can result in reduced profusion of cell populations served by the microvascular unit. The consequences of local thrombus formation and of vasoconstriction may be so severe as to produce complete thrombosis of the microcirculatory unit. Such events may be unusually severe in organs such as the liver, which have reticuloendothelial cells as resident populations within the microcirculation.

Step IX: Focal Necrosis

One can identify focal necrosis with complete thrombosis of the microcirculatory unit and in the absence of collateral perfusion of the cell populations served by that specific microcirculatory unit. Focal necrosis within those organ systems known to fail in MODS is a consistent histologic feature. The area of each identified focal necrosis increases in size with the progression of the process. The number of foci of necrosis increases in number as the severity and the duration of the process continues. Thus, the recruitment by the host of more neutrophils as part of the normal inflammatory response becomes self-destructive as additional neutrophils are recruited to injure the host's microcirculation.

Step X: The Self-Perpetuating Process

End-organ effects from systemic activation of inflammation result in clearly defined histologic necrosis of those organs known to fail in MODS.[67] The focal area of necrosis then becomes an activation signal itself to further energize and reinitialize the entire inflammatory process. Thus, a biological point of no return is reached at which the inflammatory process is perpetuated on a sustained basis even though the initial activation event of invasive infection, hemorrhagic shock or other factor has been completely eliminated. This self-perpetuating process then results in the continual loss of functional populations of cells within the affected organ systems and leads to the death of the patient.

Future Therapies Based on Mechanism

While the previous discussion detailing the specific steps of the human inflammatory response and its subsequent role in organ failure remains a hypothesis, specific therapeutic interventions have been designed based on these proposed mechanisms. For virtually every step in the preceding discussion a treatment intervention has been proposed. A growing body of knowledge of these therapies should provide even more evidence to confirm the validity of the inflammatory hypothesis of organ failure and provide information about how new therapeutic endeavors should be pursued.

Blockade of Activators of Inflammation

Several strategies have been advocated for blocking the initial activation of inflammation. Most of these strategies have been designed to address endotoxin and its effects. Endotoxin is thought to play a role in hemorrhagic shock, invasive infection and microbial gastrointestinal translocation. In theory, the blockade of endotoxin should abort the activation of systemic inflammation in many circumstances. The use of chelation agents has been advocated, and polymyxin[68] and hemofiltration[69] have been proposed. The use of bacterial permeability inducing protein is another proposed method of neutralizing endotoxin and its effects.[70,71] A soluble CD-14 receptor has been proposed as a therapy to facilitate the binding and internal elimination of lipopolysaccharide by host monocyte or macrophage cells.[72]

A generalized but nonspecific blockade of the inflammatory response has been proposed for the use of corticosteroids for the treatment of sepsis, septic shock and the associated organ failure. A litany of experimental studies over multiple decades have demonstrated some observed benefit of pharmacologic doses of corticosteroids, but usually only when given prior to the endotoxin or bacterial insult. This pretreatment benefit appears to form the rationale that corticosteroids blocked the activation process but were not of value once the inflammatory process was initiated. Two prospective clinical trials failed to demonstrate any benefit to the pharmacologic dosing in severe sepsis and septic shock.[73,74] However, more recent information has demonstrated some utility for steroids at doses less than 300 mg of hydrocortisone per day.[75] This lower dose of treatment is a physiologic supplement for a relative adrenal insufficiency rather than the traditional pharmacologic suppression of inflammation.[76]

Perhaps the most promising antiendotoxin strategy is the production of a monoclonal antibody against the lipid A moiety of endotoxin.[77] Lipid A appears to be a preserved component of endotoxin across different species of bacteria, as well as an important virulence component in endotoxin. Initial clinical trials with polyclonal antiendotoxin antibody demonstrated promise that this strategy might work.[78] However, prospective randomized clinical trials with a monoclonal antiendotoxin antibody have failed to demonstrate clinical efficacy.[79-82] Many of the problems in the trials of antiendotoxin therapy have been the consequence of our inability to clearly diagnose when endotoxin is present and when it is the driving force behind the patient's septic response. There remains hope that a future advance in bedside diagnostics combined with a high-affinity antiendotoxin antibody might result in appropriate therapy.

Inhibition of Phase I of Inflammation

Inhibition of phase I components of inflammation has been proposed and studied in many different ways. A system has been designed to accomplish neutralizing each of the five initiator events of SIRS. Because of the role of coagulation proteins and platelets as initiators of inflammation, both antithrombin III[83] and heparin[84-86] have been studied as potential neutralizing agents in these specific pathways in experimental animals. Antithrombin III investigations continue and have shown some promise, but it remains unproven to be effective therapy.[87] Inhibition of factor XII has even been advocated in experimental sepsis but its use would not seem to be prudent because of problems associated with the lack of hemostasis in this proposed therapy.[88]

The most significant recent development in using mediator-based therapy for the treatment of organ failure associated with severe sepsis has been recombinant human activated protein C. This physiologic anticoagulant has now been demonstrated in a prospective, randomized clinical trial of over 1600 patients to reduce death rates from 31% to 25%.[89] Indications for this treatment are in patients with an Acute Physiology and Chronic Health Evaluation II score that is >25, sepsis-induced multiple organ failure, septic shock or sepsis-induced acute respiratory distress syndrome. It cannot be used as treatment when patients have significant bleeding risks, but has apparent utility and safety for postoperative surgical patients.[90]

Bradykinin inhibitors have been studied in prospective randomized clinical trials after animal experimentation showed promising results.[91] Unfortunately, the prospective randomized trial in patients was unsuccessful in improving outcome.[92] Since bradykinin exerts its primary effect by stimulating the production of nitric oxide by endothelial cells, there have been efforts to use antagonists to nitric oxide production. Also, since histamine appears to have both a nitric oxide-dependent and nitric oxide-independent pathway for its physiologic effect, it was hoped that nitric oxide blockade might be of benefit in at least partially neutralizing histamine effects from mast cells as well. The use of N-methyl-arginine has not proven to be of benefit.[93] Other antihistamine therapies have been proposed, but none have been shown to be of value.[94,95] It should be emphasized again that histamine-like endotoxin has not been consistently identified in the blood of septic patients.[96] Finally, some efforts have focused on using antagonists to specific cleavage products of complement. Experimental data have been encouraging, but clinical trials have not yet been undertaken.[97-100]

Inhibition of Phase II of Inflammation

Strategies to change the phagocytic phase of inflammation have focused on attempts to modulate neutrophil margination as well as to neutralize the specific proinflammatory cytokines. Anti-CD18 monoclonal antibodies have been shown to be of benefit in animal models of shock and ischemia[101-104], but have shown potential for negative effects when infectious models have been studied.[105-107] Specific antibodies for other adhesion molecules are presently being pursued, but at present none are approaching utility.[108]

The blockade of specific proinflammatory cytokines has clearly been the focus of numerous investigations. Anti-TNF monoclonal antibody and interleukin 1 receptor antagonists have both shown promising results in animal models,[109-111] but clinical trials with both preparations have to date failed to demonstrate positive clinical effects.[112-117] A potential anti-interleukin 6 antibody is presently being explored as yet another clinical tool.[118]

Platelet activating factor (PAF) is a lipid-based inflammatory signal thought to be a very important in endothelial cell adhesion. Experimental evidence for inhibition of PAF has been encouraging.[119] A large number of PAF antagonists have been studied, but clinical trials of several of them have been unsuccessful.[120,121]

Neutralization of Effector Signals

Several experimental studies have explored the possibility of neutralizing the effector mechanisms of neutrophil-mediated damage. The use of superoxide dismutase and catalase to neutralize the effects of reactive oxygen intermediates has been explored in animal models of shock,[122,123] endotoxemia,[124,125] and acute bacterial infection.[126,127] Lazeroids have been shown to reduce lipid peroxidation in animal models.[128] Nitrones appear to be appropriate free radical scavengers of both oxygen- and nitrogen-reactive intermediates, but they are only hypothesized to be an effective therapy at this point.[129] Clinical trials of these blockers of effector signals have not been explored in patients.

Use of Counterinflammatory Cytokines

For every agonist signal in the human body, an agonist appears to exist. Recent research has identified several cytokine signals that represent counterinflammatory mediators. Interleukin 4,[130] interleukin 10,[131] and interleukin 13[132] are now being explored as endogenously-derived counterinflammatory mediators that seem to neutralize proinflammatory events. In experimental models, the use of these counterinflammatory agents appears to have a beneficial effect on animal survival and metabolic measures of septic effects.[133-141] Transforming growth factor beta is yet another counterinflammatory signal.[142] Clinical trials of these counterinflammatory agents have not been done, but it has certainly become evident that SIRS provokes an anti-inflammatory response in the host. This finding has spawned the concept of Compensatory Anti-Inflammatory Response (CARS).[143] The relationship of the proinflammatory and the anti-inflammatory responses may well explain many of the events leading to organ failure in patients in the intensive care unit (ICU). An overexuberant proinflammatory response combined with an inadequate anti-inflammatory response may well define the state of SIRS. An excessive counterinflammatory response and inadequate proinflammatory response may in fact be the basis for the immunosuppression seen in the severely ill ICU patient. The relationship of pro and counterinflammatory signaling is likely to be a major area of exploration in the future. A dysfunctional relationship may well exist in certain patients, leading to a Mixed Antagonist Response Syndrome (MARS). The concept of MARS would seem to imply the occurrence of intermittent SIRS and CARS events in the same patient over a period of time. It again emphasizes the need for a better understanding of the relationship of these various signals.

Finally, the immunosuppression attendant to systemic inflammation has been specifically addressed with particular immune modulators. Interferon-gamma,[144] levamisole,[145] muramyl dipeptide,[146] granulocyte-colony stimulating factor,[147] and granulocyte-monocyte-colony stimulating factor,[148] are all therapies under scrutiny.

Summary

The management of the patient with severe sepsis and multiple organ failure is continuing to be modified and enhanced.[149] Our current knowledge would appear to lend support to the concept that the pathogenesis of the multiple-organ dysfunction syndrome is the consequence of an overexuberant systemic inflammatory response. This hypothesis would posit that the normal salutary events of our local inflammatory response become self-destructive when activated at the systemic level. One of the clear lessons to be learned in studying the physiology of human inflammation is that it has numerous redundant pathways, thus blockade of a single mediator or a single signal is likely to be ineffective. This may mean that future therapies will focus on multimodality therapy to block the adverse effects of the inflammatory cascade. However, a drawback to multimodality therapy will be the consequences of comprehensively blocking the desirable effects of the inflammatory cascade.

More recently, anti-inflammatory cytokine signals antagonistic to the proinflammatory signals have been identified. It is likely that future directions of therapy in the patient with organ failure is going to focus on the interrelationship of these pro and counterinflammatory signals. It would certainly appear that better understanding of pro and counterinflammatory signaling, and perhaps learning to replicate our own endogenous downregulatory response at the local tissue level, will lead to a clearer understanding of why MODS occurs and how it can be better managed.

3. References

1. Skillman JJ, Bushnell LS, Goldman H, Silen W. Respiratory failure, hypotension, sepsis, and jaundice. *Am J Surg*. 1969;117:523-530.

2. Tilney NL, Bailey GL, Morgan AP. Sequential system failure after rupture of abdominal aortic aneurysms: An unsolved problem in postoperative care. *Ann Surg*.1973;178:117-122.

3. Eiseman B, Beart R, Norton L. Multiple organ failure. *Surg Gynecol Obstet*.1977;144:323-326.

4. Baue AE. Multiple, progressive, or sequential systems failure. *Arch Surg*.1975;110:779-781.

5. Fry DE, Pearlstein L, Fulton RL, Polk HC Jr. Multiple system organ failure: the role of uncontrolled infection. *Arch Surg*. 1980;115:136-140.

6. Fry DE, Garrison RN, Heitch RC, et al. Determinants of death in patients with intraabdominal abscess. *Surgery*. 1980;89:517-523.

7. Fry DE, Garrison RN, Polk HC Jr. Clinical implications in Bacteroides bacteremia. *Surg Gynecol Obstet*. 1979;149:189-192.

8. Fry DE, Garrison RN, Williams HC. Patterns of morbidity and mortality in splenectomy for trauma. *Am Surg*. 1980;46:28-32.

9. Goris RJ, Beokhorst PA, Nuytinck KS. Multiple organ failure: generalized autodestructive inflammation. *Arch Surg*. 1985;120: 1109-1115.

10. Goris RJ, Boekholtz WK, van Bebber IP, et al. Multiple-organ failure and sepsis without bacteria. An experimental model. *Arch Surg*. 1986;121:897-901.

11. Schirmer WJ, Schirmer JM, Naff GB, Fry DE. Complement activation produces hemodynamic changes characteristic of sepsis. *Arch Surg*. 1988;123:316-321.

12. American College of Chest Physicians/Society of Critical Care Medicine Consensus Conference. Definition for sepsis and organ failure and guidelines for the use of innovative therapies in sepsis. *Crit Care Med*. 1992;20:864.

13. Janeway CA Jr, Medzhitov R: Innate immune recognition. *Annu Rev Immunol*. 2002; 20:197-216.

14. Scaffidi P, Misteli T, Bianchi ME: Release of chromatin protein HMGB1 by necrotic cells triggers inflammation. *Nature*. 2002; 418: 191-195.

15. Foell DHW, Vogl T, Roth J. S100 proteins expressed in phagocytosis: a novel group of Damage Associated Molecular Pattern molecules. *J Leukoc Biol*. 2007; 81:28-37.

16. Schmitt E, Gehrmann M, Brunet M, et al. Intracellular and extracellular functions of heat shock proteins: repercussions in cancer therapy. *J Leukoc Biol*. 2007; 81:15-27.

17. Werman A, Werman-Venkert R, White R, et al. The precursor of IL-1α is an intracrine proinflammatory activator of transcription. *Proc Natl Acad Sci USA*. 2004; 101:2434-2439.

18. Bianchi ME. DAMPs, PAMPs and alarmins: all we need to know about danger. *J Leukoc Biol*. 2007;81:1-5.

19. Pasare C, Medzhitov R. Toll-like receptors and acquired immunity. *Sem Immunol*. 2004; 16:23-26.

20. Bierhaus A, Humpert PM, Morcos M, et al. Understanding RAGE, the receptor for advanced glycation end products. *J Mol Med*. 2005; 83:876-886.

21. Sundsmo JS, Fair DS. Relationships among the complement, kinin, coagulation and fibrinolytic systems in the inflammatory reaction. *Clin Physiol Biochem*.1983;1:225-284.

22. Kaplan AP, Silverberg M, Dunn JT, Ghebrehiwet B. Interaction of the clotting, kinin-forming, complement, and fibrinolytic pathways in inflammation. *Ann NY Acad Sci*.1982;389:25.

23. Cicala C, Cirino G. Linkage between inflammation and coagulation: an update on the molecular basis of the crosstalk. *Life Sci*. 1998;62:1817-1824.

24. Johnson K, Choi Y, DeGroot E, et al. Potential mechanisms for a proinflammatory vascular cytokine response to coagulation activation. *J Immunol*. 1998;160:5130-5135.

25. Gentry PA. The mammalian blood platelet: its role in haemostasis, inflammation, and tissue repair. *J Comp Path*. 1992;107:243-270.

26. Weksler BB. Roles for human platelets in inflammation. *Prog Clin Biol Res*. 1988;283:611-638.

27. Huang C, Sali A, Stevens R. Regulation and function of mast cell proteases in inflammation. *J Clin Immunol*.1998;18:169-183.

28. Metcalfe DD, Baram D, Mekori YA. Mast cells. *Physiol Rev*. 1997;77:1033-1079.

29. Gordon JR, Galli SJ. Mast cells as a source of both preformed and immunologically inducible TNF-alpha/cachectin. *Nature*. 1990;346:274-276.

30. Bressler RB, Lesko J, Jones M, et al. Production of IL-5 and granulocyte-macrophage colony-stimulating factor by naïve human mast cells activated by high affinity IgE receptor ligation. *J Allergy Clin Immunol*. 1997;99:508-514.

31. Moller A, Pippert U, Lessmann D, et al. Human mast cells produce IL-8. *J Immunol*. 1993;151:3261-3266.

32. Selvan RS, Butterfield JH, Krangel MS. Expression of multiple cytokine genes by a human mast cell leukemia. *J Biol Chem*. 1994;269:13893-13898.

33. Kaplan AP, Joseph K, Shibayama Y, et al. The intrinsic coagulation/kinin-forming cascade: assembly in plasma and cell surfaces in inflammation. *Adv Immunol*. 1997;66:225-272.

34. Hargreaves KM, Troulles ES, Dionne RA, et al. Bradykinin is increased during acute and chronic inflammation. Therapeutic implications. *Clin Pharmacol Ther*. 1988;44:613-621.

35. Ignarro LJ. Biosynthesis and metabolism of endothelium-derived nitric oxide. *Ann Rev Pharmacol Toxicol*. 1990;30:535-560.

36. Mollnes TE, Fosse E. The complement system in trauma-related and ischemic tissue damage: a brief review. *Shock*. 1994;2:301-310.

37. Kaplan AP, Silverberg N. Mediators of inflammation: an overview. *Methods Enzymol*. 1988;163:3-23.

38. Negus RPM. The chemokines: cytokines that direct leukocyte migration. *J Roy Soc Med*. 1996;89:312-314.

39. Luster AD: Chemokines—Chemotactic cytokines that mediate inflammation. *N Engl J Med*.1998;338:436-445.

40. Furie MB, Randolph GJ. Chemokines and tissue injury. *Am J Path*.1995;146:1287-1301.

41. Rollins BJ. Chemokines. *Blood*. 1997;90: 909-928.

42. Jin T, Xu X, Hereld D. Chemotaxis, chemokine receptors, and human disease. *Cytokine*. 2008; 44:1-8.

43. Brown EJ, Lindberg FP. Leukocyte adhesion molecules in host defense against infection. *Ann Med*. 1996;28:210-218.

44. Menger MD, Vollmar B. Adhesion molecules as determinants of disease: from molecular biology to surgical research. *Brit J Surg*. 1996;83:588-601.

45. Gahmberg GG. Leukocyte adhesion: CD11/CD18 integrins and intercellular adhesion molecules. *Curr Opin Cell Biol*. 1997;9:643-650.

46. Gahmberg GG, Tolvanen M, Kotovuori P. Leukocyte adhesion—structure and function of human leukocytes beta 2-integrin and their cellular ligands. *Eur J Biochem*. 1997;245:215-232.

47. Klebanoff SJ, Vedes MA, Harlan JM, et al. Stimulation of neutrophils by tumor necrosis factor. *J Immunol*. 1986;136:4220-4225.

48. Larrick JW, Graham D, Toy K, et al. Recombinant tumor necrosis factor causes activation of human granulocytes. *Blood*. 1987;69:640-644.

49. Dinarello CA. interleukin 1 and the pathogenesis of the acute phase response. *N Engl J Med*. 1984;311:1413-1418.

50. Ferrante A, Nandoskar M, Walz A, et al. Effects of tumor necrosis factor alpha and interleukin 1 alpha and beta on human neutrophil migration, respiratory burst and degranulation. *Int Arch Allergy Appl Immunol*. 1988;86:82-91.

51. Feng L, Xia Y, Garcia GE, et al. Involvement of reaction oxygen intermediates in cyclooxygenase-2 expression induced by interleukin 1, tumor necrosis factor-alpha, and lipopolysaccharide. *J Clin Invest*. 1995;95:1669-1675.

52. Rittirsch D, Flierl MA, Ward PA. Harmful molecular mechanisms in sepsis. *Nat Rev Immunol*. 2008; 8:776-787.

53. Siegel JH, Cerra FB, Coleman B, et al. Physiologic and metabolic correlations in human sepsis. *Surgery*. 1979;86:163-193.

54. Fry DE, Silver BB, Rink RD, et al. Hepatic cellular hypoxia in murine peritonitis. *Surgery*. 1979;85:652-661.

55. Deitch EA. The role of intestinal barrier failure and bacterial translocation in the development of systemic infection and multiple organ failure. *Arch Surg*. 1990;125:403-404.

56. Wilmore DW, Smith RJ, O'Dwyer ST, et al. The gut: a central organ after surgical stress. *Surgery*. 1988;104:917-924.

57. Deitch EA. Intestinal permeability is increased in burn patients shortly after injury. *Surgery*. 1990;107:411-416.

58. Rush BF, Sori AJ, Murphy TF, et al. Endotoxemia and bacteremia during hemorrhagic shock. *Ann Surg*. 1988;207:549-554.

59. Ranson JHC, Rifkind KM, Roses DF, et al. Prognostic signs and the role of operative management in acute pancreatitis. *Ann Surg*. 1974;139:69.

60. Wan S, LeClerc JL, Vincent JL. Inflammatory response to cardiopulmonary bypass: mechanisms involved and possible therapeutic strategies. *Chest*. 1997;112:67-92.

61. Deitch EA. Multiple organ failure: pathophysiology and potential future therapy. *Ann Surg*. 1992;216:117-134.

62. Biffl WL, Moore EE. Splanchnic ischaemia/reperfusion and multiple organ failure. *Brit J Anaesth*.1996;77:59-70.

63. Fearon DT, Ruddy S, Schur PH, et al. Activation of the properidin pathway of complement in patients with Gram-negative bacteremia. *N Engl J Med*.1975;292:937.

64. Schirmer WJ, Schirmer JM, Naff GB, Fry DE. Systemic complement activation produces hemodynamic changes characteristic of sepsis. *Arch Surg*. 1988;123:316-321.

65. Bernard GR, Reines HD, Halushka PV, et al. Prostacyclin and thromboxane A2formation is increased in human sepsis syndrome. Effects of cyclooxygenase inhibition. *Am Rev Respir Dis*. 1991;144:1095-1101.

66. Schirmer WJ, Schirmer JM, Townsend MC, Fry DE. Imidazole and indomethacin improve hepatic perfusion in sepsis. *Circ Shock.* 1987;21:253-259.

67. Asher EF, Rowe RL, Garrison RN, Fry DE. Experimental bacteremia and hepatic nutrient blood flow. *Circ Shock.* 1986;20:43-49.

68. Flynn PM, Shenep JL, Stokes DC, et al. Polymyxin B moderates acidosis and hypotension in established, experimental gram-negative septicemia. *J Infect Dis.* 1987;156:706-712.

69. Hirasawa H, Sugai T, Ohtake Y, et al. Blood purification for prevention and treatment of multiple organ failure. *World J Surg.* 1996;20:482-486.

70. Lechner AJ, Lamprech KE, Johanns CA, Matuschak GM. The recombinant 23-kDa Nterminal fragment of bactericidal/permeability-increasing protein (rBPI23) decreases E coli-induced mortality and organ injury during immunosuppression-related neutropenia. *Shock.* 1995;4:218.

71. Elsbach P. The bactericidal/permeability increasing protein (BPI) in antibacterial host defense. *J Leuk Biol.* 1998;64:14-18.

72. Landmann R, Reber AM, Sansano S, Zimmerli W. Function of soluble CD14 in serum from patients with septic shock. *J Infect Dis.* 1996;173:661-668.

73. Bone RC, Fisher CJ, Clemmer TP. A controlled clinical trial of high-dose methylprednisolone in the treatment of severe sepsis and septic shock. *N Engl J Med.* 1987;317:653-658.

74. The Veterans Administration Systemic Sepsis Cooperative Study Group. Effect of high-dose glucocorticoid therapy on mortality in patients with clinical signs of sepsis. *N Engl J Med.* 1987;317:659-665.

75. Annane D, Sebille V, Charpentier C, et al. Effect of treatment with low doses of hydrocortisone and fludrocortisone on mortality in patients with septic shock. *JAMA.* 2002; 288:862-871.

76. Marik PE, Zaloga GP. Adrenal insufficiency during septic shock. *Crit Care Med.* 2003; 31:141-145.

77. Burd RS, Cody CS, Raymond CS, Dunn DL. Anti-endotoxin monoclonal antibodies protect by enhancing bacterial and endotoxin clearance. *Arch Surg.* 1993;128:145-150.

78. Ziegler EJ, McCutchan JA, Fierer J, et al. Treatment of gram-negative bacteremia and shock with human antiserum to a mutant Escherichia coli. *N Engl J Med.*1982; 307:1225-1230.

79. Ziegler EJ, Fischer CJ, Sprung CL Jr, et al. Treatment of gram-negative bacteremia and septic shock with HA-1A human monoclonal antibody against endotoxin: a randomized, double-blind, placebo-controlled trial. *N Engl J Med.*1991;324:429.

80. McCloskey RV, Straube RC, Sanders C, et al. Treatment of septic shock with human monoclonal antibody HA-1A. A randomized, double-blind, placebo-controlled trial. CHESS Trial Study Group. *Ann Intern Med.* 1994;121:1-5.

81. Greenman RL, Schein RMH, Martin MA, et al. A controlled clinical trial of E5 murine monoclonal IgM antibody to endotoxin in the treatment of gram-negative sepsis. *JAMA.* 1991;266:1097-1102.

82. Bone RC, Balk RA, Fein AM, et al. A second large controlled study of E5, a monoclonal antibody to endotoxin: results of a prospective, multicenter, randomized, controlled trial. The E5 Sepsis Study Group. *Crit Care Med.* 1995;23:994-1006.

83. Dickneite G. Antithrombin III in animal models of sepsis and organ failure. *Semin Thromb Hemostas*. 1998;24:61-69.

84. Hau T, Simmons RL. Heparin in the treatment of experimental peritonitis. *Ann Surg*. 1978;187:294.

85. O'Leary JP, Malik FS, Donahoe RP, et al. The effects of a minidose of heparin on peritonitis in rats. *Surg Gynecol Obstet*.1979;148:571.

86. Schirmer WJ, Schirmer JM, Naff GB, et al. Heparin's effect on the natural history of sepsis in the rat (abstr). *Circ Shock*. 1987;21:363.

87. Eisele B, Lamy M. Clinical experience with antithrombin III concentrates in critically ill patients with sepsis and multiple organ failure. *Semin Thromb Hemostas*. 1998;24:71-80.

88. Jansen PM, Pixley RA, Brouwer M, et al. Inhibition of factor XII in septic baboons attenuates the activation of complement and fibrinolytic system and reduces the release of interleukin-6 and neutrophil elastase. *Blood*. 1996;87:2337-2344.

89. Bernard GR, Vincent JL, Laterre PF, et al. Efficacy and safety of recombinant human activated protein C for severe sepsis. *N Engl J Med*. 2001;344:699-709.

90. Fry DE, Beilman G, Johnson S, et al. Safety of drotrecogin alfa (activated) in surgical patients with severe sepsis. *Surg Infect*. 2004;5: 253-260.

91. Ridings PC, Blocher CR, Fisher BJ, et al. Beneficial effects of a bradykinin antagonist in a model of gram negative sepsis. *J Trauma*. 1995;39:81-88.

92. Fein AM, Bernard GR, Criner GJ, et al. Treatment of severe systemic inflammatory response syndromes and sepsis with a novel bradykinin antagonist, deltibant (CP-0127). Results of a randomized, double-blind, placebo-controlled trial. CP-1027 SIRS and Sepsis Study Group. *JAMA*. 1997;277:482-487.

93. Ketteler M, Cetto C, Kirdorf M, et al. Nitric oxide in sepsis-syndrome: potential treatment of septic shock by nitric oxide synthase antagonists. *Kidney Int*. 1998;53(suppl 64):S27-S30.

94. Neugebauer E, Lorenz W, Beckurts T, et al. Significance of histamine formation and release in the development of endotoxic shock: proof of current concepts by randomized controlled studies in rats. *Rev Infect Dis*. 1987;9(suppl 5):S585-S593.

95. Leeper-Woodford SK, Carey D, Byrne K, et al. Histamine receptor antagonists, cyclooxygenase blockade, and tumor necrosis factor curing acute septic insult. *Shock*. 1998:9:89-94.

96. Neugebauer E, Lorenz W, Rixen D, et al. Histamine release in sepsis: a prospective, controlled, clinical study. *Crit Care Med*. 1996;24:1670-1677.

97. Jansen PM, Eisele B, de Jong IW, et al. Effect of C1 inhibition on inflammatory and physiologic response patterns in primates suffering from lethal septic shock. *J Immunol*. 1998;160:475-484.

98. Mohr M, Hopken U, Opperman M, et al. Effects of anti-C5a monoclonal antibodies on oxygen use in a porcine model of severe sepsis. *Eur J Clin Invest*. 1998;28:227-234.

99. Lindsay TF, Hill J, Oritz F, et al. Blockade of complement activation prevents local and pulmonary albumin leak after lower torso ischemia reperfusion. *Ann Surg*.1992;216: 677.

100. Hack CE, Voerman HJ, Eisele B, et al. C1-esterase inhibitor substitution in sepsis. *Lancet*. 1992;339:378.

101. Vedder NB, Winn RK, Rice CL, et al. A monoclonal antibody to the adherence promoting leukocyte glycoprotein CD18, reduces organ injury and improves survival from hemorrhagic shock and resuscitation in rabbits. *J Clin Invest*.1988;81:939.

102. Walsh CJ, Carey D, Cook DJ, et al. Anti CD18 antibody attenuates neutropenia and alveolar capillary membrane injury during Gram-negative sepsis. *Surgery*. 1991;110:205-209.

103. Winn RK, Ramamoorthy C, Vedder NB, et al. Leukocyte-endothelial cell interaction in ischemia reperfusion injury. Ann NY Acad Sci. 1997;832:311-321.

104. Cornejo CJ, Winn RK, Harlan JM. Anti-adhesion therapy. *Adv Pharmacol*.1997;39:99-142.

105. Ramamoorthy C, Sasaki SS, Su DL, et al. CD18 adhesion blockade decreases bacterial clearance and neutrophil recruitment after intrapulmonary E coli, but not after S aureus. *J Leuk Biol*.1997;61:167-172.

106. Redl H, Schlag G, Davies J, Robinson M. Detrimental effects of the application of anti CD18 antibodies in baboon live E coli sepsis. *Circ Shock*. 1993;2(suppl):33.

107. Eichacker PQ, Hoffman WD, Farese A, et al. Leukocyte CD18 monoclonal antibody worsens endotoxemia and cardiovascular injury in canines with septic shock. *J Appl Physiol*. 1993;74:1885-1892.

108. Seekamp A, Till GO, Mulligan MS, et al. Role of selectins in local and remote tissue injury following ischemia and reperfusion. *Am J Pathol*.1994;144:592.

109. Beutler B, Milsark IW, Cerami AC. Passive immunization against cachectin/tumor necrosis factor protects mice from lethal effect of endotoxin. *Science*. 1985;229:869.

110. Tracey KJ, Fong Y, Hesse DG, et al. Anti-cachectin/TNF monoclonal antibodies prevent septic shock during lethal bacteraemia. *Nature*. 1987;330:662.

111. Wakabayashi G, Gelfand JA, Burke JF, et al. A specific receptor antagonist for interleukin 1 prevents Escherichia coli-induced shock in rabbits. *FASEB J*. 1991;5:338.

112. Abraham E, Wunderink R, Silverman H, et al. Efficacy and safety of monoclonal antibody to human tumor necrosis factor alpha in patients with sepsis syndrome. A randomized, controlled, double-blind, multicenter clinical trial. *JAMA*. 1995;273:934-941.

113. Cohen J, Carlet J. Intersept: an international, multicenter, placebo-controlled trial of monoclonal antibody to human tumor necrosis factor-alpha in patients with sepsis. International Sepsis Trial Study Group. *Crit Care Med*. 1996;24:1431-1440.

114. Reinhart K, Wiegard-Lohnert C, Grimminger F, et al. Assessment of the safety and efficacy of the monoclonal anti-tumor necrosis factor antibody-fragment, MAK 195F, in patients with sepsis and septic shock: a multicenter, randomized, placebo-controlled, dose-ranging study. *Crit Care Med*. 1996;24:733-742.

115. Fisher CJ Jr, Agosti JM, Opal SM, et al. Treatment of septic shock with the tumor necrosis factor receptor:Fc fusion protein. The soluble TNF Receptor Sepsis Study Group. *N Engl J Med*. 1996;334:1697-1702.

116. Fisher CJ Jr, Dhainaut JF, Opal SM, et al. Recombinant human interleukin 1 receptor antagonist in the treatment of patients with sepsis syndrome. Results from a randomized, double-blind, placebo-controlled trial. Phase III rhIL-1ra Sepsis Syndrome Study Group. *JAMA*. 1994;271:1836-1843.

117. Opal SM, Fisher CJ Jr, Dhainaut JF, et al. Confirming interleukin 1 receptor antagonist trial in severe sepsis. A phase III, randomized, double-blind, placebo-controlled, multicenter trial. The interleukin 1 Receptor Antagonist Sepsis Investigation Group. *Crit Care Med.* 1997;25:1115-1124.

118. Van der Poll T, Levi M, Hack CE, et al. Elimination of interleukin 6 attenuates coagulation activation in experimental endotoxemia in chimpanzees. *J Exp Med.* 1994;179:1253.

119. Fink MP. Therapeutic options directed against platelet activating factor, eicosanoids, and bradykinin in sepsis. *J Antimicrob Chemother.* 1998;41(suppl A):81-94.

120. Froon AM, Greve JW, Buurman WA, et al. Treatment with the platelet-activating factor antagonist TCV-309 in patients with severe systemic inflammatory response syndrome: a prospective, multi-center, double-blind, randomized phase II trial. *Shock.* 1996;5:313-319.

121. Dhainaut JF, Tenaillon A, Hemmer M, et al. Confirmatory platelet-activating factor receptor antagonist trial in patients with severe Gram-negative bacterial sepsis: a phase III, randomized, double-blind, placebo controlled, multicenter trial. BN 52021 Sepsis Investigator Group. *Crit Care Med.* 1998;26:1963-1971.

122. Kapoor R, Kalra J, Prasad K. Cardiac depression and cellular injury in hemorrhagic shock and reinfusion: role of free radicals. *Mol Cell Biochem.*1997;176:291-306.

123. Simon HM, Scalea T, Paskanik A, Young B. Superoxide dismutase (SOD) prevents hypotension after hemorrhagic shock and aortic cross clamping. *Am J Med Sci.* 1996;312:155-159.

124. Harris NR, Russell JM, Granger DN. Mediators of endotoxin-induced leukocyte adhesion in mesenteric postcapillary venules. *Circ Shock.* 1994;43:155-160.

125. Abello PA, Fidler SA, Bulkley GB, Buckman TG. Antioxidants modulate induction of programmed endothelial cell death (apoptosis) by endotoxin. *Arch Surg.* 1994;129:134-140.

126. Rose S, Baumann H, Jahreis GP, Sayeed MM. Diltiazem and superoxide dismutase modulate hepatic acute phase response in gram-negative sepsis. *Shock.* 1994;1:87-93.

127. Rose S, Sayeed MM. Superoxide radical scavenging prevents cellular calcium dysregulation during intraabdominal sepsis. *Shock.* 1997;7:263-268.

128. Krysztopik RJ, Bentley FR, Spain DA, Wilson MA, Garrison RN. Free radical scavenging by lazaroids improves renal blood flow during sepsis. *Surgery.* 1996;120:657-662.

129. Pou S, Keaton L, Surichamorn W, et al. Can nitric oxide be spin trapped by nitrone and nitroso compounds? *Biochim Biophys Acta.* 1994;1201:118-124.

130. Maher DW, Davis I, Boyd AW, Morstyn G. Human interleukin-4: an immunomodulator with potential therapeutic application. *Prog Growth Factor Res.* 1991;3:43-56.

131. De Waal Malefyt R, Abrams J, Bennet B, et al. interleukin 10 inhibits cytokine synthesis by human monocytes: an autoregulatory role of IL10 production by monocytes. *J Exp Med.* 1991;174:1209.

132. De Vries JE. Molecular and biological characteristics of interleukin 13. *Chem Immunol.* 1996;63:204-218.

133. Matsumoto T, Tateda K, Miyazaki S, et al. Effect of inteleukin-10 on gut-derived sepsis caused by Pseudomonas aeruginosa in mice. *Antimicrob Agents Chemother.* 1998;42:2853-2857.

134. Lubberts E, Joosten LA, Helsen MM, van den Berg WB. Regulatory role of interleukin 10 in joint inflammation and cartilage destruction in murine streptococcal cell wall arthritis. More therapeutic benefit with IL-4/IL-10 combination therapy than with IL-10 treatment alone. Cytokine. 1998;10:361-369.

135. Nicoletti F, Mancuso G, Ciliberti FA, et al. Endotoxin-induced lethality in neonatal mice is counteracted by interleukin 10 and exacerbated by anti-IL-10. *Clin Diagnost Lab Immunol*. 1997;4:607-610.

136. Mulligan MS, Warner RL, Foreback JL, et al. rotective effects of IL-4, IL-10, IL-12, and IL13 in IgG immune complex-induced lung injury: role of endogenous IL-12. *J Immunol*. 1997;159:3483-3489.

137. Muchamuel T, Menon S, Pisacane P, et al. IL-13 protects mice from lipopolysaccharideinduced lethal endotoxemia: correlation with down-modulation of TNF-alpha, IFN-gamma, and IL-12 production. *J Immunol*. 1997;158: 2898-2903.

138. Nicoletti F, Mancuso G, Cusumano V, et al. Prevention of endotoxin-induced lethality in neonatal mice by interleukin 13. *Eur J Immunol*. 1997;27:1580-1583.

139. Hogaboam CM, Vallance BA, Kumar A, et al. Therapeutic effects of interleukin-4 gene transfer in experimental inflammatory bowel disease. *J Clin Invest*.1997;100:2766-2776.

140. Inobe JI, Chen Y, Weiner HL. In vivo administration of IL-4 induces TGF-beta-producing cells and protects animals from experimental autoimmune encephalomyelitis. *Ann NY Acad Sci*. 1996;778:390-392.

141. Kato T, Murata A, Ishida H, et al. Interleukin 10 reduces mortality from severe peritonitis in mice. *Antimicrob Agents Chemother*. 1995;39:1336-1340.

142. Wahl SM, McCartney-Francis N, Mergenhagen SE. Inflammatory and immunomodulatory roles of TGF-beta. *Immunol Today*. 1989;10:258-261.

143. Bone RC, Grodzin CJ, Bulk RA. Sepsis: a new hypothesis for pathogenesis of the disease process. *Chest*. 1997;112:235-243.

144. Polk HC Jr, Cheadle WG, Livingston DH, et al. A randomized prospective clinical trial to determine the efficacy of interferon-gamma in severely injured patients. *Am J Surg*. 1992;163:191-196.

145. Meakins JL, Christou NV, Shizgal HM, MacLean LD. Therapeutic approaches to anergy in surgical patients. Surgery and levamisole. *Ann Surg*. 1979;190:286-296.

146. Brown GL, Foshee H, Pietsch J, Polk HC Jr. Muramyl dipeptide enhances survival for experimental peritonitis. *Arch Surg*. 1986;121:47-49.

147. O'Reilly M, Silver GM, Greenhalgh DG, et al. Treatment of intra-abdominal infection with granulocyte colony-stimulating factor. *J Trauma*. 1992;33:679-682.

148. Stern AC, Jones TC. Role of human recombinant GM-CSF in the prevention and treatment of leukopenia with special reference to infectious disease. *Diag Microbiol Infect Dis*. 1990;13:391-396.

149. Dellinger RP, Carlet JM, Masur H, et al. Surviving sepsis campaign guidelines for management of severe sepsis and septic shock. *Crit Care Med*. 2004;32:858-873.

4. Questions

1. Which of the following clinical parameters is not considered one of the defining criteria of the Systemic Inflammatory Response Syndrome (SIRS)?

   A. Temperature

   B. Pulse rate

   C. Breaths per minute

   D. White blood cell count

   E. Cardiac output

2. While the coagulation cascade has obvious value for hemostasis in the surgical patient, its activation also serves an important role in the initiation of inflammation. Which factor of the human coagulation cascade has the most central role in the initiation of the inflammatory response?

   A. Factor VII

   B. Factor VIII

   C. Factor IX

   D. Factor X

   E. Factor XII

3. The complement cascade is activated via both the classical and the alternative pathways. This multiplicity of activation pathways ensures that complement is activated locally in the host when any of a number of different stimuli occurs. Which of the following is the activation signal for the classical pathway of complement?

   A. Endotoxin

   B. Necrotic tissue

   C. Antigen-antibody complex

   D. Factor XII

   E. Ischemia/reperfusion

4. Cytokine signals are autocrine, paracrine, and endocrine chemical messages. Cytokines from monocytes may have proinflammatory or immunomodulatory functions. Which of the following cytokines would be considered an immunomodulatory signal?

   A. Tumor necrosis factor

   B. Interleukin 1

   C. Interleukin 4

   D. Interleukin 6

   E. Interleukin 8

5. A patient sustains a gunshot wound of the abdomen and has colon injury and massive fecal contamination of the abdominal cavity. After celiotomy, colonic resection and colostomy, he has a stormy postoperative course. On the sixth postoperative day he has a temperature of 39.8° C, a pulse of 130 beats/min, and requires ventilatory support to maintain oxygenation with an FIO_2 of 0.5 and positive end-expiratory pressure of 10 mm Hg. His arterial blood pressure is 105/72, and his urine output is 35 cc/hour. His pH is 7.33, Po_2 is 80, and Pco_2 is 28. Which of the following most accurately describes his physiologic and metabolic state?

   A. Elevated cardiac output, reduced systemic vascular resistance and respiratory acidosis

   B. Elevated cardiac output, reduced systemic vascular resistance and metabolic acidosis

   C. Normal or slightly reduced cardiac output, reduced systemic vascular resistance and respiratory acidosis

   D. Normal cardiac output, increased systemic vascular resistance and a metabolic acidosis

E. Increased cardiac output, increased systemic vascular resistance and a metabolic acidosis

6. Microbial translocation from the intestinal tract has been hypothesized as an event that can activate systemic inflammation. Which of the following statements about the current understanding of microbial translocation is false?

A. It only occurs from bacterial colonization of the intestinal tract

B. Microbes enter the portal circulation from the intestinal tract

C. Microbes enter the regional lymph nodes of the mesentery from the intestinal tract

D. Cytokine release from lymph nodes may be the principal mechanism, not microbial dissemination in blood

E. Endotoxin and not the intact microbes may be the mechanism of action

7. Bradykinin is thought to be an important mediator of the systemic inflammatory response syndrome, and blocking its effects has even been explored as a means to treat the "septic" patient. The physiologic effects of bradykinin are mediated through:

A. The autonomic release of catecholamines

B. The metabolism of arginine

C. Direct binding to vascular smooth muscle receptors

D. Activation of histamine

E. Competitive inhibition of acetylcholine

8. Which of the following statements about thromboxane A_2 is correct?

A. It is primarily produced by endothelial cells and inhibits platelet aggregation and microcirculatory vasodilation

B. It is a major product from mast cell granules

C. It is primarily produced by monocytes and stimulates the release of platelet activating factor from platelets

D. It is primarily produced by platelets, aggregates platelets, and causes microcirculatory vasoconstriction

E. It is primarily synthesized from a protein precursor in plasma

9. The failure of the antiendotoxin monoclonal antibody when studied in clinical trials was due to the fact that:

A. Endotoxin does not cause SIRS

B. Lipid A is not present in most Gram-negative bacteria

C. Study patients did not fulfill SIRS criteria

D. Endotoxin is inconsistently the cause of SIRS

E. The majority of SIRS patients don't have infection

10. The Compensatory Anti-Inflammatory Response (CARS) is the biological antagonist to the Systemic Inflammatory Response Syndrome (SIRS). Which of the following mediator signals is not a participant in CARS?

A. Interleukin 4

B. Transforming growth factor-beta

C. Muramyl dipeptide

D. Interleukin 10

E. Interleukin 13

Answers

1. E.
While changes in cardiac output are associated with SIRS, accurate measurement of this clinical variable requires invasive monitoring. The original strategy in defining SIRS was to create practical clinical evidence for outlining the entity, thus the other 4 listed clinical variables are part of the definition (Table 1). In addition, cardiac output in the SIRS patient may be elevated, reduced or normal. Cardiac output in the SIRS patient cannot be a meaningful clinical parameter without being considered along with the calculated systemic vascular resistance. The interpretation of cardiac output and vascular resistance together is important in defining the actual classification of the state of SIRS (see Figures 2A and 2B), but they cannot be determined without invasive monitoring.

2. E.
When factor XII, or Hageman factor, is activated it is important in the formation of fibrin, but it is pivotal in the initiation of inflammation. Activated factor XII appears to be important in the promotion of the other four initiators of inflammation (platelets, mast cells, the contact activating system and complement). While the intricacies of the inflammatory process remain incompletely defined and other elements of the coagulation cascade may well be important in the initiation of inflammation, it appears that factor XII has the greatest significance. The increased recognition of the role of the coagulation cascade in the initiation of inflammation has resulted in several strategies involving the use of anticoagulation as a potential treatment for SIRS and MODS.

3. C.
The antigen-antibody complex is required for activation of complement through the classical pathway. This pathway results in the activation of C-4 and the C-1 complex of complement proteins, leading to the activation of C-3. The alternative pathway bypasses these "classical" complement proteins and stimulates the activation of C-3 through properdin and other proteins. The antigen-antibody complex is thought to serve a positive purpose in the host through the actual lysis of bacteria when the host has a specific antibody for a surface antigen of the pathogen. Unfortunately, systemic activation through the classical pathway may account for SIRS and MODS occurring secondary to severe drug reactions.

4. C.
Interleukin 4, 10 and 13 are the cytokines identified as having immunomodulatory functions, and they appear to have a counterinflammatory role. Tumor necrosis factor, interleukin 1, and interleukin 6 are well identified proinflammatory cytokines. Interleukin 8 is a chemokine and is a proinflammatory signal.

5. B.
This patient is clearly experiencing a stage B systemic inflammatory response. Stage B is characterized by an elevation of cardiac output, and severely reduced systemic vascular resistance. Arterial blood pressure is sustained, but mean arterial pressure may be slightly reduced. These patients may have a slight metabolic acidosis, although lactate concentrations are significantly elevated. In this patient, the reduced Pco_2 provides compensation for the metabolic acidosis.

6. A.
The clinical situation that is clearly documented to be caused by translocation is candidemia. *Candida* spp. have been documented to translocate across the lumen of the intestine. Thus, while most research models used to study translocation have examined bacteria, and the phenomenon is commonly called bacterial translocation, it may more appropriately be called microbial gastrointestinal translocation

because bacteria are not the only microbes capable of translocating. The other four responses are hypothesized to be mechanisms responsible for activation of the systemic inflammatory response.

7. B.

Bradykinin binds to endothelial cell receptors, which results in the synthesis of inducible nitric oxide synthase. The substrate of nitric oxide synthase is arginine, which results in the production of the paracrine mediator nitric oxide. Nitric oxide then mediates the vasodilation of bradykinin.

8. D.

Thromboxane A_2 is thought to be primarily released by platelets, and causes platelet aggregation and vasoconstriction. It is produced by the action of thromboxane synthetase as part of the prostaglandin cascade. It is not thought to be produced by mast cells or monocytes, and is presynthesized in platelets.

9. D.

Our current diagnostic capability does not allow us to differentiate the cause of SIRS. SIRS may be caused by invasive infection, but dissemination of the mediator signal may actually be the cause of the syndrome, not the actual dissemination of the microbe or endotoxin. SIRS may be caused by Gram-positive bacteria or fungi, neither of which have endotoxin. Thus, the future development of more sensitive bedside diagnostic capabilities allowing the clinician to detect patients where endotoxin is present may permit effective use of this potential treatment.

10. C.

Muramyl dipeptide is a component extracted from the cell wall of mycobacteria, and it has marked immunostimulatory effects. The other four mediators are part of CARS.

Chapter 4: Hemodynamic Monitoring and Ventilator Management in the Intensive Care Unit

Matthew O. Dolich, MD

Contents

1. Introduction

As inpatient hospital-based care shifts increasingly to the critically ill, a basic understanding of techniques of hemodynamic monitoring and mechanical ventilation is crucial. Trauma, emergency surgery, and extensive operative procedures often result in physiologic derangements necessitating a stay in the intensive care unit (ICU), and it is rare to encounter a patient in the ICU who does not require some type of hemodynamic monitoring or ventilatory assistance. The surgeon must maintain a thorough working knowledge of these techniques to provide optimal patient care.

2. Hemodynamic Monitoring and Management

Arterial Blood Pressure

Arterial blood pressure may be measured indirectly (by cuff) or by direct intravascular recording. The standard indirect method of arterial blood pressure measurement is by auscultation of Korotkoff sounds, which are generated when an inflated cuff placed on an extremity is gradually decompressed. Korotkoff sounds begin when an artery, completely occluded by cuff pressure, begins to open. Although the auscultory method is quite standard, it is prone to inaccuracy in hypotensive or critically ill patients, and is thus rarely used in the modern ICU. A more commonly utilized indirect technique of arterial blood pressure measurement is the oscillometric method (eg, Dinamap®). In this technique, oscillations produced by a partially compressed artery result in pressure changes in the cuff, allowing determination of systolic and diastolic pressures. Indirect determination of blood pressure by oscillometry is generally considered more reliable than auscultation; however, no indirect method is as accurate as direct, intravascular pressure monitoring.

For these reasons, most critically ill patients require arterial catheterization for continuous blood pressure monitoring. The most common sites for insertion of these catheters are the radial and femoral arteries, in order of preference. Other sites may be used as well, including dorsalis pedis, axillary, brachial and superficial temporal arteries. Although generally considered accurate, certain characteristics inherent with this technique bear further explanation. First, systolic pressure rises as the point of measurement moves peripherally from a location close to the heart. Thus, the systolic blood pressure may be 15-20 mm Hg higher when measured at the radial artery as compared to the aortic root. Additionally, since measurement of intravascular pressure involves the use of fluid-filled, rigid-walled tubing, a resonant system is created. Artifacts may be encountered if the system is underdamped (eg, if too long a length of tubing is used) or if the system is overdamped (eg, an air bubble is present within the tubing). An underdamped system will result in overestimation of the systolic blood pressure, whereas an overdamped system will underestimate systolic pressure. It should be noted that these artifacts do not, in general, affect mean arterial pressure measurements. Thus, mean arterial pressure is the preferred parameter to utilize when making patient care decisions.

Central Venous Pressure Monitoring

Central venous pressure (CVP) monitoring provides a relatively easy way to assess the volume status of the right side of the heart since, during diastole, CVP = right atrial pressure = right ventricular end diastolic pressure (EDP). In young, healthy patients right ventricular EDP provides a reasonable approximation of left ventricular EDP, and thus systemic preload. However, in the critically ill or in patients with cardiac disease, right-sided filling pressures may not accurately predict the volume status of the left heart. Thus, pulmonary artery catheterization should be considered in such patients when more accurate assessment of volume status and cardiac performance is deemed necessary. Central venous catheterization allows measurement of central venous O_2 saturation ($ScvO_2$) via blood gas analysis or oximetry. $ScvO_2$ is a relatively reliable surrogate for mixed venous oxygen saturation (obtainable only by more invasive pulmonary artery catheterization, as detailed below), and goal-directed therapy targeting $ScvO_2 > 70\%$ has been shown to improve mortality in septic patients.[1]

Pulmonary Artery Catheterization and Monitoring

The advent of pulmonary artery catheterization in 1970 revolutionized the practice of critical care medicine. This procedure is easily performed at the bedside in the ICU, and is particularly useful in guiding the resuscitation of patients in various types of shock, as well as elderly patients with impaired cardiac function. Considerable controversy exists regarding whether pulmonary artery catheterization improves outcome in critically ill patients,[2,3] but it is important to remember that the pulmonary artery catheter is simply a diagnostic tool, not a therapy in and of itself. Pulmonary artery catheterization allows accurate measurement of pulmonary artery occlusion pressure or wedge pressure (PAOP or PCWP). This parameter is transduced distal to a balloon inflated in a proximal pulmonary artery, allowing measurement of left atrial pressure through the pulmonary circulation. During diastole, left atrial pressure is identical to the left ventricular pressure, and left ventricular end diastolic pressure (LVEDP) is generally accepted as a reasonable surrogate for end diastolic volume (EDV) or preload. Thus, the PA catheter allows a much more accurate assessment of systemic preload as compared to CVP, particularly in patients with cardiac disease.

In addition to allowing assessment of intravascular volume status, pulmonary artery catheters provide a means of measuring cardiac performance. This is accomplished either by proximal injection of saline at a known temperature, or, in newer catheters, utilizing a filament to slightly heat blood as it flows along the catheter proximal to a thermistor that measures the temperature change at the distal end of the catheter. This technique, known as thermodilution, relies on the fact that the flow rate will be inversely proportional to the amount of temperature change measured by the thermistor. A cardiac output (C.O.) monitor, connected to the pulmonary artery catheter, generates a thermodilution curve (temperature vs. time); the integral of the area under the curve is inversely proportional to C.O.

Most pulmonary artery catheters have the ability to continuously measure mixed venous oxygen saturation (SvO_2) by reflectance spectrophotometry. A light emitting diode at the tip of the pulmonary artery catheter transmits red light into the surrounding blood in the pulmonary artery. The spectrum of reflected light varies with the ratio of oxygenated and deoxygenated hemoglobin, thus permitting calculation of SvO_2. The Fick equation reveals the determinants of SvO_2:

$$SvO_2 = SaO_2 - (VO_2/C.O. \times \text{hemoglobin} \times 13.4)$$

Decreased SvO_2 usually indicates increased oxygen consumption (VO_2) or inadequate cardiac performance resulting in oxygen debt. Poor arterial oxygenation and anemia may also contribute to low SvO_2. However, in certain physiologic states (eg, septic shock), cellular uptake of oxygen from the blood may be impaired. This results in supranormal SvO_2 measurement.

New developments in pulmonary artery catheter technology allow continuous measurement of right ventricular end diastolic volume (RVEDV) and right ventricular ejection fraction (RVEF). Although the RVEDV may overestimate left ventricular EDV, several studies suggest that RVEDV may be superior to PAOP as a surrogate for left ventricular preload.

Hemodynamic Agents

Dobutamine

Dobutamine is a synthetic catecholamine that predominantly affects β1 adrenergic receptors, resulting in increased stroke volume and cardiac output. It also acts as a mild β2 receptor agonist, resulting in systemic vasodilation. Dobutamine is best used in normotensive or hypertensive patients with inadequate perfusion secondary to poor cardiac performance. Vasodilation may be problematic in patients who have not received appropriate volume resuscitation prior to dobutamine infusion. In hypotensive patients with cardiogenic shock, dobutamine should be administered in conjunction with a vasopressor, in order to ameliorate the drug's vasodilatory effects. Tachycardia may be problematic in some patients, occasionally necessitating discontinuation of the drug. Typical dose is 5-15 mcg/kg/min.

Dopamine

Dopamine is an endogenously occurring catecholamine that functions as a neurotransmitter and a precursor to epinephrine. As a pharmacologic agent, dopamine has a variety of effects that are somewhat dose dependent. Low dose dopamine (1-3 mcg/kg/min) has agonistic effects on dopaminergic receptors in the splanchnic and renal circulatory beds, resulting in increased blood flow to these areas. Although low dose dopamine improves renal blood flow and urine output, it does not appear to have a protective or therapeutic effect in renal failure, and the use of "renal dose dopamine" with the goal of averting renal failure has little scientific support.[3,4] Higher doses of dopamine (3-10 mcg/kg/min) predominantly stimulate cardiac β receptors, resulting in a positive inotropic effect. It should be noted that the relative inotropic strength of dopamine is significantly less than that of dobutamine, epinephrine or isoproteronol. High dose dopamine (>10 mcg/kg/min) has increasing α adrenergic activity and resultant vasoconstriction. At these doses, increasing afterload diminishes the β receptor-mediated inotropic effect. It is important to note that the aforementioned dose ranges vary considerably from one individual to another.

Epinephrine

Epinephrine is an endogenous catecholamine secreted by the adrenal medulla. Like dopamine, it has dose-dependent α and β receptor agonist effects. However, the inotropic action of epinephrine is significantly higher than that of dopamine, and there is significant overlap between the α and β dose range for this drug. Typical response to epinephrine involves increasing inotropy with blood pressure increase secondary to vasoconstriction. Epinephrine is indicated in cardiac arrest, anaphylaxis and, in select patients, with cardiogenic shock and hypotension. Particular care is required in the administration of epinephrine in patients with coronary artery disease, as it increases myocardial oxygen consumption and may precipitate ischemia. Tachyarrhythmias may also occur. Nonetheless, epinephrine is a powerful inotrope and a valuable tool in the treatment of certain shock states. Usual dosage is 1-4 mcg/min by continuous infusion.

Phosphodiesterase Inhibitors: Amrinone and Milrinone

Amrinone and milrinone inhibit phosphodiesterase and thus result in decreased breakdown of cyclic AMP. This action, in turn, results in both increased cardiac contractility and systemic vasodilation. These drugs do not interact with α or β receptors and do not increase myocardial oxygen consumption. Therefore, they can be used as adjuncts to dobutamine. Indications for phosphodiesterase inhibition include cardiogenic shock in the setting of myocardial ischemia, and as a second-line agent in patients who do not tolerate dobutamine. The primary difference between amrinone and milrinone lies in their respective side effect profiles; milrinone is a second-generation agent that is associated with a lower incidence of thrombocytopenia than amrinone. Amrinone is administered as a bolus of 750 mcg/kg followed by an infusion of 5-10 mcg/kg/min. Milrinone is given as a 50 mcg/kg bolus over 10 minutes, followed by continuous infusion of 0.375-0.75 mcg/kg/min.

Norepinephrine
Norepinephrine is an α and β receptor agonist that increases systemic blood pressure and coronary blood flow. It may be a useful adjunct in myocardial infarction with hypotension due to these effects, resulting in improvements in myocardial oxygenation. Reflex bradycardia may occur as blood pressure rises to normal levels during norepinephrine infusion. Norepinephrine usage is not recommended in hypovolemic or hemorrhagic shock, as hypotension in these entities is due to intravascular volume loss rather than inappropriate vasomotor tone. Usual dosage range is 1-12 mcg/min.

Phenylephrine
Phenylephrine is an α adrenergic agonist that produces vasoconstriction and increases in systolic and diastolic blood pressure. Unlike epinephrine and norepinephrine, it has little effect on β receptors and thus has no inotropic value. Indications include certain shock states (eg, septic shock or spinal shock) manifesting low systemic vascular resistance with adequate circulating volume. Phenylephrine should not be used to maintain blood pressure in hypovolemic or hemorrhagic shock, as it may produce worsening ischemia, lactic acidosis and death. Phenylephrine may be given in boluses of 50 mcg intravenously, or by continuous infusion rates of 40-80 mcg/min.

Vasopressin
Vasopressin is a hormone that is endogenously produced in the hypothalamus and stored in the posterior pituitary gland. Although its primary action is to promote water retention by the kidney, it also stimulates V_1 receptors located in vascular smooth muscle, resulting in vasoconstriction. In septic and other distributive shock states, subnormal levels of vasopressin have been observed, leading to interest in using vasopressin infusion in non-hypovolemic shock states. Although large-scale studies are lacking, it appears that vasopressin infusion decreases exogenous catecholamine requirements in septic shock, and thus may be a useful adjunct in certain circumstances. Dosage for distributive shock states is 0.01-0.08 units/min.

Fenoldopam
Fenoldopam is a selective dopamine-1 receptor agonist that produces renal vasodilation and, at higher doses, systemic vasodilation. It is currently approved by the Food and Drug Administration for treatment of hypertension and may be used as a substitute for intravenous nitroglycerin or nitroprusside. Early studies have revealed the possibility of a renal protective effect at low doses (in contrast to dopamine); however, large-scale prospective studies are lacking at this time.[4,5]

3. Mechanical Ventilation

Parameters Determining Oxygenation

FiO_2

Fractional concentration of inspired oxygen (FiO_2) may range from 21% (room air at sea level) to 100%. FiO_2 levels > 60% may be associated with oxygen toxicity; thus efforts should be made to minimize the duration of patient exposure to high FiO_2 levels. However, severe respiratory failure occasionally mandates prolonged periods of high FiO_2, lest the patient expire from hypoxemia. Generally, FiO_2 should be set at the lowest level that provides a $PaO_2 > 70$ or O_2 saturation of 93-100%. Typically FiO_2 levels of 0.3-0.4 accomplish this goal in patients without acute respiratory failure.

PEEP

Positive end expiratory pressure (PEEP) involves setting a valve in the expiratory limb of the ventilator circuit that prevents alveolar pressure from dropping back to atmospheric pressure at the end of expiration. The major physiologic effect of PEEP is to prevent alveolar collapse that tends to occur at the end of expiration. This increases the number of alveoli participating in gas exchange, improves oxygenation and increases lung compliance when the lungs are stiff (as in ARDS). Thus, PEEP may be used to allow less toxic FiO_2 levels during severe respiratory failure. Although 5 cm H_2O of PEEP is considered the physiologic equivalent of that which occurs during glottic closure in spontaneous respiration, little scientific evidence supports this theory. Despite this, 3-5 cm H_2O of PEEP is frequently applied as a minimum level and probably has little overall effect. PEEP increases mean intrathoracic pressure, which can compromise cardiac output by diminishing venous return.

Parameters Determining Ventilation

Tidal Volume (V_T)

Tidal volume is the volume of gas delivered by the ventilator during each assisted breath. Traditionally, tidal volumes have been set between 10-15 mL/kg during mechanical ventilation; however, newer research suggests that low tidal volume ventilation (eg, 6-8 mL/kg) improves survival and decreases complications in the setting of severe respiratory distress syndrome (ARDS) and acute lung injury (ALI).[6] Increasing tidal volume increases minute ventilation (defined as respiratory rate x V_T) and therefore decreases $PaCO_2$.

Respiratory Rate (RR)

Respiratory rate is simply defined as the number of full ventilator breaths/minute, and is typically set between 10-16 in a patient with no spontaneous respiratory effort. Increasing respiratory rate generally decreases arterial $PaCO_2$.

Pressure Support Ventilation (PSV)

Pressure support ventilation refers to augmented spontaneous breathing. In this mode, the negative inspiratory force associated with a spontaneous breath triggers a sensor within the ventilator circuit to augment that breath to a predetermined pressure. This pressure support level is usually set between 5-10 cm H_2O (to overcome the work of breathing associated with an endotracheal tube and ventilator circuit) although levels up to 25 cm H_2O may be required in significantly deconditioned patients. Pressure support decreases work of breathing and increases spontaneous tidal volumes, thus improving ventilation and decreasing $PaCO_2$.

Modes of Ventilation

Assist Control Ventilation (AC)

Assist control is the standard mode of volume-cycled mechanical ventilation and the easiest to understand. Parameters that may be set include FiO_2, tidal volume, respiratory rate and PEEP. In an apneic patient, the ventilator will deliver equally spaced tidal volumes at the set respiratory rate. In the non-apneic patient, a spontaneous breath triggers the ventilator to administer an "assisted" breath of the same preset tidal volume. This assisted breath is identical to the non-assisted "control" breath. Thus, spontaneously breathing patients with rapid respiratory rates may quickly develop respiratory alkalosis when on AC ventilation.

Synchronized Intermittent Mandatory Ventilation (SIMV)

This mode of ventilation was developed to ameliorate the problems associated with high respiratory rates during AC ventilation. SIMV allows spontaneous, augmented ventilation between machine breaths, and the microprocessor in the ventilator synchronizes the machine breaths to coincide with spontaneous ventilatory efforts. This prevents the ventilator from administering a machine breath when the patient is exhaling spontaneously (an occurrence which is quite uncomfortable for the patient). Basic parameters that may be set in SIMV mode are FiO_2, tidal volume, respiratory rate, PEEP and pressure support. As outlined above, the amount of pressure support will determine the amount of augmentation of spontaneous breathing. In an apneic patient, there is no functional difference between AC and SIMV.

Pressure Controlled Ventilation (PCV)
The first positive pressure ventilators worked by the technique of pressure controlled ventilation. In this mode, the ventilator delivers sufficient inspiratory flow to keep a constant, preset pressure within the circuit. This preset drive pressure, when added to the set PEEP value, defines the total peak inspiratory pressure. Thus, the tidal volume delivered varies inversely with the compliance of the lungs, as stiff lungs cause a rapid rise in pressure despite relatively small volumes of administered gas. Because pressure is held constant, inspiratory flow decreases exponentially during inflation of the lungs. This decreases overall peak pressure and may improve gas exchange. For these reasons, PCV has enjoyed renewed interest in severe ARDS, when barotrauma and volutrauma associated with high ventilatory pressures may worsen lung injury. However, ventilation may significantly decrease if the lung compliance worsens over a short period of time.

Inverse Ratio Ventilation (IRV)
Under normal circumstances, the inspiratory/expiratory (I:E) ratio during mechanical ventilation is between 1:2 and 1:4. This ratio allows adequate time for complete exhalation of alveolar gas. In cases of severe hypoxemia, this ratio can be increased to 1:1 or 2:1 by decreasing the inspiratory flow rate. This maneuver is usually performed in conjunction with pressure-controlled ventilation, and is known as PC-IRV. A longer inspiration time, like PEEP, improves alveolar recruitment and helps prevent alveolar collapse. The net result is an improvement in PaO_2; however, incomplete emptying of the lungs may occur. This phenomenon, known as auto-PEEP, may result in high intrathoracic pressures and impaired cardiac performance. Modern microprocessor-controlled ventilators allow determination of auto-PEEP, which should be considered in addition to extrinsically applied PEEP.

High Frequency Oscillatory Ventilation (HFOV)
In contrast with conventional modes of mechanical ventilation, HFOV utilizes an oscillating piston to generate very small tidal volumes at a very high frequency (eg, 5 Hz, or 300 breaths/minute). This oscillation generates a relatively high mean airway pressure that facilitates diffusion of oxygen and carbon dioxide, and therefore, alveolar gas exchange. It is believed that the characteristics of HFOV facilitate alveolar recruitment, while decreasing the incidence of ventilator-induced lung injury. For several decades, this mode of ventilation had been used successfully on neonates with respiratory distress syndrome and pediatric patients with severe respiratory failure. More recently, this technique has been utilized as a rescue mode of ventilation in adult patients with ARDS.[7,8]

Continuous Positive Airways Pressure (CPAP)
In this mode of ventilation, spontaneous respiration occurs and the pressure within the ventilator circuit is not allowed to drop below a preset value. In pure CPAP ventilation, a negative inspiratory force is not required to generate flow of gas from the ventilator. CPAP is frequently combined with pressure support ventilation to facilitate weaning patients from mechanical ventilatory support.

Criteria For Weaning and Discontinuation of Mechanical Ventilation
Multiple bedside assessment tools are available for prediction of successful weaning and extubation of mechanically ventilated patients. Patients being considered for extubation should be requiring an FiO_2 of less than 0.5 and PEEP of 5 cm H_2O or less. Minute ventilation should be less than 10 L/min. The patient should be hemodynamically stable, able to follow commands and able to maintain an airway. Pulmonary secretions should be relatively minimal. Patients who are considered ready for weaning from mechanical ventilation should undergo a 30-120 minute spontaneous breathing trial (SBT) on CPAP or T-piece ventilation, with assessment of respiratory rate/V_T ratio. This ratio, known as the rapid shallow breathing index (RSBI), is a valuable bed-

side assessment of a patient's ability to wean and separate from mechanical ventilation.[9] RSBI > 100/L suggests rapid shallow respiration consistent with ongoing pulmonary failure. Conversely, patients with RSBI < 100/L can generally be weaned from mechanical ventilation.

4. References

1. Dellinger RP, Levy MM, Carlet JM, et al. Surviving Sepsis Campaign: International guidelines for management of severe sepsis and septic shock, 2008. *Crit Care Med*. 2008;36:296-327.

2. Connors AF, Speroff T, Dawson NV, et al. The effectiveness of right heart catheterization in the initial care of critically ill patients. SUPPORT Investigators. *JAMA*. 1996;276(11):889-897.

3. Mimoz O, Rauss A, Rekik N, Brun-Buisson C, Lemaire F, Brochard L. Pulmonary artery catheterization in critically ill patients: a prospective analysis of outcome changes associated with catheter-prompted changes in therapy. *Crit Care Med*. 1994;22(4):573-579.

4. Kellum JA, Decker MJ. Use of dopamine in acute renal failure: a meta-analysis. *Crit Care Med*. 2001;29(8):1526-1531.

5. Stone GW, McCullough PA, Tumlin JA, et al. Fenoldopam mesylate for the prevention of contrast-induced nephropathy. *JAMA*. 2003;290:2284-2291.

6. The Acute Respiratory Distress Syndrome Network. Ventilation with lower tidal volumes as compared with traditional tidal volumes for acute lung injury and the acute respiratory distress syndrome. *N Engl J Med*. 2000; 342(18):1301-1308.

7. Kao K, Tsai Y, Wu Y, Huang C, Shih M, Huang C. High frequency oscillatory ventilation for surgical patients with acute respiratory distress syndrome. *J Trauma*. 2006;61:837-843.

8. Derdak S. High-frequency oscillatory ventilation for acute respiratory distress syndrome in adult patients. *Crit Care Med*. 2003;31(4):S317-S323.

9. MacIntyre N. Discontinuing mechanical ventilatory support. *Chest*. 2007;132(3):1049-1056.

5. Questions

1. Which of the following parameters is least likely to be inaccurate secondary to measurement limitations?

   A. Systolic blood pressure

   B. Diastolic blood pressure

   C. Mean arterial pressure

   D. Pulmonary capillary wedge pressure

2. Which of the following are determinants of oxygen consumption?

   A. Mean arterial pressure

   B. Hemoglobin level

   C. Pulmonary capillary wedge pressure

   D. Mixed venous oxygen saturation

   E. Systemic vascular resistance

3. An ICU patient is found to have the following hemodynamic and ventilatory parameters after sustaining a 30-foot fall and a closed head injury:

   blood pressure = 110/70 mm Hg

   PCWP = 16 mm Hg

   cardiac index = 1.9 L/min/m^2

   cardiac output = 4.1 L/min

   SaO_2 = 98%

   lactate 5.6 mmol/L

   hemoglobin = 12 mg/dL

   Which of the following would be the most appropriate intervention?

   A. Norepinephrine infusion

   B. Phenylephrine infusion

   C. Dopamine infusion

   D. Dobutamine infusion

4. With regard to the use of vasopressors and inotropes in shock, which of the following statements is/are true?

   A. In the setting of hemorrhagic shock, phenylephrine infusion should be instituted early to maintain mean arterial pressure and tissue perfusion

   B. Use of vasopressors in hemorrhage shock may be harmful

   C. Young, otherwise healthy patients do not require use of inotropic agents to support tissue perfusion

   D. Phenylephrine exerts its predominant effect on cardiac β receptors

   E. All of the above statements are true

5. A burn patient in the ICU for 2 weeks now has gram negative bacteremia, leukocytosis, and fever. Cultures are sent, and broad spectrum antibiotic coverage is begun.

   Hemodynamic parameters include:

   heart rate = 130 beats/min

   blood pressure = 70/40 mm Hg

   PCWP = 16 mm Hg

   cardiac output = 12 L/min

   cardiac index = 7 L/min/m^2

   hemoglobin = 13 mg/dL

Appropriate interventions include which of the following?

A. Dobutamine infusion

B. Esmolol infusion

C. Phenylephrine infusion

D. Calcium channel blockade

E. Vasopressin infusion

6. Which of the following may be measured by pulmonary artery catheterization?

A. Left ventricular end diastolic volume (LVEDV)

B. Right ventricular end diastolic volume (RVEDV)

C. Left ventricular ejection fraction (LVEF)

D. Right ventricular ejection fraction (RVEF)

7. Following an emergent colon resection for perforated diverticulitis, a 76-year-old man has been oliguric for two hours. Two liters of normal saline have been given intravenously, without significant improvement in urine output. The correct therapeutic measure at this point would be:

A. Pulmonary artery catheterization

B. Administration of 5% albumin solution

C. Administration of a loop diuretic

D. Administration of dopamine intravenously at 3mcg/kg/min

E. Administration of 1 additional intravenous fluid bolus

8. Renal failure in the critically ill can be prevented by which of the following maneuvers?

A. Low dose dopamine infusion

B. Low dose fenoldopam infusion

C. Strict avoidance of aminoglycoside antibiotics

D. A. and B.

E. None of the above

9. Which of the following represent appropriate ventilator settings for a 70 kg patient with moderately severe ARDS?

A. Rate = 18, $FiO_2 = 0.6$, PEEP = 12 cm H_2O, Pressure support = 10 cm H_20, Tidal volume = 0.5 liter

B. Rate = 18, $FiO_2 = 0.6$, PEEP = 12 cm H_2O, Pressure support = 5 cm H_2O, Tidal volume = 1.0 liter

C. Rate = 16, $FiO_2 = 0.4$, PEEP = 18 cm H_2O, Pressure support = 10 cm H_2O, Tidal volume = 0.5 liter

D. Rate = 16, $FiO_2 = 0.9$, PEEP = 5 cm H_2O, Pressure support = 10 cm H_2O, Tidal volume = 1.0 liter

E. CPAP = 5 cm H_20, $FiO_2 = 0.9$, Pressure support = 5 cm H_2O

10. Predictors of successful discontinuation of mechanical ventilation include which of the following?

A. RSBI = 120/min/L

B. RSBI = 60/min/L

C. PaO_2/ FiO_2 = 180

D. PaO_2/ FiO_2 = 300

E. Maximal inspiratory force = -15 cm H_2O

Answers

1. C.
All blood pressure measurements are subject to inaccuracy due to limitations of measuring equipment. However, these variations tend to cancel each other when the mean arterial pressure is calculated as (systolic blood pressure + 2 x diastolic blood pressure)/3, or when measured by direct intravascular catheterization.

2. B., D.
Oxygen consumption is determined by the Fick equation:
VO_2 = C.O. x Hemoglobin x 13.4 x (SaO_2 - SvO_2).
Thus, hemoglobin level, cardiac output, arterial oxygen saturation and mixed venous oxygen saturation affect oxygen consumption.

3. D.
The patient is in a state of compensated shock, with a relatively normal blood pressure but lactic acidosis suggesting inadequate perfusion. The patient's oxygen saturation and hemoglobin level are acceptable, but the cardiac index is abnormally low. Therefore, augmentation of the cardiac index with an inotropic agent such as dobutamine would most effectively improve oxygen delivery in this patient.

4. B.
The use of vasopressors such as phenylephrine (an α adrenergic agonist) to maintain blood pressure in the setting of hemorrhagic shock has been associated with increased mortality rates and should be avoided. Appropriate interventions include volume resuscitation with isotonic IV fluids and transfusion of blood products. Not infrequently, young, otherwise healthy patients will display poor cardiac performance during or after resuscitation from a shock state; in this circumstance, inotropic support is indicated.

5. C., E.
The patient is manifesting clinical signs of septic shock, including tachycardia, hypotension, fever and leukocytosis. In the setting of distributive shock with normal or elevated cardiac output, judicious administration of a pressor agent such as phenylephrine or vasopressin is appropriate once adequate volume status has been established.

6. B., D.
Newer pulmonary artery catheters have the capacity to measure RVEF by thermodilution, in a manner similar to cardiac output measurement. Dividing stroke volume by RVEF yields RVEDV. LVEF and LVEDV are most commonly measured by echocardiography.

7. A.
In the elderly postoperative patient, oliguria may occur for a multitude of reasons. Initial administration of crystalloid solutions may improve urine output; however, a poor response should prompt a more aggressive assessment of intravascular volume status. In this circumstance, diuresis in the setting of intravascular volume depletion may have deleterious results. Placement of a pulmonary artery catheter would facilitate fluid management in this oliguric patient with clinical signs of volume overload.

8. E.

Renal failure remains a common entity in the intensive care unit, and its prevention is based largely on adequate resuscitation principles and control of septic foci. Neither dopamine nor fenoldopam have shown definitive evidence of renal failure prevention in controlled studies to date. Aminoglycoside antibiotics, when dosed and monitored appropriately, remain a very rare cause of renal failure in the ICU.

9. A.

Patients with ARDS are hypoxemic and frequently require high PEEP and FiO_2 levels. PEEP and FiO_2 should be adjusted to minimize the deleterious effects of each; eg, compromised cardiac performance and oxygen toxicity, respectively. Thus, combinations of high PEEP and low FiO_2 or vice versa are best avoided. Additionally, low tidal volume ventilation (6-8 mL/kg) has been shown to improve survival in ARDS.

10. B., D.

Rapid, shallow breathing is suggestive of failure of weaning mechanical ventilation. A frequency/volume ratio (RR/V_T) of greater than 105 accurately predicts failure of weaning mechanical ventilation. PaO_2/FiO_2 values of 200 or less are consistent with severe respiratory failure and should prompt ongoing ventilatory support. Maximal inspiratory force, another bedside predictor of successful extubation, should be at least -25 cm H_2O (normal is greater than -90 cm H_2O).

Chapter 5: Infection in Solid Organ Transplant Recipients

David L. Dunn, MD, PhD

Contents

1. Risk Assessment

General Principles

Definition, Epidemiology and Pathophysiology

Solid organ transplantation is the cornerstone of therapy for renal, hepatic, cardiac, pulmonary, pancreatic endocrine (diabetic), and more recently, small intestinal severe dysfunction or failure. After technical advances allowed performance of kidney, liver, heart, lung, pancreas and intestinal transplantation, concurrent significant advances in two areas led to increased success as measured by decreased patient morbidity and mortality and increased allograft survival. These recent advancements consist of refinements and development of new immunosuppressive drugs and antimicrobial agents. Until recently, all immunosuppressive drugs suppressed one or more components of the host immune system, preventing rejection of the allograft, but also rendering the transplant recipient susceptible to a wide variety of microbial pathogens. With today's new agents it is possible to develop immunological tolerance to foreign tissue antigens without diminishing innate antimicrobial defenses. Several general guidelines apply regarding immunosuppressed patients: any organism can be pathogenic and cause infection, including low virulence and so-called opportunistic microbes that rarely cause disease in normal individuals; virulent organisms that cause minor infection in the normal individual can cause severe, rapidly fatal infection in immunosuppressed patients; and the signs and symptoms of infection (eg, fever, cough, pain, erythema, purulent drainage) that occur in patients with an intact immune system may be significantly diminished or absent in the immunosuppressed solid organ transplant recipient.[1] Epidemiologic data indicate that about 60%-70% of solid organ transplant recipients may develop infection requiring medical attention at some point within the first several years after the procedure.[2] Bacterial, fungal, viral and occasionally parasitic pathogens are etiologic, and some of these organisms are opportunistic pathogens capable of causing infection in these patients. Many if not all of these organisms are effectively eradicated by cellular immune mechanisms in normal individuals, particularly viral and fungal pathogens, hence the increased incidence of infection from these pathogens, as well as from certain unusual bacteria, in solid organ transplant recipients.

History

Immunosuppressed patients who develop fever (oral temperature >100.5° F), malaise, or other so-called nonspecific constitutional symptoms, or who have any specific complaints such as headache, neck pain, myalgias, lethargy, cough, abdominal pain, skin lesions or subcutaneous nodules, evidence of purulent drainage, or genitourinary or gastrointestinal symptoms must be thoroughly evaluated to exclude the presence of a serious infection. First and foremost, a thorough medical history must be obtained with particular attention paid to quantify and identify significant risk factors that predispose toward infection. These include:

- Exogenous immunosuppression (agents, dosage, temporal duration), invariably in greater use within the first 6 months post-transplant;
- Use of an organ from a cadaver source, because these recipients generally receive higher doses of immunosuppressive agents compared to patients who receive organs donated by close living relatives;
- Antirejection therapy, particularly with antilymphocyte antibody drugs or more than several courses of antirejection therapy given in close temporal association with immunosuppressive agent(s);
- Pretransplant disease processes such as dental caries, bronchitis or pneumonia, chronic cholecystitis, peptic ulcer disease, and diverticulitis, many of which are treatable and should be dealt with prior to transplantation;
- Latent infection such as from cytomegalovirus (CMV), that can reactivate during significant immunosuppression, or transmission of latent infection via donor tissue (blood transfusion, allograft), both of which can be reduced by antiviral agent prophylaxis;
- Prior post-transplant infection(s), because a number of these infections recrudesce despite apparent initial eradication; and
- Transplant patients not receiving trimethoprim-sulfamethoxazole (TMP-SMX) to prevent UTI, because they are more likely to develop infection

due to microbes sensitive to this agent *(Nocardia asteroides, Listeria monocytogenes, Legionella pneumophila, Pneumocystis carinii* and *Toxoplasma gondii)*.[3]

After initial assessment of the above factors, more detailed information related to a specific organ system that may be the target of infection, and constellations of symptoms common to particular pathogens should be elucidated. These are detailed later in this chapter.

Physical Findings

The physical examination must be thorough, encompassing all parts of the body, with particular attention directed toward those organ systems identified in the history that may harbor infection. Examination of the integument and a search for subcutaneous lesions should be undertaken, since several opportunistic pathogens cause systemic disease including vesicles, erythema nodosum and subcutaneous nodules. In addition, soft tissue infections may produce only mild erythema and surgical wound infection is not invariably associated with purulent drainage; rather, serous drainage may be observed. Mild photophobia and pain upon neck flexion even without nuchal rigidity should make one suspicious of central nervous system (CNS) infection. The oropharynx should be examined because many viral and fungal pathogens manifest infection at this site and can be readily identified. Percussion and auscultation of the chest and heart may reveal evidence of pleural or pericardial effusion or pulmonary consolidation that requires further examination. Mild abdominal tenderness, even without rebound may occur in the presence of an abdominal catastrophe such as a perforated viscus with severe fibrinopurulent peritonitis. The presence of hematuria or hematochezia mandates a thorough evaluation of the genitourinary and gastrointestinal systems, respectively, to exclude the presence of infection or other disease processes.

Laboratory Tests

Standard tests needed to establish the diagnosis of infection are extensive and include: white blood cell (WBC) count, differential, peripheral smear, hemoglobin, electrolytes, glucose, blood urea nitrogen (BUN), creatinine, bilirubin and liver enzymes, amylase or lipase, chest x-ray, and abdominal flat plate and upright x-rays if abdominal symptoms or signs are present. Samples of blood, urine, sputum, bronchoalveolar lavage (BAL) fluid, cerebrospinal fluid and any other potentially infected fluid or tissue should be sent to the microbiology laboratory for analysis with Gram's and Ziehl-Neelsen stains and KOH preparation to identify bacterial, acid-fast bacterial, and fungal pathogens, respectively, and the samples should also be cultured for the same pathogens. Additional tests to identify specific opportunistic pathogens, particularly bacteria and viruses that are difficult to identify with culture techniques in a timely fashion, are discussed below.

Management

Administration of appropriate antimicrobial therapy is critical for all infectious disease processes in immunosuppressed patients. However, many types of infection (eg, secondary bacterial peritonitis due to perforation of a hollow viscus) require surgical intervention as the primary therapeutic modality, with concurrent administration of antibiotics. In addition, the presence of serious infection in an immunosuppressed patient demands reevaluation of their immunosuppressive drug regimen; life-threatening infection or serious deterioration in condition during treatment of any infection mandates withdrawal of one or more agents, and reduction in the dose of steroids to minimal levels must also be strongly considered. For those transplant recipients for whom alternate forms of therapy to support vital functions exist (eg, kidney, hemodialysis; pancreas, exogenous insulin; intestine, hyperalimentation), the decision to reduce the level of exogenous immunosuppression and possibly increase the risk of organ rejection is less difficult than for heart, lung and liver transplant recipients, who have no alternate therapy available. However, rejection is rare after withdrawal of immunosuppression among patients who are seriously ill due to infection, probably due to the extent to which endogenous host defenses are diminished.

2. Perioperative Infections

Common Bacterial and Polymicrobial Infections

Definition, Epidemiology and Pathophysiology

During the initial 1-2 months after solid organ transplantation, patients may develop a wide variety of infections due to organisms—primarily bacteria—that cause infection in normal individuals as well. Concurrently and thereafter, these patients are subject to infection due to opportunistic pathogens. Thus urinary tract infection (UTI), pneumonia, superficial and deep surgical wound infection, and intraabdominal infection occur more frequently after solid organ transplantation. Perhaps not surprisingly, many such infections are related to the organ transplanted. Thus, renal transplant recipients are prone to develop UTIs, and liver, pancreas and bowel transplant patients are at risk for intraabdominal infection, while heart and lung transplant patients exhibit a predilection toward developing pneumonia. During the first 3-6 months after transplantation, UTIs and pneumonia may be caused by Gram-negative or Gram-positive aerobes; after 6 months fungi become more frequent pathogens.[4] Superficial and deep (intraabdominal) wound infections occur in ~1% of renal or heart transplant patients, but are more common among pancreas and kidney-pancreas, liver, and small bowel transplant patients (~10%-35%), while liver, lung and heart-lung recipients exhibit a risk of wound infection between these two extremes.[5] Intraabdominal infection due to a perforated viscus is initially caused by aerobes and anaerobes. Unfortunately, these patients frequently suffer ongoing intraperitoneal infection, called tertiary peritonitis, in which infection abscesses do not form, and organisms normally of low virulence, such as *Staphylococcus epidermidis, Enterococcus fecalis* and *fecium, Candida albicans* and *Pseudomonas aeruginosa* persist.[6] The mortality associated with this condition remains ~50%-80%. This disease process is also associated with initial periallograft infection in pancreas transplant patients. Overall, CNS infection is rare, and those cases that do occur are more commonly caused by fungi than by bacteria. Bacteremia and sepsis syndrome are associated with higher rates of mortality in this patient population (~50%-70%), so if these infections are not diagnosed and treated expeditiously, any one of them can be fatal.[7]

History

Immunosuppressive drug therapy causes a lessening of host defenses such that common symptoms and signs of infection are masked. Thus, even mild symptoms such as dysuria, cough, abdominal pain or headache should be intensively investigated, because they may be indicative of serious infection.

Physical Findings

Just as symptoms may be minimized, on physical examination signs of infection may be reduced or absent, even in the presence of life-threatening infection. For example, patients who suffer gastroduodenal or colonic perforation may show minimal voluntary and involuntary guarding during abdominal palpation, and rebound may be completely absent. Even serious, aggressive wound infection may not cause any apparent wound erythema or drainage of purulent fluid. Similarly, large, space-occupying CNS lesions due to infection may not be associated with significant mental status changes or abnormalities upon neurological examination, so findings of even minimal symptoms during physical examination of the abdomen warrants additional diagnostic studies.

Laboratory Tests

As noted above, a number of routine laboratory and radiographic studies should be obtained if infection is suspected. In addition to these routine tests, CT scans of the chest may better define pulmonary lesions, CT scans of the abdomen can provide clear evidence of serious intraabdominal or periallograft infection, and CT or MRI scans of the cranium may help identify CNS infection if intracerebral masses are present.

Management

Antimicrobial therapy should focus on the bacterial pathogens likely to be present at the site of disease, and such therapy should be administered after samples have been obtained for microbiological, immunologica and pathological analysis. However, therapy should not be withheld until the diagnosis is obtained in most patients because of the potentially life-threatening nature of many infections, and agents that are not toxic to organs (particularly the allograft) should be selected if possible. Adjustments in therapy can be made after culture and sensitivity data become available. For example, UTIs and pneumonia are often due to Gram-negative aerobes for which a fluoroquinolone can be administered; those due to *Candida albicans* can be treated with fluconazole. The presence of severe pneumonia mandates parenteral therapy, and third-generation cephalosporin or carbapenem agents often are suitable. Initial antibiotic therapy for intraabdominal infection associated with secondary bacterial peritonitis may require a single potent agent to treat Gram-negative aerobes and anaerobes (eg, carbapenem [imipenem-cilastatin or meropenem]), or an extended-spectrum penicillin plus a β-lactamase inhibitor (piperacillin-tazobactam). Antimicrobial agents typically administered for the treatment of tertiary peritonitis include one of the previously mentioned broad-spectrum agents plus vancomycin, plus either amphotericin B or fluconazole. Severe periallograft infection generally necessitates removal of the transplanted organ in kidney, pancreas, kidney-pancreas and small bowel transplant patients in whom the transplant is not lifesaving; obviously this type of disease in heart, lung, heart-lung and liver transplant recipients must be managed with the allograft *in situ*. In many cases, repeated exploration may be necessary even after initial allograft removal. Agents with a high degree of penetration (eg, ceftriaxone) should be selected for meningitis due to Gram-negative aerobes. Treatment of fungal meningitis other than that due to *Cryptococcus neoformans* may require parenteral as well as intrathecal amphotericin B; lumbar puncture should always be repeated after the termination of therapy. It is important to remember that while the patient is undergoing antimicrobial agent therapy a concurrent reduction in immunosuppressive drug therapy must be considered.

3. Opportunistic Bacterial Infections

Nocardiosis

Definition, Epidemiology and Pathophysiology

Nocardia asteroides (and rarely *N braziliensis, transvalensis, farcinica* and *otididiscaviarum*) are opportunistic bacteria that can cause serious infection in the immunosuppressed host.[8] Pulmonary, CNS, dermal, eye, joint and disseminated disease alone or in combination can occur, although the first two species listed above are the most common (80%-90% and 30%-40% of cases, respectively). Pulmonary disease is associated with a ~25%-50% incidence of mortality, while the fatality rate exceeds 50% among patients who develop CNS infection.

History

Patients who develop nocardiosis generally exhibit nonspecific clinical findings. Typical symptoms associated with pulmonary disease are fever, anorexia, productive cough, dyspnea, pleuritic chest pain and occasionally hemoptysis, while patients who develop CNS disease may present with confusion and complain of headache.

Physical Findings

Patients who harbor pulmonary nodules or small CNS abscesses may have no significant physical findings. However, patients who develop lobular or lobar pneumonia, cavitary disease, or a pleural effusion may exhibit consolidation upon percussion and decreased breath sounds upon auscultation. Absence of spontaneous venous pulsations or papilledema upon retinoscopy may indicate the presence of a large CNS lesion. Subcutaneous nodules in addition to either of the above mentioned findings associated with either pulmonary, CNS, or both types of disease should make the clinician extremely suspicious that the patient has developed nocardiosis.

Laboratory Tests

The chest radiograph may reveal the presence of nodular infiltrates and lobular or lobar consolidation, the latter with or without cavitation. A pleural effusion may be present. Bilateral disease is common in the presence of any of these findings. Among patients in whom this diagnosis is suspected, a cranial CT should be performed, and if this test is unrevealing, a magnetic resonance imaging

(MRI) study of the cranium should be undertaken. Either cranial CT or MRI may reveal the presence of numerous small ring-enhancing lesions, or less commonly a single large abscess. Sputum samples should be obtained and subcutaneous nodules should be aspirated or biopsied. In some patients, the diagnosis can only be established by limited lung biopsy via resection when small lesions are present, or percutaneous aspiration of larger (>1.5-2 cm) pulmonary lesions. Patients who develop solely CNS disease may require percutaneous sampling as well. Bacteria in long strings that resemble beaded filaments that stain blue (Gram-positive) on Gram's stain and are acid fast with Ziehl-Neelsen stain are indicative of the presence of *Nocardia* spp. The organism may take 1-3 weeks to grow in culture, so the staining results are exceedingly important to direct initial therapy.

Management

Either high-dose sulfisoxazole or TMP-SMX should be administered for 3-4 months to patients who develop nocardiosis. A second agent such as imipenem-cilastatin, amikacin or ceftriaxone should be administered during the initial 14-21 days, the particular agent being selected empirically but continued based on *in vitro* antibiotic sensitivity testing. Patients who are not allergic to sulfa drugs and who previously have not received TMP-SMX should take it daily thereafter for life. Occasionally, areas of pulmonary cavitation do not regress and may require drainage or resection of the involved portion of lung. Also, subcutaneous lesions may suppurate, necessitating incision, drainage and wound management to facilitate healing by secondary intention.

Listeriosis

Definition, Epidemiology and Pathophysiology

Listeria monocytogenes is a motile Gram-positive bacillus that requires cell-mediated immunity for eradication. The most common presentation is that associated with meningitis or cerebritis, which may be associated with pneumonia or bacteremia.[9] Although this disease process no longer commonly occurs, prior reports indicate that this infection is associated with a mortality rate of ~25%.

History

Patients may complain of headache, neck pain, and photophobia, although vague neurological complaints are not unusual. The presence of fever, malaise or cough is variable. Several risk factors for infection are invariably present. Patients for whom TMP-SMX is not prescribed, those who are unable to receive it due to allergy, or those patients who are noncompliant regarding self administration are at higher risk to develop infection due to this organism. It rarely, if ever, causes infection among patients receiving this drug.

Physical Findings

Nuchal rigidity and photophobia are the most common physical findings. No other unique manifestations occur.

Laboratory Tests

A chest radiograph and a computed tomographic (CT) study of the cranium should be obtained, following which a lumbar puncture should be performed unless there is evidence of a cerebral mass, and blood cultures should be obtained. Lumbar puncture may reveal the presence of elevated cerebrospinal fluid pressure, >100 WBCs, low glucose level, and small Gram-positive bacilli on Gram's stain. Observation of Gram-positive coccoid organisms in pairs coupled with the absence of growth in routine media should make one suspicious of the presence of this pathogen.

Management

Ampicillin plus an aminoglycoside should be administered parenterally for 14-21 days. A reduction in immunosuppressive therapy should be considered in all patients, particularly those who are seriously ill from the outset or exhibit evidence of clinical deterioration. Several days after antibiotic therapy has been halted, lumbar puncture should be repeated.

Legionella Infection

Definition, Epidemiology and Pathophysiology

Legionella pneumophila and *L micdadei* cause pulmonary infection in solid organ transplant patients on occasion.[10] Based upon reported small series of patients in the extant literature, the incidence of pulmonary infection due to these pathogens in this patient population is probably less than 1%. In most cases, a contaminated hospital water supply is responsible for an outbreak, although sporadic cases occur as well. Patients who are receiving TMP-SMX prophylaxis rarely if ever become infected.

History

The vast majority of patients who develop infection due to this organism do so within the first 3 months after transplantation or subsequent to antirejection therapy. Typically, they complain of a flu-like illness, fever, and may admit to a nonproductive cough. Few other manifestations occur.

Physical Findings

The only findings of note upon examination are rales and crackles during pulmonary auscultation. No other manifestations of this pathogen have been described.

Laboratory Tests

The chest radiograph usually reveals the presence of bilateral, patchy lobular or diffuse interstitial infiltrates. Patients with these findings should undergo bronchoscopy, bronchoalveolar lavage (BAL) specimens should be obtained, and direct immunofluorescence and cultures for *Legionella* should be performed. Because *Legionella* spp. are obligate anaerobes with fastidious growth requirements, bronchoscopy is more reliable in establishing the diagnosis, although cultures are more sensitive and will be confirmatory.

Management

In institutions where *Legionella* is endemic, empiric therapy consisting of parenteral erythromycin plus either rifampin or azithromycin, clarithromycin or ciprofloxacin should be instituted in seriously ill patients concurrent with diagnostic evaluation. Once the diagnosis is established, patients should receive these agents for 21-28 days. Depending on the severity of pulmonary disease, consideration should be given to decreasing doses of immunosuppressive agents as well.

Mycobacterial Infections

Definition, Epidemiology and Pathophysiology

Mycobacterial infections occur in ~0.1%-1% of solid organ transplant recipients, the incidence being higher in undeveloped countries. *Mycobacterium tuberculosis* accounts for ~60% of cases, while the remainder are caused by atypical mycobacteria (eg, *Mycobacterium kansasii, M avium-intracellulare* and *M chelonei*).[11] Most infections occur during the first year after transplantation, and in this same period the incidence is further increased due to antirejection therapy. Although isolated pulmonary infection is the most common manifestation, as many as 40% of patients exhibit dissemination either synchronously or metachronously in the form of pleuropulmonary infection, granulomatous hepatitis, peritonitis, osteoarthritis, meningitis or brain abscesses, soft tissue infection or miliary disease. Approximately 10% of patients exhibit only one of these latter manifestations without obvious pulmonary disease. In ~50% of cases a prior exposure history or history of infection can be elicited indicative of reactivation of mycobacterial infection, the remainder representing primary infection. Rarely, transmission via the donor organ has been reported. The mortality rate associated with mycobacterial infection is ~30%.

History

The clinician must determine whether the patient has specific risk factors for infection, including a prior history of exposure or infection due to this type of pathogen, as well as recent antirejection therapy. It should be noted that prior significant exposure or treated infection warrants consideration of isoniazid prophylaxis for 1-2 years post-transplant. Although controversial, the author recommends this approach. Patients who suffer mycobacterial infection do not invariably demonstrate symptoms such as nocturnal fever and sweats, but more often exhibit vague symptoms such as malaise, lethargy, anorexia and weight loss. Those who harbor pulmonary disease may develop cough and pleuritic chest pain that may be related to persistent coughing or pleural infection. The patient should be closely questioned regarding the presence of extrapulmonary manifestations including jaundice due to hepatic infection, monoarticular joint swelling, bone pain, headache or subcutaneous masses. Some patients have undergone percutaneous sampling of pleural or joint effusions, or examination of cerebrospinal fluid which has revealed the presence of numerous WBCs, but no organisms on Gram's stain, as well as an extremely low glucose level. Similar staining results may be obtained from fluid or tissue samples obtained via incisional biopsy of subcutaneous masses or at the time of laparotomy among patients who develop mycobacterial peritonitis. This information represents an important key to the diagnosis of this type of infection, and it is extremely important to ascertain whether or not a Ziehl-Neelsen stain and cultures for acid-fast bacilli were performed. If not, the likelihood of mycobacterial infection increases substantially.

Physical Findings
Care should be taken to determine whether pulmonary percussion or auscultatory changes compatible with consolidation or cavitation are present. The presence of jaundice should be assessed under incandescent, not fluorescent lighting, and all joints should be examined for the presence of an effusion. Any subcutaneous masses should be identified.

Laboratory Tests
The chest radiograph may reveal the presence of one or more areas of consolidation with or without cavitation, or numerous small nodules (miliary pattern) in both lung fields. Any form of pulmonary disease may be associated with unilateral or bilateral pleural effusions. Sputum samples should be obtained in the early morning on at least three separate occasions. If analysis of these samples does not immediately reveal the presence of mycobacteria, bronchoscopy and BAL should be performed. Percutaneous sampling of pleural or joint effusions or cerebrospinal fluid should be undertaken as directed by the history and initial diagnostic studies. Peritoneal fluid should be obtained at the time of laparotomy in patients who undergo this procedure to determine the source of severe abdominal pain. Analysis of fluid samples typically reveals the presence of a large number of WBCs (usually mononuclear), low or absent glucose levels, and acid-fast bacilli. Direct microscopic examination of tissue obtained via liver biopsy or incisional biopsy of subcutaneous masses for acid-fast bacilli may reveal the presence of these pathogens. Growth in culture may not occur for 4-6 weeks, and may take as long as 3 months. Speciation and *in vitro* antibiotic sensitivity determinations may require an additional 1-2 months.

Management
Once the presence of acid-fast bacilli compatible with mycobacteria has been established, treatment consists of administration of 3-4 agents in combination. Usually, isoniazid, rifampin, ethambutol or streptomycin plus pyrazinamide are selected. Treatment of atypical agents often requires alternative combinations of agents such as clarithromycin, azithromycin, amikacin, cefoxitin and/or ciprofloxacin. Liver function tests and optic field mapping should be obtained prior to instituting therapy because of the hepatic and optic nerve toxicities of isoniazid and ethambutol, respectively. Although the occurrence of isoniazid hepatic toxicity is idiosyncratic, this drug should not be administered to patients who exhibit hepatic dysfunction. Once the results of bacterial speciation and drug sensitivity testing are available, refinements in therapy can be made. Therapy should be administered for 18-24 months, and patients should be monitored closely thereafter for recrudescence.

4. Opportunistic Fungal Infections

Candidiasis

Definition, Epidemiology and Pathophysiology

Candida albicans, C glabrata, C kruseii, C tropicalis and other candidal species are yeasts that are present in small numbers as part of the autochthonous microflora of the human gut. Solid organ transplant patients who develop candidal infection may first exhibit proliferation at integumentary sites (moniliasis) or endothelial sites such as the oropharynx (thrush), which may be the harbinger of the development of invasive disease. These organisms can cause UTIs, particularly among renal transplant recipients and, less commonly, can cause esophagitis as sole pathogens. They are also frequent co-pathogens among patients who develop intraabdominal infection. In particular, pancreas, liver and small bowel transplant patients who develop this latter disease process invariably harbor *Candida albicans* as one of the components of the polymicrobial infection. Although frequently found in the sputum, candida rarely causes pneumonia as a sole pathogen. Disseminated candidal infection is diagnosed when evidence of infection is identified from 2-3 separate body sites—positive culture or hyphae upon microscopic examination, particularly from normally sterile tissue or fluid, pathognomonic physical findings such as chorioretinitis on fundoscopic examination, or fungemia. The mortality of candidemia in severely immunosuppressed neutropenic patients is in excess of 50%.

History

Proliferation of these organisms occurs during or subsequent to: 1.) poorly controlled diabetes mellitus, 2.) significant exogenous immunosuppression (eg, antirejection therapy or cancer chemotherapy), 3.) persistent neutropenia, or 4.) prolonged broad-spectrum antibacterial agent therapy. Any or all of these risk factors may be present among patients who develop invasive candidal infection, and the diagnosis should be strongly considered among patients,with the factors listed above, who concurrently provide a history of superficial colonization such as intertriginous moniliasis or thrush. Patients who develop candidal esophagitis typically are dehydrated, as it is extremely painful for them to swallow and they often complain of severe substernal chest pain that may be thought to be due to a myocardial infarction. Candidemia should be suspected in patients who harbor infection due to these pathogens at one or more sites, and then develop sepsis syndrome and clinically deteriorate.

Physical Findings

Areas of whitish superficial plaque-like disease in the intertriginous folds of the skin of the groin or on mucosal surfaces are typical findings on direct or endoscopic examination. Fluffy white retinal lesions are typically candidal chorioretinitis.

Laboratory Tests

Scrapings of superficial lesions or examination of fluid or tissue can reveal the presence of *Candida* spp. with KOH preparation or cultural analysis. Although a number of diagnostic tests have been proposed to rapidly detect the presence of this organism (eg, candida mannan, a cell wall component), as yet these have not proven clinically useful.

Management

Patients who develop superficial infection can be treated with topical therapy using miconazole cream or troches. Invasive infection due to *Candida* spp. should receive either parenteral fluconazole or amphotericin B therapy.[12] The duration of therapy is somewhat arbitrary, and generally is dictated by the severity and associated morbidity and mortality. For example, UTIs are treated with 10-14 days of oral fluconazole. On occasion, amphotericin B is administered via continuous bladder irrigation, although this approach is cumbersome and should be reserved for refractory disease. Candidal infection associated with pneumonia, intraabdominal infection, or fungemia should be treated with ~21 days of either fluconazole, caspofungin or amphotericin B (.3-.5 mg/kg/day), the latter in patients who are critically ill or who are found to harbor organisms usually resistant to fluconazole (*C kruseii, C tropicalis*, et al). In the last five years, there has been a decrease in *C albicans* and an increase in non-albicans species, (eg, *C glabrata* or *C Krusei)*. The latter two organisms have decreased susceptibility to fluconazole.[18] Potential sources of infection such as indwelling catheters should be removed promptly in patients who develop fungemia. Liposomal amphotericin B preparations can be used to treat patients who exhibit renal dysfunction, although these preparations currently are expensive. It is important to note that prolonged courses of broad-spectrum antibacterial agents should be reserved for treatment of significant, well-defined disease in solid organ transplant patients; the addition of fluconazole as prophylaxis to such therapeutic regimens does not prevent fungal infection. Instead, initial use of short courses of antibacterial agents or termination of antibacterial agent therapy and reduction of immunosuppression should candidal infection occur are key prophylactic and therapeutic maneuvers. However, fluconazole prophylaxis in certain subgroups of patients at high risk for the development of candidal infection (eg, pancreas and small bowel transplant recipients) may be useful, although this remains somewhat controversial.

Aspergillosis

Definition, Epidemiology and Pathophysiology

Infection due to *Aspergillus fumigatus, A terreus, A niger* and other species affects ~1%-4% of solid organ transplant patients, and accounts for ~1/3 of all fungal infections in this patient population. Infection at a specific site leads to dissemination in ~50% of individuals, invariably with a fatal outcome. These infections are more common during the first year posttransplant, although they can occur at any time. Interestingly, among all solid organ transplant patients, heart transplant patients are at highest risk of developing aspergillosis. The lung is the most common site of involvement; at one time the development of an "aspergilloma" in a cavity (usually due to prior tuberculosis) was common, but now this entity rarely occurs. More commonly, lobular or lobar infection or diffuse tracheobronchitis are seen.[13] *Aspergillus* spp can infect the oropharynx, sinuses, ears, eyes, and occasionally the soft tissues, particularly in severely neutropenic patients. CNS infection can cause space-occupying lesions. Blood vessel invasion can occur from any of these sites leading to endocarditis, emboli and widespread dissemination—a process that invariably is fatal.

History

Patients who develop aspergillosis typically have numerous risk factors for infection of any sort. Fever and cough are the most common presenting complaints, although patients who harbor CNS disease may complain of headache or may exhibit mild-to-moderate mental status changes. Soft tissue infection may occur in an existing surgical wound, or in the subcutaneous tissue near a site of skin breakdown, usually in the setting of severe neutropenia.

Physical Findings

Few findings on physical examination point to the diagnosis of aspergillosis. However, patients who exhibit numerous risk factors should undergo a thorough examination, with particular attention directed toward the respiratory tract and CNS: evidence of pulmonary consolidation, or papilledema or mental status changes, respectively, may be evident.

Laboratory Tests

The chest radiograph may demonstrate lobular or lobar consolidation in one or more areas of the lung, frequently bilaterally. Cavitation may occur as well, which is best delineated via chest CT. A diffuse, hazy bilateral infiltrate may be indicative of tracheobronchitis, and if the analysis of BAL fluid demonstrates numerous hyphae without yeast forms, the diagnosis of aspergillosis should be strongly considered. If BAL analysis is unrevealing, transbronchial or percutaneous CT guided sampling should be undertaken. Cranial CT may reveal the presence of CNS disease if one or more space-occupying lesions are observed. Percutaneous CT-guided biopsy may be required to establish the diagnosis. Occasionally, fungal blood cultures reveal the presence of the organism.

Management

Aspergillosis represents a serious infection and should be treated with amphotericin B. In general, pulmonary disease requires a 1.5-2 g total dose entailing a 3-4 month treatment course, and a reduction in immunosuppressive therapy is needed. Disease that does not regress may require surgical resection and additional amphotericin B therapy. This includes patients who develop pulmonary consolidation as well as CNS disease, although few patients survive the latter type of disease. Administration of liposomal amphotericin B preparations should be considered in patients who exhibit renal dysfunction initially or in whom it develops during initial therapy, or in patients whose disease is refractory to routine amphotericin B therapy. The diagnosis of aspergillosis should be considered in patients that exhibit pulmonary consolidation who are being treated with antibacterial agents and do not rapidly improve, even if fungi have not been identified. Under those circumstances, empiric administration of amphotericin B should be considered. Occasionally, itraconazole can be administered initially for milder forms of disease or later in treatment for disease that rapidly responds to amphotericin B. Surgical debridement and/or excision is often required for soft tissue infection. Invariably, patients who develop aspergillosis require significant reduction in exogenous immunosuppression and neutropenic patients should receive G-CSF.

Other Fungal Infections

Definition, Epidemiology and Pathophysiology

A number of opportunistic fungal pathogens cause infection less frequently than *Candida* and *Aspergillus* spp in solid organ transplant recipients. *Cryptococcus neoformans* can cause pneumonia and cerebromeningitis. *Histoplasma capsulatum* and *Blastomyces dermatitidis* are endemic in many areas of the central USA. Immunosuppressed patients may develop pulmonary disease after inhaling arthrospores of either organism in an endemic area, or via reactivation if they have been previously exposed. Rapid dissemination through the bloodstream can occur, and the skin often is involved. *Coccidioides immitis* can cause pulmonary as well as CNS, joint, and disseminated disease. Finally, soil fungi such as *Mucor, Rhizopus* and *Absidia* cause mucormycosis. Aggressive, invasive rhinocerebral or soft tissue infection (including the surgical wound) can occur. Because of their infrequent occurrence, infection due to any of these microbes may be difficult to diagnose.

History

Patients who develop infection due to these organisms often exhibit numerous risk factors for infection. Complaints related to infection from any of these organisms include fever, malaise and lethargy, while for those organisms that involve the lung or CNS, complaints may consist only of nonproductive cough and headache, respectively.

Physical Findings

Unique findings on physical examination are lesions that resemble erythema nodosum in histoplasmosis infection, and blackened soft tissue or wound edges (due to fungal invasion and necrosis) with a surrounding zone of erythema, both of which rapidly expand if unchecked, among patients who suffer from mucormycosis.

Laboratory Tests

Tissue should be obtained and examined histopathologically for the presence of conidiae or hyphae. Cerebrospinal fluid should be obtained in patients who develop meningitis, and the India ink preparation may reveal the presence of encapsulated yeast cells typical of *Cryptococcus neoformans*, and other typical findings include high protein, low glucose level and numerous lymphocytes. Patients who develop mucormycosis will exhibit coenocentric hyphae with 30° ramifications. Occasionally, fungal blood cultures reveal the presence of one of these organisms.

Management

Amphotericin B for 2-3 weeks followed by 4-6 weeks of fluconazole is standard therapy for cryptococcal disease. Patients who suffer cryptococcal meningitis should undergo repeat lumbar puncture after the termination of therapy. A prolonged course of amphotericin B (1.5-3 g) is required to treat the majority of these infections. Similarly to aspergillosis, pulmonary disease due to any one of a number of fungal pathogens that does not regress with therapy may require resection. Due to its aggressive nature, mucormycosis requires extensive resection without fail, plus prolonged amphotericin B therapy. Invariably, patients who develop these types of infections require significant reduction in exogenous immunosuppression and neutropenic patients should receive G-CSF.

5. Opportunistic Viral Infections

Cytomegalovirus

Definition, Epidemiology and Pathophysiology

CMV is responsible for the majority of viral infections that occur among solid organ transplant recipients. A member of the family *Herpesviridae*, it is ubiquitous in the environment but rarely causes disease in normal individuals, although >80% of the population has experienced subclinical infection as evidenced by the presence of endogenous anti-CMV immunoglobulin G (IgG) antibody. This pathogen typically causes disease ~3-6 months posttransplant or subsequent to antirejection therapy, particularly antilymphocyte antibody preparations; ~25%-30% of recipients of cadaver organs and ~10%-15% of living related transplant recipients are affected. Three types of CMV infection can occur in immunosuppressed patients, differentiated by the manner in which exogenous transmission or reactivation of endogenous virus takes place. The three types of infection are primary infection, reactivation, and superinfection. CMV disease is defined as CMV infection associated with significant clinical manifestations, and tissue invasive CMV disease (TI-CMV) is defined as disease associated with identification of CMV at one or more tissue sites (eg, lung, liver, pancreas). CMV infection can lead to disease that affects many different organ systems with protean manifestations, including pneumonitis, leukopenia, upper or lower gastrointestinal ulceration and bleeding, retinitis, hepatitis, pancreatitis and sepsis syndrome, either alone or in combination. Primary infection can occur after CMV seronegative recipients receive a blood transfusion containing WBCs or an organ from a CMV seropositive donor. Approximately 75%-80% of such patients will develop disease which often is severe, and occasionally fatal. Reactivation and superinfection occur at lower rates and are associated with less severe clinical manifestations. Although CMV disease was formerly associated with allograft loss and patient demise, these adverse events occur rarely today. However, morbidity remains common as inpatient hospitalization is often required to establish the diagnosis and implement therapy.

History

Patients who develop CMV disease generally complain of fever, malaise, lethargy, and myalgias, often associated with cough, dyspnea, nausea, vomiting, abdominal pain, diarrhea, gastrointestinal bleeding, jaundice or diminished vision. Significant risk factors for the development of CMV disease include those common to all types of infection in immunosuppressed patients, as well as the pretransplant CMV serological status (+ or –) of both donor (D) and recipient (R). The risk of CMV infection and disease is as follows: D+R– (~50%-80%) > D+R+ > D–R+ (~10%-30%) >D–R– (<5%). In addition, it should be established whether the patient received prophylaxis to prevent CMV posttransplant, and whether prior documented episodes of CMV disease occurred and the manner in which they were treated, because CMV disease recurs in ~20%-25% of patients after treatment of initial disease.

Physical Findings

There are few if any symptoms that distinguish CMV disease from other types of infections in immunosuppressed patients. Rather, the constellation of symptoms and signs as well as their temporal occurrence in relation to the transplant procedure or antirejection therapy should lead one to entertain the diagnosis.

Laboratory Tests

In addition to routine laboratory studies, patients with suspected CMV disease should undergo chest radiograph and bronchoscopy studies with BAL if pulmonary symptoms are present, and upper and/or lower gastrointestinal endoscopy and amylase determination if evidence of gastrointestinal bleeding is identified or abdominal pain or other gastrointestinal complaints are present. Liver enzyme analysis should also be obtained. Viral culture analysis has fallen into disfavor and is rarely performed, because it requires 2-3 weeks to obtain results. Rather, samples of blood and BAL fluid should be subjected to CMV "shell vial" analysis in which growth on fibroblasts and immunofluorescent staining for CMV capsid antigen occurs. This test requires 14-24 hours, and is quite sensitive and specific. Also, some transplant centers are using polymerase chain reaction (PCR)-based assays to detect CMV, but this very sensitive assay is not routinely used at present, and precise correlation with clinical disease states have not been established. In ~10%-20% of patients pathognomonic-inclusion bodies are observed upon examination of tissue.

Management

Administration of antiviral agents such as acyclovir, valacyclovir, or ganciclovir, and anti-CMV antibody preparations during the initial 3 months after transplantation significantly diminishes the incidence of posttransplant CMV disease, particularly in high-risk D+R– patients. Controversy exists over whether all patients should receive prophylaxis, and some centers use acyclovir or valacyclovir (which is less expensive, but less active against CMV *in vitro* compared to ganciclovir) for lower risk subgroups (D+R+, D–R+), and administer ganciclovir with or without CMV hyperimmune globulin to D+R– individuals.[14,15] However, ~10%-30% of individuals develop CMV disease despite prophylactic measures, and for that reason the author believes that all patients should undergo prophylaxis with a potent anti-CMV agent such as ganciclovir. Those patients who develop CMV disease should receive ganciclovir: generally, 1-3 weeks of parenteral therapy is administered, then oral drug is prescribed. Although the optimal duration of therapy that effectively treats CMV disease and reduces the incidence of recurrence has not been established, the author recommends a course of therapy totalling 6 weeks. Foscarnet is rarely used for treatment of CMV disease in solid organ transplant patients, because ganciclovir-resistant strains of CMV are uncommon, and the drug possesses substantial nephrotoxicity. Mild-to-moderate rejection and mild-to-moderate CMV disease can be concurrently treated as long as the patient is closely monitored. In all patients, if clinical deterioration or severe CMV disease occurs, the level of immunosuppression should be reduced and in some cases withdrawn, with the exception of maintenance dose corticosteroids.

Other Viral Infections

Definition, Epidemiology and Pathophysiology

A number of other herpesviruses can cause infection among solid organ transplant recipients. Infection due to herpes simplex virus (HSV) generally consists of oropharyngeal ulceration that is self limiting. Rarely, disseminated cutaneous, gastrointestinal, pulmonary, hepatic or CNS disease occur, all of which can be life-threatening. Similarly, reactivation of varicella-zoster virus (VZV) causes epidermal disease that is confined to 1 or 2 dermatomes (shingles); ~5%-25% of patients suffer this type of infection. Patients who have not previously been exposed to VZV in the form of chickenpox are at risk for more severe manifestations such as pneumonitis or encephalitis. Epstein-Barr virus (EBV) is capable of causing a spectrum of disease in allograft recipients, ranging from mononucleosis-like disease to posttransplant lymphoproliferative disorder (PTLD). Currently, it is theorized that modes of transmission and reactivation of EBV are similar to those demonstrated for CMV. However, >50% of patients who develop PTLD die, and CNS disease occurs in ~20% of individuals. Human herpesvirus 6 can cause systemic symptoms, but serious disease has not been observed. Papillomaviruses are associated with occasional ureteral stricture formation in renal transplant recipients. Adenoviruses and respiratory syncytial virus are capable of causing life-threatening pneumonia, and the former can also cause fulminant hepatitis in solid organ transplant patients. Hepatitis B and C are commonly identified pretransplant, particularly among hemodialysis patients and individuals who have developed hepatic failure due to one of these pathogens, and either or both can recur after liver transplantation and cause allograft dysfunction and eventual failure. These viruses as well as human immunodeficiency virus can be acquired post-transplant as well, causing serious manifestations including fulminant or chronic hepatic failure, and severe infection and malignancy, respectively.

History

Patients who develop infection due to these various viral agents may complain of a "prodrome" consisting of fever, malaise, lethargy, myalgias and other constitutional symptoms. Patients may complain of a "rash" that represents vesicle formation. Pulmonary (cough, dyspnea) and CNS (headache, confusion) manifestations as well as jaundice may occur on occasion as mentioned above.

Physical Findings

HSV and VZV infection may cause cutaneous vesicles. EBV infection may be associated with local or diffuse lymphadenopathy. Few other physical manifestations occur due to viral infections.

Laboratory Tests

The presence of either HSV or VZV is determined by performing a Tzanck stain on vesicle fluid. A combination of serological studies, immunoperoxidase staining, and (particularly for EBV) PCR-based analysis can reveal the presence of viral infection due to most of the above-mentioned pathogens. Patients who develop a mononucleosis-like syndrome due to EBV harbor large numbers of enlarged lymphocytes apparent on examination of a peripheral blood smear. Patients with suspected PTLD should be evaluated for EBV infection, but also should undergo an extensive staging evaluation (cranial, chest, and abdominal CT scans, bone marrow biopsy and biopsy of the suspected primary site of disease).

Management

Patients who develop HSV or VZV infection should receive acyclovir for 4-6 weeks, and primary EBV disease should be treated with ganciclovir for the same duration. PTLD localized to a single site should be resected, and a multi-drug cancer chemotherapy regimen should be administered; CNS disease should be treated with external beam irradiation as well.

6. Opportunistic Protozoal and Parasitic Infections

Definition, Epidemiology and Pathophysiology

Pneumocystis carinii can cause severe pulmonary disease, and *Toxoplasma gondii* can cause neurological disease and disseminated infection in solid organ transplant recipients.[16,17] This latter entity is more common in heart transplant patients and can be transmitted via the donor organ. In tropical environments, a number of parasites (eg, *Strongyloides stercoralis*) can cause pulmonary and visceral manifestations that can be life-threatening in immunosuppressed patients.

History

Patients who develop infection due to *Pneumocystis carinii* complain of a dry, persistent, nonproductive cough, and tachypnea may be present as well. Alterations in mentation are common among patients who develop toxoplasmosis. Infection due to either may be associated with mild fever, malaise, lethargy and myalgias. Patients who receive TMP-SMX prophylaxis rarely develop these types of infections.

Physical Findings

Bilateral rales without evidence of consolidation occur in patients with *Pneumocystis carinii* infection. Toxoplasmosis is associated with diffuse lymphadenopathy and neurological deterioration due to CNS disease.

Laboratory Tests

A chest radiograph typically demonstrates bilateral diffuse alveolar and interstitial pneumonia in patients who develop *Pneumocystis carinii* infection. Bronchoscopy and BAL and occasionally lung biopsy should be performed, and the organism demonstrates a characteristic appearance on Giemsa stain. Similarly, characteristic cysts and histopathological effects due to *Toxoplasma gondii* can be identified in samples obtained from lymph nodes or with cardiac endothelial biopsy.

Management

Patients who develop *Pneumocystis carinii* pneumonia should receive parenteral TMP-SMX or pentamidine; dapsone-TMP represents an alternative regimen. Pyrimethamine and sulfadiazine should be used to treat toxoplasmosis.

7. References

1. Acton RD, Dunn DL. Infections in solid organ transplant patients. In: Armstrong D, Cohen J, eds. *Infectious Diseases*. London, England: Mosby; 1999;4: 3.1-3.16.

2. Brayman KL, Stephanian E, Matas AJ, et al. Analysis of infectious complications occurring after solid-organ transplantation. *Arch Surg*. 1992;127:38-48.

3. Fox BC, Sollinger HW, Belzer FO, Maki DG. A prospective, randomized, double-blind study of trimethoprim-sulfamethoxazole for prophylaxis of infection in renal transplantation: Clinical efficacy, absorption of trimethoprim-sulfamethoxazole, effects on the microflora, and the cost-benefit of prophylaxis. *Am J Surg*. 1990;89:255-274.

4. Goya N, Tanabe K, Iguchi Y, Oshima T, Yagisawa T, Toma H, Agishi T, Ota K, Takahashi K. Prevalence of urinary tract infection during outpatient follow-up after renal transplantation. *Infection*. 1997;25:101-105.

5. Stephan RN, Munschauer CE, Kumar MS. Surgical wound infection in renal transplantation: outcome data in 102 consecutive patients without perioperative systemic antibiotic coverage. *Arch Surg*. 1997;132:1315-1318.

6. Everett JE, Wahoff DC, Statz C, et al. Characterization and impact of wound infection after pancreas transplantation. *Arch Surg*. 1994;129:1310-1317.

7. Dunn DL. Diagnosis and treatment of opportunistic infections in immunocompromised surgical patients. *Amer Surg*. 2000;66:117-125.

8. Palmer SM Jr, Kanj SS, Davis RD, Tapson VF. A case of disseminated infection with *Nocardia brasiliensis* in a lung transplant recipient. *Transplantation*. 1997;63:1189-1190.

9. Weston VC, Punt J, Vloebeghs M, Watson AR, Ispahani P. *Listeria monocytogenes* meningitis in a penicillin-allergic paediatric renal transplant patient. *J Infection*. 1998;37:77-78.

10. Chow JW, Yu VL. *Legionella*: a major opportunistic pathogen in transplant recipients. *Semin Resp Infect*. 1998;13:132-139.

11. Patel R, Roberts GD, Keating MR, Paya CV. Infections due to nontuberculous mycobacteria in kidney, heart, and liver transplant recipients. *Clin Infect Dis*. 1994;19:263-273.

12. Rex JH, Bennett JE, Sugar AM, et al. A randomized trial comparing fluconazole with amphotericin B for the treatment of candidemia in patients without neutropenia. Candidemia Study Group and the National Institute. *N Engl J Med*. 1994;331:1325-1330.

13. Westney GE, Kesten S, De Hoyos A, Chapparro C, Winton T, Maurer JR. *Aspergillus* infection in single and double lung transplant recipients. *Transplantation*. 1996;61:915-919.

14. Dunn DL, Gillingham KJ, Kramer MA, et al. A prospective randomized study of acyclovir versus ganciclovir plus human immune globulin prophylaxis of cytomegalovirus infection after solid organ transplantation. *Transplantation*. 1994;57:876-884.

15. Lowance D, Neumayer HH, Legendre CM, et al. Valacyclovir for the prevention of cytomegalovirus disease after renal transplantation. International Valacyclovir Cytomegalovirus Prophylaxis Transplantation Study Group. *N Engl J Med*. 1999;340:1462-1470.

16. Munoz P, Munoz RM, Palomo J, Rodriguez-Creixems M, Munoz R, Bouza E. *Pneumocystis carinii* infection in heart transplant recipients. Efficacy of a weekend prophylaxis schedule. *Medicine*. 1997;76:415-422.

17. Renoult E, Georges E, Biava MF, et al. Toxoplasmosis in kidney transplant recipients: report of six cases and review. *Clin Infect Dis*. 1997;24:625-634.

18. Gilbert DN, Doellering RC, Eliopoulos GM, Sande MA. *The Sanford Guide to Antimicrobial Therapy*. 37th ed. Sperryville, VA: Antimicrobial Therapy, Inc.; 2007.

8. Questions

1. Significant risk factors that predispose solid organ transplant patients to infection include:

A. Exogenous maintenance immunosuppression

B. Antirejection therapy

C. Cadaveric transplantation

D. Pretransplant disease processes associated with infection

E. All of the above

2. The most serious form of candidal infection is:

A. Moniliasis

B. Thrush

C. Isolation of *Candida* spp as part of polymicrobial flora from BAL

D. Candidemia

3. Significant risk factors for the development of CMV disease after solid organ transplantation include:

A. Kidney transplantation

B. Antirejection therapy

C. Serological evidence of absence of exposure of both donor and recipient to CMV

D. Serological evidence of exposure of donor, but not recipient, to CMV

E. A. and C.

F. B. and D.

4. The incidence of wound infection in renal transplant recipients is:

   A. <5%

   B. 5%-10%

   C. ~25%

   D. >30%

5. *Aspergillus* infection should be treated with which drug as first-line therapy:

   A. Fluconazole

   B. Miconazole

   C. Amphotericin B

   D. Itraconazole

6. Which of the following viruses has been closely linked with the development of post-transplant lymphoproliferative disorder (PTLD)?

   A. Cytomegalovirus

   B. Adenovirus

   C. Herpes simplex virus

   D. Epstein-Barr virus

7. Primary CMV disease occurs in which of the following donor (D)/recipient (R) CMV serological status pairs?

   A. D+R+

   B. D–R+

   C. D+R–

   D. D–R–

8. CMV disease can be treated with which of the following agents?

   A. Ganciclovir

   B. Acyclovir

   C. Foscarnet

   D. Valacyclovir

   E. A. and C.

   F. B. and D.

9. Infection due to which of the following opportunistic pathogens occurs rarely among patients receiving TMP-SMX?

   A. *Mycobacterium tuberculosis*

   B. *Nocardia asteroides*

   C. *Aspergillus fumigatus*

   D. *Pneumocystis carinii*

   E. A. and C.

   F. B. and D.

10. Antiviral agents that appear to decrease the incidence of post-transplant CMV disease include:

   A. Acyclovir

   B. Ganciclovir

   C. Valacyclovir

   D. CMV hyperimmune globulin

   E. All of the above

Answers

1. E.
Suppression of endogenous antimicrobial host defenses by exogenous immunosuppression renders solid organ transplant patients susceptible to various types of infection. Cadaveric transplant recipients generally receive higher doses of immunosuppressive drugs and exhibit a higher incidence of infection such that this factor represents a surrogate marker for exogenous immunosuppression as well. Numerous disease processes associated with infection should be dealt with prior to transplantation to avoid post-transplant complications.

2. D.
Candidemia is associated with high mortality rates (>50%) in immunosuppressed patients.

3. F.
The overall degree of exogenous immunosuppression predisposes patients to CMV infection and disease post-transplant. In addition, individuals who are CMV seronegative and who receive a donor organ from a seropositive individual are at high risk to develop serious CMV disease.

4. A.
Renal transplantation is associated with a very low risk of wound infection compared to other types of abdominal solid organ transplant procedures.

5. C.
Amphotericin B is the drug of choice for aspergillosis. Although itraconazole possesses activity against many *Aspergillus* spp, in general it does not represent a first-line therapeutic agent.

6. D.
EBV has been causally associated with the development of PTLD.

7. C.
Transmission of the donor strain of CMV to a seronegative recipient leading to primary CMV disease occurs among ~50%-80% of D+R– transplants.

8. E.
Ganciclovir and foscarnet are both used to treat CMV disease, although the latter drug is nephrotoxic and less frequently prescribed. Acyclovir, valacyclovir and ganciclovir have been used to prevent CMV disease, but among these only the latter drug is efficacious as a therapeutic agent.

9. F.
Patients who receive TMP-SMX prophylaxis are unlikely to develop infection due to microbes sensitive to this agent (*Nocardia asteroides, Listeria monocytogenes, Legionella pneumophila, Pneumocystis carinii* and *Toxoplasma gondii*).

10. E.
Each of these agents have been demonstrated to reduce the incidence of CMV disease posttransplant. Investigators continue to attempt to determine the optimal prophylactic regimen.

Chapter 6: Initial Management of the Injured Patient

Marianne E. Cinat, MD

Contents

1. Initial Assessment and Management

An organized sequential approach must be used for evaluation of all trauma patients. This consists of the primary survey, resuscitation of vital signs, a detailed secondary survey and initiation of definitive care.

Primary Survey (*ABCDEs*)

The goal and purpose of the primary survey is to identify and treat immediately life-threatening injuries. This must be carried out expediently and sequentially.

Airway Maintenance with Cervical Spine Protection (*A*)

Airway control and maintenance is the highest priority in the initial evaluation of the trauma patient. Maneuvers like the chin lift or jaw thrust should be used to help establish airway patency. Oropharyngeal and/or nasopharyngeal airways can also be used. ***C-spine precautions should always be maintained,*** but airway control should not be delayed for C-spine evaluation. Airway compromise should be considered in any patient with severe maxillofacial trauma, penetrating neck injury or laryngeal trauma (see Table 1).

Table 1

Indications for a Definitive Airway in Trauma

Indications for a definitive airway

- Apnea
- Unable to maintain a patent airway
- Impending or potential airway compromise
- Glasgow coma score (GCS) ≤ 8
- Failure to maintain adequate oxygenation by face mask supplementation

Patients at high risk for airway loss

- Laryngeal injury (hoarseness, subcutaneous emphysema, palpable fracture)
- Penetrating neck trauma with expanding hematoma
- Facial burns
- Inhalation injury
- Maxillofacial trauma (especially bilateral mandible fractures)

Patients at high risk for aspiration

- Obtundation, coma
- Bleeding oral laceration
- Massive epistaxis

Other potential indications

- Shock
- Combative patient with possible life-threatening injuries

Invasive Airway Techniques. Oropharyngeal intubation via direct laryngoscopy is the standard method for establishing an airway in the acute trauma patient. It can be rapidly performed under direct vision and it can be accomplished in both awake and apneic patients. C-spine precautions should be maintaine ***Nasopharyngeal intubation*** is rarely used in the trauma setting. It is contraindicated in patients with maxillofacial trauma, instability of the midface and suspected basilar skull fractures. It is also contraindicated in apneic patients since it is a blind technique, guided by the sound of air movement through the tube. It is also more time consuming than orotracheal intubation so is rarely used in an emergent setting. Because the neck does not need to be manipulated, this technique may be considered in a hemodynamically stable patient with C-spine injury and no respiratory distress.

Laryngeal Mask Airway (LMA). The laryngeal mask airway now has an established role in the management of a patient with a difficult airway, especially following multiple attempts at endotracheal intubation or inadequate bag mask ventilation. While the LMA does not provide a definitive airway, it does provide temporary control and a route for ventilation.

Multilumen Esophageal Airway. This device is used by pre-hospital personnel when a definitive airway is not possible. One port communicates with the esophagus, the other with the airway. Personnel using this device must be trained to identify which tube occludes the esophagus, and which will provide air to the trachea once placed. This is not a definitive airway.

Laryngeal Tube Airway (LTA). The laryngeal tube airway is an extraglottic device that can be placed for temporary airway control with minimal manipulation of the head and neck. It is not a definitve airway.

Gum Elastic Bougie. This device is a 60-cm long, 15 French, intubating stylette with a Coude tip that can be used to cannulate the trachea for an airway when visualization of the cords is difficult. An endotracheal tube can then be passed over the GEB.

Cricothyroidotomy is indicated in any patient who requires intubation and in whom orotracheal or nasotracheal intubation is unsuccessful. The technique for a surgical cricothyroidotomy is as follows:

A vertical incision is made in the neck overlying the cricothyroid membrane. Blunt dissection is carried out down to the cricothyroid membrane. The membrane is sharply incised and the opening is enlarged with a clamp or the handle of the scalpel. An endotracheal tube or tracheostomy tube is then placed into the lumen. This should be converted to a formal tracheostomy as soon as the patient is otherwise stabilized. This technique is not recommended for children under 12 years of age.

Needle cricothyroidotomy with jet insufflation can be used to provide oxygen on a short-term basis (30-45 minutes) until a definitive airway can be achieved. This technique is performed by inserting a large-caliber plastic catheter (12- or 14-gauge) through the cricothyroid membrane below the level of obstruction. The cannula is then connected to wall oxygen at 15 L/min via a Y-connector or side hole. Intermittent insufflation (1 second on and 4 seconds off) will allow adequate oxygenation with some ventilation. Urgent definitive airway management should be achieved within 30-45 minutes. This technique is appropriate for small children.

Breathing and Ventilation (*B*)
Once the airway has been secured, adequate breathing and ventilation should be assessed and oxygen should be administered. The chest should be examined, auscultated and palpated. Decreased or absent breath sounds suggests thoracic injury. Tracheal position and deviation should be assessed. Tachypnea and agitation may suggest hypoxia, while obtundation may indicate hypercarbia. A pulse oximeter should be placed. Life-threatening thoracic injuries should be identified and managed before proceeding further (ie, tension pneumothorax, open pneumothorax, flail chest, massive hemothorax).

Circulation with Hemorrhage Control (*C*)
After airway patency and adequacy of ventilation have been secured, perfusion status must be assessed. Hemorrhage is the predominant cause of death early following traumatic injury. Therefore, hypotension following injury must be considered hypovolemic until proven otherwise. Rapid assessment of organ perfusion can be determined by evaluation of level of consciousness, skin color, blood pressure, pulse rate and character. 2 large bore intravenous catheters are secured. Blood should be sent for type and cross. External bleeding should be identified and controlled (eg, scalp laceration). Intravenous fluid resuscitation is started with a 2 liter bolus of a balanced salt solution (normal saline or lactated Ringer's). If the patient remains hypotensive after this initial bolus, blood should be given (O-negative, type-specific or type- and cross-matched). All fluid and blood products should be warmed to prevent hypothermia. Hypovolemic shock should not be treated with vasopressors, steroids or sodium bicarbonate. If continued massive fluid and/or blood resuscitation is necessary, operative intervention is likely necessary to control hemorrhage (see shock section below). Major injuries affecting circulation that should be identified and addressed during the primary survey include massive hemothorax and cardiac tamponade.

Disability (Neurologic Evaluation) (*D*)
A rapid neurologic assessment should be performed at the end of the primary survey. A quick method is referred to as AVPU. This determines if the patient is *alert*, responds to *verbal* stimuli, responds to *painful* stimuli or is *unresponsive*.

Glasgow Coma Scale. The Glasgow coma score should be determined early in the evaluation of the

Table 2

Glasgow Coma Scale

Eye opening	
Spontaneous	4
To speech	3
To pain	2
None	1
Verbal response	
Oriented	5
Confused	4
Inappropriate words	3
Incomprehensible sounds	2
No speech	1
***Best* motor response**	
Follows commands	6
Localizes pain	5
Withdraws from pain	4
Decorticate (abnormal flexion)	3
Decerebrate (extension)	2
None	1

injured patient and should be continuously reassessed (see Table 2). It is quick, simple and predictive of patient outcome. In calculating the GCS, it is important to use the *best* motor response is calculating the score, even if the response is asymmetric.

Exposure and Environmental Control (*E*)
The patient should be completely exposed, with removal of all clothing and jewelry. Following the assessment, the patient must quickly be covered with warm blankets or external heating devices to prevent hypothermia. Intravenous fluids and blood products should also be warmed before infusion. Room temperature should be warmed.

Adjuncts to the Primary Survey

- **Monitors**
  - Electrocardiographic monitoring to detect cardiac dysrhythmias.
  - Pulse oximetry should be used to monitor patient oxygenation.
- **Catheters**
  - A urinary catheter should be placed to monitor volume status and to detect hematuria. Transurethral catheter placement is contraindicated if urethral injury is suspected. Signs associated with urethral injury include: 1.) blood at the meatus, 2.) perineal ecchymosis, 3.) blood in the scrotum, 4.) a high-riding or non-palpable prostate and 5.) a pelvic fracture. A retrograde urethrogram should be performed if there is blood at the meatus or if a transurethral catheter cannot be easily passed in association with the above signs.
  - A gastric catheter is placed to decrease gastric distention and reduce the risk of aspiration
- **Diagnostic Studies**
  - **Chest x-ray (anteroposterior)** — to detect potentially life-threatening injuries
  - **Pelvis x-ray (anteroposterior)** — to demonstrate pelvic fractures that may account for significant occult blood loss and need for early transfusion
  - **Focused Assessment Sonography in Trauma (FAST)** – In recent years, this screening ultrasound exam has become an adjunct to the primary survey. It is particularly useful in hypotensive patients to rapidly identify intra-abdominal or intrapericardial fluid. Ultrasound

is used to detect free fluid in 4 areas: Morrison's pouch, the pouch of Douglas, the splenorenal recess and the pericardial sac. With advanced experience and technique, recent reports have begun to describe the use of ultrasound or the identification of pleural effusions and pneumothorax. Ultrasound can be performed at the bedside in 3-10 minutes, is non invasive, and can be repeated. Disadvantages include operator variability, missed bowel and pancreatic injuries, and a limited ability to differentiate blood from other fluids. It also has limited ability to detect tamponade in penetrating trauma in the presence of a pleural effusion.

- **Other considerations**
  * Cervical spine (lateral) - This exam used to be required as part of the primary survey in blunt trauma patients. However, with the increased use, accessibility, sensitivity, and efficiency of cervical spine CT scan, plain films in the emergency department are now left to the physician's discretion and are not considered mandatory.

  * Diagnostic Peritoneal Lavage. This modality and diagnostic study has essentially been replaced by FAST. However, in a patient who remains hypotensive despite aggressive resuscitation, and a negative FAST, diagnostic peritoneal lavage may be used to detect intra-abdominal hemorrhage during the primary survey. In current practice, it is primarily used in a delayed fashion to detect intestinal injury.

Secondary Survey

The secondary survey consists of a thorough history and head-to-toe examination of the patient. The secondary survey should begin only when the primary survey (***ABCDE***s) is completed, resuscitation efforts are established and the patient's hemodynamic status is stable or improving.

Components of the secondary survey include a complete *history* (allergies, medications, past medical and surgical treatment, tetanus status, last meal and events surrounding the accident), a thorough *physical examination* (head to toe—head, maxillofacial, cervical spine and neck, chest, abdomen, perineum/rectum/vagina, pelvis, musculoskeletal, neurologic, thoracic and lumbar spine, and vascular), and additional studies as indicated (C-spine, extremity films, CT scans, angiograms and other diagnostic procedures).

Resuscitative Emergency Department Thoracotomy

Patients with penetrating thoracic injuries who arrive pulseless but with cardiac electrical activity or with a persistent SBP <60 may be candidates for immediate resuscitative thoracotomy. A left anterior thoracotomy is performed and can be extended to the right if necessary. Therapeutic maneuvers include: 1.) evacuation of pericardial tamponade; 2.) direct control of exsanguinating hemorrhage; 3.) open cardiac massage; and 4.) cross-clamping of the descending aorta to slow blood loss from below the diaphragm and increase perfusion to the heart and brain. Despite the value of these maneuvers, multiple reports confirm that emergency department thoracotomy is rarely effective for blunt trauma and cardiac arrest.

Indications for emergency thoracotomy should be based on mechanism of injury and time of arrest. Current indications include:

- Penetrating Trauma: Witness penetrating injury with <15 minutes of pre-hospital CPR

- Blunt Trauma: Witnessed arrest with <5 minutes of pre-hospital CPR

- Persistent, severe post-injury hypotension (SBP ≤60 mmHG) due to:

  * Cardiac tamponade

  * Air embolism

  * Hemorrhage (intrathoracic, intra abdominal, extremity, cervical)

Contraindications include:

- Penetrating trauma: >15 minutes of CPR, and No signs of life (no pupillary response, respiratory effort or motor activity)
- Blunt trauma: >5 minutes of CPR, and No signs of life or asystole

2. Shock

Definition

Shock is defined as inadequate organ perfusion and tissue oxygenation resulting in cellular dysfunction and cell death. A patient can be in shock with or without abnormal vital signs. The initial steps in management are to recognize its presence and then to determine its cause. The most common cause of shock in the trauma patient is ***hemorrhage***. A trauma patient in shock should be considered hypovolemic until proven otherwise. Isolated brain injuries do not cause shock. The initial treatment for shock is volume loading to restore preload. Vasopressors are contraindicated.

Classification of Hemorrhagic Shock and Physiologic Response

Hemorrhagic shock is classified by the percentage of acute volume loss and is associated with a progression of physiologic changes (see Table 3). Blood volume in a normal adult is 7% of ideal body weight (approximately 5 L in a 70-kg man). The blood volume for a child is 8%-9% of body weight (80-90 cc/kg). In general, patients require 3 cc of crystalloid for every 1 cc of blood loss.

Treatment

Initial Fluid Therapy

An initial bolus of 2 L of warmed isotonic fluid should be given to adults (or 20 cc/kg in pediatric patients). Therapeutic decisions should be based on the physiologic response. Figure 1 shows an algorithm for fluid resuscitation and management of shock.

Rapid Response. The patient's vital signs normalize and remain stable following the initial fluid bolus. Blood loss in this group is usually 10%-20%. Blood should be cross-matched, but does not need to be given immediately. Further diagnostic studies can be carried out. Surgical intervention may still be necessary.

Transient Response. Vital signs and perfusion improve following the initial fluid bolus, but then deteriorate as fluid infusion is slowed to maintenance. This indicates ongoing blood loss or inadequate resuscitation. Blood loss in this group is 20%-40%. The fluid bolus should be immediately

Table 3

Classification of Hemorrhagic Shock and Associated Physiologic Changes

	Class I	Class II	Class III	Class IV
Blood loss (cc)	Up to 750 cc	750-1500 cc	1500-2000 cc	>2000 cc
% Volume loss	Up to 15%	15%-30%	30%-40%	>40%
Pulse rate	<100	>100	>120	>140
Blood pressure	Normal	Normal	Decreased	Decreased
Pulse pressure	Normal or increased	Decreased	Decreased	Decreased
Respiratory rate	14-20	20-30	30-40	>35
Urine output (cc/hr)	>30	20-30	5-15	Negligible
Mental status	Slightly anxious	Mildly anxious	Anxious, confused	Confused, lethargic
Fluid replacement	Crystalloid	Crystalloid	Crystalloid and blood	Crystalloid and blood

Figure 1

Algorithm for fluid resuscitation and management of shock

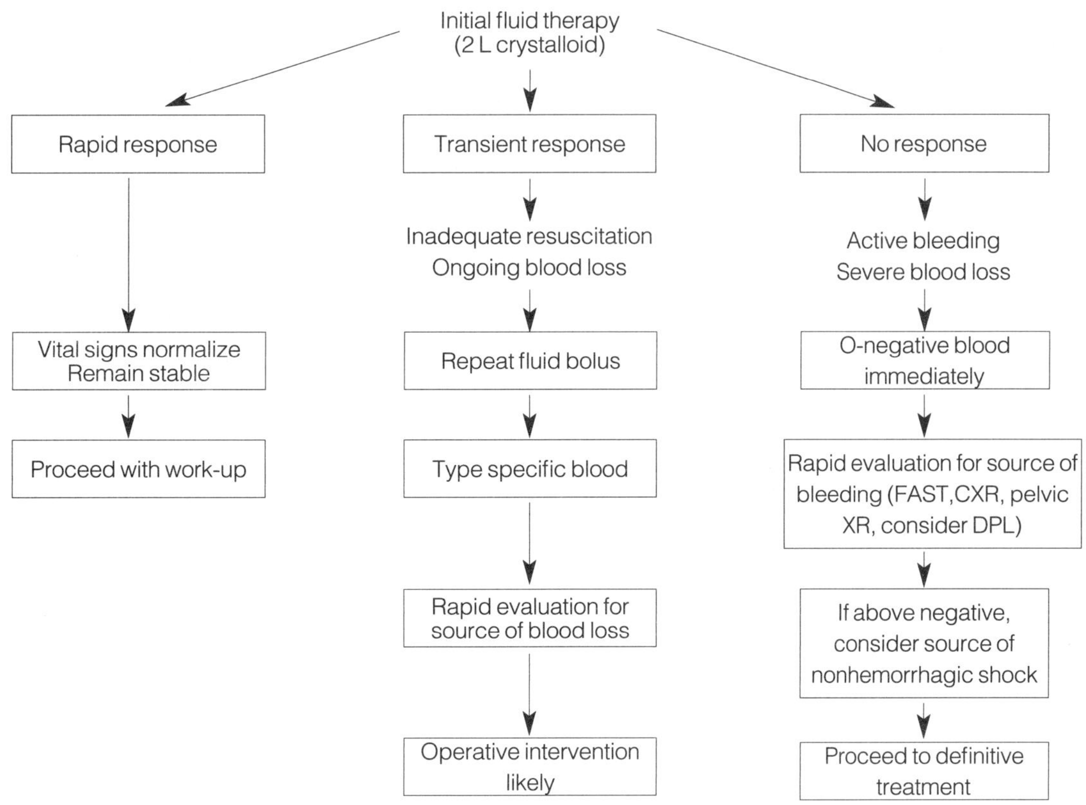

repeated. Type-specific blood should be given when available. Surgical intervention is likely to be needed.

No Response. These patients fail to respond to the initial fluid bolus, and vital signs remain abnormal. This indicates severe blood loss (>40%). Blood should be given immediately (O-negative). The need for rapid surgical intervention is highly likely. On very rare occasions, failure to respond may be due to causes of non-hemorrhagic shock (see below). Rapid evaluation and elimination of these may be necessary.

New Concepts in Resuscitation-Damage Control Resuscitation

Hypotensive Resuscitation. This strategy refers to the concept that fluid should be administered at a rate that returns the systolic blood pressure to a safe but lower than normal pressure until operative control of bleeding is achieved. The concept is that early and overaggressive resuscitation may increase blood pressure and hydrostatic pressure to such a degree that clots are dislodged and bleeding increases. Low-volume resuscitation, or "permissive hypotension", may avoid the adverse effects of early aggressive resuscitation by maintaining adequate tissue perfusion without increasing bleeding. This strategy has been suggested historically in the management of ruptured AAA. Although the concept is promising, further work needs to be done. It requires extraordinarily tight control by an experienced physician who is guiding the fluid resuscitation moment to moment. Hypotensive resuscitation should not be used in patient with traumatic brain injury and spinal cord injury, and should be used cautiously in elderly and patients with chronic hypertension.

Hemostatic Resuscitation. This strategy employs blood components early in the resuscitation process to restore both perfusion and normal coagulation function while minimizing crystalloid use. Based on retrospective military data, resuscitation and transfusion practices have moved to using thawed plasma as the primary resuscitation fluid in a ration of 1:1 or 1:2 with packed red blood cells. Massive transfusion protocols have moved to a ratio of 6 units of plasma, to 6 units of packed red blood cells, to 6 units of platelets (or one plateletpheresis) and 10 units of cryoprecipitate.

Causes of Nonhemorrhagic Shock

Tension Pneumothorax

Tension pneumothorax is a true surgical emergency. If suspected, immediate tube thoracostomy should be performed without waiting for CXR.

Cardiogenic Shock

Myocardial dysfunction causing refractory shock may be due to cardiac tamponade, blunt cardiac injury (contusion), air embolus or a myocardial infarction. Cardiac tamponade should always be suspected in a patient with penetrating injury who is refractory to fluid resuscitation. Additional information can be obtained by EKG, CVP and echocardiogram.

Neurogenic Shock

Neurogenic shock is due to the loss of sympathetic tone following spinal cord injury. The classic picture is hypotension without tachycardia or peripheral vasoconstriction (pulse pressure remains normal). Hypovolemia can compound neurogenic shock in the multiple trauma patient. Central venous pressure can be helpful in this situation. Isolated cranial injuries do not cause hypotension.

Septic Shock

Shock due to infection immediately following trauma is very uncommon. However, if arrival to the emergency department is delayed several hours, evidence of sepsis, especially from penetrating abdominal injuries, may be present.

3. Thoracic Trauma

Immediately Life-Threatening Injuries (Identified in Primary Survey)

Tension Pneumothorax

A tension pneumothorax develops when air leaks into the chest cavity but cannot escape, and is usually due to a visceral pleural injury. Air is forced into the thoracic cavity, completely collapsing the affected lung. As pressure in the thoracic cavity increases, the mediastinum is shifted to the opposite side, decreasing venous return and compressing the opposite lung. Clinical signs include hyperresonance, tracheal deviation away from the injury and hemodynamic compromise. ***Tension pneumothorax is a clincal diagnosis and treatment should not be delayed by waiting for radiologic confirmation.*** Immediate decompression can be accomplished initially by rapidly inserting a large-bore needle into the second intercostal space in the midclavicular line, followed immediately by a tube thoracostomy.

Open Pneumothorax (Sucking Chest Wound)

Large defects of the chest wall which remain open can result in an open pneumothorax. When the opening in the chest wall is greater than two-thirds the circumference of the trachea, air preferentially passes through the chest defect with each respiratory effort. Air accumulates within the pleural cavity, compressing the lung, impairing ventilation, leading to hypoxia and hypercarbia. Management consists of creating a sterile occlusive dressing that is taped on 3 sides, thus allowing a ***"flutter-type valve"*** (air can escape from the pleural cavity, but will not be sucked in). A tube thoracostomy should be placed at a site away from the wound. Definitive surgical closure of the defect will be necessary.

Flail Chest

A flail chest occurs when 2 or more ribs are fractured in 2 or more places, creating a floating segment of the chest wall. It usually occurs due to a direct impact. The unstable segment moves paradoxically during respiration. Diagnosis is usually clinical (paradoxical chest wall movement). Chest radiographs will show multiple rib fractures, but may not clearly display a flail segment. The major insult associated with flail chest is the underlying pulmonary contusion, not the chest wall instability. If the injury to the underlying lung is significant, severe hypoxia can result. Pain with breathing and splinting may also contribute to hypoxia. The cornerstones of therapy are aimed at aggressive pulmonary physiotherapy, effective analgesia (including epidural catheter), selective use of endotracheal intubation and ventilation, and close observation for respiratory decompensation. The primary indication for intubation and mechanical ventilation is respiratory decompensation.

Massive Hemothorax

Massive hemothorax is usually due to disruption of a major vascular structure and is defined as >1500 cc of blood within the chest cavity. Patients present in shock with flat neck veins due to severe hypovolemia. Breath sounds are decreased and a chest radiograph will show a large fluid accumulation. Management consists of decompression of the chest cavity with a large chest tube (36 F or larger) and aggressive fluid/blood resuscitation. If >1500 cc blood returns immediately, operative thoracotomy will likely be indicated. Persistent bleeding of >200 cc/hr for 2-4 hours may also suggest the need for operative intervention. However, this decision should be made based primarily on the patient's physiologic status, rather than solely on the rate of bleeding.

Cardiac Tamponade

Cardiac tamponade occurs when any combination of blood, fluid and air fill the pericardial sac. It is most commonly due to penetrating injury, but can occur from blunt trauma also. Because the pericardial sac is fibrous, it does not distend. Fluid within this sac causes compression of the atrial chambers and prevents blood return to the heart. Only a relatively small amount of blood is necessary to restrict cardiac activity and interfere with cardiac filling. Removal of small amounts of fluid by pericardiocentesis can dramatically improve a patient's hemodynamic status. Diagnosis can be difficult in the trauma setting. ***Beck's triad*** consists of venous pressure elevation, muffled heart tones and hypotension. Central venous pressure measurement will be elevated and an echocardiogram will show pericardial fluid. Pulseless electrical activity in the absence of hypovolemia or tension pneumothorax suggests cardiac tamponade. Treatment in hemodynamically unstable patients is pericardiocentesis or emergent/resuscitative thoracotomy for release of tamponade. Emergent surgical repair of the injury is necessary. In hemodynamically stable patients with a high likelihood of tamponade or cardiac injury, a subxiphoid pericardial window can be performed under general anesthesia to evaluate for blood in the pericardial sac. This procedure can also be performed in conjunction with a laparotomy if tamponade is suspected.

Potentially Life-Threatening Injuries (Identified in Secondary Survey)

Pulmonary Contusion

Pulmonary contusion occurs in up to 70% of patients with severe blunt chest trauma. Extensive interstitial and alveolar hemorrhage leads to a ventilation-perfusion mismatch and severe arterial hypoxemia. Pulmonary compliance decreases and work of breathing increases. Chest radiograph shows patchy infiltrates associated with rib fractures or chest trauma. These findings are present within 1 hour of injury in 70% of patients; the remainder have a delay of 4-6 hours before the contusion is visible on CXR. Treatment is primarily supportive. Supplemental oxygen should be administered. Patients with severe hypoxia (Pa_{O2}<65 on an inspired oxygen concentration of 50%) require mechanical ventilation. Contusions begin to resolve within 48-72 hours, but 2-3 weeks may be required for complete resolution.

Tracheobronchial Tree Injury

Injury to the trachea or major bronchi from blunt trauma is relatively uncommon, occurring in less than 1% of patients. It usually occurs in victims of high-speed motor vehicle accidents or results from crushing injuries with significant anteroposterior compressive forces to the chest. This causes traction injury of the trachea or mainstem bronchus, usually within 2 cm of the carina. Most patients with significant tracheobronchial injury die at the accident scene. Those who survive to reach the hospital complain of dyspnea, cough or hemoptysis. Chest radiographs reveal pneumothorax, pneumomediastinum and subcutaneous emphysema. Tube thoracostomy placement results in a persistent massive air leak without re-expansion of the lung. A second tube should then be placed. Bronchoscopy should be performed to confirm the diagnosis. If the laceration involves less than one-third of the circumference of the bronchus and the lung can be re-expanded with tube thoracostomy, conservative nonoperative management may be successful. If the laceration is one-third to one-half the circumference, early surgical intervention with primary repair is warranted to prevent late stricture.

Blunt Cardiac Injury

Blunt cardiac injury can result in myocardial muscle contusion, cardiac chamber rupture or valvular disruption.

Myocardial contusion contusion results from blunt force trauma to the chest and has been estimated to occur in up to 75% of patients with major blunt chest trauma. The incidence of myocardial contusion cannot be accurately determined because there is no consensus with regard to its definition and diagnostic criteria. Myocardial contusion results from extravasation of blood and edema in the contused area, which causes reduced local coronary microcirculation. Diminished perfusion in these localized areas may lead to tissue necrosis and infarction. Clinically significant myocardial contusions occur in fewer than 5% of patients admitted to trauma centers. Many tests have been used to diagnose myocardial contusion, but there is no universally accepted diagnostic test. Testing levels of CPK isoenzymes has been advocated, but there is poor correlation between CPK levels and conduction abnormalities. Echocardiography has also been used, but has never been proven to be superior to EKG as a predictor of arrhythmia. Nuclear medicine scans can detect abnormalities of cardiac perfusion and ventricular function but have not been fully studied. However, a number of studies have shown that the majority of clinically significant myocardial contusions are revealed by EKG abnormalities in the emergency department. The most common cause of early death from myocardial contusion is arrhythmia. Death is usually due to ventricular tachycardia or ventricular fibrillation. The most common arrythmias associated with myocardial contusion are supraventricular tachycardia, atrial flutter, and atrial fibrillation. The greatest risk of arrhythmia is the initial 24 hours following injury. Long-term follow-up following cardiac contusion is necessary due to the risk of delayed complications such as ventricular aneurysm or conduction abnormalities.

Cardiac chamber rupture is rare but can occur due to severe blunt chest trauma. The most common cause is rupture of the atrial appendage. Other reported causes are disruption of the IVC from the right atrium in severe decelerating injuries or puncture of the heart from broken ribs. Mortality is high, with most patients dying in the field.

Valvular disruption is rare but should be suspected when a new murmur is identified and/or progresses following blunt thoracic trauma.

Traumatic aortic disruption is caused by abrupt deceleration injuries (eg, high-speed head-on collisions, falls from significant heights). Shear forces act on the vessel at points of fixation, resulting in transection. The most common site is the descending aorta distal to the left subclavian artery at the ligamentum arteriosum. Approximately 50% of these patients die at the scene due to free perforation and exsanguination. Of those that survive the initial injury, the hemorrhage is contained within the adventitia and tissues of the mediastinum, forming a pseudoaneurysm. Characteristic findings on chest radiograph include: 1.) wide mediastinum (>8 cm at the level of the aortic knob in adults); 2.) obliteration of the aortic knob and aortopulmonary window; 3.) deviation of the trachea, nasogastric tube or endotracheal tube to the right; 4.) depression of the left mainstem bronchus; 5.) presence of an apical cap; 6.) widened paratracheal stripe; 7.) widened paraspinal interfaces; and 8.) a left hemothorax. Fractures of the first or second rib or scapula may also be associated with aortic rupture. Abnormal findings on CXR should prompt further diagnostic evaluation. However, because 1%-2% of patients with significant great vessel injury have no abnormality on CXR, further evaluation is warranted based on trauma mechanism alone. An anteroposterior chest film taken in the supine position tends to magnify the size of the mediastinum. Thus, an upright CXR should be obtained if it is not contraindicated. Diagnosis is usually made using CT angiography. Diagnosis can also be made using standard aortogram or transesophageal echocardiography. Treatment requires surgical repair via a left posterolateral thoracotomy. Patients undergoing repair are at risk for spinal cord ischemia and paraplegia (8%); this risk increases with crossclamp times >30 minutes. Operative mortality is 15%. Techniques of endovascular repair are rapidly evolving as an alternative approach for repair of blunt traumatic aortic injury.

Traumatic Diaphragmatic Injury

The diaphragm extends from the sternal xiphoid junction anterosuperiorly to the first 3 lumbar vertebrae posteroinferiorly. The outer muscular edges of the diaphragm surround a large central tendon that is relatively avascular.

Blunt trauma causes large radial tears of the diaphragm which leads to herniation of abdominal contents into the chest cavity. A chest radiograph will show herniation of bowel, stomach or nasogastric tube into the left chest cavity in 66% of cases. The left side is involved 5 times more often than the right, perhaps because the liver prevents herniation of contents on the right side or protects the diaphragm from rupture.

Penetrating injuries can be more difficult to diagnose. During expiration, the central dome of the diaphragm rises to the fourth intercostal space on the right, and the fifth intercostal space on the left. Thus, all penetrating injuries between the nipple and the third lumbar vertebra could potentially cause diaphragmatic injury. Chest radiograph in penetrating injury may be normal in 50% of patients with diaphragmatic injury, and the remainder will only demonstrate hemo- or pneumothorax. Diagnosis can be difficult, and no radiologic studies have proven beneficial in the acute setting. Invasive techniques include: 1.) mandatory laparotomy; 2.) diagnostic peritoneal lavage with a chest tube in place to detect communication between the abdominal and thoracic cavities (ie, peritoneal lavage fluid will come out of the chest tube with the patient in the Trendelenburg position); 3.) laparoscopy (may miss 15% of posterior injuries); and 4.) thoracoscopy. Treatment requires surgical repair with a running non-absorbable suture. Small penetrating injuries (<2 cm) on the right may be managed non-operatively. In the acute setting, all diaphragmatic injuries should be repaired via an abdominal laparotomy or laparoscopy due to the high incidence of associated abdominal injuries. In the chronic or delayed setting (ie, injuries that are diagnosed days to weeks following the acute event), associated intra abdominal injury is unlikely and repair may be approached via a thoracotomy or thoracoscopy.

Traversing Mediastinal Wounds

Penetrating injuries that traverse the mediastinum can injure any of the major mediastinal structures including the heart, great vessels, tracheobronchial tree or esophagus. Spinal cord injury must also be considered.

In the hemodynamically unstable patient, bilateral tube thoracostomies should be placed. If the patient showed signs of life in the field or on arrival to the emergency department, and then suffered acute decompensation (pulseless electrical activity or SBP <60), emergency department thoracotomy is indicated. Pericardial tamponade should be released. Urgent operative thoracotomy for massive hemothorax but with unknown injuries should be approached with a left anterolateral thoracotomy which can be extended across the sternum ("clamshell incision"). This will give access to all mediastinal structures, both chest cavities, and can be extended to the abdomen if necessary.

The hemodynamically stable patient must be thoroughly evaluated to exclude mediastinal injury. Tube thoracostomy is performed as indicated. Current evaluation using thoracic CT scanning to define the trajectory of the missile and potential injuries has allowed a more directed diagnostic approach in the hemodynamically stable patient. Following thoracic CT scan, invasive diagnostic work-up can be directed at likely injuries as indicated. Traditional management involved the diagnostic evaluation of all mediastinal structures with separate imaging modalities. Angiography was performed first to rule out great vessel injury. If negative, an esophagram was performed using water soluble contrast. Esophagoscopy increases the reliability of esophageal evaluation. Bronchoscopy would then be performed to evaluate the tracheobroncial tree. The heart/pericardium are best evaluated by echocardiography. During these tests, any acute decompensation should prompt immediate re-evaluation for tension pneumothorax, hemothorax or pericardial tamponade.

Traumatic Asphyxia

Traumatic asphyxia results from severe crushing injury to the chest by a very heavy object causing marked increases in thoracic and superior vena caval pressures. Concurrent closure of the glottis leads to even higher elevations in venous pressure, reversal of flow in the valveless veins of the head and neck, and capillary rupture. The resulting syndrome includes craniocervical cyanosis, facial edema, petechiae, subconjunctival hemorrhage and occasional neurologic sequelae (seizures, loss of consciousness, confusion, blindness). Early recognition of the physical stigmata is essential. Treatment is supportive, consisting of airway and ventilation maintenance and elevation of the head of the bed to 30 degrees. Associated injuries should be addressed. Mortality is low and is related to the severity of associated injuries and duration of asphyxia. Most neurologic sequelae clear within 24-48 hours.

Esophageal Injuries

Injury to the thoracic esophagus is rare. Blunt injuries occur in only 0.01% of all trauma patients. Penetrating injury is also uncommon and is usually associated with injuries to the adjacent structures. Early signs and symptoms include chest pain, dysphagia and a Hamman's crunch on auscultation. Late signs and symptoms include subcutaneous emphysema, fever and shock. Chest radiograph may show air in the retroesophageal space, pneumomediastinum, pneumothorax or a left pleural effusion, but it may also be normal. Diagnosis should include esophagography with water soluble contrast. Awake patients can swallow contrast under fluoroscopy. In unconscious patients, a nasogastric tube is placed into the proximal esophagus and 30-50 cc of contrast material is injected with pressure to distend the esophagus. If no leak is seen, barium is then used. Esophagoscopy should be used to follow-up suspicious or technically imperfect studies, or in a patient with a high likelihood of injury. Rigid esophagoscopy under general anesthesia is preferred. Flexible esophagoscopy does not distend the esophagus, and thus has a high rate of missed injuries. Surgical approach is dictated by location. The cervical esophagus can be approached by a collar incision, repaired primarily and drained widely. The proximal thoracic esophagus should be approached via a right posterolateral thoracotomy. Distal esophageal injuries can be approached through a left posterolateral thoracotomy. Injuries diagnosed early (<24 hours post-trauma) can be repaired primarily with wide drainage. Reinforcement with a pleural flap or intercostal muscle flap is recommended. Distal esophageal injuries can be reinforced with a circumferential or partial fundoplication. Injuries diagnosed late (>24 hours post-trauma) with established mediastinitis require esophageal exclusion with wide mediastinal drainage, cervical esophagostomy and temporary closure of the gastroesophageal junction with suture or band ligation. A proximal gastrostomy is performed for decompression and a feeding jejunostomy is performed for nutritional support. Later reconstruction is required and may be complex.

4. Abdominal Trauma

Initial Evaluation

Focused Assessment Sonogram in Trauma (FAST)
The use of ultrasound in the acute evaluation of the blunt trauma victim has become part of the primary survey in current evaluation of the trauma patient. Ultrasound is used to detect fluid in the abdomen by evaluating 4 areas: Morrison's pouch, the pouch of Douglas, the splenorenal recess and pericardial sac. Ultrasound can be performed at the bedside in 3–10 minutes, can quickly detect intraperitoneal fluid, is noninvasive, and it can be repeated. Solid organ parenchyma can be imaged to some degree, but not with as much detail as with a CT scan. Disadvantages include operator variability, missed bowel and pancreatic injuries, and a limited ability to differentiate blood from other fluids. In a hemodynamically stable patient, CT scan may be obtained even in the presence of free fluid on FAST. In a hemodynamically unstable patient, free fluid on the FAST exam necessitates emergency laparotomy to control hemorrhage.

Computed Tomography (CT)
CT scan is useful in the evaluation of the blunt trauma patient. However, CT scan should only be performed in the hemodynamically stable patient. It is noninvasive and enables the diagnostician to localize the source of intraperitoneal fluid, grade solid organ injury and identify retroperitoneal injuries. This modality allows for the option of non-operative management of solid organ injuries to the liver and/or spleen. When combined with intravenous and bladder contrast (CT cystogram), CT scan is useful in evaluating hematuria. However, CT scans may have a limited ability in detecting bowel injury. Hemodynamic instability is a contraindication to CT.

Diagnostic Peritoneal Lavage (DPL)
Diagnostic peritoneal lavage is a sensitive bedside procedure for detection of intraabdominal injury.With the increased use of FAST and increased non-operative management of solid organ injury, DPL has a limited role in the modern evaluation of a trauma patient. Its most common uses currently are for delayed identification of a bowel injury, or in the presence of a hypotensive patient with a negative FAST to rule out a false-negative FAST exam. The procedure is as follows: a

catheter is introduced into the peritoneal cavity and a syringe is used to aspirate. If more than 10 cc of gross blood or intestinal contents are aspirated, the test is considered grossly positive and the patient should be taken to the operating room for exploratory laparotomy. If this does not occur, 1000 cc (10-15 cc/kg in children) of warm crystalloid is infused into the peritoneal cavity via the catheter and then allowed to return. A positive test is defined as: 100,000 RBC/cc, >500 WBC/cc, amylase or bile level greater than serum, and/or the presence of bacteria or vegetable matter. Additionally, evidence of DPL fluid in either a Foley catheter or chest tube constitutes a positive lavage. Advantages of DPL include that it is simple, reliable, inexpensive and fast. It is extremely sensitive (98%-100%) and thus up 15% of patients who undergo exploratory laparotomy for a positive DPL have an injury that requires no specific operative therapy. Disadvan tages include its inability to identify specific organ injury and difficulty with identifying retroperitoneal injuries. The only absolute contraindication to DPL is an obvious need for exploration. Relative contraindications include a history of multiple abdominal operations, morbid obesity, and late stages of pregnancy. If bowel injury is suspected, a delayed DPL (4-8 hours following injury) will increase the sensitivity of the test.

Management of Specific Injuries

Diaphragmatic Injury
Injuries secondary to penetrating wounds are evenly divided between the right and left hemidiaphragms. Blunt rupture favors the left side (75%) over the right side (23%). Bilateral blunt rupture is uncommon (2%). Treatment is repair with a running nonabsorbable suture.

Stomach Injuries
The stomach is vulnerable to penetrating injuries of the upper abdomen and lower chest. The upper abdominal viscera underlie the lower ribs to a level as high as the fourth intercostal space. Blunt rupture of the stomach can also occur. Injuries to the stomach are usually easy to repair. Most can be repaired primarily in 2 layers, with an inner running layer of 3-0 or 4-0 absorbable sutures followed by an outer layer of 3-0 or 4-0 permanent Lembert sutures. On rare occasions, especially after shotgun wounds, large injuries of the stomach may require resection. However, because of the good blood supply, gastric injuries have excellent healing in most cases.

Duodenal Injuries
Duodenal hematomas occur due to blunt force trauma in the epigastric region. In children, this commonly occurs due to a bicycle handlebar injury. Diagnosis can be made by CT scan or upper GI series. Management is conservative with up to 2 weeks of nasogastric tube drainage and TPN. Operative decompression is rarely needed.

For penetrating or duodenal perforations, treatment is more complicated. Options include debridement of the injury with primary repair, serosal patching or resection. A Whipple procedure is indicated if the pancreaticobiliary ductal system is disrupted. The simplest technique possible should be used. External drainage is always advisable in order to create a controlled fistula should there be a leak. Duodenal bypass via a gastrojejunostomy or gastrostomy tube, with or without pyloric exclusion, is also an option, but remains controversial.

Small Intestine
The small intestine can be injured due to penetrating trauma or blunt injury and blowout. Treatment is primary repair or segmental resection.

Large Intestine
The large intestine can be injured from penetrating trauma or due to mesenteric tears leading to devascularization of portions of the colon. Right colon resection can be followed by a primary ileotransverse colon anastomosis. Primary repair or resection with primary anastomosis can also be used to treat left colon injuries. A temporary colostomy may be required if there is evidence of shock, a highly destructive injury, or multiple visceral injuries.

Rectum
Most rectal injuries are due to penetrating trauma. These can be repaired primarily with internal or external drainage. If the injury cannot specifically be identified, presacral and perirectal drains can be placed via the perineum. Rectal stump washout can then be performed with a diverting loop or end colostomy.

Liver

Most blunt liver injuries can now be managed non-operatively as long as the patient remains hemodynamically stable. Indications for operation include any evidence of hemodynamic instability or transfusion requirements of more than one-half of the estimated blood volume. Techniques in management include perihepatic packing, hepatorraphy with finger fracture technique, deep liver suturing, viable omental packing and resectional debridement. Severe hepatic trauma is frequently managed in several stages requiring multiple operations, with perihepatic packing and damage control laparotomy. The Pringle maneuver can be used to slow the rate of bleeding. If brisk bleeding persists following the Pringle maneuver, an injury to the hepatic veins or retrohepatic cava should be considered. If perihepatic packing does not arrest bleeding, an atriocaval shunt should be considered. Damage control laparotomy with repair in multiple stages is frequently required. Isolated penetrating injuries to the right upper quadrant may be safely observed in the hemodynamically stable patient without evidence of peritonitis.

Spleen

Injuries to the spleen are categorized as follows: grade I—capsular tears; grade II—lacerations not extending to the hilum; grade III—open lacerations extending to the hilum; grade IV—severe laceration involving segmental or hilar vessels; and grade V—shattered spleen or hilar vascular injury.

Management: Pediatric. Splenic injury should be observed unless the patient requires transfusion with more than one-half the estimated blood volume. Splenic salvage operation should then be attempted.

Management: Adult. CT scan will show the grade of splenic injury. Criteria for nonoperative management include: 1.) hemodynamic stability, 2.) an alert patient and the ability to perform serial abdominal examinations, 3.) absence of peritoneal signs, 4.) absence of associated intraabdominal injury and 5.) CT documentation of splenic injury not involving the hilum. Splenorraphy should only be attempted in hemodynamically stable patients, with no coagulopathy or acidosis, less than 1000 cc of blood in the abdomen and no other significant injuries. Nonoperative management should not be used in penetrating trauma due to the high incidence of associated injuries to the colon and diaphragm. Following splenectomy, patients should receive pneumococcal and H flu vaccines.

Pancreas

Most pancreatic injuries are due to penetrating trauma, and almost all are diagnosed during exploration. Blunt pancreatic injury can be more difficult to diagnose and requires a high index of suspicion and close clinical examination. Serial CT scans may be helpful. Transection usually occurs due to crush injury against the vertebral column from a blow to the epigastrium (handlebar injury). Treatment depends on the status of the pancreatic duct. Lacerations of the capsule that do not involve the duct can generally be watched and/or drained. The capsule can be repaired with nonabsorbable sutures without compromising the duct. If the pancreatic duct is disrupted, surgery is mandatory. If the duct is injured in the head of the pancreas, pancreaticoduodenectomy may be required. A midbody duct injury requires distal pancreatectomy with or without splenic preservation, or *Roux-en-Y* drainage of the distal duct with oversewing of the proximal pancreas and duct. Extensive external drainage is always recommended in order to convert leaks to a controlled external fistula.

Retroperitoneal Hematomas

For classification and management of retroperitoneal hematoma, see Table 4.

Zone 1: Central Medial. Major structures in this area include the aorta, inferior vena cava, proximal renal vascular pedicles and the pancreaticoduodenal structures. These hematomas should be explored for both blunt and penetrating injury.

Zone 2: Lateral. Zone 2 identifies the portion of retroperitoneum lateral to Zone 1 and includes the kidneys, ureters, renal vasculature, and portions of the colon and colonic mesentery. If a hematoma in this region is seen following blunt trauma and is nonexpanding, it can be observed. However, all hematomas seen following penetrating trauma must be explored.

Zone 3: Pelvic. Zone 3 includes the entire pelvis. Structures in this region include the pelvis, bones, iliac vessels, bladder, and rectum. Following blunt injury, Zone 3 injuries should be observed, but following penetrating injury, Zone 3 injuries must be explored.

Genitourinary Injuries

Bladder. Intraperitoneal bladder ruptures must be repaired operatively. Extraperitoneal bladder ruptures frequently occur in association with pubic rami fractures. These can be managed nonoperatively with catheter drainage and intravenous antibiotics. The majority will heal within 2-3 weeks. However, occasionally operative intervention and repair will be necessary. Should the patient be undergoing exploration and operative intervention for associated injuries, extraperitoneal bladder ruptures can be repaired at that time.

Urethral Injuries. The most common urethral injury is tear of the prostatic urethra due to blunt force trauma and it is usually associated with pelvic fractures. Associated signs include blood at the meatus, a high-riding prostate, or extensive perineal hematoma. If blood is noted at the meatus or if a transurethral catheter cannot easily be passed, a retrograde urethrogram should be performed. If a urethral tear is identified, a suprapubic catheter should be placed for drainage.

Table 4

Management of Retroperitoneal Hematomas

	Penetrating trauma	Blunt trauma
Zone 1 (central)	Explore	Explore
Zone 2 (lateral)	Explore	Observe
Zone 3 (pelvic)	Explore	Observe

Renal Injury. Renal parenchymal injuries occur due to blunt or penetrating trauma. In patients sustaining blunt trauma not requiring operative intervention, these can almost uniformly be observed. During operative intervention for associated injuries, however, attempted repair and renal salvage should be considered. Nephrectomy should be performed if there is extensive avulsion involving the renal hilum/collecting system, or if significant associated injuries exist.

Renovascular Trauma. Significant renal vascular injuries include pelvic avulsion, renal artery thrombosis, and segmental arterial interruption. Unfortunately, opportunities for timely revascularization in cases of pedicle injury are rare, owing to delays between the occurrence of the injury, its diagnosis and laparotomy. In general, revascularization should only be considered when the warm ischemia time can be kept under 4 hours and no other significant injuries exist. Otherwise, nephrectomy or simple observation is warranted.

Thoracoabdominal Stab Wounds

Thoracoabdominal injuries are defined as any penetrating injury between the nipple and costal margin. Injuries in this region may affect the lung, the diaphragm or intraabdominal structures. Thorough evaluation is necessary to rule out diaphragmatic injury. Diagnostic studies include diagnostic peritoneal lavage, laparoscopy or exploration.

Seat Belt Injuries

Overall, seat belt restraints save lives and decrease injuries. However, a loose lap seat belt, or one that is placed across the lower abdomen rather than over the anterior superior iliac spines of the pelvis, may cause a constellation of injuries in a frontal crash at high speed: mesenteric tears, rupture of the small bowel or colon, Chance fractures of the lumbar spine (most commonly occurring at L2), and intimal tears with dissection or thrombosis of the iliac artery or the abdominal aorta. Children in particular have an increased incidence of the combination of a Chance-type fracture and rupture of an intraabdominal viscus. Bowel injury can occur in up to 30% of patients with a seat belt sign following blunt trauma.

Damage Control Laparotomy

Damage control laparotomy refers to a systemic 3-phase approach to the multiple trauma victim requiring operative intervention. The first phase consists of an ***exploratory laparotomy*** during which there is control of exsanguinating hemorrhage, control of enteric contamination, intraabdominal packing and temporary abdominal closure. The second phase consists of ***secondary resuscitation*** which can occur in the recovery room or intensive care unit. During this phase, the patient is resuscitated in a controlled environment with strict attention to core rewarming, correction of coagulopathy, and improvement of acidosis by maximizing hemodynamics and ventilatory support. Additional diagnostic and therapeutic studies (eg, angiography) may also be utilized for injury identification. The third phase consists of ***reoperation*** for removal of packs and definitive repair of injuries. More than one reoperation may be required. The goals of damage control laparotomy are immediate survival with early recognition of physiologic limits in order to prevent irreversible cardiovascular collapse. Damage control laparotomy should be considered in patients with one or more of the following: severe metabolic acidosis (pH <7.30), hypothermia (temperature <35°C), resuscitation and/or time >90 minutes, coagulopathy as indicated by nonsurgical bleeding and massive transfusion (>10 units packed red blood cells).

5. Head Trauma

Pathophysiology

The Monroe-Kellie Doctrine

The cranial vault (calvarium) and the base of the skull represent a fixed closed space. Within this space is the brain, cerebrospinal fluid, venous blood volume and arterial blood volume. The total volume must remain constant. Thus, following injury, associated swelling and/or mass lesions begin to take up space. Venous blood and cerebrospinal fluid will be displaced, and this can be seen as small ventricles on CT scan. Intracranial pressure will remain constant until a critical point of decompensation is reached at which time the pressure will exponentially increase. This is known as the Monroe-Kellie Doctrine (see Figure 2).

Intracranial Pressure. Normal intracranial pressure (ICP) is approximately 10 mm Hg. ICP of >20 mm Hg is considered abnormal, and ICP values >40 are considered severely abnormal. The higher the ICP following injury, the worse the outcome.

Cerebral Perfusion Pressure. Cerebral perfusion pressure is the mean arterial pressure minus intracranial pressure (CPP = MAP – ICP). Cerebral perfusion pressures of less than 70 mm Hg are associated with worse outcome following trauma.

Autoregulation. Normal cerebral blood flow is approximately 50 cc/100 g brain mass/min. This remains fairly constant at MAP between 50 and 160 mm Hg. However, at MAPs <50, cerebral blood

Figure 2

The Monroe-Kellie Doctrine: volume-pressure curve for ICP

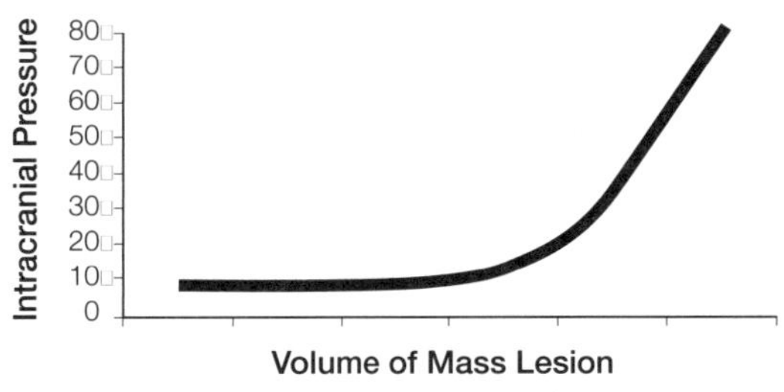

Figure 3

Autoregulation of cerebral blood flow

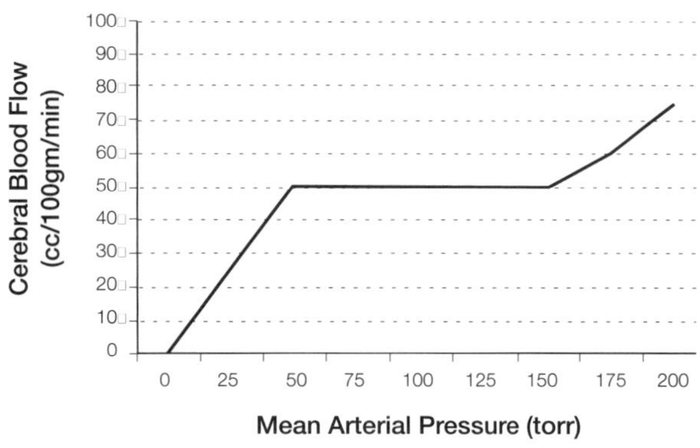

flow significantly decreases, and at MAPs >160, cerebral blood flow significantly increases (see Figure 3). These mechanisms may be disturbed in the head-injured patient.

Cushing's response refers to the hypertension and bradycardia that occurs in response to elevated intracranial pressures.

Classification (Mild, Moderate, Severe)

Mild Head Injury (GCS 14-15)

Approximately 80% of patients presenting to the emergency department are classified as having a mild head injury (GCS 14-15). Although awake and alert on arrival, patients usually report a brief loss of consciousness, amnesia to the event or severe headaches. They may also display mild confusion or repetitive questioning. Overall, 18% will have an abnormality on head CT and approximately 5% will go on to require surgery. While most patients with mild head injury recover uneventfully, 3% deteriorate unexpectedly resulting in severe neurologic consequences unless recognized and treated early. ***A CT scan should be obtained on all head injury patients who report a brief loss of consciousness, amnesia to the event, confusion or severe headache.***

Moderate Head Injury (GCS 9-12)

Approximately 10% of head-injured patients presenting to the emergency department have moderate head injury. Head CT is absolutely indicated in all moderate head injuries. Approximately 40% will have an abnormality on CT scan, 8% will require surgery, and 10%-20% will deteriorate into coma. Close serial observation and a follow-up head CT is indicated.

Severe Head Injury (GCS 3-8)

These patients are at greatest risk of developing significant morbidity and mortality. Coma is defined as a GCS <8. Secondary insults must be prevented. Head-injured patients with hypotension (SBP <95) or hypoxia (Po_2 <65 mm Hg) have significantly worse outcomes. Aggressive resuscitation is necessary.

Morphology of Injury

Skull Fractures

Skull fractures can be in the cranial vault or skull base, linear or stellate, and open or closed.

Basilar skull fractures should be suspected in any patient with periorbital ecchymosis (raccoon eyes), retroauricular ecchymosis (Battle's sign), CSF leaks (rhinorrhea or otorrhea) or cranial nerve VII palsy. Auditory problems may also occur. ***Linear skull fractures*** increase the likelihood of an intracranial hematoma by 400 times in a conscious patient and 200 times in an unconscious patient. ***Depressed skull fractures*** usually require surgical elevation when the fragments are depressed more than the thickness of the skull. ***Open skull fractures*** also usually require open surgical repair.

Focal Lesions

Epidural hematomas are classically associated with a tear in the middle meningeal artery from a skull fracture in the temporoparietal region. They are located outside of the dura but within the skull, and typically have a biconvex or lenticular shape. Occasionally, they can be associated with massive venous bleeding from skull fractures or torn venous sinuses. Patients may present with the classic "lucent interval" followed by a rapid deterioration. They are relatively uncommon (0.5% with all head injuries, 9% in comatose patients), and if recognized and treated early, prognosis is excellent because direct damage to the underlying brain is minimal. Prognosis is directly related to the neurologic status of the patient before surgery.

Subdural hematomas are the most common traumatic mass lesion in severely head-injured patients (20%-40%) and classically occur due to tearing of the bridging veins between the cerebral cortex and a draining venous sinus. These clots occur in the potential space between the dura and arachnoid meningeal layers. The underlying brain injury is usually more significant, and thus these injuries have a worse prognosis.

Cerebral contusions or hematomas occur anywhere within the brain parenchyma, but are most common in the subfrontal and anterior temporal regions. During abrupt rotational movements, the brain impacts on the rough underside of the skull in these regions, leading to small contusions which may coalesce into larger hematomas. Although initially small, these minor contusions can rapidly enlarge. Close neurologic observation with serial CT scans is necessary to follow the progression.

Diffuse Injuries

Diffuse brain injuries form a continuum of brain injury due to shearing forces associated with acceleration-deceleration injuries.

In ***mild concussion***, consciousness is preserved but there is some degree of neurologic dysfunction. Usually there is no amnesia, and complete recovery occurs. ***Classic concussion*** is usually associated with a transient loss of consciousness, and varying degrees of antegrade and retrograde amnesia, with the length of amnesia correlating with the severity of injury. ***Post-concussion syndrome*** may occur, consisting of varying degrees of memory difficulties, dizziness, nausea, anosmia and depression.

Diffuse axonal injury is the term used to describe prolonged posttraumatic coma that is not due to a mass lesion or ischemic insults. This is typically caused by shearing injury to the long axonal cylinders. The initial head CT may appear normal. Recovery is difficult to predict, and depends on the extent of axonal injury. Secondary insults must be avoided.

Subarachnoid Hemorrhage

Subarachnoid hemorrhage is common following traumatic head injury. Hemorrhage is spread diffusely, and therefore does not cause mass effect. These patients, however, are prone to cerebral vasospasm which can be detected with transcranial Doppler. If vasospasm is present, hydration and calcium channel blockers (eg, nimodipine) are indicated. Severe vasospasm can lead to cerebral infarction.

Surgical Management

In general, surgical management is indicated for significant mass effect from a hematoma or contusion. Displacement of intracranial structures by more than 5 mm has been arbitrarily used to describe significant displacement.

Medical Management

The goal of medical management following head injury is to ***prevent secondary insults***. Conditions associated with poor outcome include hypoxemia, hypotension, hypercarbia, hyperglycemia, hypercalcemia and hypermagnesemia. Care should be taken to avoid these insults.

Airway: Patients with severe head injury (GCS 3-8) should be immediately intubated and ventilated with 100% oxygen to prevent hypoxia. ***Breathing:*** Hyperventilation (P_{CO_2} 25-35 mm Hg) may be used cautiously in patients with deteriorating GCS, pupillary dilatation or other evidence of increasing intracranial pressure. However, significant hyperventilation may be detrimental by causing excessive cerebral vasoconstriction and decreased cerebral perfusion. ***Circulation:*** Aggressive fluid resuscitation to restore blood volume and prevent hypotension is necessary. Normovolemia is the goal. Dehydration is considered harmful in that it decreases cerebral perfusion. Head injury alone will ***not*** cause hypotension. An aggressive search for hemorrhage should be initiated in the hypotensive head-injured patient. ***Intravenous Fluids:*** Isotonic fluids should be used. Hypotonic and glucose-containing fluids should be avoided. Hyponatremia is associated with brain edema and should be prevented or treated aggressively.

Neurologic Evaluation. Obtain a reliable minineurologic exam prior to sedating or paralyzing the

Figure 4

Management of comatose patient with multiple injuries

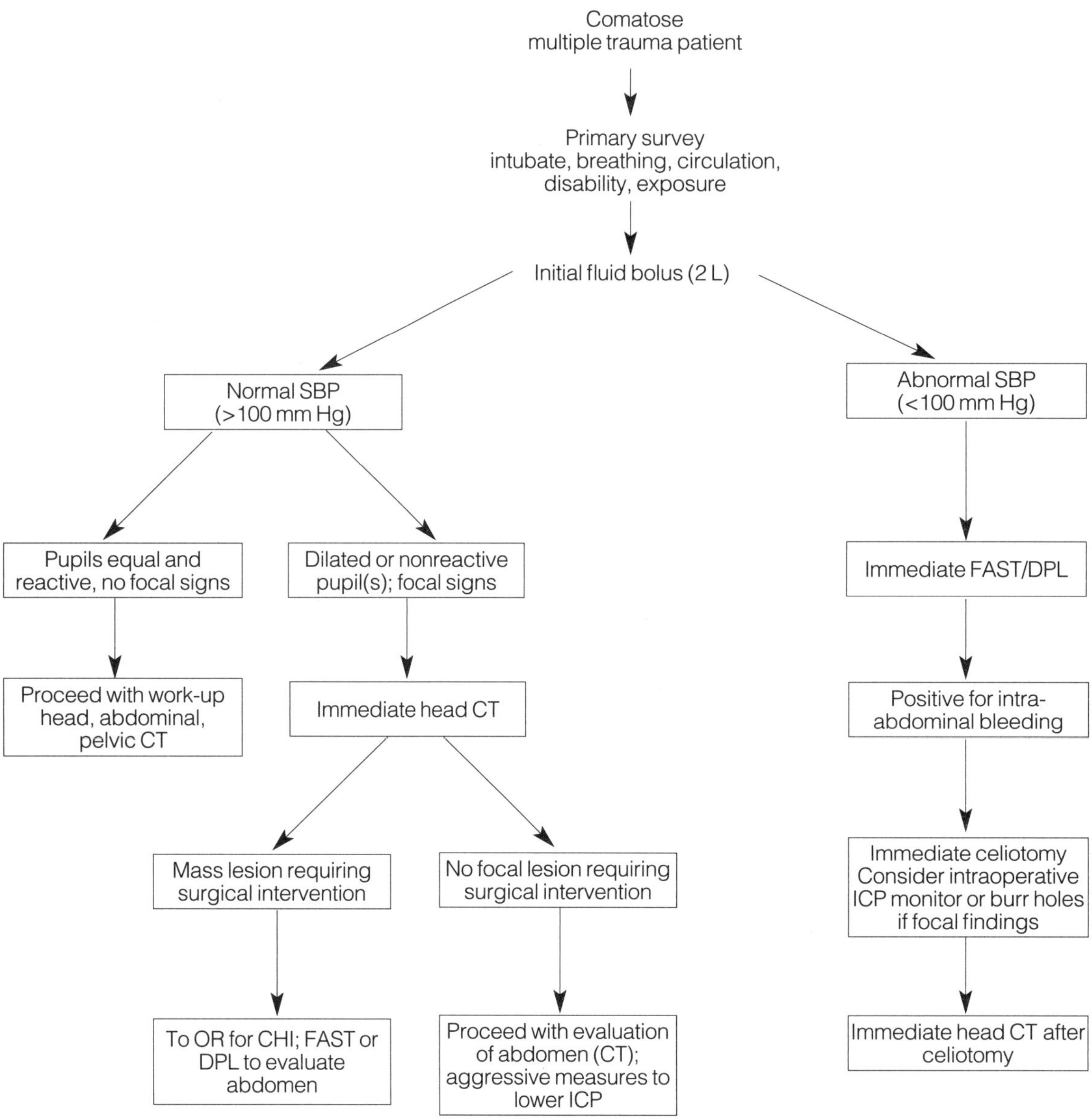

Table 5

Pupillary Abnormalities and the Associated Medical Condition

Pupillary abnormality	Associated medical condition
Bilaterally dilated (sluggish or fixed)	Inadequate brain perfusion Herniation with bilateral CN III palsy
Unilaterally dilated (no cross-reactivity)	Herniation with CN III palsy
Unilaterally dilated (cross-reactive pupil) Marcus-Gunn pupil	Optic nerve injury
Bilaterally constricted	Drugs (opiates) Pontine lesion Metabolic
Unilaterally constricted	Injured sympathetic pathway (carotid sheath)

patient. Serial evaluation including pupillary evaluation is necessary throughout the resuscitation (see Table 5).

Mannitol is an osmotic diuretic that is widely used to reduce intracranial pressure. The usual dose is 1 gm/kg. It should be given to any patient with clear evidence of elevated intracranial pressure. Care should be taken in the hypotensive patient because mannitol can exacerbate hypovolemia. Furosemide may be used as an adjunct to mannitol if diuresis is necessary.

Propofol has also been used as an adjunct to assist with sedation and to lower intracranial pressure. Advantages are that it is short-acting and can be discontinued to allow for frequent neurologic examinations. Disadvantages are that it can be associated with hypotension, bradycardia and prolonged high-dose infusions (ie >50 ug/kg/min for more than 48 hours) can be associated with propofol infusion syndrome, characterized by severe metabolic acidosis, rhabdomyolysis, hyperkalemia, lipemia, renal failure, hepatomegaly and cardiovascular collapse.

Barbituates are very effective in lowering ICP. However, they can cause hypotension and cardiovascular depression, and should not be used during acute resuscitation or in a hypotensive patient. These agents are usually used in the intensive care unit several days following injury when a patient develops intractable intracranial hypertension. Pentobarbital is infused with a loading dose of 5-10 mg/kg followed by 1-3 mg/kg/hour and is continued until 60-second burst suppression on EEG is produced. Serum levels can also be measured.

Use of anticonvulsants in head-injured patients remains controversial. Factors associated with post-traumatic epilepsy include: 1.) early seizures following injury (first week), 2.) intracranial hematoma and 3.) depressed skull fracture. Prophylactic anticonvulsants may be beneficial in the first week following injury, but have not been proven to be beneficial thereafter.

Intracranial pressure monitoring is indicated in any patient with a closed head injury and a GCS <8, or in a patient who does not have a neurologic exam that can be closely followed. Maintaining cerebral perfusion pressure at >70 mm Hg is very important in the management of head injury. This can be accomplished by lowering ICP while increasing

MAP. ICP is lowered using the methods described above. Mean arterial pressure may be increased using vasopressors once the patient has been adequately volume resuscitated.

Tentorial/Uncal Herniation

This syndrome occurs when intracranial pressure increases and the medial portion of the temporal lobe (the uncus) herniates through the tentorial notch. This leads to compression of the third cranial nerve and corticospinal tract at the midbrain. The corticospinal tract crosses over more distally at the foramen magnum. Thus, the patient exhibits an ipsilateral blown pupil (90%) and contralateral hemiplegia (60%). Occasionally the patient may exhibit ipsilateral hemiplegia (40%) if the contralateral corticospinal tract is compressed.

Emergency Burr Holes

Emergency burr holes should only be done by a nonneurosurgeon with the advice and consent of a neurosurgeon, and should only be considered when definitive neurosurgical care is unavailable. If necessary, ***the burr hole should be placed on the side of the larger pupil.***

Management of the Comatose Patient with Multiple Injuries

Priorities of the primary survey (*ABCDE*s) must be adhered to. Life-threatening injuries and hemorrhage must be dealt with first (see Figure 4).

Figure 5

Schematic of spinal cord anatomy and functional tracts

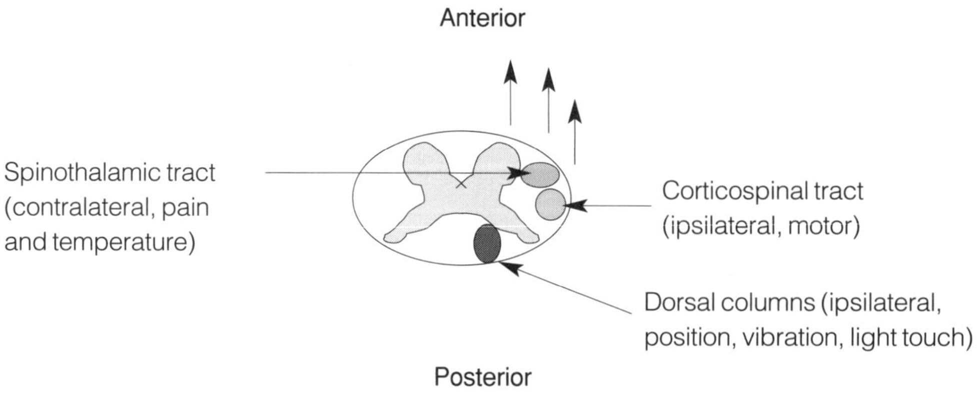

6. Spine Trauma

Anatomy and Physiology

Spinal Column (Vertebral Anatomy)

The spinal column consists of 7 cervical, 12 thoracic and 5 lumbar vertebrae, as well as the sacrum and the coccyx. The bony and ligamentous spine can be divided into 3 columns: The ***anterior column*** consists of the anterior two-thirds of the vertebral body in the anterior longitudinal ligament. The ***middle column*** comprises the posterior third of the vertebral body, the posterior longitudinal ligament and the posterior component of the annulus fibrosus. The ***posterior column*** is composed of the lamina and facet joints, the spinous processes and the interspinous ligaments. In general, disruption of 2 or more columns is required to produce an unstable injury.

Spinal Cord Anatomy

The spinal cord extends from the end of the medulla oblongata at the foramen magnum to the first lumbar vertebrae as the conus medullaris. Below this level, the spinal cord becomes cauda equina, which is more resistant to injury.

Within the spinal cord, there are 3 main functional tracts:

The ***spinothalamic tract*** is located in the anterior lateral aspect of the cord and transmits pain and temperature sensation from the contralateral side of the body. Generally, it is tested by pinprick and light touch. Within 2-3 segments of each dorsal route, the axons cross through the anterior commissure of the cord and ascend to the thalamus through this tract.

The ***corticospinal tract*** lies in the posterior lateral segment of the cord and carries motor impulses on the same side of the body. It is tested by voluntary muscle contractions or involuntary response to painful stimuli. These tracts cross the midline at the pyramidal decussation in the lower medulla.

The ***posterior (dorsal columns)*** carry sensory fibers conveying position, vibratory and light touch sensation from the same side of the body. These columns are tested by position sense in the toes and fingers, or by vibration sense using a tuning fork. These fibers cross to the opposite cerebral cortex through decussation in the brainstem (see Figure 5).

Spinal Cord Syndromes

Central cord syndrome is characterized by a greater loss of motor power in the upper extremities than in the lower extremities. Bowel and bladder function may also be impaired. This syndrome is usually seen after a hyperextension injury in a patient with preexisting cervical canal stenosis. The pathophysiology is thought to be due to vascular compromise of the cord in the distribution of the anterior spinal artery. This artery supplies the central portions of the cord. Because the motor fibers to the cervical segments are anatomically arranged toward the center of the cord, this is the region that is affected most. Function usually improves with time, but distal arm strength may remain poor.

Anterior cord syndrome syndrome is characterized by a loss of corticospinal and spinothalamic pathways with preservation of posterior column (dorsal column) function. The result is paraplegia and a loss of pain and temperature sensation distal to the level of injury. However, posterior column function (position sense, vibration and deep pressure) is preserved. The anterior two-thirds of the cord is supplied by the anterior spinal artery; therefore, occlusion or spasm of this vessel may be a cause of this syndrome. The prognosis for recovery is very poor.

Brown-Sequard syndrome results from hemisection of the cord. It is rarely seen but variations of the classical picture are not uncommon. It is usually due to a penetrating injury. In its pure form, the syndrome consists of ipsilateral motor loss and loss of position sense (due to corticospinal and dorsal column injury), and contralateral loss of pain and temperature sensation (due to spinothalamic tract injury). Some recovery is usually seen.

Spinal Cord Trauma

Vertebral column injury must always be sought and excluded in a patient with multiple trauma. Patients who are fully awake, not intoxicated, and have no distracting pain can be examined and cleared clinically. These patients do not need radiographic studies if they have no spine pain or neurologic deficits.

Other patients should have directed radiologic studies. Approximately 10% of patients with a C-spine fracture have a second associated noncontiguous vertebral column fracture and vice versa. Thus, any patient with a spinal column injury requires radiographic screening of the entire spine.

Radiographic Evaluation

Computed tomography has become the mainstay of cervical spine evaluation. If pain persists on range of motion following a normal cervical spine CT, flexion/extension views and/or an MRI of the spine should be obtained. Magnetic resonance imaging (MRI) provides the most accurate data in the presence of any neurologic deficits. However, MRI is frequently not feasible in an unstable patient. Controversy still exists as to the best way to rule out cervical spine injury in the comatose and/or pediatric patient.

Historically, cervical spine evaluation consisted of a crosstable lateral film (down to C7-T1), an open-mouth odontoid view (C1-C2) and an AP view (for detection of facet joint dislocations). A swimmer's view of the lower cervical and upper thoracic area could also be obtained if this area was not seen on the standard lateral film. A lateral C-spine film detects 85% of cervical spine injuries. The combination of lateral, AP and open-mouth x-rays increases the sensitivity for identification of a fracture to approximately 92%. Thoracolumbar spine films should be performed in any patient who has a diagnosed cervical spine fracture, who is comatose or in a patient who has significant point tenderness to examination. Any abnormality should be further investigated with CT scan through the area of interest.

Classification of Spinal Cord Injuries

Complete spinal cord injury is used to describe an injury in which there is no demonstrable sensory or motor function below a certain level.

Incomplete injury is used to describe an injury in which any motor or sensory function persists below the level of injury. The prognosis for this type of injury is significantly better than for a complete spinal cord injury. ***Sacral sparing*** may be demonstrated by preservation of sensory perception in the perianal region and/or voluntary contraction of the rectal sphincter. This may be the only sign of residual function distal to a spinal cord injury.

Table 6A

Key Sensory Points for Neurologic Examination

Nerve root	Level of sensation
C5	Area over deltoid
C6	Thumb
C7	Middle finger
C8	Little finger
T4	Nipple
T8	Xiphoid
T10	Umbilicus
T12	Symphysis
L4	Medial aspect of leg
L5	Space between first and second toes
S1	Lateral border of foot
S3	Ischial tuberosity
S4/S5	Perianal region

Examination of Spinal Cord Injury

Complete evaluation of sensory and motor function is also necessary in assessing spinal cord injuries (see Tables 6A and 6B).

Cervical Spine Injuries

Cervical spine injuries are the most common (55%) and result from one of the following mechanisms: axial loading, flexion, extension, rotation, lateral bending and distraction.

Table 6B

Key Myotomes for Neurologic Examination

Nerve root	Motor function
C3-C4	Diaphragm
C4	Shoulder shrug
C5	Elbow flexion
C6	Elbow extensors
C7	Wrist flexors
C8	Finger flexors
T1	Finger abductors
L2	Hip flexors
L3-L4	Knee extensors
L5-S1	Ankle dorsiflexors
S1-S2	Ankle plantar flexors

Atlantooccipital Dislocation. This injury is uncommon and results from severe traumatic flexion and distraction. Most of these patients die of brainstem destruction immediately. An occasional patient may survive if prompt resuscitation is available at the injury scene.

Atlas Fractures (C1). The atlas is a thin bony ring with broad articular surfaces. The most common C1 injury is a ***burst fracture (Jefferson fracture).*** The mechanism is axial loading resulting in disruption of both the anterior and posterior rings of C1 with lateral displacement of the lateral masses. This fracture is best seen on open-mouth odontoid view and can be confirmed by CT scan. In patients who survive, these fractures are usually not associated with spinal cord injury. However, they are unstable and should be treated with a cervical collar. Because of their proximity, injury to the lateral masses of the C1 vertebra is associated with vertebral artery injury.

Axis Fractures (C2). Odontoid fractures account for approximately 60% of all C2 fractures. The odontoid process is a peg-shaped bony protuberance that projects upward from the body of C2 and is normally positioned in contact with the anterior arch of C1. Odontoid fractures are best identified on lateral C-spine or open-mouth odontoid views.

- ***Type 1*** fractures typically involve the tip of the odontoid and are relatively uncommon.
- ***Type 2*** fractures occur through the base of the dens and are the most common. These do not involve the body of C2.
- ***Type 3*** fractures occur at the base of the dens and extend into the body of C2. Suspicion of this type of fracture should be confirmed with a CT scan.

A ***hangman's fracture*** (posterior element fractures of C2) represent approximately 20% of all axis fractures. This type of fracture is due to hyperextension of the neck.

Fractures and Dislocations of C3-C7. The most common level of cervical vertebral fracture is C5, and the most common level of subluxation is C5 on C6. It is at this junction at which the greatest flexion and extension of the C-spine occurs. Any abnormalities detected on cervical spine series x-rays should be followed up with a CT scan through the area of concern.

Thoracic Spine Fractures

Thoracic spine fractures can be classified into 4 categories. ***Anterior wedge*** fractures are due to axial loading with flexion. ***Burst injury*** is caused by true vertical axial compression. ***Fracture dislocations*** are relatively uncommon in T1-T10; however, when they do occur, they commonly result in complete neurologic deficits. ***Chance fractures*** are due to hyperflexion which results in a splitting injury of the vertebral column beginning posteriorly and proceeding anteriorly through the vertebral body or intervertebral disk. This is most commonly seen in the lumbar spine due to seat belt injury. Chance fractures may be associated with retroperitoneal and abdominal visceral injuries.

Thoracolumbar Junction Fractures (T11-L1)
Fractures in this region most commonly result from acute hyperflexion and rotation, and consequently are usually unstable. Because the spinal cord terminates around L1, the nerve roots that compose the cauda equina arise at the thoracolumbar junction. Injuries in this area commonly produce bladder and bowel dysfunction as well as decreased sensation and movement in the lower extremities. If a burst fracture is identified in the thoracolumbar spine, the entire thoracolumbar spine must be imaged because there is a 40% chance that a second fracture will be found caudal to the first.

Spinal Shock vs. Neurogenic Shock

Spinal shock refers to the flaccidity and loss of reflexes seen following injury to the spinal cord. This flaccidity may progress to rigidity and spasticity if the injured neurons do not recover. Alternatively, function may return in days to weeks following injury.

Neurogenic shock results from the loss of vasomotor tone due to the interruption of sympathetic stimulation associated with cervical and high thoracic spinal cord injuries. This results in pooling of blood in dilated peripheral vessels. Sympathetic tone to the heart is also lost, resulting in bradycardia and hypotension. Initial treatment is volume replacement. Once hypovolemia due to hemorrhage has been ruled out, peripheral vasoconstrictors (phenylephrine) can be used to raise the blood pressure. Atropine can be used to counteract hemodynamically significant bradycardia.

Steroids and Blunt Spinal Cord Injury

In a prospective randomized trial in 1997, steroids were shown to improve outcomes after blunt spinal cord injury. However, follow-up studies have failed to convincingly confirm these results. In addition, steroids are associated with significant adverse side effects. Therefore, recommendations for the routine use of steroids in spinal cord injury are softening and many feel there is insufficient evidence to support the routine use of steroids in blunt spinal cord injury. Steroids are *never indicated* in patients with penetrating spinal cord injury or in patients with vertebral column injury but no neurologic deficit.

The treatment protocol for blunt spinal cord injury with neurologic impairment consists of an initial intravenous bolus of 30 mg/kg of methylprednisolone followed by a 23-hour infusion at 5.4 mg/kg/hr. If treatment is started within 3 hours of injury, 24 hours of steroid treatment seems to be beneficial. Treatment is extended to 48 hours when the interval from injury to treatment is 3-8 hours. Results of clinical trials have failed to demonstrate any benefit from steroids started more than 8 hours postinjury. Side effects to steroid therapy include hyperglycemia, mental status changes and immunosuppression. In addition, extension of steroid infusion from 24-48 hours was associated with an increase in severe sepsis from 0.6%-2% and an increase in pneumonia from 2.6%-5.8%.

Penetrating Spine Injuries

Neurologic deficits from CSF leakage and contamination of the CSF space must be considered after penetrating injury to the spinal cord. The need for surgical debridement of penetrating spinal cord injuries is controversial. Debridement is currently recommended in cases of neurologic deterioration, partial neurologic deficit or cases where bone or projectile fragments impinge on nerve tissue. Broad-spectrum antibiotics are recommended. ***Steroids are not indicated.***

7. Musculoskeletal Trauma

Injuries to the musculoskeletal system occur in approximately 85% of patients who sustain blunt trauma. While they are rarely immediately life-threatening, diagnosis of potentially fatal or limb-threatening injuries must be made. Pelvic fractures can result in significant life-threatening retroperitoneal hemorrhage. In addition, femoral fractures may result in up to 3-4 units of blood loss into the thigh, producing significant shock. Blunt and/or penetrating trauma can also cause vascular injury, which may manifest itself as significant external hemorrhage, or as thrombosis with resulting limb ischemia and limb threat.

Pelvic Trauma

Pelvic fractures are classified by vector of injury: anterior/posterior compression, lateral compression, vertical shear and combined mechanical forces. Pelvic fractures are associated with an appreciable risk of death. Major pelvic hemorrhage occurs rapidly and the diagnosis must be made quickly to initiate appropriate treatment. Unexplained hypotension may be the only initial indication of major pelvic disruption. For this reason, an AP pelvic x-ray should be included during the primary survey in unstable trauma patients. If a pelvic fracture is identified, the pelvis should be temporarily stabilized (or "closed") with a sheet or commercially available pelvic binder to control bleeding. Intra abdominal sources of bleeding should be excluded or treated operatively. If the patient remains hypotensive, and intra-abdominal bleeding has been excluded, further mechanisms to control pelvic bleeding should be pursued such as angiographic embolization, surgical stabilization or direct surgical control.

In the hemodynamically normal patient, evaluation should proceed with an abdominal CT scan. Associated injuries should be treated appropriately. If persistent bleeding of >4 units of blood or hemodynamic instability develops in the absence of other significant injuries, pelvic arteriogram with embolization should be obtained.

In the hemodynamically unstable patient, a FAST exam and/or adiagnostic peritoneal lavage or ultrasound should be performed emergently to assess for intraperitoneal bleeding. If no intraperitoneal blood is identified, and again, no other injuries can explain persistent hemorrhage, pelvic arteriogram with embolization should be performed. A simple technique to stabilize the pelvis acutely is a pelvic binder. Pneumatic antishock garment (PASG) are no longer used for pre-hospital hypotension, but may be considered as a temporizing measure to stabilize pelvic fractures until an alternative method is available. External fixation can also be used for certain types of fractures.

Urethral catheterization (Foley placement) should be followed by a retrograde urethrogram if physical examination reveals a high-riding or displaced prostate, blood at the meatus or if there is difficulty passing the catheter via the urethra.

Open pelvic fractures require early surgical intervention. Conventional management of these injuries has mandated colostomy, but this may not be necessary in all open pelvic fractures. If the fracture has entered the rectum, or there is extensive perineal wounding near the anus, a colostomy is appropriate. Multiple operations for irrigation and debridement are often necessary.

Traumatic Rhabdomyolysis (Crush Syndrome)

Rhabdomyolysis and myoglobinuria occur when there is extensive injury to muscular tissue. This can be due to delayed repair of a major extremity arterial injury, sustained compression of muscle groups, invasive muscular infection, electrical injury, or a synergy of corticosteroid and nondepolarizing paralyzing agents. These conditions lead to the release of myoglobin into the circulation which is filtered in the kidneys and precipitates in the renal tubules. The intratubular casts obstruct flow, and other by-products may cause toxic injury to the tubular endothelial cells. Myoglobinuria classically produces dark amber urine that tests positive for hemoglobin yet shows no red blood cells on urinalysis. Patients with myoglobinuria can develop acute renal failure within 1-2 hours of the onset of the pathognomonic dark tea-colored urine. Diagnosis is usually made by clinical suspicion or the appearance of dark urine. Myoglobin concentrations in the urine are diagnostic, but frequently results are delayed. A creatine phosphokinase (CPK) level above 10,000 IU/cc is a sensitive but not specific laboratory test that indicates patients at risk for acute renal failure (ARF) from myoglobinuria. Treatment should be started early to avoid renal failure in any patient considered to be at high risk. Aggressive hydration with a balanced salt solution to establish urine flow rates >200 cc/hour keeps the renal tubules flushed. Because myoglobin solubility increases at a higher pH, urine should be alkalinized to a pH >6 using intravenous sodium bicarbonate. Intravenous mannitol may also be used to augment urine flow. Diuretics that decrease urine pH (furosemide) should be strictly avoided. The preferred diuretics are carbonic anhydrase inhibitors (acetazolamide) which increase urine pH. While most clinicians agree that aggressive hydration to maintain urine output is necessary, controversy exists over the role of mannitol and sodium bicarbonate to alkalinize of the urine.

Compartment Syndrome

Compartment syndrome results from elevated pressures within a closed fascial compartment resulting in microvascular compromise, and ultimately muscle and nerve necrosis. The most common causes of compartment syndrome include acute trauma, crush injuries, reperfusion after prolonged ischemia and electrical burns. Patients with tibial and forearm fractures are at particular risk. A high degree of awareness is important, especially if the patient has an altered mental sensorium. The signs and symptoms of compartment syndrome include: pain greater than expected given the injury, that increases with passive stretching of the muscles; paresthesia; decreased sensation or functional loss of the nerves involved; and tense swelling of the involved region. A palpable distal pulse is usually present in compartment syndrome. Weakness, paralysis or loss of pulses are late signs of compartment syndrome. A high index of suspicion must be maintained for patients at risk. Compartmental pressures should be measured, and patients with initial ***compartment pressures over 30 mm Hg*** should be decompressed surgically by fasciotomy.

Fasciotomy of the lower extremity is performed most commonly due to complex tibial fractures or secondary to reperfusion following repair of a vascular injury. The double incision technique is performed by making a longitudinal incision from the knee to the ankle over the anterior and lateral compartments. This incision should be placed directly over the fibula starting just distal to the head of the fibula and extending just proximal to the lateral malleolus. Care should taken to avoid the common peroneal nerve as it wraps around the neck of the fibula proximally. The anterior and posterior compartments can be released by longitudinally incising their fascial coverings. The second incision extends from the knee to the ankle and is centered 1-2 cm posterior to the posterior medial border of the tibia. The fascia overlying the gastrocnemius and soleus muscles is identified and incised. The deep posterior compartment is visualized in the distal third of the leg. To adequately decompress the deep compartment, it is necessary to detach part of the soleus muscles from the posterior tibia. Wounds are left open and dressing changes are performed. Every attempt to close the wounds primarily within 7 days should be attempted. If this is not possible, split thickness skin grafts can be used. Following need for fasciotomy, the patient should be well hydrated and monitored closely for signs of myoglobinuria or renal failure.

Late sequelae of lower extremity compartment syndrome include equinus contracture (gastrocsoleus contracture), varus foot (posterior tibial infarct), claw toes with ankle dorsiflexion (flexor digitorum longus infarct) and drop foot (anterior compartment infarct).

Immobilization

The goal of fracture immobilization is to realign the injured extremity in as close to anatomic position as possible. This will prevent excessive fracture site motion and may also decrease the amount of hemorrhage. All fractures should be splinted prior to patient transport. Early definitive operative reduction of fractures is associated with improved patient outcomes and earlier mobilization. Early fixation should be pursued once the patient is hemodynamically stable and other life-threatening injuries have been ruled-out or controlled.

8. Vascular Trauma

Vascular trauma can be life- or limb-threatening. Combined injuries are particularly treacherous and may require meticulous prioritization, using a staged repair approach. An organized approach to evaluation, control, exposure and repair improves the chance for successful outcome.

Evaluation

Hard signs for peripheral arterial injury include external bleeding, expanding hematoma, murmur, thrill, pulselessness or overt ischemic changes. These signs are sufficient to justify immediate operative exploration without additional studies. Arteriography may play an adjunctive role in a hemodynamically stable patient when the level of injury is unclear or multiple injuries are suspected. ***Soft signs*** of arterial injury include proximity to a major vascular structure, a nonexpanding but significant hematoma, or a history of prehospital hemorrhage. A Doppler ankle/brachial index of <0.9 is indicative of abnormal arterial flow secondary to injury or peripheral vascular disease. Thus, further arterial workup is necessary with an ABI of <0.9.

Techniques for Control

Temporary control of hemorrhage is best obtained by direct pressure. Blind clamping should be avoided. Tourniquets may be used selectively. Balloon catheter tamponade or intraluminal balloon occlusion may be valuable in difficult-to-access regions such as the neck, groin or axilla.

Exposure

The basic concept for exposure is to make an incision that allows for proximal and distal control. The incision should be placed close to, but outside, the region of a traumatic hematoma. A summary of incisions for vascular exposure is shown in Table 7.

Repair

Options for repair depend on the severity of injury, surrounding tissue destruction, and patient hemodynamics. Options include simple techniques such as ligation, lateral suture and temporary intraluminal shunts. More complex techniques include primary anastomosis, resection with placement of vein interposition graft and extraanatomic bypass. The ***greater saphenous vein*** is the most frequently harvested autologous graft material. Depending on size considerations, it can be taken from below the knee or from the thigh and should be harvested from the leg ***opposite*** the injury. ***Acute complications*** of vascular injuries include hemorrhagic shock, ischemic limb loss and reperfusion injury leading to compartment syndrome. ***Late complications*** include arteriovenous fistula or pseudoaneurysm formation, stenosis or occlusion. Major arterial repairs should be followed by noninvasive examination at 3, 6 and 12 months following repair.

Table 7

Incisions for Vascular Exposure

Vessel	**Incision**
Ascending aorta Innominate artery Proximal right subclavian Right common carotid artery	Median sternotomy ± right supraclavicular extension ± resection of medial head of clavicle
Right proximal subclavian artery	Supraclavicular incision ± extension to a median sternotomy ± resection of medial head of clavicle
Left proximal subclavian artery	Left lateral thoracotomy or Supraclavicular incision ± extension to a "trapdoor" ± resection of medial head of clavicle
Descending aorta Left subclavian	Left lateral thoracotomy
Distal subclavian or axillary	Transverse infraclavicular
Carotid artery (Zone 2)	Anterior sternocleidomastoid
Brachial	Medial triceps Antecubital
Radial and ulnar	Longitudinal volar forearm
Abdominal aorta and vena cava	Laparotomy with medial visceral rotation
Iliac vessels (common, internal, external)	Oblique suprainguinal
Femoral (common, superficial, deep)	Longitudinal femoral
Distal femoral and proximal popliteal	Medial supracondylar
Distal popliteal and trifurcation	Medial infracondylar
Popliteal	S-shaped posterior popliteal

9. Penetrating and Blunt Neck Trauma

Anatomy

The anterior neck is divided into 3 zones defined by horizontal planes numbered from the bottom up (see Figure 6).

Zone 1 represents the base of the neck and is variably defined as extending from the sternal notch to the cricoid cartilage or the top of the clavicles. Injuries here carry the highest mortality rate because of the risk of major vascular and intrathoracic injury.

Zone 2 represents the central and largest portion of the neck. It extends from the top of Zone 1 (cricoid cartilage) to the angle of the mandible. Zone 2 injuries are most common, but carry a lower mortality rate because surgical exposure of vital structures is readily accomplished. The carotid arteries, esophagus and upper airway structures (larynx, hypopharynx and trachea) are all at risk in this area.

Zone 3 represents the area of neck above the angle of the mandible. Risk of injury to the distal common carotid artery, salivary glands and pharynx is greatest in this zone. Exposure can be difficult.

Figure 6

Anatomic zones of the neck

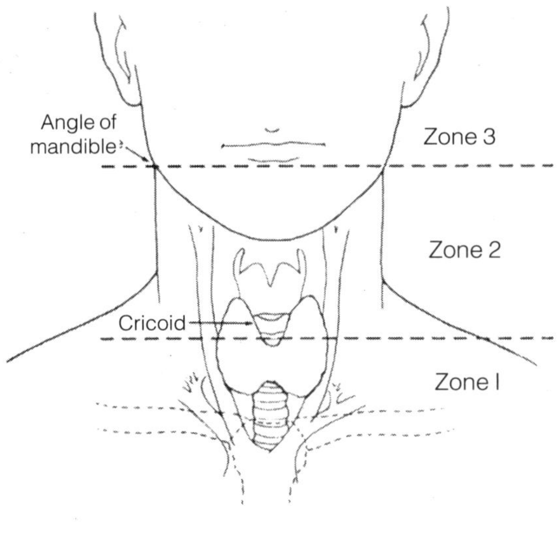

Initial Management and Evaluation

The major landmark in the neck is the platysma muscle. Penetration of this muscle must be considered a serious surgical problem that mandates hospital admission and further evaluation.

Initial management includes securing the airway and ensuring adequate ventilation. Rapid assessment of air movement, crepitus, hoarseness and subcutaneous emphysema should be made. A patient with significant swelling or hematoma should have the airway secured with endotracheal intubation immediately. Major neck hemorrhage should be treated with direct pressure. Blind clamping of vessels is discouraged to avoid inadvertent injury to the esophagus or nerves. Cervical spine injuries should always be considered in a patient with significant blunt or penetrating neck injury.

Management of Stable Patients

Zone 1

Management is selective. These injuries are treated like traversing thoracic wounds. Work-up is aimed at identifying possible injury to the great vessels, esophagus, trachea, phrenic nerve and brachial plexus. CT scanning with CT angiography to define the trajectory of the missile and delineate potential injuries has become the preferred initial imaging modality in stable patients with penetrating trauma to the neck. Following CT, additional studies can be ordered if necessary to further delineate suspected injuries. ***Angiography*** is performed to identify potential vascular injury and to allow better preparation for the operative approach. ***Cinefluoroesophagography***, first with water soluble contrast, then with barium, is performed after angiography. ***Endoscopy*** is considered a complementary examination and should be performed if there is any question of abnormality. ***Bronchoscopy*** should be performed to rule out tracheal injury.

Zone 2

Management is controversial. Selective management mandates a diagnostic work-up to rule out potential injuries to the vessels, trachea, esophagus and nerves. Historically, this evaluation consisted of angiography, cinefluoroesophagography, rigid endoscopy and bronchoscopy. Recent evidence supports the use of CT of the neck with or without CTA to evaluate potential injuries. Duplex scanning can also be used to rule out an arterial injury of the neck in Zone 2. Others support mandatory exploration through an anterior sternocleidomastoid incision. The tract of the missile is followed through its course to exclude vascular, tracheal, esophageal or neurologic injury. Endoscopy can be performed in the operating room if an injury is suspected but cannot be identified.

Zone 3

Management is selective. Angiography is performed to identify injury to the distal internal carotid artery or to demonstrate the need for anticoagulation. Vascular injuries identified at the base of the skull are usually managed by interventional radiology. Esophageal studies are not done for Zone 3 injuries.

Management of Unstable Patients

The unstable patient should be taken directly to the operating room. The incision should be made to allow full exposure of the tract of the injury.

Unilateral injury (Zone 2 or 3): anterior sternocleidomastoid incision.

Bilateral neck injury (Zone 2 or 3): transverse collar incision extending to both sides or bilateral anterior sternocleidomastoid incisions.

Thoracic outlet injuries (Zone 1): supraclavicular incision with extension to a median sternotomy or book thoracotomy as necessary.

Exposure for Specific Vascular Injuries

Innominate artery or proximal right subclavian artery: anterior sternocleidomastoid incision or supraclavicular incision with extension to a median sternotomy.

Left subclavian artery: options depend on operative circumstances: left anterior thoracotomy; extension of left anterior sternocleidomastoid or supraclavicular incision to a "trapdoor" incision; or 2 incisions, a left anterior sternocleidomastoid or supraclavicular incision and a left anterolateral thoracotomy with the patient bumped anteriorly. Resection of the medial head of the clavicle can also assist in exposure of the subclavian artery on either the right or left side.

Management of Specific Injuries

Carotid Injury

Penetrating Carotid Injury. A carotid artery injury should be suspected in any patient with a Zone 2 injury and an expanding hematoma, extensive external hemorrhage, bradycardia or a neurologic deficit. An anterior sternocleidomastoid incision should be made. Treatment should consist of debridement with primary repair or interposition graft with vein, PTFE or ligated ipsilateral external carotid artery. Ligation of the carotid artery is indicated in the comatose patient with no prograde flow, in the presence of uncontrollable hemorrhage, severe associated injuries or if technical reasons prohibit repair. Ligation results in neurologic deficit in 20% patients.

Blunt Carotid Injury. This is a difficult diagnosis to make. It should be suspected in any trauma patient who develops neurologic deficits unexplained by associated head injuries. Early recognition and treatment may reduce the risk of stroke. These injuries are usually caused by hyperextension of the neck, but can be caused by a direct blow. Endothelial flaps with dissection are most common, followed by endothelial flaps with thrombosis. The injury usually extends quite far distally, and is therefore treated nonoperatively with anticoagulation. CT angiography, MRA, duplex or formal angiography may be used for diagnosis. Suggested criteria for screening include: 1.) C1-C3 fracture; 2.) C-spine fracture with subluxation; and 3.) fractures involving the foramen transversarium.

Vertebral Injury. Vertebral artery injuries are rare but are now more commonly diagnosed with the liberal use of angiography. Unilateral vertebral occlusion rarely results in a neurologic deficit. Blunt vertebral artery occlusions are treated nonoperatively with anticoagulation if possible. Penetrating injuries should be treated with embolization by interventional radiology if possible. Surgical exposure and ligation is difficult, but may occasionally be necessary.

Internal Jugular Vein Injury. These injuries can usually be treated with primary repair, resection and reanastomosis, or vein patch. If necessary, ligation can be performed if the contralateral vein is intact.

Esophageal Injury. Signs associated with esophageal injury include hemoptysis, hematemesis, subcutaneous emphysema, odynophagia and retropharyngeal air. Treatment includes exploration, debridement and primary repair with drainage. If the injury is extensive or diagnosis has been delayed >24-48 hours, esophageal diversion and drainage are recommended.

Tracheal/Laryngeal Injuries. Signs associated with airway injuries include hemoptysis, dysphonia, subcutaneous emphysema or airway obstruction. Initial signs may be subtle, followed by rapid deterioration and loss of airway. Endotracheal intubation should be attempted. Sometimes emergent cricothyroidotomy or direct intubation of the trachea through the wound is necessary to obtain control of the airway. In this instance, urgent conversion to formal tracheostomy is required. Diagnosis is made with fiberoptic endoscopy and neck CT. Treatment is debridement and repair of the open wound. Occasionally very small or minor injuries can be observed.

Combined Tracheoesophageal Injuries. Treatment is primary repair with interposition muscle flap (sternocleidomastoid or strap muscle) and wide drainage.

10. Pediatric Trauma

Anatomic and Physiologic Characteristics

Pediatric Airway

The pediatric airway should be optimized by placing the child's head in the sniffing position and using the chin lift or drop draw thrust maneuver.

Oral tracheal intubation is the most reliable means of establishing an airway and ventilating the child. Uncuffed tubes of appropriate size should be used. The cricoid ring forms a natural seal around the endotracheal tube, because this is the narrowest area of the child's airway. Endotracheal tube size can be approximated by the diameter of the external nares or the child's little finger, or by the formula (age/4) + 4. Nasotracheal intubation should not be performed in children under the age of 12 years due to a relatively acute angle in the nasopharynx which makes this route particularly difficult. Because the child's airway is short (5-7 cm), the endotracheal tube should be positioned 2-3 cm below the level of the vocal cords. Frequent assessment is necessary during resuscitation to ensure appropriate placement of the endotracheal tube.

Surgical cricothyroidotomy is rarely indicated for the infant or small child and can safely be performed in children older than 11 years of age. If necessary, needle cricothyroidotomy is the preferred method.

Breathing

An infant requires 40-60 breaths per minute, whereas the older child breathes 20 times per minute (Table 8). Tidal volumes are 6-10 cc/kg. Hypoventilation is the most common cause of cardiac arrest in the child.

Circulation

Pediatric patients have an increased physiologic reserve. Blood loss of 25% is required to manifest even minimal signs of shock in the pediatric patient. Subtle signs of shock include a decreased pulse pressure, skin mottling, decreased capillary refill, cold extremities compared to torso skin and a decreased level of consciousness with dull response to pain. Increased physiologic reserve in children allows maintenance of normal vital signs followed by an acute decompensation.

Table 8

Normal Pediatric Vital Signs

Age Group	Weight (kg)	Heart rate	SBP	RR	Urine (cc/hr)
0-6 months	3-6	160-180	60-80	60	2.0
Infant	12	160	80	40	1.5
Preschool	16	120	90	30	1.0
Adolescent	35	100	100	20	0.5

Hypotension represents uncompensated shock and indicates severe blood loss of >45% of the circulating blood volume. Heart rate is the major determinant of cardiac output in the child. ***Tachycardia changing to bradycardia is an ominous sign in the pediatric patient.***

Fluid Resuscitation. A child's blood volume can be estimated at 80 cc/kg. When shock is suspected, an initial fluid bolus of isotonic warmed crystalloid solution of 20 cc/kg is given, and this should be repeated 1 time. If the patient continues to show evidence of shock, a third bolus should be started and consideration should be given to the use of packed red blood cells. Packed red blood cells should be given in the volume of 10 cc/kg of warmed packed red blood cells.

Venous Access. The preferred sites for venous access in children are: percutaneous peripheral lines (2 attempts); intraosseous infusion (children ≤ 6 years of age); venous cutdown (saphenous vein at the ankle); percutaneous placement (femoral vein or subclavian vein); percutaneous placement (external jugular vein) (do not use if cervical collar is applied); and internal jugular vein. The common femoral vein should be avoided in infants and children whenever possible, due to the high incidence of venous thrombosis and possibility of ischemic limb loss or other growth discrepancies.

Indications for Intraosseous Infusion. Use of intraosseous infusion is limited to children 6 years of age or younger. It should be used in children for whom venous access is impossible due to circulatory collapse or for whom percutaneous peripheral venous cannulation has failed on 2 attempts. The preferred site for intraosseous cannulation is the proximal tibia, below the level of the tibial tuberosity. This method is safe, efficacious and requires less time than does a venous cutdown. Complications include cellulitis and, rarely, osteomyelitis. Intraosseous infusion should not be performed distal to a fracture site.

Urinary Output

Urinary output is an excellent measure of adequate resuscitation, however, urine output varies with age. For the newborn and infant (up to 1 year old) the goal is 2 cc/kg/hour. The toddler has a urinary output of 1.5 cc/kg/hour, and the older child requires a urinary output of 1 cc/kg/hour through adolescence.

Thermal Regulation

Due to the high ratio of body surface area to body mass, the pediatric patient has an increased evaporative heat loss and caloric expenditure. To prevent hypothermia, overhead heat lamps, heaters and thermal blankets may be necessary.

Chest Trauma

Rib fractures are uncommon in childhood. The compliant chest wall causes a high frequency of pulmonary contusion in the absence of associated rib fractures. The mobility of mediastinal structures also makes the pediatric patient more sensitive to tension pneumothorax in final segments.

Abdominal Trauma

Evaluation of pediatric abdominal injuries should proceed similarly to adult evaluation. FAST can be used to screen pediatric patients for the presence of intraperitoneal fluid. Computed tomography (CT) scan can be used for the identification of intraabdominal injuries in the hemodynamically normal pediatric patient. Although not utilized frequently, diagnostic peritoneal lavage (DPL) can be used to detect intraabdominal bleeding. The technique is as follows: warmed Ringer's lactate solution in a volume of 10-15 cc/kg is infused over a 10-minute period. Aspiration of >100,000 RBC/cc is considered a positive result. Because of the increased utility of nonoperative management of blunt solid organ injury in the pediatric patient, the presence of blood in the peritoneal fluid does not in and of itself mandate celiotomy in a child. However, the presence of glucose, feces, fibers or bile in the lavage does mandate celiotomy.

Nonoperative Management

Nonoperative management of solid organ injury has been very successful in the pediatric population. Serial abdominal examination and measurement of hematocrit is necessary. ***Children who require transfusion of more than one-half of their blood volume (40 cc/kg) within 24 hours of injury will almost always require operative intervention.*** Those who develop hemodynamic instability should also undergo immediate operative intervention.

Specific Visceral Injuries

Certain abdominal visceral injuries are more common in children. ***Duodenal hematomas*** result from a bicycle handlebar or an elbow striking the child in the upper abdomen. This injury is most often treated nonoperatively with nasogastric suction and parenteral nutrition. ***Pancreatic injuries*** occur from the same mechanism. Small bowel perforations at or near the ***ligament of Treitz*** are more common in children than adults. ***Bladder rupture*** is also more common in children than in adults. ***Bowel perforation*** is more common in children who are restrained by a lap belt, especially if they sustain a flexion disruption (Chance fracture) of the lumbar spine. Any pediatric patient with this constellation of symptoms should be assumed to have a bowel injury until proven otherwise.

Pediatric Head Trauma

Outcome in children suffering severe head injury is better than in adults. The pediatric brain is more susceptible to parenchymal structural damage from momentum due to an increased water content and decreased subarachnoid space. Because of the open fontanel and mobile cranial suture lines, signs of an expanding intracranial mass may be hidden until rapid decompensation occurs. A bulging fontanel should be treated as a severe injury and aggressive neurosurgical evaluation obtained. In addition, significant intracranial blood loss can lead to hypotension in infants due to their low circulating blood volume and expanding cranial suture lines. Treatment is appropriate volume resuscitation and attention to the intracranial injury. Pediatric patients are more susceptible to secondary brain injury, and aggressive prevention of hypotension, hypoxia, seizures and hyperthermia is warranted. In small children less than 4 years of age, a modified Glasgow coma score is used for the verbal component.

Spinal Cord Injury

Fortunately, spinal cord injury in children is uncommon, accounting for only 5% of all spinal cord injuries.

Pseudo-subluxation occurs in approximately 40% of children <7 years of age, and 20% of children up to 16 years of age. It is represented by an anterior displacement of C2 on C3. To correct this radiographic abnormality, the child's head should be placed in the sniffing position and the x-ray repeated.

Spinal cord injury without radiographic abnormality (SCIWORA) occurs more commonly in children than in adults. A normal spine series is seen in up to two-thirds of children suffering spinal cord injury. If spinal cord injury is suspected based on history or neurologic examination, normal x-rays do not exclude injury. Cervical spine precautions should be maintained until appropriate neurosurgical or orthopedic consultation is obtained. MRI of the spine should be obtained in any child with a high-risk mechanism and an unreliable exam.

Steroids should be used for blunt spinal cord injuries with neurologic deficits in pediatric patients at the same dosage as that recommended for adults. The use of steroids for the treatment for spine trauma in childhood remains controversial and studies are currently underway to evaluate this.

Musculoskeletal Trauma

Radiographic diagnosis of fractures in the pediatric patient is difficult due to the lack of mineralization of the bones. Thus, history and observation of patient behavior are of vital importance in distinguishing some skeletal trauma. ***Green stick fractures*** are incomplete fractures with angulation maintained by cortical splinters on immature pliable bone. A ***torus or buccal fracture*** involves angulation due to cortical impaction with a radiolucent fracture line. ***Supracondylar fractures*** at the elbow or knee have a high propensity for vascular injury.

Blood loss associated with long bone and pelvic fractures is proportionately greater in the child than in the adult. A small child can lose 1-2 units of blood into the muscle mass of a thigh.

Child Abuse

In the United States, doctors are bound by law to report incidents of child abuse to authorities, even when abuse is only suspected and not proven. Approximately 50% of abused children who are released back to those who abused them return to the hospital dead. ***Child abuse should be suspected if:*** a discrepancy exists between the history and degree of physical injury; a prolonged interval has passed between time of injury and the seeking of medical advice; the history includes repeated trauma, treated in different emergency departments; parents respond inappropriately or do not comply with medical advice; the history of injury changes between parents or guardians. ***Findings on physical examination*** which suggest child abuse include: multiple subdural hematomas; retinal hemorrhage; perioral injuries; ruptured internal viscera without antecedent major blunt trauma; trauma to the genital area; old scars or healed fractures on x-ray; fractures of long bones in children younger than 3 years of age; bizarre injuries (bites, cigarette burns, rope marks); sharply demarcated second and third degree burns (submersion injuries).

Pitfalls in Childhood Injuries

Unique characteristics which must be kept in mind during pediatric trauma include the small size of the endotracheal tube which may present difficulty with clearing secretions. Uncuffed tubes can easily be dislodged, so frequent reassessment is necessary. Because of the pediatric patient's ability to compensate in the early phases of blood loss, inadequate fluid resuscitation may lead to rapid deterioration which is often precipitous. Subtle signs of hypovolemia must be recognized. Abdominal examination and detection of solid organ injury or hollow viscus injury may be difficult. Orthopedic injuries may be difficult to detect on radiologic examination alone due to lack of mineralization of the bone.

11. Trauma and Pregnancy

Although the treatment priorities remain the same in the pregnant trauma patient, there are several anatomic and physiologic alterations during pregnancy which must be considered during resuscitation.

Anatomic Variations

During the ***first trimester***, the uterus remains a thick-walled structure within the pelvis. During the ***second trimester***, the uterus begins to enlarge. At 20 weeks, the uterus is at the level of the umbilicus. Although the uterus is now enlarged beyond its protected intrapelvic location, the small fetus is protected and cushioned by a relatively large amount of amniotic fluid. During the ***third trimester***, the uterus continues to enlarge and expands to the level of the costal margin. The uterus becomes a large, thin-walled structure. The placenta is largest at 36-38 weeks and becomes devoid of elastic tissue. Thus, during the third trimester the placenta is more susceptible to abruption. These anatomic changes in the size and structure of the uterus can have an impact on both the maternal and fetal response to injury.

Changes in Blood Volume

Blood volume increases by 50% during pregnancy. There is a physiologic anemia of pregnancy which is secondary to a relatively greater increase in plasma volume versus red cell volume. The average hematocrit for a patient at term gestation is approximately 34%. This increased blood volume is important because ***the pregnant patient can lose up to 35% of her circulating blood volume (1200-1500 cc) before any signs of tachycardia, hypotension or other signs of hypovolemia occur***. However, despite the lack of physiologic signs of shock in the mother, blood is being diverted away from the placenta and the fetus may be in severe distress. This fact must be kept in mind during early resuscitation of the pregnant trauma patient. There is also a change in blood composition resulting in a decreased PT and PTT, and increased WBC and fibrinogen levels. The bleeding time and clotting time remain normal.

Physiologic Variations

Hemodynamic: increased cardiac output, increased heart rate, decreased systolic blood pressure, associated EKG changes. ***Respiratory:*** increased minute ventilation. ***Gastrointestinal***: decreased gastric emptying. ***Genitourinary***: increased GFR, increased renal blood flow, hydroureter (right < left). ***Endocrine***: 50% increase in pituitary mass, thus shock may cause pituitary necrosis during pregnancy (Sheehan's syndrome). ***Neurologic***: eclampsia is a complication of late pregnancy that may mimic head injury, and should be considered if seizures occur with associated hypertension, hyperreflexia, proteinuria and peripheral edema. ***Musculoskeletal***: symphysis pubis widens 4-8 mm by the seventh month, sacroiliac joint spaces increase.

Assessment and Management

All treatment priorities are the same for the pregnant trauma patient as for nonpregnant patients. The primary survey consists of rapid evaluation of the *ABCDE*s. In addition, the patient should be positioned with her ***left side down.*** This lifts the uterus off the inferior vena cava which improves venous return without impairing essential perfusion. ***Radiographs*** should be performed as indicated. Less than 10 rads is considered to be low risk. A standard chest x-ray causes 0.003 rads of exposure, and a pelvic x-ray 0.31 rads. The abdomen and fetus should be shielded as much as possible. ***Ultrasound*** may also be useful. ***Diagnostic peritoneal lavage*** can be performed as indicated via an open technique above the fundus of the uterus. ***Aggressive fluid resuscitation*** is necessary to ensure adequate perfusion of the fetus and placenta. Close monitoring of volume status via urine output and the recognition of subtle signs of shock are necessary. ***Vasopressors must be avoided at all costs because the placenta is very sensitive to these agents and severe vasoconstriction will result.*** The placenta and fetus are also very sensitive to hypoxia. Tetanus toxoid is safe.

Seat belt restraints decrease maternal injury and death by preventing ejection. Use of both lap and shoulder belts have the best results. The lap belt should be worn low, across the pelvis. If worn too high over the uterus, it can cause uterine rupture or placental abruption.

Penetrating injury: As the gravid uterus increases in size, the maternal viscera are relatively protected from penetrating injury. The fetus, however, is at increased risk and exposure. While there is generally excellent maternal outcome in penetrating wounds of the gravid uterus, the fetus generally fares poorly.

Fetal Assessment

Obestetric consultation should be obtained early. Fetal complications and premature labor can occur even with very minor trauma. Any fetus beyond 20-24 weeks gestation should be monitored continuously to ensure early recognition of fetal demise.

Fetal assessment consists of an ***ultrasound*** study, which can assess fetal movement, uterine-placental status and yields a biophysical profile. A ***continuous fetal heart rate monitor*** should also be utilized. A normal fetal heart rate should be 120-160 beats per minute. Studies show that ultrasound with external fetal monitoring reliably detects all complications. Most complications are manifested within 6-24 hours. The exact duration of required fetal monitoring remains controversial. ***The current recommendation is that any fetus beyond 24 weeks gestation should be monitored for at least 6-24 hours following injury.***

Syndromes Associated with Blunt Trauma

Uterine rupture rarely occurs, but it has an increased incidence in later gestation due to the large, thin-walled uterus. The clinical picture varies. Radiologic examination of the abdomen may show extended fetal extremities, abnormal fetal position, or free air in the abdomen. Treatment is immediate exploration, delivery of the fetus and repair of the uterine rupture.

Placental abruption occurs in 38% of major trauma injuries and 2.5% of minor trauma injuries. Although the maternal mortality rate is only 1%, fetal demise is estimated at 25%. This syndrome most typically occurs during the third trimester when the placenta is large and devoid of elastic tissue, increasing its susceptibility to shearing forces and disruption from the uterine wall. Diagnosis is by ultrasound and external fetal monitoring. Classic signs on physical examination include vaginal bleeding, uterine cramping, maternal hypovolemia and fetal heart rate abnormalities.

Consumptive coagulopathy may occur following placental disruption due to release of thromboplastin and/or plasminogen activator from the myometrium. This can result in widespread DIC. Diagnosis is clinical. Serial evaluation of fibrinogen level may be useful. Treatment is immediate uterine evacuation.

Fetal-maternal hemorrhage: Rh isoimmunization occurs when Rh-positive blood from the fetus escapes into maternal circulation. As little as 0.01 cc of Rh-positive blood will sensitize 70% of Rh-negative patients. The resulting maternal antibody formation will result in fetal anemia and death. A Kleihauer-Behtke test is a citric acid elusion smear of the maternal blood for detection of fetal cells in the maternal circulation. Due to this risk, ***all Rh-negative trauma patients should be treated with Rh immunoglobulin within 72 hours unless the injury is remote from the uterus (eg, isolated distal extremity injury).*** The dose is 300 mcg for every 30 cc of fetomaternal hemorrhage.

Perimortem Cesarean Section

There are few data to support perimortem cesarean section in pregnant trauma patients suffering from hypovolemic cardiac arrest. Fetal distress can be present even when the mother is hemodynamically normal. Thus, progressive maternal instability compromises fetal survival. For other causes of sudden maternal cardiac arrest, a perimortem cesarean section occasionally may be successful if performed within 4-5 minutes.

12. Burn and Cold Injury

Classification of Burn Depth

First-degree burns are characterized by erythema, pain and the absence of blisters. They are not life-threatening, and generally do not require intravenous fluid replacement.

Second degree or partial thickness burns are characterized by a red or mottled appearance and associated swelling and blister formation. The surface may have a wet appearance and is painfully hypersensitive, even to air currents.

Third degree or full thickness burns usually appear dark and leathery. The skin may appear translucent, mottled, or waxy white. Because this depth of burn extends through the epidermis and dermal layers, all pain fibers and sensation fibers are destroyed. Thus, the surface is painless and generally dry.

Estimating Total Body Surface Area

The *Rule of Nines* is the standard guide used to determine the extent of the burn (see Figure 7). The adult body is divided into anatomic regions, each of which represents a multiple or fraction of 9% of the body's total surface area. There is variation in children, with the infant or young child's head representing a larger proportion of the surface area and the lower extremities a lesser proportion. The patient's palm (excluding fingers) represents approximately 1% of the patient's total body surface area (TBSA).

Fluid Resuscitation

The Parkland formula for fluid resuscitation is 4 cc/kg/%TBSA burned. The consensus formula for fluid replacement is 24 cc/kg/%TBSA with second and third degree body surface burns. The calculated volume is then replaced with one-half given in the first 8 hours post-burn, and the remaining half administered over the following 16 hours. It is important to remember that this volume replacement is calculated from the *time of burn injury*. Any resuscitation formula provides only an estimate of fluid need. Hourly volume rate is titrated to maintain an average urinary output of $^{1}/_{2}$-1 cc/kg/hr. Increased volume requirements are seen in electrical injury, inhalation injury and in patients who have a delay in resuscitation.

Figure 7

Rule of Nines—a useful estimate of the distribution of surface area by anatomical region

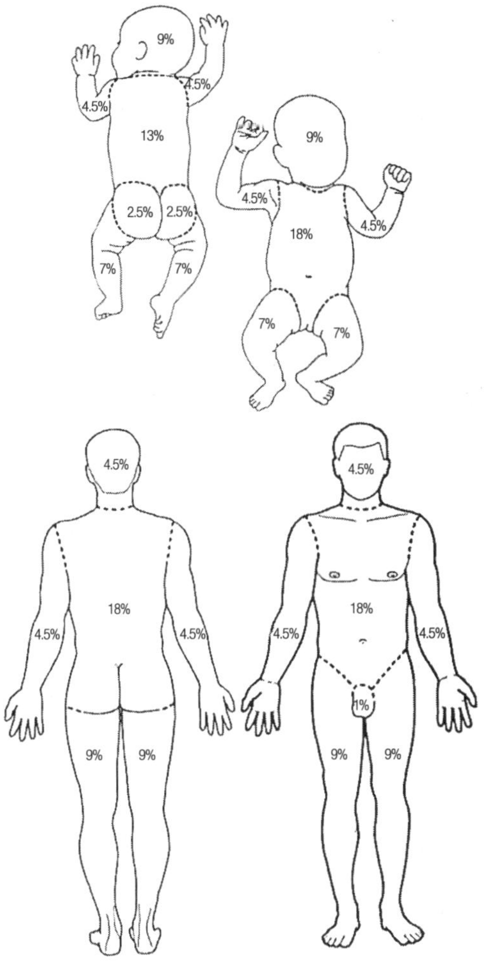

Inhalation Injury

There are 2 types of inhalational injury. ***Supraglottic injuries*** occur due to heat exposure of the oropharynx and supraglottic airway. This leads to supraglottic airway edema, swelling and potential obstruction. ***Infraglottic inhalational*** injury occurs not due to heat or burn of the upper airway, but rather is caused by the inhalation of toxic substances that cause alveolar dysfunction. This can occur due to smoke inhalation.

Clinical signs of inhalation injury include facial burns, singeing of the eyebrows and nasal hairs, inflammatory changes in the oropharynx, carbonaceous sputum, history of impaired mentation and/or confinement in a burning environment, explosion with burns to head and torso, and a carboxyhemoglobin level >10%.

Carbon monoxide exposure should be considered in patients burned in enclosed areas. Carbon monoxide has an affinity for hemoglobin 240 times that of oxygen. Thus, it displaces oxygen from the hemoglobin molecule, and shifts the oxyhemoglobin dissociation curve to the left. The half-life of carbon monoxide in the blood is 250 minutes while breathing room air. However, by increasing the inspired oxygen to 100%, carbon monoxide can disssociate within 40 minutes. Therefore, patients suspected of exposure to carbon monoxide should receive high-flow oxygen via a nonrebreathing mask. Patients with carbon monoxide levels of <20% usually have no symptoms. However, higher levels result in headache and nausea (20%-30%), confusion (30%-40%), coma (40%-60%) and death (>60%). Cherry-red skin color is rare.

Chemical Burns

Chemical burns should be treated with copious irrigation for a minimum of 20-30 minutes. Alkali burns are generally more serious than acid burns because the alkalis penetrate more deeply. Removal of the chemical with prolonged irrigation is the immediate treatment.

Electrical Burns

Electrical burns result from a source of electrical power making contact with the patient's body and then exiting at a remote site. Although only a small surface area may be affected externally, deep tissue and muscle burns occur as the current passes through tissues. Fluid requirements should be based on urine output and vital signs rather than on the amount of external skin affected. Complications include cardiac arrhythmias and rhabdomyolysis. Electrocardiographic monitoring is indicated. Precautions against myoglobinuria should be taken, including aggressive hydration, administration of mannitol, and alkalinization of the urine to a pH of >6.0.

Cold Injury

Frostbite is injury due to freezing of tissue with intracellular ice crystal formation and microvascular occlusion with subsequent tissue anoxia. Tissue damage may also result from a reperfusion injury that occurs on rewarming. Treatment should be immediate to decrease the duration of tissue freezing. The injured part should be placed in a circulating water bath at 40ºC until the pink color and reperfusion return (usually 20-30 minutes). Avoid dry heat and do not rub or massage the area. Rewarming can be extremely painful and use of adequate analgesics is essential. Cardiac monitoring during rewarming is advised.

Hypothermia

Hypothermia is defined as a core body temperature below 35ºC. Treatment depends on the patient's temperature. Treatment of mild and moderate exposure hypothermia (30º-35ºC) can be treated with passive external rewarming in a warm room using blankets, clothing and warmed intravenous fluids. Severe hypothermia (<30ºC) requires active core rewarming with invasive surgical rewarming techniques such as peritoneal lavage, gastric and pleural lavage, hemodialysis or cardiopulmonary bypass. All should be done in a critical care or operative setting. Ventricular fibrillation in severe hypothermia should be treated with bretyllium.

13. References

American College of Surgeons Committee on Trauma. *Advanced Trauma Life Support*. 8th ed. Chicago, IL; 2008.

Eastern Association for the Surgery of Trauma (EAST) - Trauma Practice Guidelines. Available at http://www.east.org. Accessed April 3, 2009.

Moore EE, Feliciano DV, Mattox KL. *Trauma*. 5th ed. New York, NY:McGraw-Hill Professional;2003.

Trunkey DD, Asensio JA. *Current Therapy of Trauma and Surgical Critical Care*. Philadelphia, PA:Mosby-Elsevier;2008.

Trunkey DD, Lewis FR. *Current Therapy of Trauma*. St. Louis, MO: Mosby; 1999.

Cantor RM, Leaming JM. Evaluation and management of pediatric major trauma. *Emerg Med Clin North Am*. 1998;16:229-256.

Bracken MB, Shepard MJ, Holford TR, et al. Administration of methylprednisolone for 24 or 48 hours or tirilazad mesylate for 48 hours in the treatment of acute spinal cord injury. Results of the Third National Acute Spinal Cord Injury Randomized Controlled Trial. National Acute Spinal Cord Injury Study. *JAMA*. 1997;277:1597-1604.

Gerndt SJ, Rodriguez JL, Pawlik JW, et al. Consequences of high-dose steroid therapy for acute spinal cord injury. *J Trauma*. 1997;42:279-284.

Morris JA Jr, Eddy VA, Rutherford EJ. The trauma celiotomy: the evolving concepts of damage control. *Curr Prob Surg*.1996;33:611-700.

Murray JA, Demetriades D, Colson M, et al. Colonic resection in trauma: colostomy versus anastomosis. *J Trauma*. 1999;46:250-254.

Guidelines for the management of severe traumatic brain injury. Brain Trauma Foundation; American Association of Neurological Surgeons; Congress of Neurological Surgeons. *J Neurotrauma*. 2007;24 (Suppl 1): S1-S106.

Muench MV, Canterino JC. Trauma in pregnancy. *Obstet Gynecol Clin N Am*. 2007;34:555-583.

14. Questions

1. A 56-year-old man is involved in a head-on MVA and sustains an open mandibular fracture, chest trauma and evidence of head injury. The patient is apneic on arrival to the emergency department. The best initial method for immediately obtaining an airway is:

   A. Needle cricothyroidotomy.

   B. Nasal tracheal intubation.

   C. Oral tracheal intubation.

   D. Intubation over a bronchoscope.

   E. Surgical cricothyroidotomy.

2. A patient presents to the emergency department after being assaulted with a bat. He has multiple facial contusions. He opens his eyes to deep painful stimuli, grunts, withdraws his right arm to pain and localizes with his left arm. His Glasgow coma score is:

   A. 6.

   B. 7.

   C. 8.

   D. 9.

   E. 10.

3. Each of the following is true regarding chest trauma *except:*

   A. Massive hemothorax as defined is >1500 cc of blood within the chest cavity, or >200 cc per hour of chest tube output for 2-4 consecutive hours.

   B. Patients with flail chest should be intubated early to stabilize the chest wall and facilitate healing.

   C. The major insult associated with flail chest is the underlying pulmonary contusion.

   D. Pulmonary contusions are evident on the initial chest x-ray in the majority of patients.

   E. An open pneumothorax should be treated with an occlusive dressing that is taped on three sides (flutter-type valve), and a chest tube should be inserted at a remote site.

4. A 29-year-old man is found on the ground in a park, having fallen out of a tree. He is unresponsive, with pulseless electrical activity. He is immediately intubated, given atropine and epinephrine, and his pulse returns. On arrival to the emergency department, his pulse is 40, blood pressure 90/40 mm Hg, and temperature 31°C. He opens his eyes spontaneously, but has right lateral gaze, does not move his extremities and has no sphincter tone. His initial hemoglobin is 12.9. Cervical spine series shows fractures of cervical vertebrae 2-4. Each of the following is true *except:*

   A. The patient's hypotension and bradycardia are likely due to spinal shock.

   B. The patient should receive a fluid bolus of lactated Ringer's for hypotension.

   C. Head CT is indicated.

   D. An ultrasound study can be performed to rule out intraabdominal hemorrhage.

   E. The patient is at risk for aortic transection.

5. A 17-year-old man sustains a gunshot wound to the chest at the level of T4. An entrance wound is seen in the right chest in the midaxillary line with an exit wound in the left posterior chest. Bilateral chest tubes are placed with return of 200 cc of blood from each. Chest x-ray shows good placement of the chest tubes with a fracture of T4. The patient has no movement of his lower extremities, but does demonstrate sacral sparing. Appropriate initial management includes:

A. Methylprednisolone bolus of 30 mg/kg followed by a 23-hour infusion of 5.4 mg/kg per hour.

B. Methylprednisolone bolus of 10 mg/kg followed by a 23-hour infusion of 5.4 mg/kg per hour.

C. Hydrocortisone bolus of 10 mg/kg followed by a 23-hour infusion of 5 mg/kg per hour.

D. Methylprednisolone.

E. Esophagram with water-soluble contrast.

6. A 24-year-old man sustains a stab wound to the left chest in the midclavicular line just below the nipple. He is awake and alert with a pulse of 130, and a systolic blood pressure of 80. There is no jugular venous distention, trachea is midline, his tones are normal and there are decreased breath sounds on the left. Which of the following are possible diagnoses? (Please include all):

A. Pericardial tamponade.

B. Massive left hemothorax.

C. Open pneumothorax.

D. Tension pneumothorax.

E. Diaphragmatic tear.

7. Appropriate management of the patient in question 6 includes which of the following? (Please include all):

A. Subxiphoid pericardial window.

B. Chest x-ray.

C. Emergency department thoracotomy.

D. Left tube thoracostomy.

E. Needle decompression of the left chest in the second intercostal space in the mid clavicular line.

8. An 18-year-old woman is involved in a high-speed MVA. She sustains multiple injuries to her head, chest and abdomen. On arrival at the emergency department, her Glasgow coma score is 6, and she has agonal respirations and decreased breath sounds on the left. Her initial pulse is 160 and her initial systolic blood pressure is 80 mm Hg. She is immediately intubated, a left chest tube is placed and 2 L of lactated Ringer's is given. Repeat vital signs show a pulse of 140 and a systolic blood pressure of 80 mm Hg. The most appropriate management sequence includes:

A. Repeat fluid bolus, chest x-ray, pelvic x-ray, immediate head CT.

B. Repeat fluid bolus, chest x-ray, pelvic x-ray, cervical spine series, head CT.

C. Blood transfusion (O negative), chest x-ray, pelvic x-ray, DPL, if positive, head CT, then operating room.

D. Blood transfusion (O negative), chest x-ray, pelvic x-ray, DPL, if positive, then operating room.

E. Blood transfusion (O negative), chest x-ray, pelvic x-ray, complete cervical spine series, DPL, if positive, then operating room.

9. A 37-year-old farm worker (weight 80 kg) is injured following the explosion of his tractor at 6:00 a.m. He is seen at a local community hospital, given pain medication and intravenous fluids are started at 200 cc per hour. He arrives at your hospital at 10:00 a.m. Evaluation shows the patient to have multiple burns, including 10% first degree, 40% second degree and 10% third degree to his chest, arms, back and legs. Appropriate fluid resuscitation should be:

A. 1000 cc per hour of lactated Ringer's for 8 hours, followed by 500 cc per hour for 16 hours.

B. 1800 cc per hour of lactated Ringer's for 4 hours, followed by 500 cc per hour for 16 hours.

C. 667 cc of normal saline per hour for 24 hours.

D. 2200 cc per hour of lactated Ringer's for 4 hours, followed by 600 cc per hour for 16 hours.

E. 1200 cc per hour of lactated Ringer's for 8 hours, followed by 600 cc per hour for 16 hours.

10. With regard to the pregnant trauma patient, each of the following is correct except:

A. Circulating blood volume is increased by 50% in the pregnant patient.

B. Pregnant patients are at increased risk for disseminated intravascular coagulation following trauma.

C. All RH-negative women with significant blunt trauma should be treated with RH immunoglobulin.

D. The pregnant patient should be positioned on her right side during transport and resuscitation.

E. Ultrasound and external fetal monitoring should be used to monitor a fetus of 24 weeks gestation for at least 6 hours following trauma.

Answers

1. C.
Oral tracheal intubation can be attempted in any trauma patient with indications for an invasive airway. C-spine precautions should be maintained at all times. Nasotracheal intubation is contraindicated in an apneic patient. Surgical cricothyroidotomy may be indicated in a patient with massive facial trauma if an oral tracheal airway cannot be obtained. Fiberoptic intubation with a bronchoscope cannot be performed quickly enough in an apneic patient with an airway emergency. Needle cricothyroidotomy with jet insufflation is an appropriate technique in small children, however, hypocarbia occurs rapidly using this technique in the adult.

2. D.
Glasgow coma score is calculated by adding together the patient's eye response, verbal response and best motor response. In this example, the patient receives a 2 for eye opening to pain, a 2 for grunting noises and a 5 for localizing pain with his left arm.

3. B.
The major insult associated with flail chest is the underlying pulmonary contusion. Chest x-ray will show patchy infiltrates within 1 hour of injury in 70% of patients. Intubation is indicated only for respiratory failure (A PaO_2 of <65 on an inspired oxygen concentration of 50%).

4. A.
The patient described displays signs and symptoms consistent with neurogenic shock, not spinal shock. Spinal shock refers to the flaccidity and loss of reflexes seen following injury to the spinal cord. Recovery from spinal shock is variable. Neurogenic shock, on the other hand, results from the loss of vasomotor tone due to the interruption of sympathetic stimulation to the heart and peripheral blood vessels. The initial treatment of neurogenic shock is fluid resuscitation. Once hemorrhage has

been excluded, vasopressors and/or atropine may be indicated for symptomatic bradycardia and hypotension. Associated injuries must still be ruled out. CT scan of the head is indicated to evaluate for intracranial injury from the fall. The abdomen should be evaluated with ultrasound, diagnostic peritoneal lavage or CT scan. Aortic transection occurs following deceleration injuries. These can include high-speed MVAs or falls from significant heights.

5. E.

Steroids are not indicated for penetrating spinal cord injury. This patient sustained a transthoracic gunshot wound which should be evaluated with angiography, esophagram, esophagoscopy, bronchoscopy and echocardiography. Steroid therapy is only indicated following blunt spinal cord injury. Treatment protocol for blunt spinal cord injury with neurologic impairment consists of an initial intravenous bolus of 30 mg/kg of methylprednisolone followed by a 23-hour infusion at 5.4 mg/kg per hour. Treatment is extended to 48 hours when the interval from injury to treatment is 3-8 hours. No benefit is gained when steroids are started more than 8 hours after injury.

6. A, B, D, E.

This patient sustained a penetrating injury to the chest and displays evidence of shock. An open pneumothorax is not possible, because in an open pneumothorax the chest wall defect measures >2/3 of the diameter of the trachea, creating a sucking chest wound so that air is sucked into the chest cavity during inspiration. While classic signs of pericardial tamponade include systemic hypotension, distended neck veins and muffled heart tones, these are frequently not seen in the acute setting.

7. A, B, D, E.

If pericardial tamponade is suspected and the patient is stable, an intraoperative subxiphoid pericardial window can be performed under general anesthesia. If positive, the incision can be extended to a median sternotomy and the heart repaired. Chest x-ray will show evidence of pneumo- or hemothorax. A left tube thoracostomy can be placed when there is penetrating chest trauma and evidence of decreased breath sounds. Other diagnostic modalities to assist in the diagnosis of pericardial tamponade include echocardiogram, central venous pressure or pericardiocentesis. Emergency department thoracotomy is not indicated in this patient. ED thoracotomy is only indicated in the patient with penetrating thoracic injuries who arrives pulseless, but with cardiac electrical activity or a persistent systolic blood pressure of <60.

8. D.

This patient shows evidence of multiple injuries to the head, chest and abdomen. Immediate intubation and left tube thoracostomy are indicated. However, following an initial fluid bolus, the patient remains in shock. This suggests continued and ongoing blood loss. Appropriate management includes immediate blood transfusion with O negative blood, chest x-ray and pelvic x-ray should be obtained to rule out massive hemorrhage from these sources, and immediate evaluation of the abdomen for bleeding. This can be done with diagnostic peritoneal lavage or ultrasound. If positive for intraperitoneal bleeding, immediate exploratory laparotomy is indicated. In an unstable patient, cervical spine films should be deferred and resuscitation continued maintaining C-spine precautions at all times. Head CT in the unstable patient should be deferred until exsanguinating hemorrhage is controlled. An intracranial pressure monitor can be placed in the operating room to assist in management of intracranial pressure until a head CT can be performed. Emergency burr holes can be performed in the operating room should the patient develop signs of herniation.

9. B.

The consensus formula for fluid resuscitation is 2-4 cc/kg/%TBSA burned. This resuscitation should occur from the ***time of injury*** and applies to ***second and third degree burns*** only. Increased fluid needs are required for inhalation injury, electrical injury, and delay in resuscitation. This patient was underresuscitated for the initial 4 hours following injury. During that time, he received only 200 cc per hour (800 cc total). Because of the delay in resuscitation, 4 cc/kg/hour should be used to calculate fluid resuscitation. This calculation would be 4 x 80 x 50 = 16,000 cc. Half of this should be given over the first 8 hours (8000 cc) from the time of injury. This patient received 800 cc in 4 hours, therefore he should receive 7200 cc over the next 4 hours, or 1800 cc/hour x 4 hours. The second half of the resuscitation (8000 cc) should be given over the next 16 hours at 500 cc/hour.

10. D.

The pregnant trauma patient should be positioned on her left side during transport and resuscitation. This will lift the uterus up off the inferior vena cava, thus allowing for improved venous return and resuscitation.

Chapter 7: Hernias of the Groin and Abdominal Wall

F. Charles Brunicardi, MD
Herminio F. Ojeda, MD
Lisa Hawkins, MD

Contents

1. Anatomy

An understanding of inguinal and abdominal wall anatomy is essential to properly treat patients with hernias. The posterior wall of the inguinal canal is composed of transversalis fascia and transversus abdominis muscles while the anterior aspect is formed by the aponeurosis of the external oblique muscle. Relatively unprotected, Hesselbach's triangle (defined by the borders of the rectus sheath, inguinal ligament, and inferior epigastric vessels) is subjected to the strain of abdominal pressure. The inferolateral margin thickens where it becomes the iliopubic tract. Medial to the internal ring, the posterior wall of the inguinal canal thickens as it becomes the interfoveolar ligament. The wedge-shaped posterior wall of the inguinal canal is bordered superiorly by the transversus abdominis and internal oblique, inferiorly by the iliopubic tract and medially by the rectus. The spermatic cord and its associated structures enter the inguinal canal through the superolateral portion of the posterior wall.

Other important structures of the inguinal region include the structures of the spermatic cord (vas deferens, testicular artery and vein, lymphatics and autonomic nerves) and the nerves that run in the area. The main nerves of concern are the ilioinguinal nerve, iliohypogastric nerve and the genital branch of the genitofemoral nerve. Division of the ilioinguinal and/or iliohypogastric nerves (which intermingle) leads to sensory deficits in the area of the groin, base of the penis and the medial upper thigh. Division of the genital branch of the genitofemoral nerve (which has motor fibers to the cremasteric muscle) leads to sensory deficits on the side of the scrotum or labia. It is also important to realize that the femoral nerve, artery and vein run directly below the posterior wall of the inguinal canal. Stitches placed too deeply during an open repair have the potential to damage any of these structures.

2. Diagnosis of Inguinal Hernias

History

A patient with an inguinal hernia often presents with a bulge in the inguinal region, but some patients may be unaware of the presence of a hernia. Most symptomatic hernias present with a variety of nonspecific complaints relating to the contents of the hernia sac and pressure on surrounding structures. The discomfort associated with a hernia often worsens throughout the day and is relieved with reclination, which can reduce the hernia. Extreme pain related to the hernia in the absence of incarceration or without evidence of strangulation is unusual and should raise the possibility of another etiology for the pain. Most hernias develop slowly over time with gradual enlargement and increased symptoms; however, some are precipitated by a single instance of strenuous exertion.

Physical Examination

The physical examination of the groin is conducted with the patient standing and facing the physician. Visual inspection may reveal an asymmetry or a distinct visible bulge. Typically, the hernia enlarges with straining and coughing and these maneuvers may make the hernia more visible. After palpation of the abdominal wall, which the physician performs by placing fingers over the inguinal region, the patient is instructed to strain or cough. A finger can also be placed into the inguinal canal via the scrotum and the maneuvers repeated. These techniques allow the physician to palpate the hernia bulge. Differentiating direct from indirect inguinal hernias is difficult on physical examination alone. A femoral hernia can sometimes be differentiated by its location, since it occurs below the inguinal ligament. Since hydroceles transilluminate and hernias do not, differentiating a hernia from a hydrocele is easily achieved by transilluminating the groin mass. Auscultation of the hernia contents may disclose bowel sounds, an indication that intestines are in the sac.

Diagnostic Imaging in Inguinal Hernias

Sensitivity, specificity and predictive values of abdominal wall sonography vary according to pathology. Reports show that inguinal hernias have a sensitivity of 82% and a specificity of 98.9%;

femoral hernias have a sensitivity of 72% and 97%, respectively. The use of ultrasonography in the evaluation of hernias is recommended; the procedure is free of complications, time-efficient, low-cost and the results are of reproducible quality.[1]

In a consecutive study of 642 children, the sonographic evidence of the dimensions of the inguinal canal were compared to the operative findings. The operative findings correlated the width of the inguinal canal as follows: a normal inguinal canal measures 3.6 ± 0.8 mm; in patent processus vaginalis the width is 4.9 ± 1.1 mm; in inguinal hernia the width is 7.2 ± 2.0 mm; and in a large hernia the width is 12.8 ± 3.6 mm.2 These results suggest that ultrasound evaluation in children may be useful in cases of equivocal clinical diagnosis.

Computed tomography (CT) scans are especially useful in evaluating obese patients, assessing patients postoperatively and locating hernias in unusual places. Furthermore, CT scans may detect incidental intraabdominal pathology, may be used to evaluate the content of the hernia and can help identify postoperative complications such as abscesses or seromas.[3] Magnetic resonance imaging (MRI) is appropriate in cases of abdominal wall relaxation and is also helpful in differentiating femoral from inguinal hernias (over 95% sensitivity and specificity).[4]

Herniography is performed by instilling a non-irritant contrast agent into the abdominal cavity in order to look for the outline or pooling of contrast within a hernia sac. Some authors consider that potential complications of herniography due to direct puncture of the abdominal cavity and the injection of contrast material and radiation unnecessary due to the availability of other less invasive imaging techniques.[5]

Initial evaluation of abdominal wall and inguinal hernias should be based on the patient's clinical history. Proceed with clinical examination and ultrasound, followed by CT/MRI if indicated. The use of ultrasound after laparoscopic inguinal hernia surgery may help to verify mesh placement, diagnose fluid collections and assess swelling of the spermatic cord (and blood flow to the testicle).[6]

Differential Diagnosis

Developing an accurate differential diagnosis of groin masses may be difficult; however, the differentiation of a hernia from other groin masses is often achieved by a thorough physical examination. If the presence of a hernia has been ruled out, further workup and evaluation may be needed to determine the nature of the groin mass (Table 1).

Table 1

Differential Diagnosis of Groin Masses

Major
Inguinal hernia
Femoral hernia
Inguinal lymphadenopathy
Femoral lymphadenopathy
Hydrocele
Lipoma
Ectopic testicle
Varicocele
Hematoma
Psoas abscess
Lymphoma
Tuberculosis
Metastatic disease
Epididymitis
Testicular torsion
Femoral aneurysm or pseudoaneurysm
Sebaceous cyst
Hidradenitis of inguinal apocrine glands
Endometriosis
Torsion of appendix testis

Townsend CM, Beauchamp DR, Evers BM, Mattox KL. Sabiston Textbook of Surgery. *16th ed. Philadelphia, PA: WB Saunders; 2000.*

3. Classification of Hernias

Hernias are generally classified by type, location, volume of the sac and diameter of the neck. There are several different systems in use to classify prevalent groin hernias. 5 of these classification systems are as follows: Halverson and McVay, Gilbert (modified by Rutkow and Robbins), Nyhus, Bendavid, and Schumpelick-Aachen. The most recent and comprehensive system, the Unified Classification, has been described by Zollinger and reviewed by Nyhus (Table 2). By using a consistent method of describing hernias, the Unified Classification system allows comparison to be made with a common frame of reference.[7]

Inguinal Hernias

Direct inguinal hernias compose 25% of inguinal hernias. They originate through the floor of the inguinal canal. They are usually diffuse and involve the entire canal floor. Rarely do they have small necks and/or diverticular sacs. If they become large enough, direct hernias can descend through the external ring and into the scrotum. The bladder is the organ most commonly involved in a sliding direct inguinal hernia.

Table 2

Unified Classification by Zollinger

I	Indirect, small
II	Indirect, medium
III	Indirect, large
IV	Direct, small
V	Direct, medium
VI	Direct, large
VII	Combined pantaloon
VIII	Femoral
IX	Other[a]

[a]Any not classified by number above; femoral + indirect or direct; massive, >6 cm (4 fingers) inguinal defect; prevascular.

Zollinger RM Jr. Unified Classification for Inguinal Hernias. Hernia. *1999;3:195-200.*

Indirect inguinal hernias, referred to as persistent processus vaginalis, make up 50% of all hernias. This sac travels through the internal ring that is anterior and lateral to the spermatic cord and may extend into the scrotum. Properitoneal fat associated with the hernia sac is often referred to as a lipoma of the cord and can be confused with an indirect inguinal hernia on physical examination.

Femoral Hernia

Femoral hernias, which occur through a defect on the medial side of the femoral sheath, make up 3% of all hernias. The space occupied by a femoral hernia is defined superiorly by the iliopubic tract, inferiorly by Cooper's ligament, laterally by the femoral vein and medially by the insertion of the iliopubic tract into Cooper's ligament. A femoral hernia produces a mass below the inguinal ligament that can be detected on careful physical examination. Femoral hernias occur more commonly in females.

Umbilical Hernia

An umbilical hernia occurs at the umbilicus, a weak area of the abdominal wall. In children, umbilical hernias are usually congenital and the majority spontaneously close by age 2. In adults, umbilical hernias are considered acquired and are associated with conditions that increase intraabdominal pressure, eg, pregnancy, ascites or acute abdominal distension. Strangulation of omentum and intestine frequently occur. Rupture of an umbilical hernia in patients with chronic ascitic cirrhosis may require an emergency portal decompressive procedure.

Epigastric Hernia

An epigastric hernia occurs between the umbilicus and the xiphoid process in the midline. It is the result of properitoneal fat and perironeum protruding through decussating fibers of the rectus sheath.

Spigelian Hernia

Spigelian hernias occur along the semilunar line below the level of the umbilicus. They usually occur along the lateral edge of the rectus muscle inferior to the semicircular line of Douglas, where the lack of a posterior rectus sheath causes weakness.

Lumbar Hernia

There are 2 types of lumbar hernias: Grynfelt's hernia, which occurs in the superior lumbar triangle (bounded by the twelfth rib, internal oblique muscle and sacrospinalis muscle), and Petit's hernia, which occurs in the inferior lumbar triangle (bounded by the latissimus dorsi muscle, external oblique muscle and the iliac crest).

Obturator Hernia

Obturator hernias are characterized by a weakening of the obturator membrane that often leads to intestinal incarceration and strangulation within the obturator canal. This type of hernia is most often seen in cachetic elderly patients, especially women. The patient may present with pain in the region of the hip, knee and inner thigh due to compression of the obturator nerve. This characteristic symptom is known as the Howship-Romberg sign and is seen in approximately one half of all patients with obturator hernias.

Sciatic Hernia

Sciatic hernias are extremely unusual. They occur in the greater or lesser sciatic foramen and are often difficult to diagnose until intestinal obstruction occurs. Some patients present with gluteal or infragluteal masses and discomfort when standing. Compression of the sciatic nerve can also cause sciatica-like pain.

Ventral (Incisional) Hernia

Ventral or incisional hernias make up 10% of all hernias. They result from the breakdown of an abdominal wall incision due to incomplete, inadequate healing or excessive strain on the incision site. They can occur anywhere an incision has been made in the abdominal wall. Factors contributing to ventral hernia formation include obesity, malnutrition, pregnancy, ascites and other conditions that increase stress on the abdominal wall. The most common factor contributing to ventral hernia formation, ie, postoperative wound infection, impairs wound healing and subsequently decreases the strength of the healed incision.

Epigastric Hernia

Epigastric hernias occur in the crossing fibers of the linea alba above the level of the umbilicus. They tend to be small and are frequently multiple.

Perineal Hernia

A perineal hernia occurs through the pelvic diaphragm and may develop anterior or posterior to the superficial transverse perineal muscle. The anterior perineal hernia, which occurs only in women, passes into the labia majora. In men the posterior perineal hernia enters the ischiorectal fossa; in women, close to the vagina. Perineal hernias may occur after an abdominoperineal resection, prostatectomy, or removal of pelvic organs.

Sliding Hernia

A sliding hernia occurs in the event that an internal organ forms a portion of the hernia sac. The most commonly involved organs are the bladder or a segment of intestine.

Richter's Hernia

A Richter's hernia, in which the antimesenteric border of the intestine is involved in the hernia sac, never involves the entire circumference of the intestine.

Littre's Hernia

A Littre's hernia is one in which a Meckel's diverticulum is the only organ involved with the hernia sac. It is frequently difficult to diagnose since there are no obstructive symptoms. Strangulation may occur and present as an abscess or fistulization.

Cloquet's Hernia

A Cloquet's hernia is a femoral hernia that penetrates the pectineus muscle fascia.

Serafini's Hernia

A Serafini's hernia is a femoral hernia that travels underneath the femoral vessels.

Cooper's Hernia

A Cooper's hernia involves the femoral canal that tracts into the scrotum or labia majora.

Valpeau's Hernia

A Valpeau's hernia is a hernia through Gimbernat's ligament (Laugier's hernia).

Internal Hernias

There are 2 types of internal hernias: congenital and acquired. Congenital internal hernias include paraduodenal hernias, transmesenteric hernias and pericecal hernias. The paraduodenal hernias are induced by abnormal intestinal rotation. Transmesenteric hernias occur through an opening within the mesentery, often the transverse mesocolon. Lastly, pericecal hernias occur through defects in the ileocecal mesentery.

Other congenital internal hernias occur through the gastrocolic ligament, gastrohepatic ligament (and greater omentum) and the foramen of Winslow. Acquired hernias occur through mesenteric defects created by surgery or trauma. Approximately 0.8% of small bowel obstructions have an internal hernia as their etiology.

4. Etiology

Although the etiologies of hernias are considered to be multifactoral, they are generally classified as congenital or acquired. In infants, preterm and persistence of the processus vaginalis have been claimed as determinants for the development of indirect inguinal hernias. Birthweights between 500 and 1000 g are associated with a 30%-40% incidence of hernias; birthweights between 1500 and 2000 g are associated with only a 3% incidence of hernias. The incidence of bilateral hernias is also higher in premature babies (about 50%).[8,9] At birth, 80% of male babies are born with a patent processus vaginalis. This number decreases to 25%-35% by age 4.[4] Spontaneous closure more often will occur on the left side. The lifetime risk of the development of groin herniation has been reported by some authors to be 24%.[10] Some indirect inguinal hernias are associated with congenital pelvic deformities such as exstrophy of the bladder, which can cause abnormal development of the inguinal canal and subsequent development of an indirect inguinal hernia. Direct inguinal hernias are generally attributed to normal wear and tear.

In 1804, Cooper listed factors causing disparity between intraabdominal pressure and the resistance of the abdominal wall (ie, abdominal herniation): cough, obesity, constipation, ascites, pregnancy and unusual exertion (only 7% of patients recall such an incident). Today, other factors have been identified, eg, prostatic hypertrophy, erect posture, aging, carcinomatosis, peritonitis, smoking and genetic influences.

Biochemical alterations in leukocytes and collagen may play a role in hernia development. The suspected etiology of groin hernias linked to smoking may be due to alterations in the levels of neutrophil elastase activity.[11,12] A decreased ratio between collagen I/III, which affects fiber bonding, has been observed in patients with hernias.[13-15] In fascia samples from patients with hernias, Bellon demonstrated lower levels of proline and lysine hydroxylation in addition to higher levels of metalloproteinase-9. It has been proven that the activity of this enzyme is uninhibited in patients with recurrent hernias.[16] These observations are associated with a decreased deposition of collagen in patients with hernias. Also, several studies demonstrate altered leukocytes and proteases in patients with abdominal aortic aneurysms, which may be responsible for a higher incidence of hernias in this particular population.[17]

Aging has also been indicated as a factor contributing to the potential cause of hernias. Rodriguez and colleagues reported a progressive weakening of elastic and elastin-related fibers in the transversalis fascia of elderly patients.[18]

A familial tendency to develop groin hernias has been well documented in a number of conditions, eg, polycystic disease of the kidney (in which up to 40% of patients develop hernias), joint hypermotility and other connective tissue disorders.[19]

5. Incidence

It is estimated that 700,000 inguinal hernia repairs are performed in the United States annually. The lifetime risk of inguinal hernia is 25% for men and 5% for women.[20] The associated costs from lost work days, medical treatment and surgery are considerable.

The true incidence of hernias is not known, but it is estimated that the overall incidence of inguinal hernias in the Western hemisphere is between 10% and 15%. The male to female ratio is 9.121. Approximately 75% of all hernias are inguinal; 50% are indirect inguinal hernias and 25% are direct inguinal hernias. Incisional and ventral hernias make up about 10% of all hernias, femoral hernias account for about 3% and other, more unusual types of hernias account for the remaining 12%.[22]

The most common hernia in both males and females is the indirect inguinal hernia. Inguinal hernias tend to occur on the right side, since the left processus vaginalis closure is more common. Femoral hernias occur more frequently in females by a ratio of 4:1.[13]

6. Indications for Surgery

Hernia management can be stratified into conservative, elective and emergent. Hernias continue to increase in size over time, making surgical repair the definitive treatment. However, the need for surgical repair of an asymptomatic hernia has been questioned. In a randomized multicenter trial involving 720 patients with asymptomatic or minimally symptomatic hernias, the study group was randomized to either surgery or watchful waiting. The primary outcomes, namely pain and function, were equal in both groups at 2 years, and the risk of incarceration was found to be 0.3%, concluding that conservative management of asymptomatic hernias is safe. All symptomatic hernias should be repaired unless a patient has contraindications for surgery. Given the low risks associated with hernia surgery however, it should be strongly considered in elderly persons, regardless of any concomitant conditions. Emergency repair of a neglected hernia is associated with markedly increased morbidity and mortality. Absolute indications for emergent repair of a hernia are incarceration and strangulation of hernia contents.

7. Open Repair of Inguinal Hernias

Many different hernia operations have been described for hernia repair, eg, open tissue repair, tension-free repair using mesh and, most recently, laparoscopic repair. Surgical repair of a groin hernia can be simple, but in some cases the normal anatomy can be so distorted as to present a significant technical challenge.

Bassini Repair

The Bassini procedure is frequently used to repair indirect inguinal hernias and small direct hernias. The Bassini repair begins with a skin incision 2 cm above and parallel to Poupart's ligament, ie, between the anterosuperior iliac spine and the pubic symphysis. Then a transverse incision is made in the external oblique fascia and the spermatic cord is encircled. The cremaster muscle is carefully dissected off the medial aspect of the cord to identify an indirect sac. If a sac is found, it is dissected free to the level of the abdominal wall and its contents are reduced. The neck of the sac is ligated at the level of the abdominal wall. The remaining distal sac is then amputated. Nonabsorbable interrupted sutures are used to approximate the conjoined tendon and internal oblique muscular edge to the shelving edge of the inguinal ligament. The spermatic cord is returned to its normal anatomic position and the external oblique fascia is approximated over the cord structures. The overall recurrence rate after a Bassini repair is reported to be between 5% and 9%.[23]

McVay (Cooper's Ligament) Repair

In 1942, McVay demonstrated that the normal insertion of the transversalis fascia and the transversus abdominis muscle was to the ligament of Cooper, not Poupart.[24] The McVay repair is a popular procedure for the correction of large inguinal hernias, direct inguinal hernias, recurrent hernias of the groin and femoral hernias. The skin incision is likened to that of other hernia repairs, ie, it is carried down to the external oblique aponeurosis, which is opened in the direction of its fibers. Any indirect hernia sac is identified and high ligation is performed. Cooper's ligament is then exposed, and after a relaxing incision is made in the anterior rectus sheath, the transversus abdominis arch is sutured to Cooper's ligament (beginning at the pubic tubercle).

A transition suture is made that encompasses Cooper's ligament, the transversalis fascia, and Poupart's ligament. The suture line is continued until the internal inguinal ring will admit a fingertip alongside the spermatic cord. The cord is placed in its anatomic position within the inguinal canal and the external oblique aponeurosis is closed. In a large personal series by Rutledge, he reported a 2% overall recurrence rate for a McVay repair, with an average follow-up of 9 years.[23]

Shouldice (Canadian) Repair

The Shouldice (Canadian) repair is used for direct as well as indirect hernias. It emphasizes a multilayer imbricated repair with running sutures of the floor of the inguinal canal. The groin anatomy is carefully dissected and the indirect sac is ligated as described above. The transversalis fascia is opened and the inferior epigastric vessels may be divided to facilitate opening the internal ring. The lateral cut edge of the transversalis fascia is sutured medially to the undersurface of the internal oblique muscle. The medial superior edge is then sutured to the inguinal ligament. The conjoined tendon is sutured to the inguinal ligament, providing a firm repair. The external oblique aponeurosis is closed over the cord, leaving the external ring loose. Proponents of the Shouldice repair report a recurrence rate of less than 1%.[25]

Lichtenstein (Tension-Free) Repair

One of the most commonly performed open herniorrhaphy techniques is the tension-free repair popularized by Lichtenstein. Lichtenstein demonstrated that when performed with mesh reinforcement of the inguinal floor, a tension-free hernia repair significantly decreases the recurrence rate. The repair is performed by careful dissection of the inguinal canal, high ligation of any indirect hernia sac and inferior retraction of the spermatic cord structures. A sheet of mesh is fashioned to fit the inguinal canal. A slit is made in the lateral aspect of the mesh and the spermatic cord is placed between the 2 tails of the mesh. The mesh is secured to the aponeurotic tissue overlying the pubic tubercle using a running suture. The suture is continued laterally by suturing the inferior edge of the mesh to the shelving edge of the inguinal ligament to a point just lateral of the internal inguinal ring. A second suture is placed at the level of the pubic tubercle and continued superiorly and laterally, thereby securing the mesh to the internal oblique aponeurosis. The lower edges of the 2 mesh tails are sutured to the shelving edge of the inguinal ligament to create a new internal ring. The spermatic cord structures are placed within the inguinal canal overlying the mesh and the external oblique aponeurosis is closed over the spermatic cord. The Lichtenstein Hernia Institute series reported 4 recurrences out of 3125 consecutive patients, a follow-up rate of 87%, and a follow-up period of 1-8 years.[26]

Plug-and-Patch Repair

Another popular tension-free open hernia repair is the plug-and-patch technique. This technique is similar to the Lichtenstein repair described above except that it also incorporates the use of a mesh plug placed into the inverted, reduced hernia sac. The plug may then be secured with individual sutures to hold it in position. An onlay patch of mesh is then placed as in the Lichtenstein repair. In addition to being technically straightforward to perform, the plug-and-patch technique has also produced good long-term results. In one study of 3268 patients, 2861 patients (88%) underwent this repair for primary hernias and 407 (12%) underwent the repair for recurrent hernias. With follow-up extending to 5 years, it was reported that less than 1% of patients who underwent this repair for a primary hernia had a recurrence. In patients who underwent this procedure for a recurrent hernia, 3% had another recurrence. Furthermore, there were only 19 patients (less than 1%) who required treatment for local wound infections and no other significant complications were reported.[27] The plug-and-patch method of open hernia repair demonstrates good overall results. Its relative ease in performance is likely to contribute to its popularity as an open hernia repair technique.

Prolene Hernia System (PHS)

The PHS was developed to take advantage of the anterior and preperitoneal repair using an open approach. The mesh consists of an onlay and underlay patch with an intervening connecter. The underlay portion is positioned in the preperitoneal space, while the onlay flap rests above the inguinal floor. The underlay portion is placed through the internal ring, or through the transversalis fascia in the case of direct defects. The overlay portion reinforces the floor of the canal in a similar fashion to a tension-free repair. The greatest advantage to this technique is that it provides a preperitoneal reinforcement to a tension-free repair.

Open Mesh Repairs Vs. Nonmesh Repairs

Although tension-free techniques of hernia repair (using synthetic mesh) have produced encouraging results, the single best method of inguinal hernia repair is still unclear. When attempting to measure postoperative pain and analgesia, a prospective randomized study by Zieren showed that tension-free methods were superior to Shouldice repairs. Furthermore, the laparoscopic repair had significantly longer operating times and was more expensive than the Shouldice operation.[28] A large review in Denmark that included 26,304 herniorrhaphies found that non-mesh repairs had higher secondary operative rates than open mesh repairs. Similar results have been observed in other studies.[29,30]

8. Laparoscopic Repair of Inguinal Hernias

In addition to the open repairs described previously, inguinal hernias may also be repaired via a laparoscopic approach. The 2 most commonly performed minimally-invasive hernia operations are the trans-abdominal preperitoneal (TAPP) repair and the totally extraperitoneal hernia repair. Laparoscopic repair was first described by Ger in 1982 when he closed an indirect sac with a metal clip.[31] Intraperitoneal onlay mesh repairs used by Schultz resulted in high recurrence rates.[32] The TAPP repair was first reported by Arregui and Spitz in 1991. In 1993, Phillips et al and Mc Kernan introduced the totally extraperitoneal (TEP) repair.[33,34]

For the diagnosis of concurrent, asymptomatic or rare hernias, or for the repair of bilateral and recurrent hernias, this technique should be the procedure of choice. It has a distinct advantage in that a number of previously undiagnosed bilateral hernias that warrant repair are discovered during the course of laparoscopic hernia repair. Although the procedure is somewhat more expensive to perform due to the equipment required, proponents argue that these costs are offset significantly by early return of the patient to his or her job.

The potential advantages to the laparoscopic approach include a reduction in both postoperative pain and level of disability.[35,36] The laparoscopic approach also decreases the risk of nerve injury, seroma formation, dysejaculation, hypospermia, infection or ischemic orchitis in recurrent hernias. One disadvantage of the laparoscopic approach is the need for general anesthesia, which may exclude patients with significant underlying illnesses. Another is the use of expensive instrumentation, which increases the overall cost of the procedure. Short-term recurrence rates for various techniques of laparoscopic inguinal herniorrhaphies range from 0%-5% over a follow-up period of 13-23 months.[37-39] Between 1993 and 1995, 13 series of noncomparative trials with laparoscopic inguinal herniorraphy using TAPP showed a recurrence rate of 0%-3.5% with a follow-up time of 18-30 months.[40] In collected series comparing TAPP to TEP, TEP showed a lower recurrence rate that varied from 0%-1.5% and a lower complication rate.41 The true long-term recurrence rate of laparoscopic inguinal hernia repairs is not known because adequate follow-up data are not yet available.

In 2004, a meta-analysis of randomized controlled trials (RCT) of endoscopic procedures vs. Lichtenstein and other open mesh techniques for inguinal hernia repair per Schmedt, Sauerland and Bittner[42] reviewed over 34 RCT. This study included 7223 patients and included reports from Europe, Asia and the U.S. This meta-analysis included the VA hernia study of 2004 from Neumayer et al that compared TEP vs. Lichtenstein repair. The study acknowledged that endoscopic repairs did have some advantages in terms of local complications and pain-associated parameters, but again concluded that well-structured trials with improved standardization of hernia type, operative technique and surgeon's experience were necessary.

We believe that the general surgeon should do the repair he or she is most comfortable with, and recommend they have a personal tracking system for outcomes. The average general surgeon should have mastered 1 or 2 open techniques for hernia repairs and should have the adequate training in the laparoscopic repairs to obtain the best results. We believe that laparoscopic repairs constitute one of the hardest operations in laparoscopy to teach and to learn.

Transabdominal Preperitoneal (TAPP) Hernia Repair

Definition
The TAPP repair approaches the groin through a traditional intraperitoneal laparoscope. The preperitoneal inguinal region is inspected through an incision in the peritoneum. Synthetic mesh prosthesis is secured over the posterior abdominal wall covering the hernia defect. The peritoneum is then closed and used to cover the mesh.

History
The TAPP hernia repair was first reported by Arregui in 1992.[42]

Technique
In this procedure, a pneumoperitoneum is established and trocars are placed. The peritoneum is incised cephalad to the inguinal floor and the hernia defects are dissected. Synthetic mesh is secured to Cooper's ligament and the underside of the conjoined tendon. Small indirect hernia sacs are mobilized and reduced. Large hernia sacs may need to be divided distal to the internal ring, thereby leaving the distal sac in situ. Mesh should cover the direct, indirect and femoral spaces. One technical variation is to mobilize the spermatic cord, slit the mesh laterally and place the mesh around the cord structures in the preperitoneal space. However, recurrences have been reported through these slits.

Indications
The transabdominal preperitoneal (TAPP) repair is indicated for incarcerated hernias, as it allows reduction and inspection of the involved bowel. The TAPP repair is also indicated when the preperitoneal space has been obliterated by prior surgery such as prostatectomy. As well, the TAPP approach is useful when a patient is undergoing a laparoscopic procedure for an unrelated abdominal issue. Surgeon preference or experience may also dictate the choice of TAPP repair. This technique is easier in that there is more room to operate than in other procedures. It is more difficult, however, in that the peritoneum must be closed at the completion of the procedure. This also adds the risk of exposing the mesh to the bowel, and hernias may occur if the closure fails or is incomplete. Absolute contraindications are peritonitis and intraabdominal infection.

Results
One disadvantage to the TAPP approach is that the peritoneal cavity is violated and a pneumoperitoneum is required. Kald compared 339 TAPP repairs with 87 TEP repairs.[43] He found recurrence rates of 2% with TAPP and 0% with TEP at 23 and 7 months follow-up, respectively. Felix compared 733 TAPP repairs and 382 TEP repairs in a retrospective, nonrandomized study.[44] This study found 9 complications and 2 recurrences with the TAPP approach vs. no complications and 1 recurrence with the TEP approach.

Totally Extraperitoneal (TEP) Hernia Repair

Definition
The TEP hernia repair provides access to the groin through the preperitoneal space, specifically avoiding the peritoneal cavity. Synthetic mesh prosthesis is then secured over the hernia defect and to the posterior abdominal wall as in the TAPP repair.

History
McKernan initially described the TEP hernia repair as laparoscopically-performed, preperitoneal, prosthetic mesh repair based on the open preperitoneal repairs of Stoppa.[45]

Technique
In this procedure, the space between the rectus muscle and the posterior rectus sheath is entered on the side of the hernia. After the balloon dissector is passed through the incision and traverses the preperitoneal space to the pubic symphysis, the balloon is inflated. After it is deflated and removed, the dissected space is insufflated. 3 trocars are then placed in the midline (or lateral lower abdomen). As with the TAPP repair, the cord structures and hernia sac are identified and dissected free. Synthetic mesh is then placed to cover Hesselbach's triangle, which fixes the mesh to Cooper's ligament, the pubic tubercle, posterior rectus muscle and transversalis fascia. Gentle counterpressure should be applied to the tacker or stapler against the anterior abdominal wall to avoid nerve injury. This ensures that the tacks are being placed above the level of the iliopubic tract, away from inguinal nerve courses.

Indications
The totally extraperitoneal (TEP) repair may be used for any groin hernia. In contrast to the TAPP, it obviates the need to enter the peritoneal cavity, thereby decreasing the risk of intrabdominal organ injury. Its greatest advantage in treating bilateral inguinal hernias is that the number and size of the incisions are the same as those used for unilateral repair. In addition, little time or cost is added to the procedure. Since the TEP approach is through a new tissue plane, it may be used in reoperative hernia repairs as well.

Results
In the TEP approach, the abdominal cavity is intentionally avoided. Also, TEP affords easy examination of bilateral inguinal and femoral regions. Although the TEP approach is technically more difficult, in experienced hands it is associated with fewer complications and recurrences than the TAPP approach. Tetik showed the TEP repair to have a recurrence rate of 0.4% in 457 repairs over a mean follow-up period of 13 months.[37] Phillips showed a 0% recurrence rate in 578 repairs over a 22-month mean follow-up period.[33] Fitzgibbons also reported a 0% recurrence rate in 87 patients over a follow-up period of 23 months.[40]

Intraperitoneal Onlay Mesh (IPOM) Hernia Repair

Hernia Repair
The intraperitoneal onlay (IPOM) mesh repair was initially advocated by Fitzgibbons.[46] In this procedure, using a transperitoneal approach, polytetrafluoroethylene (PTFE) mesh is fixed directly to the peritoneum and Cooper's ligament with staples or sutures. Although Fitzgibbons has abandoned the technique to avoid complications related to possible mesh erosion into the intestine, Franklin et al continued to obtain good results with it.[46] Other indications for IPOM include repeat recurrence of inguinal hernia, where distortion of the peritoneum may have resulted from previous laparoscopic repairs.

Complications
The risks of laparoscopic inguinal hernia repair are comparable to those of open hernia repair. Felix has shown that the complication rate of laparoscopic hernia repair is significantly influenced by the experience of the surgeon.[47] Potential complications of the laparoscopic inguinal herniorrhaphy include the risks associated with general anesthesia and laparoscopy in addition to the risks of hernia repair. Complications from anesthesia and pneumoperitoneum, however, are rare.

Other potential complications include major vascular injury, injury to hollow viscera, urinary tract complications, nerve injury, mesh complications, vas deferens and testicular complications, seromas/hematomas and recurrence.

Wound infection is reported in between 0.5% and 9% of cases and most likely results from primary contamination at the time of the procedure. Surgeon's gloves, patient's skin, environment and surgical instruments are the sources of most contaminations.[48] The presence of multiknot sutures, redundancy and/or crinkled mesh edges also increases the risk of infection. Antibiotic prophylaxis with a first-generation cephalosporin is commonly used; however, in a large multi-institutional, prospective randomized study by Platt, it was demonstrated that cephalosporin afforded no appreciable difference in infection incidence compared to placebo.[49] Mesh infection generally will require removal and usually can be tracked to a mesh fold or suture. Although rare, necrotizing fasciitis can occur.[48]

Vascular injury typically involves the inferior epigastric or spermatic vessels but may involve the external iliac, circumflex iliac, profunda or obturator vessels. A multi-institutional survey shows that the incidence of bleeding complications following totally extraperitoneal (TEP) herniorrhaphy ranges from 0%-0.7%.[50]

Urinary tract complications associated with repair include urinary retention (2%-18% incidence with TEP), infection and hematuria. Bladder injury is less common (0%-0.3%). Prior surgery in the space of Retzius, eg, in prostatectomy, is a relative contraindication to laparoscopic hernia repair due to increased technical difficulty of the procedure and increased risk of injury to the bladder.

Nerve injury most frequently involves dissection or stapling of the femoral branch of the genitofemoral nerve, lateral cutaneous nerve of the thigh or the intermediate cutaneous branch of the anterior branch of the femoral nerve. Neuroma, deafferentation and projected pain can be the result of complete, partial transection of the nerve or an entrapped nerve, respectively. Chronic pain is also more common than realized and should be incorporated as a possible outcome of the surgery;[51] recent series report 10% incidence of chronic pain at 2 years. Geis et al reviewed chronic inguinal pain after herniorrhaphy and suggested the evaluation and management of pain after inguinal repair.[52]

Testicular complications are usually short-lived and include testicular pain and swelling, orchitis and epididymitis (0%-5% incidence in TEP repairs). Out of 4114 patients undergoing groin hernia repairs, Wantz reported testicular ischemia in 0.61% and testicular atrophy in 0.34% of patients. Prevention is the best method to avoid these events. Minimal mobilization of the cord avoiding removal of the testicle from the scrotum are essential. Unless it is small, the distal sac should be avoided and left cut open after ligation of the proximal end.[53] Other potential complications include pubic and pelvic osteitis and seroma or hematoma formation (1.2%-10% incidence). Mesh complications include mesh migration, infection, erosion into other organs and adhesions.

Open Vs. Laparoscopic Hernia Repairs

Critics of laparoscopic herniorrhaphy argue its disadvantages, ie, the need for general anesthesia, high operative costs, violation of the peritoneal cavity in the TAPP repair and lack of long-term recurrence data.[54] However, in a cost-analysis study between open and laparoscopic repair in the United Kingdom, the cost was less of an issue when reusable equipment was utilized.[55]

In a prospective, randomized trial comparing 52 patients who had a Lichtenstein tension-free open hernia repair to 48 patients who had totally TEP or TAPP laparoscopic repairs, Payne reported that open and laparoscopic-repair patients have similar postoperative times to discharge. TAPP was associated with shorter time periods needed to be able to return to work, eg, patients with TAPP patients returned to work after 8 days, TEP patients returned after 9 days and open repair patients returned after 17 days. He reported 1 recurrence each for TEP and TAPP. His complication rates were 18% for the open approach, 12% for TAPP and 7% for TEP.[56]

Kozol studied 62 hernia patients in a randomized, prospective, blinded trial comparing open repair to laparoscopic repair.[57] Although he found no difference in the complication rate, the laparoscopic group reported less postoperative pain. Liem compared recovery following open hernia repair to recovery following TEP in 105 patients in a prospective randomized trial.[58] The laparoscopic group returned to normal activities sooner (6 days vs. 10 days), were able to perform more sit-ups and straight leg raises, and had better scores on activities of daily living questionnaires. He later reported a separate large, multicenter prospective randomized trial of 994 patients comparing recovery after open hernia repair to recovery after TEP (all unilateral hernias).[59] The laparoscopic group demonstrated more rapid recovery and fewer recurrences.

In a prospective randomized trial, Heikkinen compared 18 patients who had laparoscopic hernia repair to 20 patients who had open hernia repair.[60] The laparoscopic repair group took longer to recover and had higher operative costs but had less postoperative pain, decreased analgesic consumption, a quicker return to work and fewer complications. Johansson compared 3 groups of patients: those who had open repair, those who had open repair with mesh and those who had TAPP.[61] The TAPP group had shorter recovery time and returned to work faster, but at greater cost than the other groups.

Between 1990 and 2002, a meta-analysis of 10 randomized trials including 3212 patients was conducted comparing outcomes associated with TEP to those associated with open inguinal repair. Compared to the open repair group, TEP group demonstrated a statistically significant lower wound complication rate (P <0.001), less postoperative pain at 1 week and earlier return to normal activities. Although the recurrence rate associated with both procedures was similar, TEP patients had lower recurrence rates.[62]

The VA Cooperative Study encompassed the largest randomized controlled trial of inguinal hernia repair to date. A total of 1983 patients underwent either a laparoscopic (TAPP or TEP) or open (Lichtenstein tension-free) repair. One of the most significant findings was a significantly increased recurrence rate at 2 years in the laparoscopic group compared to the open group (10.1% vs. 4.9%). This was attributed to the steep learning curve associated with laparoscopic inguinal hernia repair. However, the study also discerned that pain was significantly lower in the laparoscopic group. Furthermore, there was a faster return to normal activities in those patients who underwent a laparoscopic inguinal hernia repair.

Laparoscopic repair is superior to open when treating a bilateral inguinal groin hernia. In patients presenting with an inguinal hernia recurrence following a previous open repair, the laparoscopic approach is also useful since it takes advantage of a virgin tissue plane. Other considerations which make the laparoscopic approach superior include less postoperative pain and a shorter return to work and normal activities.[56,63]

As many surgeons are becoming more familiar with the laparoscopic technique and overcoming the learning curve, further randomized trials may be needed to compare long-term outcomes. The laparoscopic repair of inguinal hernias remains controversial because the procedure has not definitively been shown to be cost-effective and the true long-term recurrence rate is unknown.

9. Abdominal Wall Hernias

Ventral hernias are hernias that arise in the anterior abdominal wall. There are several inherent weaknesses of the abdominal wall predisposed to the development of hernias. Epigastric hernias are confined to the upper abdomen along the linea alba above the umbilicus, where the aponeurotic decussations of the linea alba above the umbilicus can vary in strength and thickness (ie, it is vulnerable to herniation). An umbilical hernia arises at the umbilicus, the thinnest portion of the anterior abdominal wall. Lumbar hernias form in the superior and inferior triangles of the lumbar zone, where the anterior wall laterally joins the flank. The abdominal wall, as it extends caudally toward the groin and onto the extremities, forms the inguinofemoral zone where inguinal and femoral hernias can occur.

Once a diagnosis of an abdominal wall hernia is made and the patient is a suitable surgical candidate, an operation is indicated. With the introduction of laparoscopic techniques, the number of options for hernia repair has increased. The advantages and disadvantages of laparoscopic repair vs. open repair are still being defined.

Epigastric Hernia

Most epigastric hernias are considered to be acquired hernias of the linea alba. They occur in the midline above the umbilicus in 0.5%-10% of the population, are 2-3 times more common in men, and are most commonly seen in the third to fifth decade of life.[64] The linea alba is the line of decussation between the digastric rectus sheaths. Nearly all epigastric hernias occur in patients with a single midline decussation of the aponeurotic fibers, unlike patients with complete 3-layer decussation.

Ventral hernias have been classified by origin and are described as congenital, acquired, incisional or traumatic.[65,66] Hernias of the infraumbilical linea alba are rare unless they are of the incisional type. Congenital epigastric hernias regress spontaneously. Expectant therapy is acceptable management for patients up to 5-6 years of age.

Epigastric hernias are frequently multiple. At the time of surgery there may be more defects identified along the linea alba that were not apparent on physical examination. It is often necessary to extend the original incision in order to fully expose all hernia defects found during intraoperative examination of the abdominal wall. These herniations frequently contain only preperitoneal fat with no sac.[67] Since epigastric hernias often present with sharp pain in the region of the hernia, a diagnostic workup is indicated.[1]

Open repair of an epigastric hernia begins with an upper midline incision over the region of the suspected hernia. Once the hernia is identified, its contents are reduced and the rest of the abdominal wall is inspected. 1-2 cm of fascial edge are cleared for proper closure. Nonabsorbable interrupted stitches are then used for primary closure, or prosthetic mesh can be used for repair. Recurrence rates with the open technique have been reported to be between 7%-9.4%.[68]

Laparoscopy can also be a good approach for epigastric hernias. In cases of multiple occult defects, it allows complete examination and repair of the anterior abdominal wall, whereas in a regular open repair these defects are not exposed.[69] Laparoscopy is also a helpful diagnostic tool in patients with chronic epigastric pain and can aid in the diagnosis of occult epigastric hernias.

With the laparoscopic repair, pneumoperitoneum is located and ports are placed. The abdominal wall is carefully inspected to document the presence, location, and number of hernias. Any adhesions are taken down and the hernia is reduced. A single piece of prosthetic material that is at least 3-4 cm larger than the identified defect is circumferentially applied to the abdominal wall. The prosthetic is secured in place with suture and endoscopic tacks.[70,71]

Umbilical and Paraumbilical Hernias

Most umbilical hernias in children are true congenital hernias that present at birth. The majority spontaneously resolve by age 4. Umbilical hernias are up to 8 times more common in infants of African descent than white infants.[72,73] In adults, 90% of umbilical hernias are acquired and only 10% are considered to be congenital.[74] They occur more frequently in multiparous women, patients with ascites and in other conditions which chronically increase abdominal pressure.[75]

The umbilicus is the thinnest portion of the abdominal wall. Since 80% of paraumbilical hernias occur in patients that have single midline aponeurotic decussation, they are associated with an inherent weakness of the fascia. The remaining 20% are found in those with triple midline aponeurotic decussation.[66] At the umbilicus, there is further weakening of the fascia by the insertion of the round ligaments in the inferior aspect, the obliterated course of the urachus and umbilical arteries, and the tendinous inscriptions of the rectus abdominis muscle that insert just above the umbilicus.

In children less than 4 years old, umbilical hernias are observed for a time prior to surgical intervention since the majority close spontaneously.[76,77] Laparoscopic surgery to repair umbilical hernias should generally be avoided in children less than 14 years old. The "vest over pants" method of repair has been largely abandoned in favor of simple closure with nonabsorbable suture.[78] Small umbilical hernias (less than 3 cm) should be closed with open repair, not laparoscopically.[79] Prosthetic material can still be used to repair the smaller defects if needed. If mesh is used, it should be placed preperitoneally whenever possible to avoid contact with the bowel.

The technique for open repair is generally as follows. A curved infraumbilical incision is made with preservation of the umbilicus. The hernia sac is isolated and detached from the overlying umbilical skin. The sac contents are reduced and 1 cm of the fascial edge is cleared circumferentially. Interrupted nonabsorbable suture is generally used to approximate the fascial edges, either primarily or with intervening prosthetic material. Laparoscopic repair is performed in the same manner described for epigastric hernias. Recurrence of these hernias appears to be extremely uncommon when repaired properly by either method.[80]

Incisional Hernia

Incisional hernias, the most common ventral hernias, are iatrogenic defects occurring in 2%-11% of patients undergoing abdominal operations. They account for 90,000-100,000 operations in the United States annually. Open repair defects greater than 4 cm have a recurrence rate of 41%; defects less than 4 cm carry a significant recurrence rate of 25%.[81-83] 50% of incisional hernias occur within 1 year of the date of surgery, and another 35% are found within 5 years of the date of surgery. The incisional hernia rate has been reported to be greater than 40% after a wound infection.84 Once an incisional hernia has occurred it remains a significant problem even after attempted repair, because many of the factors that lead to its development persist at the time of the repair. Recurrence rates after open incisional hernia repairs have been reported to be as high as 30%-50%. Some authors report a recurrence rate of 44% for small hernias (less than 10 cm) vs. a recurrence rate of 6% when these same hernias were repaired with mesh.[85-87] Imaging may be helpful in the determination of recurrences easily detected by CT scan.[3]

Predisposing factors for the development of an incisional hernia include obesity, prolonged ileus or bowel obstruction, ascites, malnutrition, old age, poor surgical technique or anatomical knowledge, postoperative pulmonary complications, male gender, jaundice, pregnancy, cancer, straining, persistent coughing and, most importantly, wound infection. Chemotherapy, radiation and steroid use have also been implicated as contributing factors to incisional hernia development.[81,88-90]

Successful incisional hernia repair is dependent on approximation of healthy tissue under minimal tension and reduction of the previously described risk factors. The most important factor contributing to the recurrence of an incisional hernia is a wound infection. Meticulous surgical technique and use of prophylactic antibiotics are necessary measures in order to reduce the chance of developing a wound infection.[91]

Obesity is also a major factor in the development of incisional hernias. The bulk associated with the fatty omentum and excessive subcutaneous tissue increases the strain on the operative wound during the early healing phase. The loss of muscle mass and muscle tone associated with obesity may also provide inadequate support to overcome the added strain of the excess weight on wound healing.

The timing of the repair of an incisional hernia should be individualized. Medical conditions should be stabilized prior to surgery. Weight loss, cessation of smoking, rigid control of diabetes and avoidance of medications that impair wound healing can reduce recurrence and complication rates. The surgical options for the treatment of incisional hernias include primary repair or simple closure, repair with flaps or component separation, and prosthetic repair that is either open or laparoscopic. Specific details of these repairs can be obtained from any surgical textbook.

In the open technique of incisional hernia repair, an incision is made through the previous incision and dissection is carried down to the fascial borders around the hernia sac. The sac contents are safely reduced and excess sac is excised or inverted. The fascial defect is then cleared circumferentially 3-4 cm and closed in a single transverse layer with permanent interrupted suture placed evenly, ie, 1 cm from the edge and 1 cm apart. This type of repair is generally limited to small incisional hernias since the closure of large defects may place tension on the repair.

If it appears that the primary repair will be under tension (even with smaller hernias), prosthetic mesh should be utilized. Polypropylene, as opposed to PTFE mesh, should not be placed in direct contact with the bowel since studies have demonstrated an increased risk of obstruction and fistulization.[92] Advantages of polypropylene mesh are its strength, low cost and ease in handling laparoscopically. It may be used if omental coverage is available; if it is not, ePTFE may be the better choice. The ePTFE mesh promotes good tissue ingrowth with low adhesive potential and no reports of fistula or bowel obstruction; however, it is somewhat difficult to handle laparoscopically. Biological products based on bovine pericardium, cadaveric skin and small intestine submucosa are other options, but are generally reserved for clean contaminated cases.

The laparoscopic technique of ventral hernia repairs has supplanted the traditional open technique, mainly owing to a decreased recurrence rate, less pain and faster recovery. The laparoscopic technique is the same as the one described previously for epigastric hernia repairs. The approach avoids going through the previous incision; the entire abdominal wall can be visualized and the defect is clearly defined. If the hernia is larger than 15 cm in diameter, however, trocar placement may be difficult. Recurrence and infection rates are lower in laparoscopic repair than in traditional open techniques.[93-95] For example, Heniford reported a 3.4% recurrence rate with a mean of 23 months follow-up (range 1-60 months).[96-97] Other studies have estimated the recurrence rate following laparoscopic repair to be anywhere from 4%-13%.[69,102] Furthermore, the length of hospital stay was reduced from 5-7 days for open repairs to 1-2 days for laparoscopic repairs. Also, a faster return of bowel function was observed.[69,98-102]

The mesh infection rate after a laparoscopic incisional hernia repair has been reported to be from 0.5% to 12%. Presence of a wound infection after the mesh repair of an incisional hernia does not necessarily mandate mesh removal. Medical management should first be attempted if the infection is localized and amenable to good local wound care and antibiotics. The enterotomy rate has been reported to be 1.5% to 6%.[69] Operative time can be increased, especially if adhesiolysis is required. Special care should be taken when placing sutures and/or spiral tacks in the mesh, since recurrences have been noted to be less frequent when more sutures are placed. Recent retrospective studies have concluded that transfacial fixation sutures placed 4-5 cm apart, along the circumference of the mesh, limit the recurrence rate. The overall morbidity after a laparoscopic repair is approximately 23% compared to 31% for open repairs.[102]

Finally, recent data on a retrospective cohort of 716 patients at the Cleveland Clinic seemed to demonstrate a lower incidence of ventral hernia and small bowel obstruction when laparoscopy and not laparotomy was used for bowel resection.[103]

Obturator Hernia

An obturator hernia occurs through the obturator canal located in the anterior pelvis. It is the most common of the pelvic hernias, but only 550 cases are reported in the literature.[104] It is a rare type of hernia with a high associated mortality rate, mainly due to the patient population in which it occurs and the vague symptoms it produces until incarceration and strangulation occur. Obturator hernias are considered to be acquired hernias occurring secondary to progressive laxity of the pelvic floor associated with multiparity and increasing age.[105] It occurs with a female:male ratio of 9:1, multiparity and a wider pelvis. Larger triangular obturator rings have been implicated as possible reasons for higher incidence in females.

Symptoms of obturator hernias tend to be vague and intermittent. Pain and intestinal obstructive symptoms predominate later in the clinical course. Pain in the medial thigh with occasional radiation to the hip joint can occur secondary to obturator nerve compression within the canal by the hernia sac. This characteristic discomfort is known as the Howship-Romberg sign. The hernia tends to occur more frequently on the right side and is usually not visible. Occasionally it can be palpated in the upper medial thigh on careful physical examination. This is best appreciated with the thigh flexed, externally rotated and abducted. The hernia may also be palpated on a vaginal or rectal examination.[106-108] Repeated herniation can lead to scarring and eventual incarceration with possible strangulation of the hernia contents. Ileum is the most common herniating organ and often presents as a Richter's type hernia. Mortality rates as high as 30% have been reported.[105,108] Diagnosis is by history and physical examination. Plain radiography is rarely helpful. Computed tomography or ultrasound scans can confirm the diagnosis. Patients with vague obstructive symptoms who require operation often have their hernias diagnosed intraoperatively.

The treatment of obturator hernias is surgical. If the hernia is not incarcerated and the diagnosis of an obturator hernia has been made preoperatively, the hernia can be repaired laparoscopically in the preperitoneal space.[109] Many open surgical approaches have been proposed, but the transabdominal approach is used most frequently.[106,110] This approach provides good exposure and allows for easy reduction of bowel and bowel resection when required. After the obturator hernia is identified and exposed, gentle traction is usually adequate to reduce the hernia. If the obturator membrane needs to be incised to reduce sac contents, it should be done along the inferior or medial border of the foramen to avoid vessel and nerve injury. The obturator vessels lie lateral to the sac in about 59% of cases. The repair requires a patch of prosthetic mesh to be implanted in the preperitoneal space over and beyond the borders of the parietal defect in the obturator canal. Suture fixation is not always necessary if a soft, pliable polyester mesh is used. The contralateral side should also be examined since obturator hernias may be bilateral in 6% of cases or may be associated with femoral hernias.[62] Regardless of the method of closure, recurrence is rare.[112,113] If the hernia sac and defect are not closed, however, there is a 10% chance of recurrence.

Lumbar Hernia

A lumbar hernia is an interstitial type of hernia through the lumbar zone. 20% are congenital, one half are considered primary (spontaneous and acquired) and the remaining number are attributed to trauma. Congenital lumbar hernias can be associated with the lumbo-vertebral syndrome, a syndrome more common in middle-aged persons characterized by vague discomfort to severe, localized pain over a tender nodule in the lumbar region. Strangulation occurs in about 10% of cases.[114] Presence of a mass in the lumbar region is usually sufficient to make the diagnosis. The differential diagnosis of a mass in this region includes abscess, soft tissue tumor, renal tumor and hematoma. The natural history of a lumbar hernia is gradual progression to larger size. Early repair is recommended since the larger hernias are technically more difficult to repair. Given the difficulty of diagnosis by history and physical examination alone, ultrasound and computed tomography (CT) scans are often needed to make the diagnosis.

Lumbar hernias can occur anywhere between the twelfth rib and iliac crest in the posterior abdominal wall. The lumbar zone boundaries are defined superiorly by the twelfth rib, inferiorly by the iliac crest, posteriorly by the erector spinae (sacrospinalis) muscles and anteriorly by the posterior border of the external oblique muscle. The hernia defect occurs in the attenuated transversalis fascia (lumbar zone) that overlies this region. The most frequent sites of herniation are the superior and inferior lumbar triangles.[115]

The superior triangle (Grynfelt's) is below the twelfth rib where the subcostal neurovascular bundle enters anterior to the serratus inferior posterior muscle. The base of the superior triangle is the twelfth rib and serratus posterior inferior muscle. It is delineated anteriorly by the posterior border of the internal oblique muscle and posteriorly by the anterior border of the sacrospinalis muscle. The floor of the superior triangle is defined by the aponeurosis of the transversus abdominis muscle; the roof is defined by the external oblique and latissimus dorsi muscles.[116]

The inferior triangle (Petit's) is defined laterally by the latissimus dorsi tendon immediately above the iliac crest with the iliac crest as its base. The anterior border is defined by the posterior edge of the external oblique and the posterior border by the anterior edge of the latissimus dorsi muscle. The floor and roof of the inferior triangle are the internal oblique muscle and the superficial fascia and skin, respectively.[117]

Grynfelt's triangle has an inverted apex and the apex of Petit's triangle is upright. The superior triangle is larger and is covered by the latissimus dorsi muscle. In contrast, the inferior triangle is covered only by superficial fascia and skin. The floor of the superior triangle is weaker because it consists only of the aponeurosis of the transversus abdominis arising from fibers of the thoracolumbar fascia. Thus, lumbar hernias are more common in Grynfelt's triangle. Petit's triangle, on the other hand, is a union of 3 layers: the thick thoracolumbar fascia, the internal oblique muscle and the transversus abdominis muscle.

Lumbar hernias are difficult to repair successfully without the use of prosthetic mesh or a myoaponeurotic flap. Rotational flaps of fascia lata, gluteal fascia or latissimus dorsi muscle have fallen out of favor. Tissue repairs in general have had recurrence rates reported as high as 20%.[118] The success of a lumbar hernia repair is improved by utilizing the Rives-Stoppa technique, ie, using a large piece of mesh and extending it well beyond the hernia edges. The prosthesis should be implanted well into the retroperitoneal space. The iliac fossa should be implanted laterally and inferiorly. Anteriorly, it is placed behind the rectus muscle and superiorly it is fixed to the rib cage (intraperitoneally). Larger hernia repairs often require closed suction drainage postoperatively because extensive dissection is involved in the mesh placement.[98]

The patient is positioned in the lateral decubitus position over a kidney rest to afford better exposure for the surgical repair of a lumbar hernia. An oblique or vertical incision is made over the mass. Care should be taken in making an incision over an inferior triangle hernia since there is no muscle layer, only superficial fascia between the skin and the hernia. The prosthesis is then laid out after reduction and ligation of the sac. The latissimus dorsi muscle should then be approximated to the external oblique muscle as much as possible without tension. Primary closure of lumbar hernias is usually difficult because of the rigidity of the tissues involved. Occasionally, holes may need to be drilled through the bone to permit fixation if insufficient soft tissue is available for suture fixation next to the bone.[119]

Spigelian Hernia

Spigelian hernias usually occur in the fourth to seventh decades of life. They are more common in obese women who have had significant weight loss. In men they are associated with groin hernias.

Spigelian hernias occur inferior to the umbilicus, but above the epigastric vessels lateral to the termination of the posterior rectus sheath (linea semicircularis) where the Spigelian fascia is the weakest.[120] Hence, most Spigelian hernias occur within an approximated 5 cm "belt" situated just below the umbilicus and above an imaginary line connecting the anterior superior iliac spines.[121] The parallel arrangement of the fibers is weaker than crisscrossing fibers and results in potential slit defects.[121,122] Almost uniformly, Spigelian hernias have an interparietal hernia sac dissecting beneath the external oblique muscle and aponeurosis that make palpation difficult. Most Spigelian hernias are small (less than 2 cm in diameter) and herniate laterally and inferiorly because they are constrained medially by the external oblique insertion. The neck of these hernias tends to be narrow and rigid with a tendency to originate a partial or complete intestinal obstruction.[119]

Herniation usually begins with preperitoneal fat passing through defects in the transversus abdominis and internal oblique aponeurosis (Spigelian zone) dissecting beneath the external oblique muscle, which remains intact beneath the skin. The medial border of the Spigelian zone is the lateral margin of the anterior lamina of the rectus sheath, and the lateral border consists of the muscular fibers of the internal oblique muscle. The semilunar line (of Spiegel) marks the lateral border of the rectus sheath and extends from the pubic tubercle to the tip of the costal cartilage of the ninth rib. The semicircular line (arcuate line, line of Douglas) marks the caudal end of the posterior rectus sheath below the umbilicus and above the pubis. It is composed of the approximation and fusion of the internal oblique and transversus abdominis aponeuroses. The external oblique aponeurosis remains intact over the hernia.[123]

Spigelian hernias usually present with localized tenderness and are exacerbated by muscular tension of the abdominal wall. Because Spigelian hernias are difficult to diagnose on physical examination, the diagnosis is often established with imaging studies such as ultrasound scans, cross-table lateral plain films with gastrointestinal contrast studies, and computed tomography.[119,124]

Surgical repair of Spigelian hernias is usually made by a transverse or vertical incision through the aponeurosis of the external oblique muscle over the palpable mass or suspected region of the hernia. If the hernia is incarcerated, the ring should be incised medially toward the rectus abdominis muscle, which retracts the external oblique and reveals the internal oblique and the hernia sac. For reduction of the hernia contents, the rectus sheath can be incised and the rectus muscle retracted medially if necessary. The defects in the transversus abdominis and the internal oblique muscles are then closed with nonabsorbable interrupted suture as is the aponeurosis of the external oblique muscle.[76] Primary closure of Spigelian hernias is often possible since these defects are small and the use of prosthetic mesh is rarely required. Laparoscopic repair of these hernias has been described but should only be employed by experienced and advanced laparoscopic surgeons.[119,125]

Spigelian-like hernias in which the visceral contents lie between the abdominal wall muscle layers may occur at laparoscopic trocar sites, particularly at larger trocar sites not closed during the original operation. Depending on where on the abdominal wall they are located, the repairs described above should be adequate.

10. References

1. Truong SN. Value of ultrasound in the diagnosis of undetermined findings in the abdominal wall and the inguinal region. In: Shumpelick V. Inguinal hernia repair. *Expert meeting on hernia surgery*. St. Moritz, Basel: Karger; 1995:29-43.

2. Erez I. Preoperative ultrasound and intraoperative findings of inguinal hernias in children: A prospective study of 642 children. *J Pediatr Surg*. 2002;37(6):865-8.

3. Lin BHJ. CT findings after laparoscopic repair of ventral hernia. *Am J Roenterol*. 1999;172 389-392.

4. Van der Berg JC. Detection of groin hernia with physical examination, ultrasound and MRI compared with laparoscopic findings. *Invest Radiol*. 1999;34 (12):739-743.

5. Son Ngoc. Diagnostic imaging in the evaluation and management of abdominal wall hernia. In: Fitzgibbons RJ Jr. and Greenburgh AG. *Nyhus and Condon's Hernia*. 5th ed. Philadelphia, PA: Lippincott Williams & Wilkins; 2002:81-94.

6. Bittner R. Ultrasound examination in laparoscopic/endoscopy hernia surgery. In: Fitzgibbons RJ Jr. and Greenburgh AG. *Nyhus and Condon's Hernia,* 5th ed. Philadelphia, PA: Lippincott Williams & Wilkins; 2002:95-102.

7. Zollinger RM Jr,. Unified classification for inguinal hernias. *Hernia*. 1993;195.

8. Rescorla F. Inguinal hernia repair in the perinatal period and early infancy: Clinical considerations. *J Pediatr Surg*. 1984;19(6): 832-7.

9. Rowe MI, et al. The other side of pediatric inguinal hernia. *Surg Clin N Am*. 1971;(51):1371.

10. Abramson JH. The epidemiology of Inguinal Hernia. A survey in Western Jerusalem. *J Epidemiol Comm Hlth*. 1978;32:59-67.

11. Weitz JL. Increased neutrophil elastase activity in cigarette smoking. *Ann Intern Med*. 1987;107:608-612.

12. Read RC. Cigarette smoking and recurrence. *Surgery*. 1998;124;942.

13. Abrahamson J. Hernias. In: Zinner MJ, et al. *Maingot's Abdominal Operations*. Stamford, CT: Appleton & Lange; 1997.

14. Pans A. Adult groin hernias: a new insight into their biochemical characteristics. *Eur J Clin Invest*. 1997; 27:1-6.

15. Sorensen LT. Biochemical aspects of abdominal wall, hernia formation and recurrence. In: Fitzgibbons RJ Jr. and Greenburgh AG, eds. *Nyhus and Condon's Hernia*. 5th ed. Philadelphia, PA: Lippincott Williams & Wilkins; 2002:9-16.

16. Bellon JM. Fibroblasts from the transversalis fascia of young patients with direct inguinal hernias show constitutive MMP-2 overexpression. *Ann Surg*. 2001;233:287-291.

17. Read RC. Why do human beings develop hernias? In: Fitzgibbons RJ Jr. Greenburgh AG. *Nyhus and Condon's Hernia*. 5th ed. Philadelphia, Pa: Lippincott Williams & Wilkins; 2002:3-7.

18. Rodrigues AJ. Electron microscopic study on the elastic related fibers in the human fascia transversalis at different ages. *Gengenbaurs Morphol Jahrb*. 1990;136-645.

19. Read RC. Recent advances in the repair of groin herniation. *Curr Probl in Surg*. 2003;40(1)13-79.

20. Schumpelik, et al. Inguinal hernia repair in adults. *Lancet*. 1994;(8919):

21. McIntosh A, et al. Evidenced-based management of groin hernia in primary care—a systematic review. *Fam Pract*. 2000;17:442.

22. The biological basis of modern surgical practice. In: Townsend CM, et al. *Textbook of Surgery: The Physiologic Basis of Modern Surgical Practice*. 16th ed. Philadelphia, C: WB Saunders; 2000;1215-1233.

23. Rutledge RH, et al. The Cooper ligament repair of groin hernias. In: Fitzgibbon RJ, Greenberg AG, eds. *Nyhus and Condon's Hernia*. 5th ed. Philadelphia, Pa: Lippincott Williams & Wilkins; 2002:139-148.

24. Khoury N, et al. A comparative study of laparoscopic extraperitoneal and transabdominal preperitoneal herniorrhaphy. *J Laparoendosc Surg*. 1995;5:349-355.

25. Bendavid R, et al. The Shouldice repair. In: Fitzgibbon RJ, Greenberg AG, eds. *Nyhus and Condon's Hernia*. 5th ed. Philadelphia, PA: Lippincott Williams & Wilkins; 2002.

26. Toy KF, et al. Smoot laparoscopic hernioplasty. *Del Med J*. 1992;1:4-11.

27. Robbins AW, et al. Mesh and plug repair and groin hernia surgery. *Surg Clin N Am*. 1998;78:1007-1023.

28. Mc Gillicuddy JE, et al. Prospective randomized comparison of the Shouldice repair and Lichtenstein repair procedures. *Arch Surg*. 1998;133:974-978.

29. Scott NW, et al. Open mesh versus non-mesh repair of inguinal hernia. *Cochrane Database Syst Rev*. 2001;(4):CD002197.

30. Bay Nielsen, et al. Quality assessment of 26304 herniorrhaphies in Denmark: A prospective nationwide study. *Lancet*. 2001;358:1124.

31. Ger R, et al. The management of certain abdominal herniae by intraabdominal closure of the neck of the sac. *Ann R Coll Surg Eng*. 1982;64:342-344.

32. Schultz JD, et al. Laparoscopic herniorrhaphy: a clinical trial, preliminary results. *J Laparoendoscopic Surg*. 1990;1:41-45.

33. Phillips EH, et al. Laparoscopic preperitoneal inguinal repair without peritoneal incision. *Surg Endosc*. 1993;7:159-163.

34. Mc Kernan JB, et al. Laparoscopic repair of inguinal hernias using totally extraperitoneal prosthetic approach. *Surg Endosc*. 1993;7:26-28.

35. Mac Fayden BV, et al. Complications of Laparoscopic herniorrhaphy. *Surg Endosc*. 1993;7:155-158.

36. Paganini AM, et al. A randomized, controlled, clinical study of laparoscopic vs. open tension free inguinal hernia repair. *Surg Endosc*. 1998;12:979-986.

37. Tetik C, et al. Complications and recurrences associated with laparoscopic repair of groin hernias. A multi-institutional retrospective analysis. *Surg Endosc*. 1994;8:1316-1323.

38. Phillips EH, et al. Incidence of complications following laparoscopic hernioplasty. *Surg Endosc*. 1995;9:16-21.

39. Fitzgibbons RJ Jr, et al. Laparoscopic inguinal herniorrhaphy. Results of a multicenter trial [comments]. *Ann Surg*. 1995;221:3-13.

40. Fry D.Wound infection in hernia repair. In: Fitzgibbon RJ, Greenberg AG, eds. *Nyhus and Condon's Hernia*. 5th ed. Philadelphia, Pa: Lippincott Williams & Wilkins; 2002:279-290.

41. Platt R, et al. Perioperative antibiotic prophylaxis for herniorrhaphy and breast surgery. *N Engl J Med*. 1990;322:153-160.

41a. Schmedt CG, Sauerland S, Bittner R. Comparison of endoscopic procedures vs. Lichtenstein and other open mesh techniques for inguinal hernia repair. *Surg Endosc*. 2005;19:188-199.

42. Arregui ME, et al. Laparoscopic mesh repair of inguinal hernia using a preperitoneal approach: a preliminary report. *Surg Laparosc Endosc*. 1992;2:53-58.

43. Kald A, et al. Transperitoneal or totally extraperitoneal approach in laparoscopic hernia repair: results of 491 consecutive herniorrhaphies. *Surg Laparosc Endosc*. 1997;7: 86-89.

44. Felix EL, et al. Laparoscopic hernioplasty. TAPP vs. TEP. *Surg Endosc*. 1995;9:984-989.

45. McKernan JB, et al. Laparoscopic repair of inguinal hernias using a totally extraperitoneal prosthetic approach. *Surg Endosc J*. 1993;7: 26-28.

46. Franklin ME. The intraperitoneal onlay mesh procedure for groin hernias. In: Fitzgibbon RJ, Greenberg AG, eds. *Nyhus and Condon's Hernia*. 5th ed. Philadelphia, Pa: Lippincott Williams & Wilkins; 2002:269-276.

47. Felix EL, et al. Laparoscopic hernioplasty: significant complications [comments]. *Surg Endosc*. 1999;13:328-331.

48. Fry D. Wound infection in hernia repair. In: Fitzgibbon RJ, Greenberg AG, eds. *Nyhus and Condon's Hernia*. 5th ed. Philadelphia, PA: Lippincott Williams & Wilkins; 2002.

49. Platt R, et al. Perioperative antibiotic prophylaxis for herniorrhaphy and breast surgery. *N Engl J Med*. 1990;322:153-160.

50. Crawford DL, et al. Laparoscopic repair and groin hernia surgery. *Surg Clin N Am*. 1998;78:1047-1062.

51. Cunningham J. The physiology and anatomy of chronic pain after inguinal herniorrhaphy. In: Fitzgibbon RJ, Greenberg AG, eds. *Nyhus and Condon's Hernia*. 5th ed. Philadelphia, PA: Lippincott Williams & Wilkins; 2002:297-306.

52. Geis, et al. An algorithm for the treatment of chronic groin pain after inguinal herniorrhaphy. In: Fitzgibbon RJ, Greenberg AG, eds. *Nyhus and Condon's Hernia*. 5th ed. Philadelphia, PA: Lippincott Williams & Wilkins; 2002;307-316.

53. Richards A. Cord and testicular complications of groin herniorrhaphy. In: Fitzgibbon RJ, Greenberg AG, eds. *Nyhus and Condon's Hernia*. 5th ed. Philadelphia, PA: Lippincott Williams & Wilkins; 2002;291-296.

54. Collaboration EH. Laparoscopic compared with open methods of groin hernia repair: systematic review of randomized controlled trials. *Br J Surg*. 2000;87:860-867.

55. O'Boyle CJ, et al. Cost-utility analysis of open versus laparoscopic groin hernia repair: results from a multicenter randomized clinical trial. *Br J Surg*. 2001;(11):1543-1545.

56. Payne JH Jr, et al. Laparoscopic or open inguinal herniorrhaphy? A randomized prospective trial [comments]. *Arch Surg*. 1994;129:973-981.

57. Kozol R, et al. A prospective, randomized study of open vs. laparoscopic inguinal hernia repair. An assessment of postoperative pain. *Arch Surg*. 1997;132:292-295.

58. Liem MS, et al. A randomized comparison of physical performance following laparoscopic and open inguinal hernia repair. The Coala Trial Group. *Br J Surg*. 1997;84:64-67.

59. Liem MS, et al. Comparison of conventional anterior surgery and laparoscopic surgery for inguinal-hernia repair [comments]. *N Engl J Med*. 1997;336:1541-1547.

60. Heikkinen TJ, et al. A prospective randomized outcome and cost comparison of totally extraperitoneal endoscopic hernioplasty versus Lichtenstein hernia operation among employed patients. *Surg Laparosc Endosc*. 1998;8: 338-344.

61. Johansson B, et al. Laparoscopic mesh versus open preperitoneal mesh versus conventional technique for inguinal hernia repair: a randomized multicenter trial (SCUR Hernia Repair Study). *Ann Surg*. 1999;230:225-231.

62. Lau H et al. Systematic review and meta-analysis of clinical trials comparing endoscopic totally extraperitoneal inguinal hernioplasty with open repair of inguinal hernia. *Ann Coll Surg Hong Kong*. 2003;(1):2-10.

63. Kald et al. Laproscopic hernia repair in patients with bilateral groin hernia. *Eur J Surg*. 2000;166:210-212.

64. Iason AH. *Hernia*. Philadelphia, PA: Blakistan; 1941.

65. Askar OM. Surgical anatomy of the aponeurotic expansions of the anterior abdominal wall. *Ann R Coll Surg Engl*. 1977;59:313.

66. Askar OM. Aponeurotic hernias. *Surg Clin North Am*. 1984;64:315-333.

67. Bennett D. Umbilical, Epigastric and Spigelian hernia. In: Nyhus L, London RE, eds. *Hernia*. Philadelphia, PA: JB Lippincott; 2002:389-415.

68. McCaughan JJ. Epigastric hernia. Results obtained by surgery. *Arch Surg*. 1956;73:972.

69. Koehler RH, et al. Recurrences in laparoscopic incisional hernia repairs: a personal series and review of the literature. *J Soc Laparoend Surg*. 1999;3:293-304.

70. Piskun G, et al. Simplified technique of mesh fixation during laparoscopic repair of abdominal ventral hernia. *J Laparoendosc Adv Surg Tech*. 1999;9:193-196.

71. Barie PS, et al. A technique for laparoscopic repair of herniation of the anterior abdominal wall using a composite mesh prosthesis. *Am J Surg*. 1995;170:62-63.

72. Evans AG. The comparative incidence of umbilical hernias in colored and white infants. *J Natl Med Assoc*. 1941:3:158.

73. Crump E. Umbilical hernia: Occurrence of the infantile type in Negro infants and children. *J Pediatr*. 1952;40:214.

74. Jackson O, et al. Umbilical hernia: a retrospective study. *Calif Med*. 1970;113:8.

75. Morgan W, et al. Prophylactic umbilical hernia repair in childhood to prevent adult incarceration. *Surg Clin North Am*. 1970;50:839.

76. Woods G. Some observations on umbilical hernia in infants. *Arch Dis Child*. 1953;28:450.

77. Sibley WI, et al. A 25-year study of infantile umbilical hernia. *Surgery*. 1964;55:462.

78. Farris J, et al. Umbilical hernia: An inquiry into the principle of imbrication and a note on the preservation of the umbilical dimple. *Am J Surg*. 1959;98:256.

79. Larson G. Laparoscopic repair of ventral hernia. In: Scott-Conner C, ed. *The SAGES Manual*. New York, NY: Springer-Verlag; 1999:379-385.

80. Pollak R. Epigastric, umbilical, and ventral hernias. In: Cameron J, ed. *Current Surgical Therapy*. Philadelphia, PA: BC Decker; 1984:284.

81. Hesselink VJ, et al. An evaluation of risk factors in incisional hernia recurrence. *Surg Gynecol Obst*. 1993;176:228-234.

82. Santora TA, et al. Incisional hernia. *Surg Clin North Am*. 1993;73:557-570.

83. Larson GM, et al. Approaches to repair of ventral hernia and full-thickness losses of the abdominal wall. *Surg Clin North Am*. 1984;64:335-349.

84. Mudge M, et al. Incisional hernia: A 10-year prospective study of incidence and attitudes. *Br J Surg*. 1985;72:70-71.

85. Vander Linden FT, et al. Long-term results after correction of incisional hernia. *Neth J Surg*. 1988;40:127-129.

86. Langer S, et al. Long-term results after incisional hernia repair. *Acta Chir Scand*. 1985;151:217-219.

87. Luijendijk RW, et al A comparison of suture repair with mesh repair for incisional hernia. *N Engl J Med*. 2000;343:392-398.

88. Cleveland RD, Zitschin RP, Laws HC. Incisional closure in morbidly obese patients. *Am Surg*. 1989;55:61-63.

89. Blomstedt B, Welin-Berger T. A comparison between midline, oblique, and transrectal incisions. *Acta Chir Scand*. 1972;138:275-278.

90. Guillou PJ, et al. Vertical abdominal incisions-A choice? *Br J Surg*. 1980;67:395-399.

91. Bucknall TE, Cox PJ, Ellis H. Burst abdomen and incisional hernia: prospective study of 1129 major laparotomies. *Br Med J*. 1982;284:931-933.

92. Leber GE, et al. Long-term complications associated with prosthetic repair of incisional hernia. *Arch Surg*. 1998;133:378-382.

93. Heniford T, et al. Laparoscopic ventral and incisional hernia repair in 407 patients. *J Am Coll Surg*. 2000;190(6):645-650.

94. Robbins SB, et al. Laparoscopic Ventral hernia repair reduces wound complications. *Am Surg*. 2000;67(9): 896-900.

95. LeBlanc KA, et al. Laparoscopic incisional and ventral herniorrhaphy in 100 patients. *Am J Surg*. 2000;180(3):193-197.

96. LeBlanc KA, et al. Current Considerations in Laparoscopic Incisional and Ventral Herniorrhaphy. *J Soc Laparoendosc Surg*. 2000;4: 131-139.

97. Costanza MJ , et al. Laparoscopic repair of recurrent ventral hernias. *Am Surg*. 1998;64(12):1121.

98. Stoppa RE. The treatment of complicated groin and incisional hernias. *World J Surg*.1989;13: 545-554.

99. Wantz G. Incisional hernioplasty with Mersilene. *Surg Gynecol Obstet*. 1991;172(2): 129-137.

100. Ramshaw BJ. Comparison of laparoscopic and open ventral herniorrhaphy. *Am Surg*. 1999;65(9):827-831.

101. Carbajo MA, et al. Laparoscopic treatment versus open surgery in the solution of major incisional and abdominal wall hernias with mesh. *Surg Endosc*. 1999;13:250-252.

102. Park A, et al. Laparoscopic and open incisional hernia repair: a comparison study. *Surgery*. 1998;24:816-822.

103. Duepree H, et al. Does means of access affect the incidence of small bowel obstruction and ventral hernia after bowel resection? Laparoscopy versus laparotomy. *Journal of Am Coll Surg*. 2003; 97:177-181.

104. Cali RL, et al. Rare pelvic floor hernias: report of a case and review of the literature. *Dis Colon Rectum*. 1992;35:604-612.

105. Bjork KJ, ct al. Obturator hernia. *Surg Gynecol Obst*. 1988;167:217-222.

106. Wakely C, Wakely J. Rare types of external abdominal hernias. In: Schwartz SI, Ellis H, Husser WC, eds. *Maingot's Abdominal Operations*. Norwalk, Conn: Appleton & Lange; 1989:1650-1660.

107. Carter J. Sciatic, obturator, and perineal hernias: a view from the gynecologist. In: Nyhus LM, Condon RE, eds. *Hernia*. Philadelphia, PA: JB Lippincott; 2002:539-549.

108. Arbman G. Strangulated obturator hernia: a simple method for closure. *Acta Chir Scand*. 1984;115:408-410.

109. Srivastava KP, Racela IG, Pohl JJ. Strangulated hernia of the obturator canal as a cause of acute abdomen: report of two cases. *Int Surg*. 1972;566-570.

110. Temple DF, Miller RE. Incarcerated obturator hernia: two case reports and review of the literature. *JAMA*. 1980;72:513-515.

111. Rogers FA. Strangulated obturator hernia. *Surgery*.1960;48:394-403.

112. Schackelford RT. *Surgery of the Alimentary Tract*. Philadelphia, PA: WB Saunders; 1955.

113. Watson LF. *Hernia*. 3rd ed. St Louis, MO: Mosby;1948.

114. Swartz W. Lumbar hernia. In: Nyhus L, Condon RE, eds. *Hernia*. Philadelphia, PA: JB Lippincott; 1978;409-425.

115. Richter MH, Nyhus ML, et al. Lumbar and Obturator Herniation. In: Cameron JL, ed. *Current Surgical Therapy*. 7th ed. St. Louis, MO: Mosby; 2001:616-620.

116. Grynfelt J. Quelques mots sur la nerie lombaire. *Montpellier Med*. 1866;16:323.

117. Petit JL. Traite des maladies chirurgicals, et des operations qui leur conviennent. *TF Didot*. 1774;2:256-258.

118. Champion J, McKeernan JB. Epigastric, umbilical, and ventral hernias. In: Cameron J, ed. *Current Surgical Therapy*. Philadelphia, PA: BC Decker;1998; 568-575.

119. Scott-Conner CEH. Hernia repairs, operations for necrotizing fasciitis and drainage of subphrenic abcess. In: Scott-Conner CEH, ed. *Chassin's Operative Strategy in General Surgery*. 3rd ed. New York, NY: Springer; 2002;747-815.

120. Spangen L. Spigelian hernia. *Acta Chir Scand Suppl*. 1976;462:1-47.

121. Zimmerman L, Anson BJ, Morgan EH, McVay CB. Ventral hernia due to normal banding of the abdominal muscles. *Surg Gynecol Obstet*. 1944;78:535.

122. Zucker K, et al. *Surgical Laparoscopy*. Philadelphia, PA: Lippincott Williams & Wilkins; 2001.

123. Skandalakis JE. *Surgical Anatomy and Technique*. London, England: Springer-Verlag; 1995.

124. Spangen L. Spigelian hernias. *World J Surg*. 1989;13:573-580.

125. Kasirajan K, Lopez J, Lopez R. Laparoscopic technique in the management of Spigelian hernias. *J Laparoendosc Adv Surg Tech*. 1997;7:385-388.

11. Questions

1. In descending order of frequency, which is the correct order:

A. Spigelian, indirect, direct, femoral

B. Indirect, direct, incisional, lumbar

C. Direct, indirect, incisional, femoral

D. Lumbar, ventral, direct, Spigelian

2. Correlate both columns:

A. Littre's hernia	1. Femoral canal
B. Cloquet's hernia	2. Pectineus muscle
C. Serafini's hernia	3. Meckel's diverticulum
D. Cooper's hernia	4. Underneath femoral vessels

3. Hernia repairs that involve placement of prosthetic mesh are:

A. Bassini repair

B. Shouldice repair

C. Lichtenstein repair

D. Totally extraperitoneal (TEP)

4. Disadvantages of the transabdominal preperitoneal (TAPP) hernia repair compared to the totally extraperitoneal (TEP) hernia repair include:

A. Decreased visualization of anatomic structures

B. Entrance into the peritoneal cavity is required

C. Closure of the peritoneum over the mesh repair is required

D. TAPP cannot be done in patients with a previous prostatectomy

5. Complications of hernia repairs include all of the following except:

A. Nerve injury

B. Vascular injury

C. Intestinal injury

D. Testicular injury

E. Bladder injury

F. All are potential complications

6. Advantages of laparoscopic hernia repairs over open hernia repairs reportedly include:

A. Decreased cost

B. Need for general anesthesia

C. Quicker return to work

D. Decreased wound complications

7. Abdominal wall hernias that can reasonably be approached laparoscopically are:

A. Epigastric hernias

B. Umbilical hernias

C. Ventral incisional hernias

D. Lumbar hernias

E. All of the above

F. Only A. and B.

8. A hernia that occurs inferior to the umbilicus, but above the epigastric vessels lateral to the termination of the posterior rectus sheath with preperitoneal fat passing through a defect in the transversus abdominis and internal oblique aponeurosis and dissecting beneath the external oblique muscle is a:

A. Obturator hernia

B. Femoral hernia

C. Lumbar hernia

D. Spigelian hernia

9. Risk factors for the recurrence of an incisional hernia after surgical repair include:

A. Obesity

B. Malnutrition

C. Steroid use

D. Infection

10. A 48-year-old, healthy, white male who had a right inguinal hernia repair 10 years ago presents with a recurrent right inguinal hernia and a questionable left inguinal hernia. Which surgical approach is most appropriate for this patient?

A. Transabdominal preperitoneal (TAPP) repair

B. Totally extraperitoneal (TEP) repair

C. Open hernia repair

D. Intraperitoneal onlay mesh (IPOM)

11. A 64-year-old Hispanic male with hypertension and coronary artery disease and a history of prior radical prostatectomy presents with a right inguinal hernia. Which surgical approach is appropriate for repair of this patient's hernia?

A. Transabdominal preperitoneal (TAPP) repair

B. Totally extraperitoneal (TEP) repair

C. Open hernia repair

D. A. and C.

E. B. and C.

Answers

1. B.

75% of all hernias are inguinal hernias (50% indirect, 25% direct). 3% of all hernias are femoral hernias, 10% are ventral or incisional hernias, and the remainder are rare hernias such as lumbar, Spigelian and obturator hernias.

2.

A. – 3

Littre's hernia is one in which a Meckel's diverticulum is the only organ involved with the hernia sac.

B. – 2

Cloquet's hernia is a femoral hernia that penetrates the pectineus muscle fascia.

C. – 4

Serafini's hernia is a femoral hernia that travels underneath the femoral vessels.

D. – 1

Cooper's hernia is a hernia involving the femoral canal that tracts into the scrotum or labia majora.

3. C., D.

Both the Lichtenstein and TEP repair require a sheet of prosthetic mesh. Both the Bassini and Shouldice repairs involve approximation of native tissue and do not incorporate mesh.

4. B., C.

The transabdominal preperitoneal (TAPP) repair is indicated when the preperitoneal space has been obliterated by prior surgery such as prostatectomy. The TAPP repair is easier in that there is more room to operate. However, it is more difficult in that the peritoneum must be closed at the completion of the procedure. This also adds the risk of exposing the mesh to the bowel and of recurrence of hernias if the closure fails or is incomplete. Another disadvantage to the TAPP approach is that the peritoneal cavity is violated and a pneumoperitoneum is required.

5. F.

The potential complications of the laparoscopic inguinal herniorrhaphy include the risks of general anesthesia and laparoscopy in addition to the risks of hernia repair. However, anesthetic complications and complications from pneumoperitoneum are rare. Other potential complications include major vascular injury, injury to hollow viscera, urinary tract complications, nerve injury, mesh complications, vas deferens and testicular complications, and recurrence.

6. C., D.

Proponents of laparoscopic herniorrhaphy cite the advantages of better visualization and magnification of anatomy, better cosmesis, less postoperative pain, quicker return to work and fewer wound complications. Critics of laparoscopic herniorrhaphy argue its disadvantages are the need for general anesthesia, higher operative costs, violation of the peritoneal cavity in the TAPP repair and lack of long-term recurrence data.

7. A., B., C.

Epigastric, umbilical and ventral incisional hernias are all reasonably approached laparoscopically, unless they are so large as to prevent adequate trocar placement. Lumbar hernias are not approached laparoscopically because their location is not amenable to the laparoscopic approach.

8. D.

Spigelian hernias occur inferior to the umbilicus but above the epigastric vessels lateral to the termination of the posterior rectus sheath (linea semicircularis) where the Spigelian fascia is the weakest. The surface landmark is usually two thirds of the way up on a line from the anterior superior iliac spine to the umbilicus where the transversus and internal oblique muscle aponeuroses do not intersect, as above the umbilicus, but instead become almost parallel. The parallel arrangement of the fibers is weaker than crisscrossing fibers and results in potential slit defects. Herniation usually begins with preperitoneal fat passing through defects in the transversus abdominis and internal oblique aponeurosis (Spigelian zone), and dissecting beneath the external oblique muscle, which remains intact beneath the skin. The medial border of the Spigelian zone is the lateral margin of the anterior lamina of the rectus sheath and the lateral border consists of the muscular fibers of the internal oblique muscle. The semilunar line (of Spiegel) marks the lateral border of the rectus sheath and extends from the pubic tubercle to the tip of the costal cartilage of the ninth rib. The semicircular line (arcuate line, line of Douglas) marks the caudal end of the posterior rectus sheath, below the umbilicus and above the pubis. It is composed of the approximation and fusion of the internal oblique and transversus abdominis aponeuroses. The external oblique aponeurosis remains intact over the hernia.

9. A., B., C., D.

Predisposing factors for the development and recurrence of an incisional hernia include obesity, prolonged ileus or bowel obstruction, ascites, malnutrition, old age, poor surgical technique or anatomical knowledge, postoperative pulmonary complications, male gender, jaundice, pregnancy, straining, persistent coughing and, most importantly, wound infection. Chemotherapy and steroid use have also been implicated as contributing factors to incisional hernia development. Successful incisional hernia repair is dependent on approximation of healthy tissue under minimal tension and reduction of the previously described risk factors. The most important factor contributing to the recurrence of an incisional hernia is a wound infection. Meticulous surgical technique and the use of antibiotics are necessary to reduce the chance of a wound infection developing. Obesity is also a major factor in the development and recurrence of incisional hernias. The bulk associated with the fatty omentum and excessive subcutaneous tissue increases the strain on the operative wound during the early healing phase. The loss of muscle mass and muscle tone associated with obesity may also provide inadequate support to overcome the added strain of the excess weight on wound healing.

10. B.

The TEP repair is the most appropriate repair. In this approach, the right inguinal hernia may be repaired through fresh tissue planes avoiding the scar tissue and mesh from the first repair. Also, the left inguinal region may be examined for the presence of bilateral hernias, and, if needed, repaired with no added incisions and minimal additional operative time.

11. C.

Any approach through the preperitoneal space of Retzius may be difficult, if not impossible, after a prostatectomy. Both the TEP and TAPP repairs are carried out in this space; only the approach to the space is different. The open technique under local anesthesia is probably most appropriate for this patient if he is at high risk for general anesthesia. The TEP and TAPP repairs are not appropriate because the preperitoneal space has been violated by the prior prostatectomy.

Chapter 8: Benign and Malignant Breast Disease

John A. Butler, MD

Contents

1. Breast Diseases

Anatomy and Physiology

Embryologically, the human breast develops from the ectodermal primitive milk streak which courses from the axilla to the pubis in early fetal life. Late in the first trimester, all but the thoracic portion regresses. This subsequently develops into an epithelial bud with 15-25 mammary ducts. Parenchymal differentiation occurs in the third trimester with the development of lobular-alveolar structures that contain colostrum. In the neonate, the stimulated mammary tissue secretes colostral milk, but this activity tapers and ends over a 3-4 week period postpartum, due to involution of the breast after withdrawal of placental hormones. Failure of milk streak regression leads to the most common congenital breast anomaly, accessory breast tissue, which is most frequently manifested as an accessory nipple, a condition called polythelia.

At puberty, the female breast undergoes a series of changes initiated by ovarian estrogen synthesis during early menarche. The early anovulatory cycles are then replaced by ovulatory cycles which, governed by progesterone secretion of the corpus luteum, allow the later phases of breast maturation to occur. Estrogen and progesterone together act to produce the ductal-lobular-alveolar development of mammary tissues.

Adult breasts extend from the second to the sixth ribs vertically and between the sternal edge and the midaxillary line horizontally. The breast has a teardrop shape with projection into the axilla as the axillary tail of Spence. The parenchyema itself is divided into 15-20 segments which converge into 5-10 major milk collecting ducts just beneath the nipple. The breast tissue is enveloped by the superficial pectoral fascia, which is contiguous with Camper's fascia. Posteriorly, the breast lies in the deep pectoral fascia which covers the pectoralis major and anterior serratus muscles. Connecting these fascial layers are fibrous bands called Cooper's suspensory ligaments which provide architectural support for the breast.

The primary blood supply to the breast is derived from anterior perforating branches of the internal mammary artery and branches of the lateral thoracic artery. The pectoral branch of the thoracoacromial artery, as well as intracostal arteries, also provides blood supply to the breast.

The lymphatics of the breast drain primarily to the axillary lymph nodes. In addition, a small amount of lymphatic flow courses to the internal mammary nodes, which lie adjacent to the internal mammary vessels in the parasternal region. Radioactive tracer studies demonstrate over 90% of lymphatic flow to the axilla, however, these studies also show that drainage to the internal mammary nodes can originate from anywhere in the breast tissue.[1] The axillary boundaries consist of the axillary vein superiorly, the subscapular muscle posteriorly, the chest wall medially and the medial border of the latissimus dorsi laterally. The inferior border of the axilla is where the serratus and latissimus dorsi are juxtaposed. The lymph nodes of the axilla are divided into three levels: level 1 comprises all nodes lateral to the pectoralis minor muscle, level 2 nodes are beneath the pectoralis minor, and at level 3 are the nodes, usually few in number, medial to the pectoralis minor muscle. In addition, Rotter's nodes are located between the pectoralis major and minor muscles.

2. Benign Breast Disorders

Mastalgia

Mastalgia or breast pain is a common problem for which women seek medical consultation. It is experienced at some point in their lives by over 50% of women. The single most important factor in the evaluation of breast pain is to determine whether it is cyclic or constant. Cyclic pain can be present throughout the entire menstrual cycle, but typically is greatest just prior to onset of menses. This type of pain is almost always physiologic. Noncyclic pain is most often idiopathic. Reassurance that pain is not a presenting symptom of carcinoma as well as an explanation of the physiologic causes of breast pain are often all that is required in treating these patients. In certain situations hormonal treatment with either antiestrogens or androgens is indicated. The vast majority of cases resolve with menopause.

Nipple Discharge

Nipple discharge in a nonlactating woman is another common breast problem. It is rarely a presenting sign of breast carcinoma. It is important to determine if the discharge is bilateral or unilateral, and if unilateral, if it is coming from a single duct. Milky discharge, while common, is only rarely associated with a prolactin-secreting tumor. Spontaneous nipple discharge from a single duct requires surgical attention, particularly if it is bloody. While this is most often due to a solitary intraductal papilloma, carcinoma is also part of the differential diagnosis and surgical excision is required. Unilateral or multiduct discharge is a common finding in postmenopausal women and is almost always secondary to duct ectasia.

Fibrocystic Changes

In the past this entity has been called fibrocystic disease, but it is not a distinct clinical or pathologic abnormality. The term is usually used to describe patients who have fluctuating nodularity of both breasts with associated tenderness. Fibrocystic changes may be secondary to an exaggerated response of the breasts' epithelium and stroma to the individual's hormonal milieu. There is no specific association between fibrocystic changes and breast cancer. In an attempt to clarify this issue, Dupont and Page developed a system for classifying benign breast lesions, often grouped under the heading of fibrocystic disease, into three groups with different relative risks for the development of breast cancer. Nonproliferative lesions, which carry no increased risk of breast cancer, include adenosis, apocrine change, duct ectasia and mild epithelial hyperplasia. Proliferative disease without atypia includes hyperplasia of the usual type, moderate or florid, papilloma and sclerosing adenosis. This carries with it a slightly increased risk of cancer development of 1.5-2 times normal. The third category, atypical hyperplasia, includes both atypical ductal hyperplasia and atypical lobular hyperplasia. These diagnoses carry with them an increased cancer risk of 4-5 times normal. Dupont also found that a biopsy demonstrating atypia, when combined with a positive family history, increased the risk of subsequent development of cancer to nearly 9 times that of the general population.[2]

The Vanderbilt group also lists *in situ* diseases, both ductal and lobular, in the high-risk category, with an 8-10 times increased risk of subsequent development of invasive cancer. These two lesions will be discussed subsequently in the section on breast cancer.

Breast Abscess and Inflammation

Breast abscess and inflammation occur infrequently and usually involve the subareolar breast tissue. Lactation and periductal mastitis are risk factors for the development of breast infections, with *Staphylococcus aureus* being by far the most common pathogen. Many infections begin with inflammation and will not go on to develop an abscess cavity. Treatment should be conservative because the condition usually responds to antibiotics. If the process progresses to frank abscess formation, then surgical drainage is indicated.

Fat Necrosis

Fat necrosis occurs in large pendulous breasts. While a history of trauma may sometimes be elicited it can also occur in situations in which the patient is unaware of any prior injury. The importance of this lesion is that it may mimic carcinoma on physical examination, mammography and even fine-needle aspiration cytology. Histologic examination of the biopsy tissue will provide an accurate diagnosis.

3. Diagnosis of Breast Masses

Mondor's Disease

In 1939, Mondor described "string phlebitis of the chest wall."[3] This condition can occur after trauma, breast biopsy, cosmetic surgery and radiation therapy. Clinically, the patient presents with pain and tenderness along the course of the thoracoepigastric vein, which runs from the axilla to the subareolar area and then medially toward the epigastrium. The phlebitic vein is usually visible and can cause dimpling of the skin. It can sometimes be confused with carcinoma. Its course is self-limited and requires no specific treatment other than anti-inflammatory medication.

Gynecomastia

Gynecomastia is benign, progressive enlargement of the male breast. It may be unilateral or bilateral and may be caused by hormonal or drug-related stimulation, secondary to other systemic disorders, or idiopathic in origin. Puberal gynecomastia, often seen in teenage boys, is very common and frequently bilateral. It will almost always regress and should be treated with reassurance. Hypertrophy in older men is frequently unilateral and often causes the patient to complain of discomfort. Medications such as digoxin, thiazide diuretics and phenothiazine are commonly implicated. Endocrine abnormalities such as hyperthyroidism and failing liver function, as well as chronic renal failure, have also been implicated. Gynecomastia in older men is primarily treated nonsurgically, with treatment instead directed at the underlying cause. Surgery is reserved for patients who are persistently symptomatic, or in cases where male breast cancer is suspected.

The single most common problem for which surgeons are consulted is evaluation of breast masses. Nodularity is a frequent finding in the otherwise normal breast exam, particularly in premenopausal women, as well as in postmenopausal women on hormone replacement. When an abnormality is detected, differentiating benign from malignant masses can often be difficult. The "triple test," which combines physical examination, mammography/ultrasound and fine-needle aspiration/core biopsy, is a highly accurate methodology which can be successfully used to determine which masses may be watched and which require either further evaluation or definitive treatment.

Physical Examination

Inspection of the breast is carried out with the patient's hands on her hips, and then with her hands over her head. Signs to look for are asymmetry of the breast architecture, nipple-areolar abnormalities and skin dimpling. Physical examination of the breast is also carried out with the patient in the sitting, then the lying position. In patients presenting with a mass it is best to examine the contralateral breast first to get an appreciation of the patient's normal mammary glandular architecture. Dominant masses that are either clearly demarcated or ill-defined, but that are different from the remainder of the breast tissue, are searched for. Areas typically difficult to evaluate include the periareolar breast tissue, tissue at the inframammary ridge, and the tissue where the axillary tail of Spence merges with the axillary fat. The breast tissue beneath the nipple should be compressed to evaluate for nipple discharge. The axillary tissue should be examined with the arm supported in the limp position to rule out the presence of axillary adenopathy.

Mammography and Ultrasound

Mammography should be performed in all patients over age 35 being evaluated for a palpable breast mass. In women under this age who have a mass of questionable significance that cannot be successfully diagnosed with physical examination or aspiration, mammography is usually unrewarding and should be supplanted by ultrasound. With the increasing use of screening mammography, a greater percentage of breast lesions are now being identified on the basis of mammography alone. Findings highly suggestive of malignancy include stellate lesions, microcalcifications, particularly if they are in a linear, branching pattern, and areas of increased density associated with architectural distortion.

Aspiration Cytology and Core Biopsy

This is the procedure providing the most relevant information in terms of need for subsequent treatment. Consultation with an experienced cytopathologist is mandatory if aspiration cytology is going to be used to define further therapy. While core biopsy provides tissue for histologic interpretation, the multiple passes made with aspiration cytology can provide a more complete evaluation of the mass in question. Close cooperation between the surgeon, pathologist and mammographer is required no matter what method of tissue procurement is used.

In evaluating breast masses we consider three distinct categories: a dominant palpable mass, a nondominant mass and a nonpalpable mammographic abnormality. Our algorithms for working up lesions in each category are depicted in Figures 1, 2 and 3.

Figure 1

Algorithm for diagnosis and treatment of dominant palpable lump

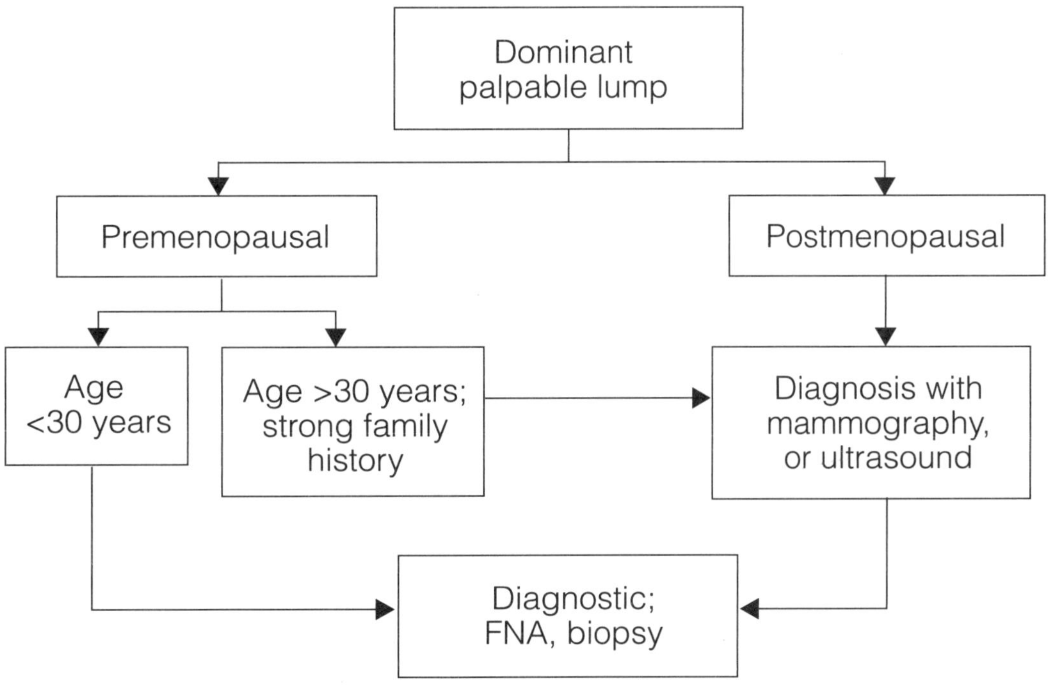

Figure 2

Algorithm for treatment of nondominant palpable lump

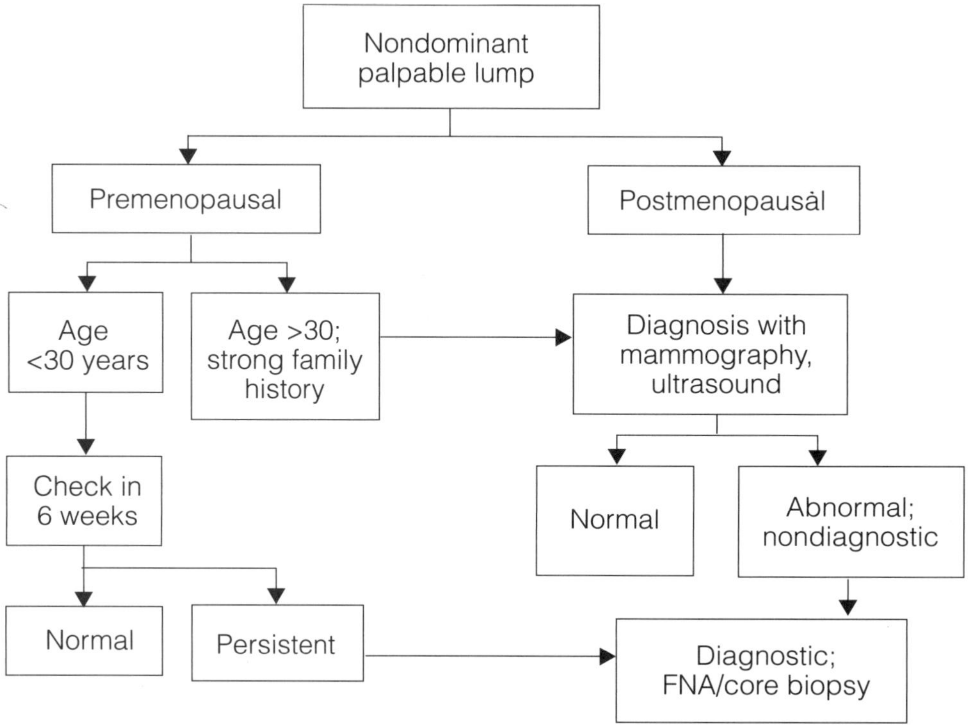

Figure 3

Algorithm for treatment of mammographic nonpalpable lesion

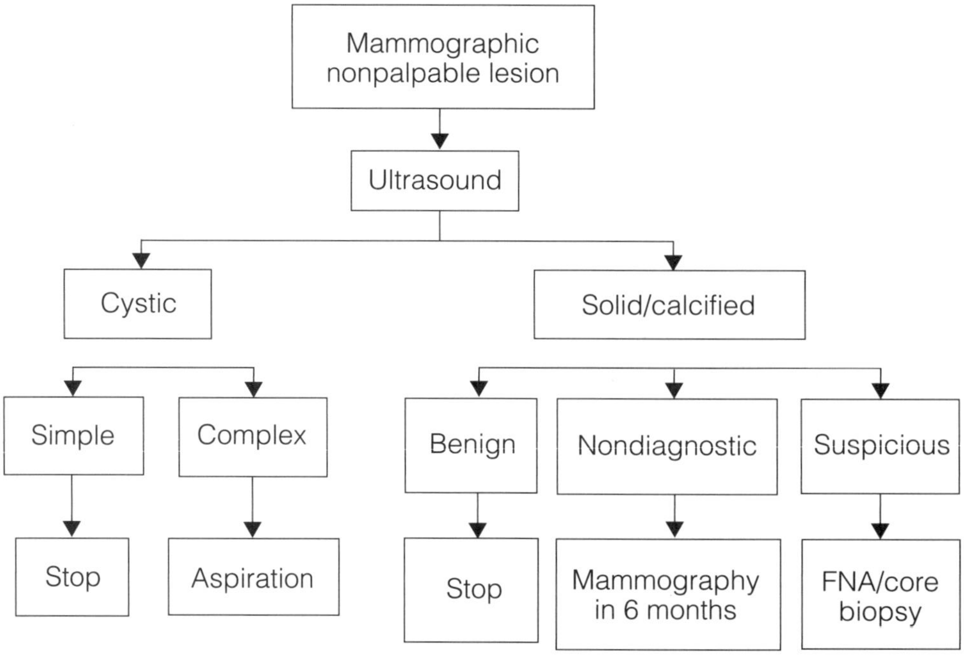

4. Breast Cancer

Epidemiology

Breast cancer is a common disease in American women and is responsible for approximately 30% of all female-related malignancies. The lifetime risk of developing breast cancer is now one in six, and one in eight for invasive disease.[2] It is estimated that there were 182,460 new cases of breast cancer diagnosed in the United States in the year 2008.[4] This represents a slight decrease in incidence compared to previous years. More importantly, breast cancer-related mortality is clearly decreasing. The reduction in mortality for the 5-year period from 1989 through 1993 was estimated to be approximately 6%. This decrease, however, is confined primarily to Caucasian females, and is thought to be due to early diagnosis as well as improved treatment.

5. Risk Factors

Age

The risk of breast cancer is exceedingly small in women under the age of 25. Data concerning increasing incidence in premenopausal women are somewhat inconsistent, due in part to improvements in diagnosis and staging. The risk of breast cancer continues to rise until the eighth decade of life, at which time it plateaus.

Family History

Positive family history for breast cancer is associated with increased risk. Women with a relative who has been diagnosed with breast cancer have twice the relative risk as women who do not. The risk of breast cancer is even higher when the affected relative is diagnosed at an earlier age.

Early Menarche, Late Menopause

It is currently thought that these factors play a role in increasing the risk of breast cancer due to unopposed estrogen stimulation.

Prior Radiation Therapy

Patients with previous exposure of their breasts to radiation therapy are at increased risk for developing cancer. As with other radiation-induced cancers, there is a considerable lag time of approximately 15-25 years between the exposure and subsequent development of cancer. Women who received mantle radiation therapy for Hodgkin's disease are a classic example of this increased risk.

Alcohol

Numerous studies demonstrate conflicting results regarding the association between alcohol consumption and breast cancer. A pooled analysis of data demonstrated that women who consumed 2-5 drinks per day had a relative risk of 1.4 in comparison to women who did not drink.[5]

Exogenous Hormones

This continues to be a source of considerable controversy. The preponderance of evidence suggests that there is no increased risk for premenopausal women who take oral contraceptives. A slight increased risk was detected in women who used birth control pills for a prolonged period at an earlier time when the hormonal content of these pills was substantially greater than it is today.

The more difficult question concerns the risk of developing breast cancer in postmenopausal patients receiving hormone replacement therapy. The most recent data available tend to support an association between increased risk and long-term use of HRT.[6] The Women's Health Initiative randomized 16,000 women to either estrogen and progestin or placebo, and an additional 11,000 women who had a prior hysterectomy to either estrogen or placebo to determine the risks and benefits of HRT on the overall health of postmenopausal women. The study found an increased risk of breast cancer in patients taking the combination of estrogen and progestin but not in patients taking estrogen alone. The overall conclusion, however, was that the risk of hormone replacement outweighs the benefits. On that basis, hormone replacement therapy is currently recommended only for the short-term relief of perimenopausal symptoms.

Dietary Factors

Differences in the prevalence of breast cancer among different populations have led to the evaluation of dietary factors as a possible risk factor for breast carcinogenesis. The amount of fat in the diet, and particularly the amount of calories derived from fat, is the factor most frequently cited. The results of current studies are conflicting, although obesity is now recognized as a risk factor.

Prior Breast Biopsy

In the past, a diagnosis of fibrocystic disease was felt to represent a significant risk factor in the development of breast cancer. As was discussed in the earlier section on benign disease, however, this is really only true for patients with proliferative lesions, and in particular those with epithelial hyperplasia with atypia. The other benign processes that have been implicated pose, at most, a slightly increased risk.

6. Inherited Breast Cancer

Hereditary breast cancer accounts for approximately 5% of all cases. Syndromes associated with an increased risk of breast cancer are listed in Table 1. In comparison with sporadic cases, hereditary breast cancer tends to appear at a much earlier age and has a tendency to be both multifocal and bilateral. These tumors arise as a result of inherited constitutional or germ-line mutations, as opposed to sporadic cancers in which the genetic mutation is acquired somatically in the epithelial tissue at risk. While the list of mutations associated with breast cancer is growing, it is felt that the vast majority of truly inherited breast cancer cases are due to mutations in the BRCA I and BRCA II genes. Both of these genes are tumor-suppressor genes. Despite the elucidation of these risk factors, the majority of patients diagnosed with breast cancer have no discernible risk factors prior to the diagnosis of their disease.

Table 1

Genetic Syndromes Associated with Breast Cancer

BRCA I and BRCA II
Li-Fraumeni syndrome
Lynch syndrome II
Cowden disease
Muir-Torre syndrome
Ataxia-telangiectasia
Klinefelter's syndrome

7. Breast Cancer Screening

The three components of breast cancer screening are: breast self-examination performed monthly approximately 7 days after the onset of menses, a physician's physical examination and mammography. Although 10-15% of all breast cancers will not be visible on screening mammography, it is abundantly clear that mammography holds the greatest potential for establishing an early diagnosis. The routine application of yearly screening mammography in women over the age of 50 will result in a 30% reduction in breast cancer-related mortality. An area of considerable controversy, however, concerns the benefits of annual screening in patients between the ages of 40 and 50. To date, no study examining this question has demonstrated a significant improvement in survival in this age group. When these patients are followed beyond the age of 50, however, some benefit does accrue. A consensus conference convened to specifically address this question concluded that the evidence does not support yearly mammography in this age group.[7] Having said that, however, the current recommendation of various cancer groups includes yearly mammography after the age of 40. The high incidence of false positives from mammography necessitating further testing in this age group highlights the need for a definitive answer to this question.

For patients at high risk for the development of breast cancer on the basis of strong family history, or a BRCA1 or BRCA2 mutation, magnetic resonance imaging is being evaluated for earlier detection. Patients typically begin screening 10 years prior to the age at which the youngest relative developed breast cancer.

8. Pathology of Breast Cancer

Noninvasive Disease

There are two forms of noninvasive breast cancer: ductal carcinoma *in situ* (DCIS) and lobular carcinoma *in situ* (LCIS). The fact that these tumors do not penetrate the basement membrane of either the duct or terminal lobule means they do not have access to lymphovascular channels, and precludes the possibility of systemic spread. The vast majority of these patients are cured with their initial management.

DCIS

Prior to the advent of mammographic screening, DCIS was a rare tumor which presented as a palpable mass. With increasing use of mammography and the realization that mammographic microcalcifications are often associated with DCIS, the incidence increased dramatically. In areas where screening is religiously practiced, DCIS can account for up to 40% of newly diagnosed breast cancers. There were 68,000 cases of DCIS diagnosed in 2008.[4] A tumor typically appears in the sixth decade of life and may be one of several histologic subtypes. It tends to be multifocal and, to a lesser extent, multicentric. The risk of subsequent development of invasive carcinoma is largely confined to the ipsilateral breast, and has an overall incidence of 20%-50%. When cancer recurrence is invasive, it is almost always of ductal histology.

LCIS

In comparison to DCIS, LCIS is usually diagnosed approximately a decade earlier, in the fifth decade of life. There are no clinical or mammographic signs of LCIS, and it is frequently found inadvertently in histologic sections of biopsy specimens. It has a very high incidence of both multicentricity and bilaterality. The risk of subsequently developing invasive cancer is variously estimated to be between 25% and 40%. Interestingly, the tumor is equally likely to be in the opposite breast as in the breast in which the LCIS was initially diagnosed. In addition, the interval to diagnosis of subsequent cancer tends to be prolonged, with a lag time of approximately 10-15 years. Finally, the histology of subsequent cancers is more frequently invasive ductal rather than invasive lobular cancer. On the strength of this observation, LCIS is now treated as a marker of increased risk for the subsequent development of breast cancer.

Invasive Cancer

Invasive Ductal Carcinoma
This entity, also known as infiltrating ductal carcinoma, represents 75%-80% of all breast cancers. There are several variants of invasive ductal carcinoma. Medullary carcinoma is the most common and represents approximately 6% of all invasive cancers. These tumors tend to be characterized by a marked lymphocytic infiltrate and have a better prognosis than infiltrating ductal cancer.

Tubular carcinoma is another well-differentiated form of ductal carcinoma with a favorable prognosis that is found in approximately 2% of all breast cancers. Mucinous or colloid carcinoma represents another 1%-2% of breast cancers. The diagnosis is made histologically on the basis of extracellular mucin found around the tumor cells.

Invasive Lobular Carcinoma
Approximately 5%-10% of all invasive breast cancers are lobular in histology. These tumors have a high incidence of bilaterality, the opposite breast being involved either simultaneously or at a later time. Lobular cancers tend to be diffusely infiltrative, making them difficult to diagnose both clinically and on mammographic examination. Magnetic resonance imaging, however, has been useful in determining the extent of breast involvement in lobular carcinoma.

Inflammatory Breast Carcinoma
This is a clinical diagnosis made on the basis of a characteristic appearance of the overlying skin called *peau d'orange*. The skin is usually markedly thickened and a breast mass is difficult to palpate. The appearance is secondary to plugging of the subdermal lymphatics with tumor cells. This entity is almost always associated with both axillary and distant disease necessitating neoadjuvant treatment prior to consideration of surgical therapy.

9. Staging

Staging is important from a prognostic as well as a therapeutic standpoint. This is particularly relevant in breast cancer, in which adjuvant therapy is known to be efficacious. The staging system used for breast cancer is the TNM system depicted in Table 2. The American Joint Committee on Cancer (AJCC) staging schema based on the TNM system is listed in Table 3. On the basis of this system, stages 3A and 3B are recognized as locally advanced disease.

Table 2

TNM Staging for Breast Cancer

Tumor	
T0	No evidence of primary tumor
Tis	Carcinoma *in situ*
T1	Tumor 2 cm or less in greatest dimension
T2	Tumor more than 2 cm but not more than 5 cm in greatest dimension
T3	Tumor more than 5 cm in greatest dimension
T4	Tumor of any size with direct extension into chest wall, skin edema, skin ulceration or satellite skin nodules confined to the same breast or inflammatory carcinoma
Regional Lymph Nodes	
N0	No regional lymph node involvement
N1	Metastasis to movable ipsilateral axillary lymph node(s)
N2	Metastasis to ipsilateral axillary lymph node(s) fixed to one another or to other structures
N3	Metastasis to ipsilateral internal mammary lymph nodes
Distant Metastasis	
M0	No distant metastasis
M1	Distant metastasis present (including ipsilateral supraclavicular lymph nodes)

Table 3

AJCC Classification for Breast Cancer Based on TNM Criteria

Stage	Tumor	Nodes	Metastases
0	Tis	N0	M0
I	T1	N0	M0
IIA	T0,1 T2	N1 N0	M0 M0
IIB	T2 T3	N1 N0	M0 M0
IIIA	T0, 1, 2 T3	N2 N1, 2	M0 M0
IIIB	T4 Any T	N1, 2 N3	M0 M0
IV	Any T	Any N	M1

10. Treatment

Invasive Breast Cancer

The surgical treatment of local and regional disease has been a source of considerable controversy over the past 30 years. Surgical treatment has been predicated on prevailing theories of how breast cancer spreads and the ability to surgically interdict those routes of spread. At the turn of the 20th century, Halsted proposed the first cogent theory of breast cancer dissemination. He believed that it was an orderly process in which there was a significant local tumor burden prior to dissemination through the breast lymphatics to the axillary lymph nodes, and only after significant axillary involvement was there spread to metastatic sites throughout the body. His theory concerning breast cancer dissemination, combined with the fact that he was confronted with patients with locally advanced disease, made Halsted's radical mastectomy an appropriate surgical approach. Half a century later, the modified radical mastectomy replaced the radical mastectomy as tumors were found at an earlier stage at the time of diagnosis. It was, however, the pathologic staging of the tumors found in specimens from radical and modified radical mastectomies that allowed surgeons to challenge Halsted's original hypothesis. In particular, the finding that a significant percentage of patients with negative axillary lymph nodes went on to develop systemic disease suggested an alternative hypothesis of the means of breast cancer dissemination. This "biologic theory" championed by Bernard Fisher and the National Surgical Adjuvant Breast and Bowel Project (NSABP) stated that in the vast majority of cases breast cancer is a disseminated disease at the time of diagnosis, and that local therapies are only important in their ability to control local disease. While the presence of axillary nodal disease is predictive of metastatic spread, it is not a necessary prerequisite in the development of distant disease. In the 1970s and 1980s, six major randomized trials compared some form of mastectomy versus breast conservation surgery involving either lumpectomy or quadrantectomy, usually with the addition of radiation therapy. Each of these trials demonstrated that radical and conservation surgery have equivalent results with respect to overall survival.

The largest randomized trial was the NSABP B-06 trial comparing total mastectomy and lumpectomy with or without breast radiation.[8] This trial was restricted to patients with tumors less than 4 cm in size. There was no difference in survival between the three treatment arms. Of particular interest was the fact that survival was equivalent despite a 40% incidence of local recurrence in patients treated with lumpectomy alone.

On the basis of these trials, a National Institute of Health Consensus Development Conference, convened in 1992, wrote that "breast conservation treatment is an appropriate method of primary therapy for the majority of women with Stage I and II breast cancer and is preferable because it provides survival equivalent to total mastectomy and axillary dissection while preserving the breast."[9]

Radiation therapy is an integral part of breast conservation therapy. Whole breast irradiation to a total dose of 4500-5000 cGy is a mainstay of the standard protocol for breast conservation therapy. An additional boost dose to the primary site raises the total dose to approximately 6000-6600 cGy. Accelerated partial breast irradiation is currently being evaluated as an alternative to whole breast irradiation, with promising short-term results in carefully selected patients.[10] In addition, studies of patients with favorable tumors (small, receptor positive) are being conducted to determine if certain patients can forego radiation therapy as part of their treatment algorithm.[16]

There are both absolute and relative contraindications to breast conservation therapy. The absolute contraindications include pregnancy (if radiation therapy cannot be delayed until after delivery), proven multicentric disease and/or diffuse malignant-appearing microcalcifications, a history of prior irradiation of the breast, and persistently positive surgical margins after several attempts at lumpectomy. Relative contraindications include multiple tumors in the same quadrant and indeterminate microcalcifications, a history of collagen vascular disease and large tumor size. There is no absolute size which rules out the possibility of breast conservation therapy; the size of the tumor in relationship to the size of the breast is the determining factor. If removal of the tumor with a rim of surrounding normal tissue will significantly deform the breast, the patient is probably better served with mastectomy and immediate reconstruction. A tumor just below the nipple is also regarded as a relative contraindication. However, lumpectomy with excision of the nipple areolar complex can be considered.

For patients with locally advanced or Stage III disease, immediate surgical therapy is contraindicated. A course of neoadjuvant chemotherapy is indicated, with the expectation that approximately 70%-80% of patients will respond with decrease in the size of the tumor. This may allow the use of breast conservation therapy in selected patients. There is, however, an increased risk of local recurrence following breast conservation therapy in patients who present with initial bulky disease.

DCIS

The surgical treatment of DCIS has evolved over the last 10-15 years. The therapy initially mandated when DCIS presented as palpable disease was a simple mastectomy. While this resulted in curative resection in the vast majority of patients, the argument has been made that if mastectomy is no longer required for invasive disease its role should be minimal in noninvasive disease. Lumpectomy alone will result in a recurrence rate of approximately 25%-35%, with half of those recurrences being invasive carcinomas. NSABP trial B-17 demonstrated that the addition of radiation therapy will reduce the recurrence rate from 25% to 13%.[11] A follow-up study, NSABP B-24, compared lumpectomy and radiation to lumpectomy, radiation and tamoxifen.[12] It was found that the addition of tamoxifen further reduces the recurrence rate from 13% to 8%. On the basis of these studies, the current recommendation is to treat DCIS with lumpectomy, radiation therapy and tamoxifen for receptor positive tumors. For receptor positive tumors, studies are currently underway to identify patients who can be treated without radiation therapy. The subset of patients for whom this might be applicable is patients with small, mammographically-detected tumors which are low grade and whose resection margins are clearly negative. Patients with comedo carcinoma or high grade DCIS require wide resection, radiation therapy and tamoxifen. In addition, some surgeons advocate axillary lymph node sampling in this subset of patients, to identify patients with microinvasion which might be missed on histologic examination.

LCIS

The facts that LCIS is frequently multicentric, often bilateral, and has a significant lag time before subsequent development of invasive cancer, suggests that a nonsurgical approach may be warranted in the treatment of this disease. The finding that patients with a prior diagnosis of LCIS who subsequently develop invasive disease develop invasive ductal as opposed to invasive lobular disease, led surgeons to view LCIS as a marker for increased risk of developing breast cancer. The only method to totally obviate this risk would be bilateral mastectomy with immediate reconstruction. Consideration of this approach should be reserved for a small subset of patients with LCIS who have either a very strong family history of breast cancer or documented BRCA I or BRCA II mutations. Other management options include chemoprevention, which will be discussed later in this chapter, and close clinical follow-up.

Treatment of the Axillae

Identification and treatment of axillary disease has also undergone recent changes. Clinical assessment of axillary disease is inaccurate in approximately 25% of cases, evenly distributed between false positives and false negatives. In 1971, NSABP protocol B-04 was initiated.[13] Women with breast cancer and clinically negative axillae were randomized to either radical mastectomy, total mastectomy with radiation to the regional lymph nodes or total mastectomy alone with subsequent removal of axillary nodes in patients who developed suspicious adenopathy. Women with clinically positive nodes were randomized to either radical mastectomy or total mastectomy with local regional radiation. There were no differences in survival among the three groups of node-negative patients or the two groups of node-positive patients. These results suggested that the removal of clinically-negative nodes was of no therapeutic benefit. It would, however, be of prognostic benefit, particularly if it changed the type of therapy received in an adjuvant setting. These findings led surgeons to change their surgical strategy for the axilla from radical axillary dissection involving removal of all three levels of lymph nodes to a level 1 and 2 dissection, often with sparing of the intercostal brachial nerve.

The development of axillary sentinel lymph node biopsy, however, has had the greatest impact on the treatment of the axilla over the past 5 years. The sentinel lymph node is defined as the first lymph node encountered by the lymphatics draining the cancer. This technique, while first described for penile cancer, was popularized in the treatment of malignant melanoma. Lymphatic mapping utilizes either blue dye (Lymphazurin™), technetium-labeled sulfur colloid, or a combination of both. The dye and/or colloid is injected at multiple sites around the periphery of the tumor, into the subdermal lymphatics just anterior to the tumor or subareolarly. With this technique, sentinel nodes can be found in approximately 95% of patients. Sentinel lymph nodes are resected and subjected to rigorous pathologic examination with multiple histologic sections and immunohistochemistry staining for cytokeratins. Negative sentinel lymph nodes are predictive of a negative axillary dissection with an accuracy approaching 100%. Because over two-thirds of patients are currently being diagnosed with node-negative breast cancer, this technique spares those patients from the morbidity associated with formal axillary dissections. Patients with a positive sentinel node should undergo axillary dissection, although in almost 50% of cases the sentinel node will be the only positive lymph node encountered. While the finding of micrometastasis in the sentinel nodes improves the accuracy of surgical staging, the need for further axillary dissection and the impact of this finding as a prognostic factor remains to be determined.

Adjuvant Systemic Therapy

In addition to the replacement of mastectomy with lumpectomy and the more recent conversion from axillary nodal dissection to sentinel node sampling, perhaps the most significant advance in breast cancer management in the past 30 years has been the successful application of adjuvant systemic therapy. From early trials in the 1960s and 1970s first testing single agents and subsequently multiple drug regimens, adjuvant systemic therapy has become a mainstay for the majority of patients diagnosed with breast cancer. Breast cancer is the second leading cause of cancer-related mortality among women and is responsible for approximately 16% of all cancer-related deaths. The recent improvement in breast cancer mortality, first demonstrated in the early 1990s, is partly attributable to the advances made in adjuvant treatment. While its application is universally accepted, controversies remain concerning the optimal treatment regimen and indications for treatment in patients with node-negative Stage I breast cancer.

Indications for Adjuvant Therapy

Patients with locally advanced Stage IIIA and IIIB disease require other treatment in addition to adjuvant therapy. In the absence of advanced disease, however, the best indicator of risk of subsequent relapse is the axillary lymph node status. Patients with involved nodes have a 60%-70% risk of recurrence within 5 years without additional therapy, with a particularly poor prognosis for patients with 10 or more positive nodes.

For patients with node-negative disease, however, the risk of recurrence is only 30% and the need for adjuvant therapy is less clear. In patients with Stage I disease the risk of recurrence has to be assessed, not only in terms of expected benefit, but also in conjunction with the morbidity associated with adjuvant therapy. As an example of this, most oncologists would be more likely to suggest tamoxifen as an adjuvant therapy in patients with a limited risk of recurrence, partly due to its excellent side effect profile and efficacy, as opposed to an intensive course of chemotherapy involving a cardiotoxic agent such as doxorubicin. Patients with tumors ≥3 cm in size have a 30%-50% chance of recurrence and universally require adjuvant therapy. This is probably also true for patients whose tumors are between 1 and 3 cm in size, although there is some controversy over patients with receptor positive tumors in this category. For patients with tumors less than 1 cm, however, the impact of adjuvant therapy will be exceedingly small since their overall risk of recurrence is on the order of <10%.

There has been an intensive search for prognostic factors that might identify patients with node-negative disease who are destined to have a recurrence. In addition to tumor size, histologic grade is a well-established prognostic marker. Other prognostic markers routinely assessed include estrogen and progesterone receptors, markers of proliferation, such as Ki-67 expression identified by immunohistochemistry, S-phase fraction by flow cytometry, oncogene amplification such as HER-2 NEU, and tumor suppressor genes such as p-53. Of these markers ER and PR are the most widely accepted, both in terms of indicating a less aggressive course in patients who are receptor positive, and more importantly in identifying patients who are likely to benefit from hormonal therapy. The association of the HER-2 gene amplification, noted in approximately one-quarter of invasive breast cancers, and indicating a poor prognosis in Stage I patients, is still controversial. Prognostic markers still being studied include markers of invasion such as cathepsin D, as well as angiogenesis markers assessed by either microvessel count or immunohistochemical staining for vascular endothelial growth factor. The most recent development of a multigene assay to predict recurrence, and the need for adjuvant therapy, in patients with node-negative breast cancer, is a major advance in this field and will be employed in the future to determine not only the need for additional therapy but specific drug regimens of benefit.[14]

The National Comprehensive Cancer Network, in conjunction with the American Cancer Society, has recently established treatment guidelines for adjuvant therapy of breast cancer. Adjuvant chemotherapy is recommended for patients with node-positive hormone receptor negative disease. For node-positive hormone receptor positive disease, adjuvant chemotherapy together with tamoxifen is the current recommendation. For node-negative disease, no adjuvant chemotherapy is currently recommended for tumors less than 1 cm in size, except for patients with unfavorable prognostic features, in which case adjuvant therapy can be considered. For tumors larger than 1 cm that are hormone receptor positive, tamoxifen is indicated, with the addition of chemotherapy if the tumor is larger than 3 cm. For tumors larger than 1 cm that are hormone receptor negative, adjuvant chemotherapy is recommended in all cases.

The reduction in mortality risk associated with the use of chemotherapy is on the order of approximately 30%-35%. Currently accepted regimens include multiple drugs given for a period of 3-6 months. A combination of cyclophosphamide, methotrexate and 5-fluorouracil has been the standard therapy, but is being supplanted by a combination of doxorubicin and cyclophosphamide. The role of the taxanes is also being evaluated, as is the use of dose-dense treatment regimens. At present there is no role for high-dose chemotherapy with autologous stem cell transplantation, although it is under investigation in patients with 10 or more positive nodes. The addition to chemotherapy of trastuzumab, an antibody directed against the HER-2 receptor, for tumors overexpressing the HER-2 gene has resulted in a significant improvement in both disease free and overall survival in the adjuvant setting.[17] Other biologic agents are also being tested, based on results achieved in metastasis.

Treatment of Metastatic Disease

Although the majority of patients currently being diagnosed with breast cancer are cured of their disease, approximately 20% of node-negative and 60% of node-positive patients will develop recurrent disease. Recommendations for follow-up of patients after their primary treatment usually involve visits every 3-4 months for the first 2 years, followed by visits every 6 months until year 5, from which point patients are followed annually. Although a number of chemistry tests and imaging studies can be performed in an attempt to make an early diagnosis of recurrent disease, studies have never shown an impact of this aggressive approach in terms of improved survival. These tests should be employed, however, when symptoms or physical findings merit further investigation. In addition, monthly breast self-examination, as well as annual mammography and pelvic examinations should be continued.

The majority of patients who develop metastatic disease will do so within five years of their initial diagnosis. Breast cancer, however, can recur 15, 20, and even 30 years after the original diagnosis. The risk of recurrence depends on the stage at initial presentation, but no patient can be considered risk-free for recurrence. Once a diagnosis of recurrence is made, the patient is incurable. The most common sites of recurrence include bone, soft tissue, lung and pleura, and liver.

Despite the fact that patients with metastatic disease will almost all die of their disease, significant long-term palliation can be achieved in this setting. This is particularly true of postmenopausal women who have estrogen receptor positive disease. Once the diagnosis of metastatic disease has been made, imaging studies should be performed both to determine the extent of disease and to establish a baseline to evaluate efficacy of planned therapy. The treatment modalities used in an adjuvant setting—chemotherapy, hormonal therapy and radiotherapy—are also effective in the palliative treatment of metastatic disease. It must be emphasized that since this therapy is never curative, treatment decisions must be made from the standpoint of providing relief of symptoms and prolongation of life where the quality of life is of primary importance.

For patients with hormone-responsive disease that is not life-threatening, hormonal therapy should be instituted with the expectation of an objective response in up to 80% of patients. Tamoxifen has long been considered the first-line endocrine therapy of choice. Its response can be expected to last for a period of 12-18 months. Following progression, second-line hormonal agents such as megestrol, a progestational agent, can be used successfully. Evidence is accumulating that aromatase inhibitors, which block estrogen biosynthesis in the peripheral tissues, is proving more efficacious than tamoxifen, with an improved safety profile. In addition, other new agents collectively known as selective estrogen receptor modulators (SERMs) are also being tested.

For patients with hormone unresponsive or life-threatening disease, chemotherapy should be initiated. Recent trends in this area include switching from multiple-drug regimens with their increased toxicity to single-agent treatment. The taxanes have shown particular promise in this area. Capecitabine, a new oral fluoroparemidine, is also being tested. Finally, the monoclonal antibody trastuzumab in combination with paclitaxel is also being studied in the treatment of metastatic disease. Reported results with high-dose chemotherapy with stem-cell rescue have been disappointing and these treatments should only be pursued in a protocol setting.

Radiation therapy is also an important modality in treatment of metastatic disease. It is particularly useful in the treatment of metastasis to weight-bearing bones to prevent pathologic fractures, and in relieving pain from bony metastasis. Radiotherapy is effective in treating brain metastasis, as well as spinal cord compression secondary to metastatic disease. Bisphosphonates, which are potent inhibitors of osteoclastic activity, also show efficacy in both the prevention and treatment of bony metastasis.

11. Prevention

In evaluating the effects of hormonal therapy in an adjuvant setting, it was found that tamoxifen decreased the risk of a second primary breast cancer in the opposite breast by a factor of 50%. This led the NSABP to initiate the P1 Trial, a randomized, double-blind study comparing tamoxifen versus placebo in patients judged to be at high risk for the development of breast cancer.[15] Almost 14,000 patients were randomized to the study, and results reported in 1998 showed tamoxifen provided a 50% reduction in the incidence of both invasive and non-invasive breast cancer. The reduction in incidence of breast cancer was apparent in all age groups and at all risk levels. Furthermore, tamoxifen was found to be effective in patients whose increased risk was detected by a prior biopsy demonstrating epithelial hyperplasia with atypia. Despite this impressive reduction in risk, there were toxicities associated with tamoxifen use. In particular, patients on tamoxifen had an approximately 2-1/2 times increased risk of developing uterine cancer as did patients on placebo, and were also at higher risk for development of deep venous thrombosis and pulmonary embolism. These events, however, were few in number and restricted to patients over age 50. All of the tamoxifen-associated uterine cancers were Stage I disease.

The results of this study establish tamoxifen as an effective chemopreventive agent. The fact that the reduction in risk occurred as early as 1 year following initiation of treatment, however, suggests that part of the improvement may be due to treatment of preclinical disease. While the treatment duration in the trial was 5 years, the optimal duration of therapy also remains in question. The second-generation study, also administered by the NSABP, tested tamoxifen versus raloxifene, a new selective estrogen receptor modulator, which in trials as a treatment for osteoporosis demonstrated efficacy in the reduction of risk for the development of breast cancer. The study demonstrated equal efficacy of the two drugs with different toxicity profiles.[18] Adjuvant studies utilizing aromatase inhibitors strongly suggest an advantage over tamoxifen. This is also being investigated.

12. Breast Centers

In an effort to incorporate rapidly changing strategies directed at the prevention, early diagnosis, and treatment of breast cancer, ***breast centers*** have been created to address the multidisciplinary aspects of treatment of both benign and malignant breast disease. Surgeons, genetic counselors and radiologists are closely aligned in both the identification of high-risk patients, and the possible roles of chemoprevention, prophylactic surgical strategies such as the skin-sparing mastectomy with immediate reconstruction, and intensive screening algorithms which may play a role in the management of these high-risk women. As breast cancer therapy in particular has evolved into a multidisciplinary regimen, breast centers afford patients the opportunity to be evaluated by the surgeon, medical oncologists, radiation therapists and, when appropriate, a plastic surgeon, in one clinic visit. Treatment regimens can then be devised on the basis of both the patient's clinical stage at presentation as well as her desire for breast conservation or, when indicated, immediate reconstruction. Decisions concerning the need for and timing of chemotherapy and radiation therapy in relation to the primary surgical procedure are of a critical nature in the management of both early stage as well as locally advanced breast cancer. As a corollary to breast centers, breast-specific tumor boards are necessary to ensure the implementation of recent advances in breast cancer management such as sentinel node sampling, post-mastectomy radiation and sequential combination chemotherapy.

Finally, breast centers play an important role in providing the educational material necessary for patients to make truly informed decisions as to the treatment choices best suited for their own personal needs. Involvement of social workers, psychologists, support groups and former patients can do much to enhance the quality of life for patients confronted with this disease. The psychosocial health of both the patient and her family is an area of critical importance which has only recently received attention; breast centers provide an ideal forum for addressing these concerns.

13. Conclusions

The treatment of breast cancer has rapidly evolved over the past 25 years. New treatment modalities have improved our ability to successfully manage advanced disease for prolonged periods. For patients with early stage disease, who now represent an increasing majority of newly diagnosed patients, recent refinements have limited the extent of surgery required in the primary management of the disease and sharply lessened the side effects previously associated with surgical therapy. An improved understanding of *in situ* disease, together with the successful application of chemoprevention strategies, suggest that we are likely to see further reductions in both incidence and mortality from this disease. Finally, advances in genetic molecular biology coupled with a more sophisticated appreciation of the gene-host-environment interactions responsible for breast carcinogenesis will provide a means to more precisely define risk for breast cancer development and offer therapeutic options to minimize that risk.

14. References

1. Hultborn KA, Larsen LG, Rahgnult I. The lymph drainage from the breast to the axillary and parasternal lymph nodes: studies with the aid of colloidal 198Au. *Acta Radiol.* 1955;43:52.

2. Dupont WD, Page DL. Risk factors for breast cancer in women with proliferative breast disease. *N Engl J Med.* 1985;312:146.

3. Mondor H. Tonculite sous-cutanee subaigue de la paroi thoracique antero-laterale. *Mem Acad de Chir.* 1939;65:1271.

4. Jemal A, Siegel R, Ward E, et al. Cancer statistics, 2008. *CA Cancer J Clin.* 2008; 58:71.

5. Smith-Warner SA, Spiegelman D, Yaun S-S, et al. Alcohol and breast cancer in women: a pooled analysis of cohort studies. *JAMA.* 1998;279:535-540.

6. Schairer C, Lubin J, Troisi R. Menopausal estrogen and estrogen-progestin replacement therapy and breast cancer risk. *JAMA.* 2000;283:485-491.

7. NIH Consensus Development Panel. National Institutes of Health Consensus Development Conference statement: Breast cancer screening for women ages 40-49, January 21-23, 1997. *J Natl Cancer Inst.* 1997;89:1015-1026

8. Fisher B, Bauer M, Margolese R, et al. Five-year results of a randomized clinical trial comparing total mastectomy and segmental mastectomy with or without radiation in treatment of breast cancer. *N Engl J Med.* 1985;312:665-673.

9. NIH Consensus Development Conference. Consensus statement. Treatment of early-stage breast cancer. *J Natl Cancer Inst Monogr.* 1992;11:1-5.

10. Hughes KS, Schanaper LA, Berry D, et al. Lumpectomy plus Tamoxifen with or without irradiation in women 70 years of age or older with early breast cancer. *N Engl J Med.* 2004;351:971-977.

11. Fisher ER, Costantino J, Fisher B, et al for The National Surgical Adjuvant Breast and Bowel Project Collaborating Investigators. Pathologic findings from the National Surgical Adjuvant Breast Project (NSABP) Protocol B-17. Intraductal carcinoma (ductal carcinoma in situ). *Cancer.* 1995;75:1310-1319.

12. Wolmark N, Dignan J, Fisher B. The addition of tamoxifen to lumpectomy and radiotherapy in the treatment of ductal carcinoma in situ (DCIS): Preliminary results of NSABP protocol B-24. *Breast Cancer.* 1998;50:227.

13. Fisher B, Redmond C, Fisher E, et al. Ten year results of a randomized trial comparing radical mastectomy and total mastectomy with or without radiation. *N Engl J Med.* 1985;312:674-681.

14. Paik S, Shak S, Tang G, et al. A multigene Assay to predict recurrence of Tamoxifen-treated, node-negative breast cancer. *N Engl J Med.* 2004;351:2817-2825.

15. Fisher B, Costantino JP, Wickerham DL, et al. Tamoxifen for prevention of breast cancer: Report of the National Surgical Adjuvant Breast and Bowel Project P-1 Study. *J Natl Cancer Inst.* 1998;90:1371-1388.

16. Hughes KS, Schnaper LA, Berry D, et al. Lumpectomy plus tamoxifen with or without irradiation in women 70 years of age or older with early breast cancer. *N Engl J Med.* 2004; 351:971.

17. Romond EH, Perez EA, Bryant J, et al. Trastuzumab plus adjuvant chemotherapy for operable HER2-positive breast cancer. *N Engl J Med.* 2005; 353:1673.

18. Vogel VG, Constantino JP, Wickerham DL, et al. Effects of tamoxifen vs raloxifene on the risk of developing invasive breast cancer and other disease outcomes. *JAMA.* 2006; 295:2727.

15. Questions

1. Which of the following statements concerning breast development are true?

A. The human breast develops from the ectodermal primitive milk streak

B. The thoracic portion of the milk streak regresses during the third trimester

C. The neonate will often produce milk as a result of placental hormones

D. Polythelia is the most common congenital breast abnormality

E. Breast development during early menarche is primarily governed by progesterone secretion

2. The following statements are true concerning lymphatic drainage of the breast:

A. Breast lymphatics drain primarily to the axillary lymph nodes

B. Lymphatic drainage is equally distributed between the axillary and internal mammary nodes

C. The axillary lymph nodes are divided into three levels in relation to their proximity to the pectoralis major muscle

D. Rotter's nodes are located between the pectoralis major and minor muscles. For purposes of dissection the boundary of the axilla is the axillary artery

3. Benign breast lesions which confer an increased risk of subsequent development of breast cancer include:

A. Duct ectasia

B. Apocrine metaplasia

C. Sclerosing adenosis

D. Atypical ductal hyperplasia

E. Mild epithelial hyperplasia

4. The work-up of a patient with a breast mass would include:

A. Bilateral mammogram

B. An ultrasound done either initially in a younger woman or as a follow-up to mammography in selected cases

C. Fine-needle aspiration cytology, but only after the noninvasive procedures have been performed

D. Core biopsy of a palpable lesion

E. All of the above

5. Suspicious abnormalities which are nonpalpable and only detectable on mammography should:

A. Be taken to the operating room for needle localized breast biopsy

B. Undergo observation with a follow-up mammogram after 3-4 months

C. Be evaluated by ultrasound to determine if the lesion is cystic or solid

D. Be sampled by a stereotactic core biopsy under mammographic guidance

E. All of the above

6. Inherited breast cancer is:

A. Responsible for approximately 25% of all diagnosed breast cancers

B. Diagnosed at an earlier age than most cases of sporadic breast cancer

C. More likely to be both multifocal and bilateral

D. Most often caused by mutations in the BRCA I and BRCA II genes

E. All of the above

7. In comparison to ductal carcinoma *in situ*, lobular carcinoma *in situ*:

A. Occurs at an earlier age

B. Has a more prolonged time lag between diagnosis and subsequent development of invasive cancer

C. Is a predictor of risk of subsequent development of cancer in both breasts

D. Is currently considered a marker for increased risk of the development of breast cancer rather than a cancer itself

E. All of the above

8. Contraindications to breast conservation therapy include:

A. Tumors greater than 3 cm in size

B. A tumor which is noted to be 3 cm posterior to the nipple

C. A 1 cm lower inner quadrant tumor with malignant-appearing calcifications in the upper outer quadrant of the same breast

D. A 2 cm cancer in a previously irradiated breast

E. All of the above

9. Which of the following cases should be considered for adjuvant chemotherapy?

A. A 9 mm cancer with negative lymph nodes and positive ER and PR

B. A 2 cm node-negative breast cancer with positive PR and ER

C. A 5 mm node-negative cancer which is receptor negative

D. All of the above

10. Drug prophylaxis of breast cancer is:

A. Considered an experimental technique

B. Associated with a 50% reduction in risk

C. Associated with no significant side effects

D. Effective when given for at least 1 year

E. All of the above

Answers

1. A., C. and D.
All but the thoracic portion of the primitive milk streak regresses late in the first trimester and maturation during early menarche is initially regulated by estrogen synthesis.

2. A., D.
The three levels of the axillary nodes are based on their relationship to the pectoralis minor muscle. The axilla is bordered superiorly by the axillary vein.

3. C., D.
Duct ectasia, apocrine metaplasia and mild epithelial hyperplasia are considered nonproliferative with no increased risk of breast cancer. Sclerosing adenosis is a proliferative lesion which confers only a slightly increased risk. Atypical hyperplasia, however, is a proliferative lesion which confers a definite increased risk, particularly in patients with a positive family history.

4. E.
All of these procedures are indicated in the work-up of a breast mass. Invasive procedures such as FNA and core biopsy should be delayed until after mammography because bleeding secondary to these procedures may cause otherwise benign lesions to appear suspicious on both mammogram and ultrasound.

5. D.
A 3-month follow-up mammogram would not be appropriate in a lesion characterized as suspicious on initial mammography. While open biopsy is a possibility, a stereotactic core biopsy would provide a diagnosis that, if malignant, would allow the patient to undergo definitive therapy with their initial surgical procedure. Ultrasound can be used to differentiate solid from cystic lesions, but tissue diagnosis is mandatory on the basis of a suspicious mammographic report.

6. B., C. and D.
Hereditary breast cancer is responsible for, at most, 10% of all disease. Early age at diagnosis and a predisposition toward multifocal bilateral disease are hallmarks of truly inherited breast cancer. BRCA I and BRCA II are felt to be responsible for 80%-90% of inherited breast cancers.

7. E.
All of the facts listed above are true about LCIS.

8. C., D.
A finding of multicentric tumors is considered an absolute contraindication to breast conservation therapy. A lesion deep to the nipple which can be excised with negative margins should not preclude breast conservation therapy. In addition, there is no absolute size cut-off for breast conservation therapy, but rather the size of the tumor in relation to the size of the remainder of the breast is the determining factor.

9. B.
All node-positive patients should be considered for adjuvant chemotherapy, and node-negative tumors larger than 1 cm, even if they are receptor positive, should at minimum be considered for chemotherapy in conjunction with tamoxifen. For tumors smaller than 1 cm, if they are receptor positive, tamoxifen would be the treatment of choice. A 5 mm tumor should not receive adjuvant therapy regardless of hormone receptor status.

10. B.
On the basis of the results of the NSABP P-1 trial, tamoxifen is now clinically indicated in patients who are at high risk for breast cancer, with an expected reduction in incidence of approximately 50%. There are, however, side effects, including an increased risk of uterine cancer as well as possible thromboembolic effects. The time period for which tamoxifen has been demonstrated to be efficacious is over a 5-year course of therapy.

Chapter 9: Benign Diseases of the Esophagus, Stomach and Duodenum

Hernan I. Vargas, MD

Contents

1. Disorders of Esophageal Motility

Achalasia

Definition and Epidemiology

Achalasia is a motor disorder of the esophagus characterized by a functional obstruction of the distal esophagus due to incomplete relaxation of the lower esophageal sphincter (LES).[1] Consequently there is lack of progressive peristalsis in the body of the esophagus.

The incidence of achalasia is about 0.5-1 case/100,000 population, and is most prevalent between the ages of 20 and 50, but also occurs in the elderly and during childhood.[2] It has no gender predilection.

Pathophysiology

The etiology of idiopathic achalasia remains unclear. Histologically, there is loss of ganglion cells in the myoenteric plexus of Auerbach, in particular the inhibitory neurons that secrete vasoactive intestinal polypeptide and nitric oxide synthase. These changes cause increased resting pressure of the LES and incomplete relaxation upon swallowing. Disordered esophageal body motility follows with lack of progressive peristalsis.[3]

Secondary achalasia (pseudoachalasia) may be of neuropathic origin (Chagas disease, postvagotomy and diabetes mellitus), or may be caused by distal obstruction (carcinoma, lymphoma or infiltrative disorders). Esophageal carcinoma can cause pseudoachalasia or occur secondary to chronic longstanding esophagitis and dysplasia in patients with achalasia (there is a 7-fold higher incidence of esophageal squamous cell carcinoma in patients with achalasia[4]).

Clinical Presentation

The typical patient, an adult between 20 and 50 years of age, usually complains of a long history (frequently several years) of progressive dysphagia to liquids and solids. Initially the dysphagia may be intermittent and may be worsened by emotional stress or ingestion of cold liquids. Patients tend to eat slowly, and in an effort to seek relief drink liquids, extend the neck, elevate the chin and do Valsalva maneuvers. Regurgitation is common, particularly in the recumbent position, as a consequence of large volumes of saliva and food retained in the esophagus. Respiratory symptoms also occur due to frequent aspiration. Weight loss follows in the more advanced stages of disease. Although pain occurs with some frequency, a subset of patients suffers from vigorous achalasia that is characterized by severe retrosternal pain associated with esophageal contractions.

Assessment and Diagnosis

Initial evaluation should include a chest x-ray. In advanced stages a sigmoid esophagus with retained liquids may show a widened mediastinal silhouette with an air-fluid level in the posterior mediastinum. Evidence of aspiration may be seen in the lung fields. A subtler finding is the absence of a gastric bubble.

A barium swallow may be normal in the early stages of disease. It characteristically shows a dilated esophagus with evidence of tertiary waves and narrow tapering distally that has the appearance of a bird's beak as shown in Figure 1. In advanced stages of disease, a tortuous, sigmoid esophagus may be present. Barium swallow is also valuable in evaluating other possible causes of obstructive symptoms, such as a tumor or benign strictures.

Figure 1

Barium esophagogram of a patient with achalasia. The bird's-beak appearance of the esophagus is apparent.

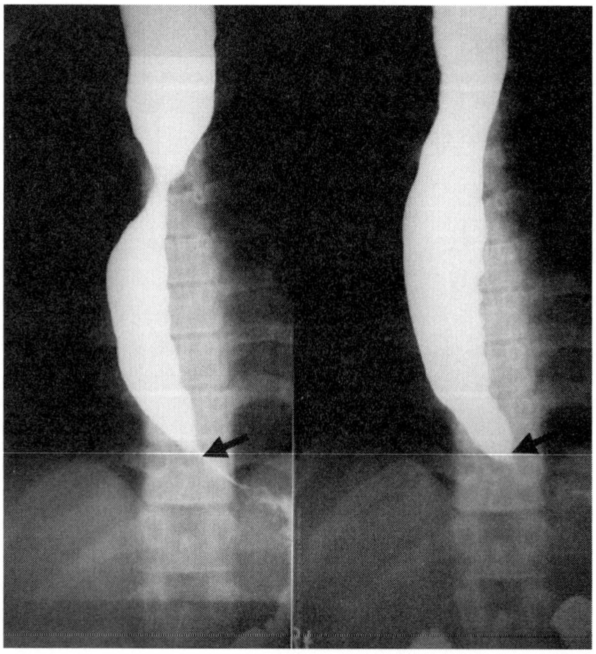

Esophageal manometry is used to confirm the diagnosis. Elevated LES pressure, incomplete relaxation of the LES upon swallowing and lack of progressive peristalsis of the body of the esophagus are the hallmarks of achalasia on esophageal manometry.[1]

Retention esophagitis is seen frequently on upper endoscopy. Examination may be difficult due to retained food and inflammatory or fibrotic changes. In either case, esophageal examination must be thorough with careful attention paid to the cardia in a retroflexed view.

Management

The treatment of achalasia is directed toward relieving the obstruction caused by the nonrelaxing LES. A practical treatment approach for patients with achalasia is presented in Figure 2. Medical therapy using diet or behavioral changes is futile. Nitrates, given either orally or sublingually, can cause temporary relief in mild cases of achalasia, but are associated with significant side effects of headache and postural hypotension. Calcium channel blockers (nifedipine, verapamil) taken before meals may also be effective. These drugs cause short-lived symptomatic relief and may be useful for short periods of time in patients awaiting definitive therapy.[5] Long-term medical therapy is generally reserved for elderly patients who are not candidates for more permanent forms of therapy or as an adjunct in those who have partially or completely failed them.

Intersphincteric injection of botulinum toxin can be done endoscopically with or without the aid of endoscopic ultrasound. This agent acts by blocking cholinergic excitatory nerves in the sphincter causing relaxation of the LES. It is effective for short-term relief of

Figure 2

Practical approach to the management of achalasia

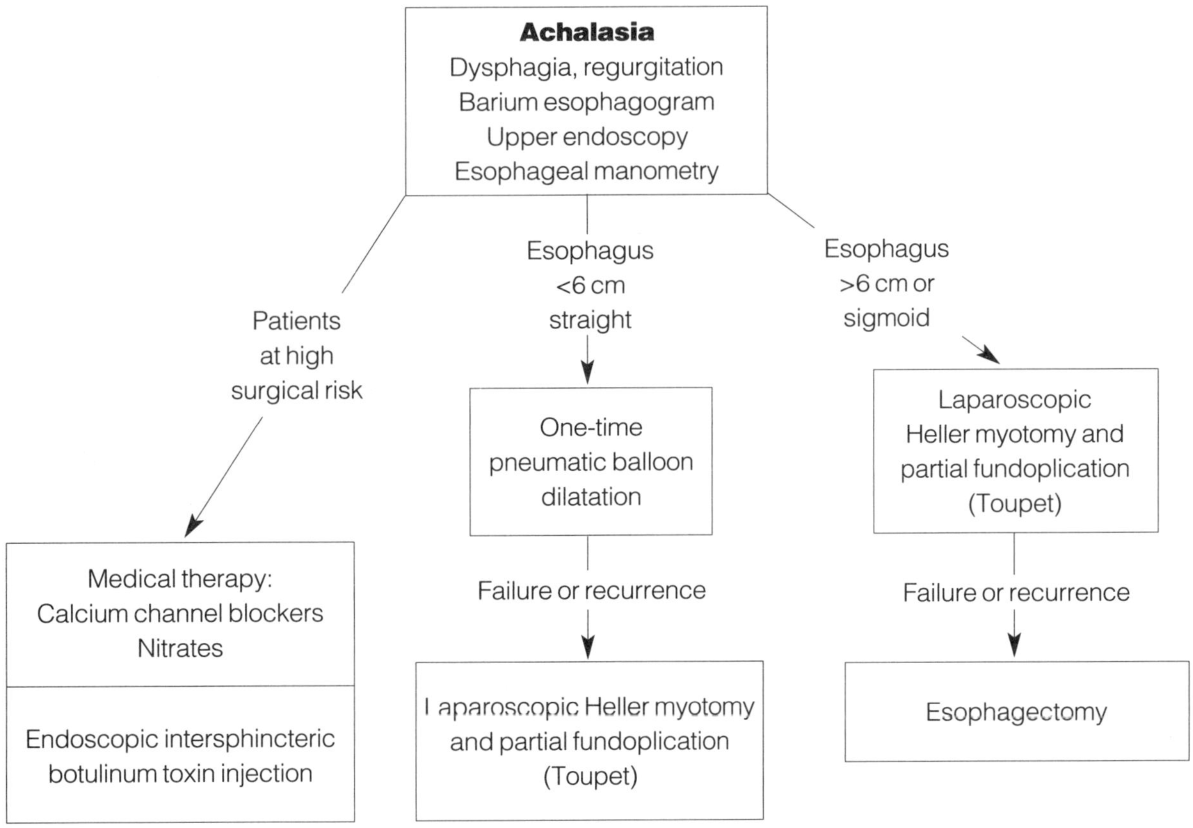

symptoms in 60% of patients; clinical improvement lasts from 2-6 months.[6] Long-term follow-up data are limited, but available data suggest that the majority of patients require repeat therapy. The major advantages of botulinum toxin are its ease of use and lack of significant complications. Only 20% of patients complain of transient chest or epigastric pain.

Pneumatic balloon dilatation of the LES is an effective means of relieving LES obstruction by causing disruption of the muscular layer of the sphincter. Approximately two-thirds of patients experience symptomatic relief after a single dilatation, and after multiple dilatation sessions the effectiveness approaches 65%-85%.[7,8] This procedure is performed by placing a balloon at the level of the LES under fluoroscopic guidance. Once at the appropriate level, the balloon is insufflated to a pressure slightly higher than is necessary to cause disappearance of the gastroesophageal waist under fluoroscopy, generally to a pressure no higher than 10 psi. The duration of dilatation is variable from a few seconds up to 2 or 3 minutes. A serious complication of this technique is esophageal perforation, and it occurs in 5% of patients.[1] Patients with an intramural or contained perforation can frequently be managed nonoperatively by the use of intravenous antibiotics and by abstaining from oral intake. Patients with noncontained perforation in the thoracic or peritoneal cavity should be treated surgically, at which time definitive surgical therapy for achalasia should be seriously considered in addition to repair of the perforation. The results of an aggressive surgical approach to repair of the perforation and esophagomyotomy are comparable to those of elective surgical myotomy.[9] Other complications of balloon dilatation occur in up to 30% of patients, and include esophageal hematoma, diverticula, chronic pain and reflux. Though not universally accepted, elderly patients, young children, patients with a sigmoid esophagus and those with hiatal hernia or esophageal diverticula are thought to be at higher risk for complications.

Surgical esophagomyotomy is highly successful in the treatment of achalasia, and between 75% and 90% of patients enjoy long-term symptomatic relief.[10] Most variants of esophagomyotomy are modifications of the Heller myotomy. It can be performed through a thoracic or an abdominal approach using either open or laparoscopic techniques with minimal morbidity. An important aspect of the surgical procedure, regardless of whether it is laparoscopic or open, transthoracic or transabdominal, involves the incision through the circular and longitudinal muscle fibers, across the LES. An initial incision is enlarged longitudinally to involve the distal 6 cm of the esophagus and distally 1 or 2 cm towards the gastric cardia. During this procedure, the mucosa and submucosa are spared and typically protrude through the myotomy. Attention must be paid to confirm the division of all muscle fibers, and the sectioned muscle edges generally spread about 1 cm apart.

Gastroesophageal reflux occurs as a long-term complication of surgery in 8%-50% of patients.[11,12] The primary factors contributing to postoperative reflux are the extent of dissection in the esophageal hiatus and diaphragmatic crura and the degree to which the myotomy is extended into the cardia. Gastroesophageal reflux occurs more often after a transabdominal operation due to more extensive dissection of the esophageal hiatus and disruption of the phrenoesophageal ligament. Some authors advocate routine use of a partial fundoplication (Dor, Touppet) in order to decrease the incidence of gastroesophageal reflux when the operation is done transabdominally.[13] A limited myotomy that extends into the gastric cardia only minimally has been proposed as a means of decreasing postoperative reflux. However, there is a 10%-20% higher failure rate due to incomplete myotomy.[14]

The use of minimally invasive techniques has dramatically changed the postoperative recovery of patients undergoing esophagomyotomy. Early results are comparable to those of open surgery.[15] The use of a laparoscopic or thoracoscopic approach is primarily based on the training and experience of the surgeon. Both methods offer comparable success with equally good outcomes, although the postoperative recovery is better after laparoscopy.

Single institution and multicenter studies support that pneumatic balloon dilatation and surgical myotomy are effective means of treatment for patients with achalasia. These studies also support the concept that esophagomyotomy is more reliable, providing good to excellent relief of dysphagia. Csendes,[16] in the only prospective randomized study, has compared these 2 methods. 95% of patients treated by surgery improved, compared to 65% in the pneumatic dilatation group.

Due to the higher efficacy, esophagomyotomy is recommended for young patients with achalasia. Nevertheless, we cannot ignore the benefit of pneumatic dilatation in that it is an outpatient procedure that does not require surgery. From a practical point of view, we offer elderly or infirm patients with achalasia a single pneumatic dilatation and follow the subjective and objective outcome of this therapy. If there is significant persistent or recurrent symptoms, we proceed to a laparoscopic esophagomyotomy with a partial fundoplication. Patients who present with a sigmoid megaesophagus are initially treated by laparoscopic esophagomyotomy with a partial fundoplication rather than pneumatic dilatation. If this approach fails and patients have persistent symptoms, the decision to perform a transhiatal esophagectomy is individualized.

Diffuse Esophageal Spasm

Definition and Pathophysiology

This is a functional disease of the esophagus of muscular and neurologic origin characterized by the presence of simultaneous esophageal contractions that correlate with episodes of chest pain and dysphagia.

The pathophysiology of DES is poorly understood. The pain and dysphagia that occur are attributed to repetitive, simultaneous, high-amplitude esophageal contractions. Symptoms may be exacerbated during periods of emotional stress or with the ingestion of cold liquids or solids.

Clinical Presentation

Patients typically complain of retrosternal chest pain that is described as oppressive and may radiate to the jaw, arms and through to the back. Symptoms may be worse during periods of stress and are intermittently associated with dysphagia.

Assessment and Diagnosis

Initial evaluation is directed at investigating angina pectoris and coronary artery disease as possible sources of pain. Having excluded a cardiac source, a thorough and carefully directed history may elicit associated gastrointestinal complaints. Esophageal evaluation includes a barium esophagogram that may reveal a corkscrew esophagus that represents simultaneous contractions of the circular muscle layer. A pulsion diverticulum in a symptomatic patient is diagnostic of diffuse esophageal spasm.

The diagnostic test of choice is esophageal manometry. It is difficult to interpret because simultaneous, multiphasic, repetitive, high amplitude contractions after a swallow in the presence of otherwise normal peristalsis are also seen in asymptomatic individuals, causing a significant degree of overlap between symptomatic individuals and normal volunteers. Stricter criteria to discriminate patients with diffuse esophageal spasm and correlation with the patient's symptoms have been proposed. These include a high frequency of contractions (2 standard deviations above normal volunteers) and involvement of at least 60% of the length of the esophagus.

Management

Initial management of DES consists of reassurance that the pain is not cardiac in origin. Patients' symptoms may decrease in severity and frequency through avoidance of any precipitating factors. Diet and behavioral modification may play a significant role in the improvement of symptoms. Pharmacologic management consists of sublingual nitroglycerine when symptoms develop. In those patients with reproducible symptoms during or after meals, preprandial medication may be effective.

Long esophagomyotomy has been proposed as an option for patients with severe symptoms that are refractory to medical management. This operation involves a left thoracotomy with a myotomy of the esophagus that extends from the aortic arch proximally to 1 cm into the cardia distally. Frequently, a partial fundoplication such as a Belsey-Mark IV is added. Careful documentation of the esophageal motility disorder and correlation with symptoms is essential in patient selection. The success rate is approximately 50%-60%, but in highly selected series following strict criteria for diagnosis, the success rate is on the order of 80%-90%.[17]

Scleroderma

Definition and Epidemiology

Esophageal motility disorders may occur in several of the collagen vascular diseases, such as dermatomyositis, polymyositis, and lupus erythematosus, but are more common in scleroderma. Gastrointestinal involvement occurs in up to 80% of patients with scleroderma.[18] The esophagus is the most frequently affected, but functional problems of the ano-rectum, small bowel, colon and stomach may occur.

Pathophysiology

Smooth muscle atrophy and, to a lesser degree fibrosis, cause a loss of esophageal peristalsis, a defect of the lower esophageal sphincter and gastric hypomotility, thus predisposing to severe reflux esophagitis. Peptic strictures occur in up to 40% of patients with scleroderma.[19]

Clinical Presentation

The initial symptom may be dysphagia if involvement begins in the esophageal body. As the disease progresses, the LES is involved and reflux symptoms predominate. Evidence of gastric outlet obstruction is common and patients also complain of epigastric discomfort and pain.

Assessment and Diagnosis

Initial assessment in patients with dysphagia should include a barium esophagogram that frequently reveals esophageal atony or tertiary waves. Upper endoscopy reveals findings consistent with reflux disease and manometry typically shows decreased peristalsis in the distal two-thirds of the esophagus with diminished contraction amplitude. The LES is atonic.

Management

Lifestyle changes, prokinetic drugs and long-term use of proton pump inhibitors (PPI) are the mainstays of therapy. Patients with intractable symptoms or persistent esophagitis should be considered for antireflux surgery. Due to the esophageal motility disorder, a partial wrap is preferred, and in cases of esophageal shortening, a Collis gastroplasty is necessary. Antireflux surgery, gastrectomy and esophagectomy have been used in patients with scleroderma with good results in highly selected subsets of patients.[20] The goals of therapy are obtaining symptomatic relief and the prevention of strictures.

2. Gastroesophageal Reflux Disease (GERD)

Definition

GERD is the involuntary, repeated or prolonged, migration of gastric contents from the stomach to the esophagus. Consequently, it gives rise to symptoms and anatomic changes in the esophagus.

Epidemiology

GERD is prevalent in the Western hemisphere, however epidemiological data of documented GERD are not well defined. Reflux symptoms occur along a continuum of severity. It is estimated that 36% of a presumably normal population experiences heartburn at least once a month. Daily heartburn occurs in up to 7% of adults.[21] The actual prevalence of the disease is not fully known because symptoms do not reliably correlate with abnormal gastroesophageal reflux measured by prolonged pH monitoring.

GERD occurs equally in both sexes and prevalence increases with age. Reflux symptoms occur commonly during pregnancy, likely due to the increased abdominal pressure from the enlarging uterus and as a consequence of the relaxing effects of the pregnancy hormones on the LES.

Pathophysiology

The etiology of gastroesophageal reflux disease is multifactorial. A number of anatomic and physiologic factors contribute to reflux of gastric contents and the symptoms and anatomic consequences of GERD.

Lower Esophageal Sphincter (LES). Relaxation of the LES is the most significant factor in the occurrence of reflux. The LES physiologically relaxes after swallowing and following distension of the fundus of the stomach. Episodes of relaxation also occur postprandially and because of the presence of fat in the duodenum. DeMeester proposes that the resting sphincter pressure and the total and abdominal length of the sphincter determine LES competence.[22,23]

Diaphragmatic Hiatus. Electromyographic studies show that the striated muscle of the diaphragmatic crura participates in esophageal continence. Its action is particularly noticeable upon sudden increases in abdominal pressure in preventing "stress reflux." The causal role of hiatal hernia on gastroesophageal reflux is controversial. Approximately 2%-5% of individuals in the general population have a hiatal hernia and do not suffer from significant GERD.[24] On the other hand, 85% of patients with GERD suffer from a hiatal hernia.[24] A larger hiatal hernia (more than 2 cm in length) may play a more significant role in the pathophysiology of GERD. Hiatal hernia may contribute to GERD by 3 possible mechanisms: decreased acid clearance, altered constricting function of diaphragmatic crura and decreased effect of intraabdominal pressure on the distal esophagus.

Esophageal Motility and Clearance. Clearance of esophageal contents is accomplished through the action of gravity, peristalsis, and salivary secretions. A number of studies have shown that esophageal peristaltic contractions have lower amplitude in patients with GERD than in normal individuals.[25] Furthermore, the severity of the esophagitis seems to correlate with the peristaltic dysfunction. However, acid clearance times in patients with GERD seem to be close to those in normal individuals.

Once the reflux has occurred, the extent of damage to the esophageal mucosa depends on several factors. The action of the refluxed chyme leads to erosion of the mucosal barrier by the action of acid and pepsin. Patients with bile reflux suffer from more severe esophagitis. Normal mechanisms of clearance include neutralization of acid by the salivary bicarbonate and elimination of the esophageal contents by peristalsis. The severity of esophagitis may correlate with the degree of peristaltic dysfunction.

Clinical Presentation

Patients often complain of a retrosternal burning sensation radiating to the neck, and may also report episodes of regurgitation. Some patients suffer from a retrosternal pressure-like pain that radiates to the shoulders and arms. The differential diagnosis includes cardiac disease, and this should be ruled out first. The refluxate in some cases reaches the hypopharynx and may cause reflux laryngitis and episodes of bronchospasm. The possibility of reflux disease should be entertained in nonallergic patients with nocturnal episodes of asthma that are difficult to control. Advanced cases of reflux esophagitis may present with severe pain and dysphagia due to esophageal ulceration or difficulty swallowing secondary to obstruction by a peptic stricture. Weight loss and malnutrition may ensue in these patients.

Assessment and Diagnosis

The diagnostic evaluation should be tailored to the presenting symptoms. Patients who present with heartburn should have a therapeutic trial of lifestyle changes and acid-reducing therapy with proton pump inhibitors as the initial diagnostic intervention. If this trial of therapy is successful, the treatment is maintained and no other diagnostic evaluation is necessary. Patients who fail initial treatment should undergo upper endoscopy.

Some patients present with symptoms secondary to complications of GERD, such as odynophagia, dysphagia, upper gastrointestinal bleeding, weight loss or anemia. These patients should undergo endoscopic and radiologic evaluation soon after presentation in order to make a prompt diagnosis and to evaluate for other causes of these symptoms, such as achalasia, tumors or strictures.

Upper endoscopy is the initial preferred test in patients suffering from uncomplicated GERD that is recurrent or does not respond to initial medical therapy. It provides important diagnostic information that guides subsequent evaluation and therapy. The range of endoscopic findings includes:

- Normal esophagus: approximately 50% of patients with heartburn or regurgitation have no anatomic evidence of esophageal mucosal damage, but this does not exclude the diagnosis of GERD. 24-hour pH monitoring should be done to document the presence of significant reflux.

- Esophagitis: in the presence of appropriate symptoms in the immunocompetent patient, esophagitis is a reliable indicator of GERD.[26] Redness, linear erosions or ulceration of the mucosa characterizes it. Immunocompromised patients must have biopsy of the abnormal areas for culture and Gram's stain analysis.

- Ulcer/stricture/shortened esophagus: these represent a more advanced degree of mucosal damage with chronic changes. These findings are highly diagnostic of GERD.

- Barrett's esophagus: this is a premalignant condition resulting from chronic irritation by the refluxate. Histologically, the native squamous epithelium of the esophagus is replaced by metaplastic columnar epithelium. In practical terms it is diagnosed when specialized epithelium (ie, intestinal type, containing goblet cells) is identified above the gastroesophageal junction. It is characterized by the endoscopic finding of gastric-like mucosa ascending into the esophagus with a squamocolumnar junction that is located more than 2 cm above the gastroesophageal junction.

Barium esophagogram is a test done in conjunction with upper endoscopy to delineate anatomic and physiologic abnormalities of the esophagus. Barium esophagogram is recommended as the first test in patients complaining of obstructive symptoms of dysphagia or regurgitation of esophageal contents. Some authors have suggested that this test be used for screening and even as a diagnostic method for GERD.[27] However, numerous reports document 25%-30% false positive and false negative rates, making it unreliable.[27] Its primary value is to determine the presence of a large hiatal hernia, a stricture, other obstructing lesion or a shortened esophagus.

Quantitative documentation with a ***24-hour pH study*** of reflux is helpful in the management of patients who suffer from reflux symptoms without anatomic changes of esophagitis, ulceration or Barrett's metaplasia. This study also contributes to the assessment of patients with atypical presentations of GERD, such as noncardiac chest pain, adult-onset asthma or chronic laryngitis, and in patients who have failed medical management. pH monitoring provides a measurement of the period of time the esophageal mucosa is exposed to acid. There is no threshold value of esophageal acid exposure that unequivocally represents a diagnosis of GERD because esophageal acid exposure is just 1 factor in this multifactorial disease.[28]

The test is performed by placing a pH probe 5 cm above the LES. H_2 (histamine 2) receptor antagonists and prokinetics should be stopped 72 hours prior, and PPIs should be stopped for 1 to 2 weeks before the procedure. The time of exposure to acid measured by 24-hour pH monitoring loosely predicts esophageal injury and correlates with the severity of damage. An esophageal pH less than 4.0 is considered a reflux episode. Normal acid exposure time is between 4% and 7% during a 24-hour period. Patients with erosive esophagitis have an average of 12%-15% acid exposure time, and patients with Barrett's metaplasia have an average of 25% acid exposure time. However, approximately 10%-15% of patients with evidence of peptic esophagitis on endoscopy have normal 24-hour pH studies, but it has been reported to be as high as 40%.[29] The degree of reflux varies with the recumbent or upright position of the patient. Furthermore, episodes of continuous and prolonged exposure may cause more esophageal damage than more frequent shorter episodes. In order to improve the accuracy of this technique, a composite score has been developed. DeMeester developed a composite score in order to improve the accuracy of this technique. It takes into account 6 criteria:

- Total number of episodes of reflux
- Number of episodes longer than 5 minutes duration
- Duration of the longest episode
- Percentile time of pH less than 4
- Differential time of percentile upright time of pH less than 4
- Supine percentile time of pH less than 4

Esophageal manometry is used to evaluate limited aspects of esophageal function, such as LES function and the integrity of esophageal primary peristalsis. Manometric findings in patients with GERD include decreased length, increased transient relaxation and hypotension of the LES, and in some cases, impaired esophageal peristalsis. From a surgeon's perspective, it is useful to obtain manometric studies in patients who are contemplating antireflux surgery. Some data indicate that manometric assessment of the LES predicts the likelihood of response to medical therapy and the outcome of surgery, but this idea is not universally accepted.[28] However, it is important to exclude other esophageal pathology, because misguided antireflux surgery may compound other problems, such as achalasia or esophageal spasm. Furthermore, the presence of a motility defect in the esophageal body changes the operative strategy in patients with GERD.

The test is performed by advancing a manometric catheter into the esophagus, through the LES and into the stomach. Pressure recordings are obtained at different levels and plotted over time. The response of esophageal motility and LES function is measured in the basal state, during and after swallowing.

Management

The natural history of GERD is one of recurrent symptoms that persist in long-term follow-up,[30] therefore chronic therapy is required. Complications of GERD develop in as high as 50% of patients, and include esophagitis, esophageal ulcer, esophageal stricture and Barrett's esophagus.

The initial assessment and treatment of patients who suffer from GERD must be tailored to the patient's symptoms and functional assessment, along with a clear understanding of the objectives of therapy. The goals of treatment are relief of symptoms, healing of esophagitis, and treatment of complications.

Figure 3

Upper endoscopy of a patient with Barrett's esophagus. Note the erythematous "salmon patches."

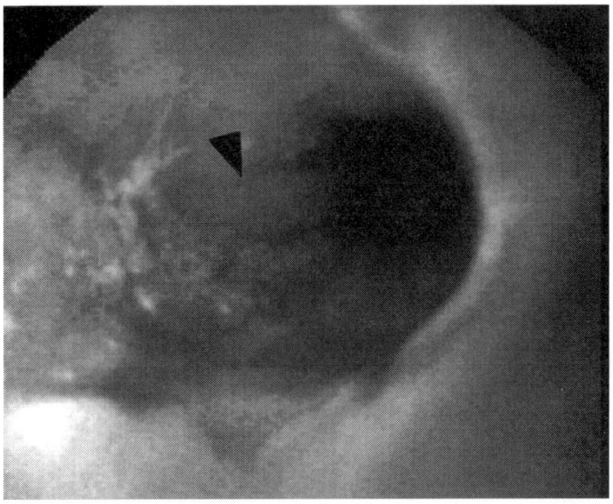

A practical approach to the management of patients with GERD is presented in Figure 4.

Barrett's esophagus is a premalignant condition induced by severe, chronic reflux. Endoscopically, areas of erythematous patches in the esophagus called salmon patches are seen (see Figure 3). It is characterized histologically by columnar metaplasia of the squamous epithelium of the esophagus.

Medical Therapy. The majority of patients with symptoms of uncomplicated GERD receive a trial of medical therapy that includes lifestyle modification. Esophageal acid exposure is decreased by cessation of smoking, decreasing fat intake, and avoiding coffee, chocolate and alcohol. Elevation of the head of the bed and avoiding recumbence for 3 hours after meals facilitate esophageal clearance by gravity.[31] Antacids, H_2 receptor antagonists (cimetidine, ranitidine, famotidine), and PPIs improve the symptoms of GERD and are superior to placebo in controlled trials.[32] Unfortunately, GERD is a chronic disease and patients require long-term therapy. A majority of individuals improve, accept lifestyle modification and use medication intermittently.

A subset of patients with GERD suffers from very frequent, severe or recurrent symptoms. These patients should undergo upper endoscopy as an initial evaluation in order to make a diagnosis and to exclude other pathology. Furthermore, stratification of reflux patients into those with tissue damage and complications and those without tissue damage has important diagnostic and therapeutic implications.

Symptomatic patients without tissue damage should undergo 24-hour pH study to establish a diagnosis of GERD and be treated symptomatically. In addition to lifestyle changes, frequently-used protocols implement H_2 receptor antagonists alone or in combination with prokinetic agents (ie, cisapride). PPIs may be used as well. Patients with evidence of esophagitis should receive a trial of medical therapy with PPIs. It is expected that 80% of patients will have symptomatic relief, and the esophagitis will heal in more than 75% of patients within a 4-8 week period. H_2 receptor antagonists have been used in the treatment of esophagitis with limited success (healing in 45% of patients after 4-8 weeks of ther-

Figure 4

Practical approach to the management of gastroesophageal reflux disease (GERD)

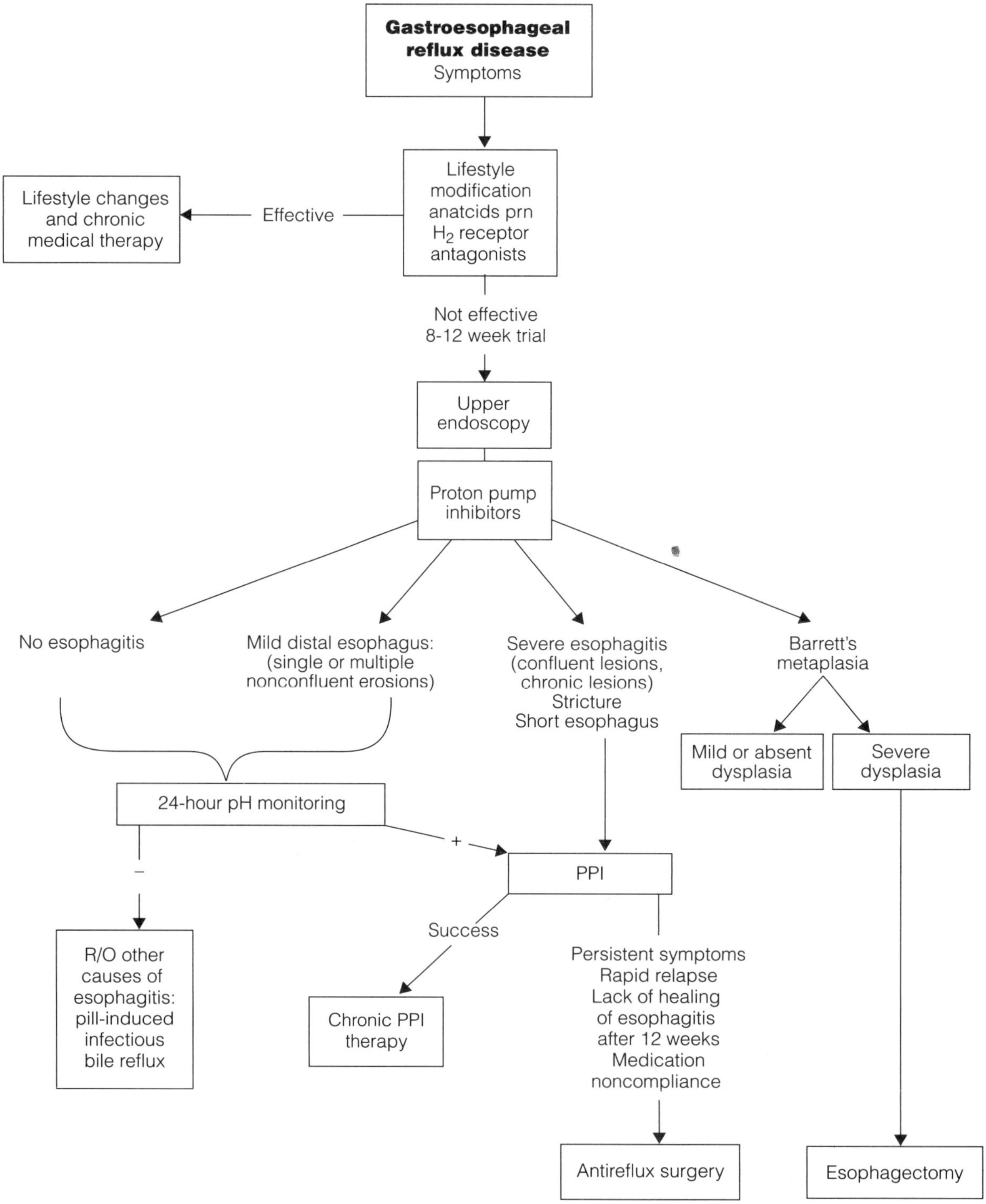

apy).[33] The addition of cisapride improves the efficacy of H_2 receptor antagonists.[34]

Surgical Therapy. Surgery is of tremendous help in the management of GERD in selected groups of patients. Some studies estimate that 10%-25% of patients experience recurrent or progressive disease and are candidates for surgery.[35] Surgical therapy is considered when:

- Patients suffer from a significant disturbance in lifestyle
- Patients' symptoms do not respond to medical therapy
- Patients have persistent esophagitis after best medical therapy including PPIs
- Patients have complications of reflux such as peptic stricture or ulceration
- Patients have reflux laryngitis or nocturnal aspiration and asthma-like symptoms

Patient selection is based on these factors and an objective assessment of the physiologic status of the gastroesophageal junction. If typical peptic esophagitis is not seen on endoscopy, ambulatory 24-hour pH study should be performed to confirm the diagnosis. Evaluation of LES function and esophageal motility is of vital importance in planning antireflux surgery. The results of esophageal manometry change the operative plan in approximately 10% of patients.[36]

A prospective controlled trial has compared medical therapy to surgery, and a significant benefit from surgery was found.[37] However, PPIs as medical therapy vs. laparoscopic antireflux surgery were examined, making this study obsolete for current standards of therapy. The objective of surgery is to restore cardioesophageal competence. Objectives of reconstruction are:

- Reduction of hiatal hernia and closure of the diaphragmatic hiatus
- Abdominal positioning of the gastroesophageal junction and distal esophagus
- Construction of a cardia fundoplication that functions as a valve
- Avoidance of any undesirable sequelae from fundoplication, such as dysphagia or inability to burp

The different surgical procedures done for GERD are described in Table 1. The primary considerations in selecting the operative approach are:

- Minimally invasive vs. open approach: a number of studies have confirmed that patients subjected to laparoscopic or open approaches have similar symptomatic improvement and functional outcomes. In addition, the laparoscopic approach offers the advantages of minimal postoperative pain and shorter hospitalization and convalescent periods. Laparoscopic techniques are the approach of choice in patients with uncomplicated reflux.[38,39]
- Thoracic vs. abdominal approach: the thoracic approach can be selectively used in patients who have a shortened esophagus, particularly if extensive mobilization of the esophagus is anticipated or if a Collis gastroplasty is planned to place the repair in the abdominal position.
- Need for esophageal lengthening procedure: patients with a short esophagus present a challenge in positioning the distal esophagus and fundoplication in the abdomen. A number of adverse outcomes have been reported with an intrathoracic position of the reconstruction, and they include gastric ulceration, progressive herniation and gastric strangulation. A lengthening procedure, such as a Collis gastroplasty, allows for esophageal lengthening and intraabdominal positioning of the reconstruction. This operation is most commonly performed through a thoracic approach, but it can also be done using a transabdominal exposure.
- Type of fundoplication, complete vs. partial: in patients with otherwise uncomplicated reflux, without significant esophageal dysmotility or shortening, the choice of repair depends primarily on the experience of the surgeon. Options include the Nissen fundoplication, Belsey-Mark IV repair, Hill repair, and Toupet or Dor partial fundoplication. Patients with significant loss of peristaltic amplitude in the esophagus may have difficulty

Table 1

Description of Operations Commonly Used in the Management of Gastroesophageal Reflux Disease (GERD)

Operation	Description	Approach	Advantages	Disadvantages/ Complications
Nissen fundoplication	Total (360°) wrap of gastric fundus on the distal esophagus	Laparoscopic transabdominal	Widely used. Gold standard. Good/excellent results in over 90% of cases	Persistent/recurrent reflux in 10%. Dysphagia in 5%-15%. Gas bloat in 10%-20%
Toupet fundoplication	Partial (270°) wrap of gastric fundus on the distal esophagus. Anchoring to the esophageal crux	Laparoscopic transabdominal	Success compar- ableto Nissen fundoplication. Used when esophageal motility is impaired	
Hill gastropexy	Anchoring of the gastroesophageal junction to aortic fascia and median arcuate ligament	Laparoscopic transabdominal	Good to excellent results in over 90% of patients	Lack of familiarity with anatomy and procedure. Dysphagia in 10% Gas bloat in 5%
Belsey-Mark IV antireflux procedure	Construction of 240° two-layer antireflux mechan- ism as a "partial intussusception" of the esophagus into the stomach	Transthoracic	Good to excellent results in over 90% of cases. Commonly used as antireflux repair in transthoracic approach or in con- junction with Collis gastroplasty. Also in patients with impaired esophageal motility	
Collis gastroplasty	Lengthening of short esophagus by the construction of a "neoesophagus" using a stapled gastric cardia tube. It is coupled with a Nissen or Belsey- Mark IV antireflux procedure.	Transthoracic transabdominal laparoscopic/ thoracoscopic	Good/excellent results in 75%-80% of cases. Allows for intraabdominal placement of the gastroesophageal junction and con- structed antireflux mechanism	Esophageal leak in 3%. Outcome is dependent on the severity of strictures and esophageal motility impairment

Figure 5

Endoscopy of a patient with severe peptic stricture

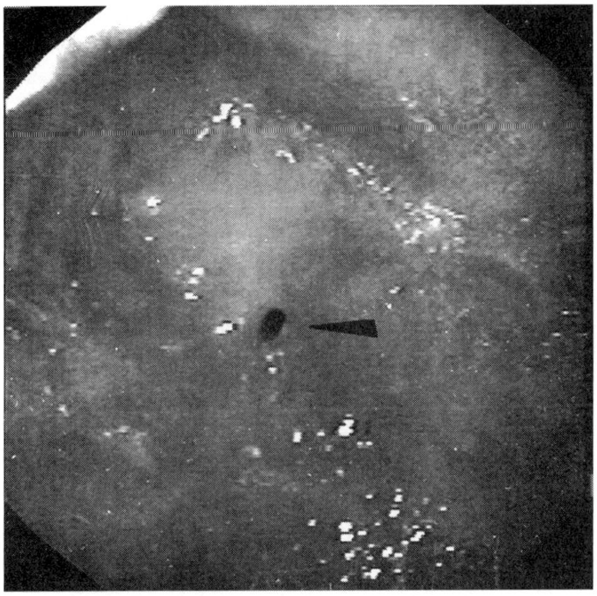

overcoming the newly created cardioesophageal valve when there is a complete wrap of the fundus on the distal esophagus. They should have a partial fundoplication of the Toupet, Dor or Hill type.

Management of Complications

Peptic Stricture. Peptic strictures can occur as a consequence of GERD (see Figure 5). Patients with dilatable peptic strictures can be treated with esophageal dilatation followed by partial fundoplication. This approach is successful in more than 70% of cases.[40] Patients with difficult-to-dilate strictures and those requiring multiple or frequent dilatations should be considered for endoscopic stricturoplasty or stent placement. Non-dilatable esophageal strictures, or those refractory to medical/endoscopic therapy may require resection and reconstruction with gastric-pull-up, jejunum or colonic interposition.

Barrett's Esophagus. In cases of metaplastic epithelium without evidence of dysplasia, endoscopic surveillance is important. Neither surgical techniques[41] nor medical therapy[42] in GERD have convincingly demonstrated a reduction in the rate of progression to high-grade dysplasia or in the incidence of adenocarcinoma. Therefore, uncomplicated Barrett's metaplasia is not considered an indication for surgery, unless the patient suffers from ulcer, esophagitis with stricture, or symptoms that are difficult to treat. An important goal in the management of Barrett's esophagus is to diagnose the presence of severe metaplasia associated with carcinoma of the esophagus in as many as 40% of cases. These patients require esophagectomy. Endoscopic methods for treatment of Barrett's esophagus have been recently developed and long-term follow-up is unavailable. These methods include thermal ablation (monopolar/bipolar cautery, argon plasma coagulation, laser therapy), photodynamic therapy or endomucosal resection.

3. Injuries to the Esophagus

Esophageal Perforation

Esophageal perforation is a serious condition with a high morbidity and mortality. The resulting mediastinitis requires rapid diagnosis and swift treatment.

Epidemiology, Etiology and Pathophysiology

The epidemiology of esophageal perforation has changed as the number of invasive procedures used in the practice of medicine has increased. Iatrogenic perforation of the esophagus accounts for approximately 60% of cases, 20% are the result of external injuries or foreign bodies and 15% are barogenic (Boerhaave's syndrome).[43] The remaining cases are secondary to a variety of conditions, such as carcinoma and infectious esophagitis.

Iatrogenic perforation of the esophagus is seen in less than 0.1% of patients subjected to endoscopy. Injuries occur in the intrathoracic esophagus (80%) or cervical esophagus (20%). The esophagus can also be perforated during dilatation or bougienage at or above the level of the procedure. Procedures involving placement of other devices in the lumen of the esophagus such as use of Sengstaken-Blakemore tubes, endotracheal intubation, placement of nasogastric tubes or feeding tubes, and sclerotherapy are also associated with perforation.

Penetrating injuries to the esophagus occur most commonly at the cervical or thoracic level, and should be investigated in the evaluation of patients with cervical or mediastinal penetrating injuries.

Boerhaave's syndrome occurs as a consequence of a sudden increase in intraluminal esophageal pressure.[44] It can occur in any age group or either sex, but it is more common in middle-aged men who relate a history of vomiting after excessive eating and alcohol consumption. It can take place during retching, vomiting, laughing fits, weightlifting or after blunt abdominal trauma. The full-thickness tear of the distal esophagus frequently develops a communication into the left pleural cavity. In some cases the rupture may be contained in the mediastinum. Communication and contamination of the right pleural cavity or abdomen is seen less commonly, but correlates with rupture of the esophagus in unusual places (upper esophagus or intraabdominal segment).

Whatever the cause of esophageal perforation, the enzyme-laden saliva and gastric juices contaminate the mediastinum causing a severe inflammatory reaction. In addition, the negative intrathoracic pressure contributes to significant contamination of the pleural cavity by this "culture broth" that encourages rapid growth of bacteria. The consequences are a septic picture with massive third-spacing.

Clinical Presentation

Patients with an iatrogenic perforation of the esophagus complain of sudden-onset pain during or immediately after the procedure. Dysphagia is common. Subcutaneous crepitance may be the only finding on early physical examination.

An esophageal injury should be suspected in patients with penetrating injuries to the neck, chest or upper abdomen, based on the trajectory of the penetrating object or missile. A missed injury has dire consequences because patients may progress to sepsis within hours of presentation. The proximity of the esophagus to vital organs, such as the heart, great vessels and airway, contributes to the morbidity and mortality of these injuries. It emphasizes the importance of making an accurate and prompt diagnosis, because these patients are subjected to extensive evaluation to determine the need for immediate surgery.

Patients with Boerhaave's syndrome present with complaints of precordial chest or epigastric pain following an episode of retching or vomiting. An initial physical exam may be normal or may reveal subcutaneous emphysema. A radiographic evaluation of the esophagus is mandatory in patients with such a history because the physical examination may be normal and misleading.

If an esophageal perforation is not suspected, diagnosed and treated early, regardless of the cause, patients develop progressively worsening pain, fever and even signs and symptoms of sepsis from mediastinitis, pleural empyema or peritonitis.

Assessment and Diagnosis

A chest x-ray is essential in the initial evaluation, since it may reveal cervical, mediastinal or pericardial emphysema, evidence of a hydropneumothorax or free air under the diaphragm. Even after a normal

Figure 6

CT scan showing free extraluminal contrast in the left pleural cavity in a patient with Boerhaave's syndrome

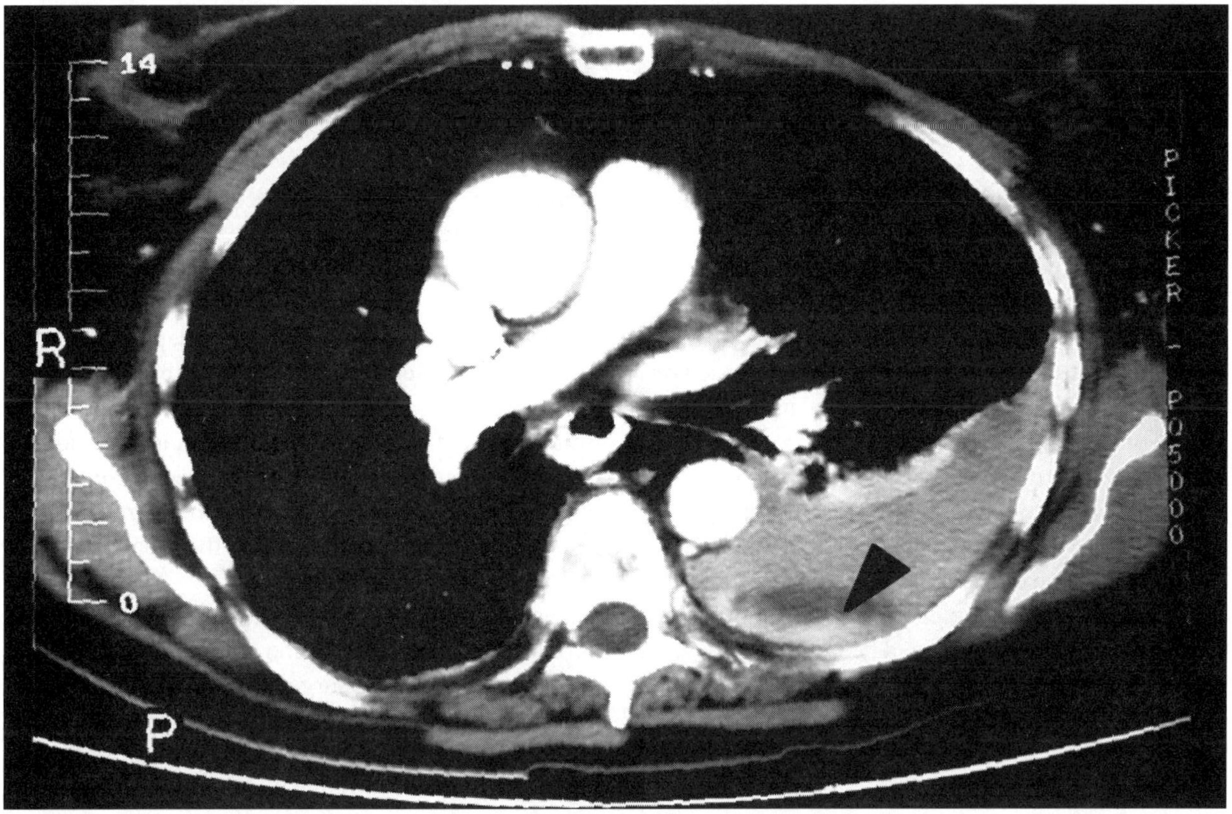

chest x-ray, a study of the esophagus with water-soluble contrast is mandatory in patients with suspected esophageal perforation. If an injury is identified, prompt institution of therapy is essential. An esophagogram with barium contrast should be performed following a negative study with water-soluble contrast because it may detect up to 20% of injuries.[43] In addition to being a diagnostic procedure, this study provides valuable information, such as the site and severity of the injury, that assist in the determination of a therapeutic plan and when indicated, the operative approach. Computed tomography has a complementary role in the diagnosis of esophageal perforation as seen in Figure 6. It is commonly used in the trauma setting, but it may be particularly helpful in the early period after an esophageal injury or in case of minimal injury, when the only findings are esophageal thickening or extraluminal mediastinal air.

Management

Early diagnosis and appropriate treatment are essential for decreased morbidity and mortality. The mortality from esophageal perforation has improved with increased awareness, early recognition, better critical care and superior operative techniques. It is likely that these changes reflect the higher incidence of iatrogenic injuries seen since the advent of endoscopy. Iatrogenic injuries are generally less severe and are usually recognized early.

The mortality of esophageal injury is strongly correlated to the interval of time from the onset of symptoms to the institution of effective therapy. Patients who receive treatment, including operative intervention within 24 hours, suffer a mortality rate of about 10%-25%, whereas in patients with delayed presentation the mortality ranges from 25%-90%.[45,46]

There is a spectrum of severity of injuries to the esophagus. Therefore, the management of individual patients should be tailored to the characteristics of the perforation, underlying esophageal disease and overall condition. Initial efforts are directed to fluid resuscitation and administration of antimicrobial agents. Diagnostic evaluation takes place simultaneously.

Patients without evidence of clinical sepsis who on radiographic studies have a contained perforation with spontaneous drainage into the esophagus may be treated nonoperatively.[47] The clinical course must be followed expectantly because any indication of sepsis or deterioration should prompt operative treatment. The success of this therapy is based on proper patient selection. Reports primarily based on postendoscopic iatrogenic esophageal injuries, dilatation or bougienage indicate a success rate of 90%-100%. Active intervention is indicated in those patients who have any evidence of sepsis or those who have evidence of noncontained extraluminal contrast on esophagography.[48] The preferred approach and the principles of operative approach are debridement of injured and necrotic tissue, repair of the esophageal injury, and irrigation and drainage of the mediastinum and pleural spaces.

The surgical approach is tailored to the level of the injury and the body cavity involved. The segment of esophagus involved must be defined on radiographic studies in order to plan the operative approach. Injuries to the cervical esophagus are approached through a longitudinal incision anterior to the sternocleidomastoid muscle. Injuries to the upper thoracic esophagus require a right thoracotomy, while a low (seventh intercostal space) left thoracotomy is used for perforation of the distal esophagus. The rare injuries to the short abdominal esophagus are approached through an upper midline laparotomy.

After adequate and wide exposure has been obtained, extensive debridement of the nonviable tissue in the esophagus and mediastinum is done in order to clearly identify the limits of the perforation. It is often necessary to extend the traumatic myotomy superiorly and inferiorly in order to define the extent of the mucosal injury, particularly in cases of barogenic rupture. The esophageal defect can be closed, generally in the longitudinal direction over a 42F or larger dilator within the esophagus. The repair must use viable esophageal tissue and be tension free. Numerous techniques with purportedly similar success have been described for closure, including single layer closure with absorbable sutures, double layer closure with absorbable and/or nonabsorbable sutures, or a stapled technique. The suture line can be reinforced with tissue on a vascularized pedicle. Most commonly parietal pleura, pericardium, intercostal muscle or even omentum are used. The fundus of the stomach as a partial fundoplication is ideal for reinforcement of distal esophageal repairs as long as the stomach can be replaced into the abdomen.

The success of esophageal repair is dependent on the nutritional and immune status of the patient, the underlying disease of the esophagus, adequate identification of the extent of the mucosal injury and quality of the repair, and on the degree of contamination and inflammatory reaction in the mediastinum and pleura at the time of the repair.

The severity of mediastinitis and pleural irritation worsens as a function of time after an injury. This concept has led some surgeons to propose that the esophageal perforation should not be repaired in patients who present more than 24-48 hours after the onset of symptoms due to a high failure rate of the repair. An array of alternative procedures has been proposed for patients with very large esophageal tears or massive tissue injury and contamination.

After the initial exploration and debridement, the esophageal perforation can be drained with an intraluminal T tube with the intention of creating a controlled fistula to avoid continuous leakage into the mediastinum and pleura. The mortality using this approach varies from 36%-50%.[43] Another method of decreasing continuous contamination is by exclusion of the esophageal perforation. This can be accomplished by stapling or oversawing the esophagus proximal and distal to the perforation while a nasogastric tube is placed in the proximal stump. Some surgeons advocate proximal diversion through a cervical esophagostomy as an alternative. Long-term sequelae of these methods commit the patient to subsequent surgery for closure of the esophagostomy and dilatation or surgery for the likely stricture at the level of the banding.

Patients with underlying severe esophageal disease and a large perforation treated at a late stage may be candidates for resection therapy with immediate or delayed esophageal conduit reconstruction.

Recent literature supports the view that repair of esophageal injuries, even after a 24-48-hour delay before presentation, yields good success rates, even comparable to that of repairs done within the first 24 hours.[49,50] Therefore, the decision to repair the perforation is based on a careful intraoperative assessment of the injury and the degree of contamination of the pleura, as well as the overall nutritional and septic status of the patient, and not solely on the time interval since the perforation. A changing pattern of injuries with lesser degrees of severity and improved intensive care most likely play an adjunctive role in the better results seen with repair after the first 24 hours.

Stent placement as a means of esophageal perforation exclusion has been reportedly used in patients in whom resection is not feasible.[51] We have used endoluminal covered stents with success in rare patients who present very late after an esophageal perforation, are poor operative risks and have an adequately drained pleural cavity through the use of thoracostomy tubes.

Caustic Ingestion

Caustic ingestion causes severe acute injury and debilitating chronic sequelae due to chemical injury of the esophageal and gastric mucosa.

Epidemiology and Pathophysiology

Ingestion of caustic agents is bimodal in its incidence: young children may accidentally swallow a caustic agent, and adults attempting suicide are the second group affected by this ailment.[52] The degree of damage caused by caustic ingestion is related to the physical characteristics of the compound (solid versus liquid), pH (acid or alkaline), the volume ingested and the time the mucosa are exposed to the substance. Solid caustics tend to adhere to the oropharyngeal mucosa, causing localized damage. Liquids on the other hand rapidly travel through the esophagus to the stomach, causing damage to both organs. Alkaline substances tend to rapidly injure the esophagus and stomach, whereas acids do less damage to the esophagus. Upon reaching the pylorus, pylorospasm occurs and the caustic liquid pools in the antrum. It subsequently causes relaxation of the LES and refluxes into the distal esophagus. Esophageal and gastric atony immediately follow.

Direct tissue damage occurs and may be only superficial or may involve full-thickness necrosis of the esophagus or stomach. The initial degree of penetration and tissue damage determines the potential for acute life-threatening complications and for long term sequelae. If full-thickness necrosis takes place, superinfection and sepsis occur. Patients with partial thickness injury may suffer from long-term complications such as stricture formation. Patients with superficial injuries generally recover uneventfully.

Clinical Presentation

Clinical manifestations vary according to the sites and severity of injury. The most dramatic cases present with severe airway compromise due to edema of the hypopharynx and larynx. More often symptoms are related to mucosal and tissue injury of the esophagus when patients complain of retrosternal pain, odynophagia or dysphagia, or injury to the stomach with epigastric or abdominal pain, nausea and vomiting. Patients who suffer from full-thickness necrosis of viscera will experience signs and symptoms of mediastinitis, peritonitis or sepsis characterized by severe chest or abdominal pain, severe third-spacing and sepsis.

Assessment and Diagnosis

Initial steps are directed at assessment and management of the airway and fluid resuscitation. Early upper endoscopy after initial resuscitative measures is important in guiding further management. Endoscopic appearance of the injured mucosa may reveal erythema, edema, blistering or ulceration in the acute setting. Caution must be exercised in the use of endoscopy due to the fragility of the injured tissues. A pediatric flexible endoscope is frequently used.

In cases of suspected early perforation a Gastrografin esophagogram is indicated. If negative, thin barium should be used for better definition of the mucosa and more sensitive identification of a perforation. Chest and abdominal series, or the more sensitive CT scan may reveal early evidence of perforation if extraluminal air is seen in the mediastinum or abdomen.

Management

Caustic injury takes place in the span of seconds to a few minutes, therefore there are no specific measures directed at minimizing direct tissue damage once the patient is seen. Induction of emesis is contraindicated because it can cause further exposure of the esophagus, and more importantly, of the larynx. Prospective studies have proven that corticosteroids are not useful and may have potential adverse effects.[53] If endoscopy reveals minimal or no mucosal injury, no further therapy is necessary. If there is evidence of partial-thickness injuries, the patient must be closely followed for the risk of perforation or full-thickness necrosis.

Patients with clinical or radiologic evidence of full-thickness necrosis and perforation should undergo immediate laparotomy, resection and debridement of the damaged tissue. If necrosis of the stomach is seen, a gastrectomy should be done. A transhiatal esophagectomy can be done if there is any evidence of esophageal necrosis or mediastinitis. Reconstruction of the alimentary tract should not be attempted at this operation. The cervical esophagus is then exteriorized as a stoma in the neck or upper chest. Nutritional support via enteral feeding should then be begun.

After the acute phase, patients with partial-thickness injuries suffer from a high incidence of stricture formation. Initial options for management are nonsurgical, with dilatation therapy either with a bougie or a pneumatic balloon. Recent data suggest that placement of Silastic® stents early in the course of caustic injury may prevent the development and decrease the severity of strictures.

Patients who cannot be dilated, those who fail repeated dilatation, patients who require esophageal dilatations 6 months after the injury, and patients who suffer from perforation during dilatation of strictures should undergo esophageal reconstruction. The ideal substitute for the esophageal tissue is stomach tissue, however in a significant proportion of these patients the stomach is partially injured by the caustic agent. Therefore, a colonic interposition graft is commonly used as a conduit. Esophageal resection should be performed at the same time to allow for placement of the conduit in the posterior mediastinum and avoid the long-term risk of malignancy (these patients havc a 1000-fold increased risk of malignancy compared to the general population).

4. Esophageal Diverticula

Esophageal diverticula are pouches arising from the esophageal lumen. They are classified based on their location, pathophysiology and histology. Based on these factors the clinician can gain an understanding of their origin, natural history and appropriate management.

Pharyngoesophageal (Zenker's) Diverticulum

Definition

This is a diverticulum occurring through Killian's triangle in the posterior pharyngoesophageal junction, defined inferiorly by the upper border of the cricopharyngeus muscle and superolaterally by the right and left thyropharyngeus muscles.

Epidemiology and Pathophysiology

Zenker's diverticulum is the most commonly recognized form of esophageal diverticulum, and it affects middle-aged and elderly patients. It is a pulsion diverticulum caused by lack of coordination of the swallowing mechanism. The pharyngeal musculature contracts after constriction of the cricopharyngeus, causing markedly increased pressures in the hypopharynx that are transmitted to the weakest point, the triangle of Killian.[54]

Clinical Presentation

Dysphagia localized to the neck is the main complaint, and it varies with the degree of motor dysfunction. As the diverticulum enlarges, patients notice gurgling sounds in the neck and regurgitation of undigested food, and they suffer from episodes of aspiration. As these symptoms impair their ability to acquire nutrition, the patient experiences weight loss.

Assessment and Diagnosis

A barium esophagogram is the study of choice for detecting Zenker's diverticulum. Upper esophageal sphincter manometry is difficult to perform and interpret due to the interference of laryngeal excursion and movement during swallowing. Upper endoscopy must be undertaken with caution in patients with suspected Zenker's diverticulum, particularly a large one, due to the potential risk of perforation.

Management

Relief of the functional distal obstruction with a cricopharyngeal myotomy is the mainstay of treatment.[55] The diverticulum and cricopharyngeus muscles are exposed through a left cervical incision along the sternocleidomastoid muscle. An avascular plane is developed by dissection of the strap muscles, thyroid, trachea and esophagus medially, and the sternocleidomastoid muscle and carotid sheet contents laterally. The recurrent laryngeal nerve must be identified and protected. After ligation and division of the inferior thyroid artery, the diverticulum is uncovered anterior to the prevertebral fascia, generally extending to the left side of the neck. Once the diverticulum has been dissected, a longitudinal myotomy extending for 3-4 cm is carried out posteriorly starting at the base of the diverticulum.

Small diverticula (<3 cm) do not require any further intervention. In addition to a myotomy, larger diverticula are resected to avoid continuous accumulation of food residua and the associated risk of continued aspiration. The primary risk of excision of the diverticulum is a postoperative leak, particularly in a nutritionally depleted patient. If a cricopharyngeal myotomy is not performed, the risk of suture line dehiscence is very high. An alternative is to suspend the diverticulum, suturing it to the prevertebral fascia as a diverticulopexy. This approach may be useful in malnourished patients. An endoscopic technique has been in use for 3 decades.[56] The wall of the diverticulum may also be stapled to the esophageal lumen, creating a side-to-side anastomosis. This is done with an endo-GIA stapler introduced per mouth. Several reports indicate good results with this technique. It is worth considering as an alternative for debilitated patients or patients with a high operative risk.

Epiphrenic and Other Pulsion Diverticula

Pathophysiology

Epiphrenic diverticula arise within the distal 10 cm of the thoracic esophagus. These are pulsion diverticula by nature, caused by segmental increases of intraluminal pressure, particularly above the LES. Histologically these are pseudodiverticula and are formed only by the mucosa and submucosa.

Clinical Presentation, Assessment and Diagnosis

Although some patients are asymptomatic and diverticula are incidental findings, most patients are symptomatic. Dysphagia, regurgitation and pain are the common complaints. However, symptoms are often nonspecific and may be the result of an associated esophageal motility disorder.

Barium esophagogram is the initial and most relevant diagnostic tool in the evaluation of the diverticulum, associated esophageal abnormalities and complications. The typical pulsion diverticulum has a globular shape with a small opening that communicates with the esophagus. Manometric evaluation of midthoracic or epiphrenic pulsion diverticula usually shows an associated motility disorder and may influence treatment decisions.

Management

Asymptomatic or minimally symptomatic patients with a diverticulum smaller than 3 cm should be followed periodically for enlargement of the diverticulum. Patients who are symptomatic, those with a pouch larger than 4 cm and those who show enlargement should undergo operative treatment.

Surgical treatment consists of resection or imbrication of the diverticulum. A longitudinal esophagomyotomy that extends from the aortic arch superiorly, to 1 cm into the cardia distally, addresses the underlying motility disorder.[57] A partial fundoplication of the Belsey-Mark IV type is added in order to prevent reflux from the disruption of the LES. Some surgeons advocate doing the esophagomyotomy only if objective disturbances of esophageal motility are detected during manometry. The traditional surgical approach was done through a left thoracotomy. Most recently, several reports have validated the use of laparoscopic and thoracoscopic techniques in the treatment of these patients.[58]

Traction Diverticula

This type of diverticulum results from inflammatory conditions of the mediastinum (tuberculosis) and are located in the midthoracic esophagus. These are histologically true diverticula, containing all layers including mucosa, submucosa and muscle. It is commonly diagnosed on barium esophagogram incidentally. The typical radiographic image is that of a triangular-shaped diverticulum with its base resting on the esophageal wall. Most mid-esophageal diverticula are small, cause no specific symptoms and no therapy is necessary. It is important to differentiate it from the more common pulsion diverticulum that is associated with a motility disorder of the esophagus.

5. Stress Gastritis

Superficial erosions of the gastric mucosa that occur in acutely ill patients are known as stress gastritis.

Epidemiology and Pathophysiology
Stress gastritis occurs in nearly 100% of patients in the intensive care unit, particularly those in a high-stress clinical situation, such as sepsis, after burns or trauma, and in ventilator-dependent patients.[59] It is complex and multifactorial, a consequence of the overactivity of aggressors (acid) and disruption of the stomach's protective mechanisms (gastric mucosal lining). Some acid production must occur for the development of acute erosive gastritis, however patients do not suffer from a hypersecretory state.

Mucosal ischemia plays a critical role in the development of acute gastritis. Ischemia most likely occurs at the microcirculatory level as a consequence of the metabolic and hormonal response to stress. Mucosal ischemia leads to decreased clearance of hydrogen ions, which impairs the buffering capacity of the mucosa.[60]

Clinical Presentation, Assessment and Diagnosis
Though acute erosive gastritis is common, the main clinical manifestation is acute upper gastrointestinal bleeding. This can manifest as bleeding through the nasogastric tube, hematemesis, melena or acute anemia. Bleeding in the ICU patient should prompt initial gastric lavage. The decision to perform upper endoscopy is individualized. Emergency upper endoscopy is indicated if:

- The bleeding persists after gastric lavage
- There is a large amount of bleeding or clots
- The patient experiences hematemesis
- There is evidence of hemodynamic changes

Management
If the blood loss manifests as bleeding through the nasogastric tube, is estimated to be less than 200 mL, and stops after the gastric lavage, the treatment of erosive gastritis is primarily pharmacological. The regimen involves the use of intravenous H_2 receptor antagonists and monitoring of the gastric fluid pH in the absence of blood via the nasogastric

tube. In patients with more significant bleeding, diagnostic and therapeutic endoscopy is indicated. A number of endoscopic techniques can be used to control the bleeding, such as injection of epinephrine, electrocoagulation or laser photocoagulation. The success rate of endoscopy is approximately 90%.[61] When endoscopic means fail, use of vasopressin (systemic or selective intraarterial) and somatostatin analog have been used with some success.

Surgical control of the bleeding site is used as a life-saving measure in infirm patients with persistent, significant bleeding. If diffuse bleeding is found, a total gastrectomy is necessary. Less radical operations are done when feasible, including gastrotomy with oversawing of the bleeding area or partial gastrectomy.

The most important intervention is prophylaxis.[62] Maintaining hemodynamic homeostasis, adequate nutritional support and oxygenation are primary factors in the prevention of acute erosive gastritis. In addition, a number of controlled studies have documented the benefit of H_2 receptor antagonists and antacids in decreasing its incidence in ICU patients.[63] The routine use of these drugs has been challenged due to cost issues and potential side effects. The best policy seems to be the use of pharmacologic prophylaxis selectively in patients who are nutritionally depleted, on a ventilator, or in high-stress situations like sepsis, trauma or burns.

6. Peptic Ulcer Disease

A peptic ulcer is a lesion in the mucosa of the stomach or duodenum induced by the proteolytic effects of pepsins and gastric acid.

Duodenal Ulcer (DU)

Definition and Epidemiology

Duodenal ulcer is a lesion of the mucosa and deeper layers of the duodenum that is typically chronic and recurrent. DU affects approximately 10% of individuals in western populations during their lifetime and the prevalence is approximately 1.8%.[64] It affects males and females equally and can occur in any age group, but is most commonly seen in young adults, and rarely occurs during childhood. The incidence of DU has steadily decreased during the last three decades. DU occurs in the first portion of the duodenum in 95% of patients.

Pathophysiology

The pathophysiology of DU is multifactorial and not completely understood. The Dragstedian principle of "no acid no ulcer" is still valid today, and acid must be present during the genesis of peptic ulcers. However in recent years, indirect evidence emphasizing the critical role of *Helicobacter pylori* infection in the pathogenesis of this disease has been mounting.[65,66] Approximately 95% of patients with DU have *H pylori* in the mucus layer of the gastric mucosa, but the prevalence in healthy subjects is as high as 15%-25%, supporting the theory of a multifactorial etiology of DU. *H pylori* produces urease, proteases and phospholipases that may directly damage the protective layer of the mucosa, disrupting the balance between the acid/pepsin and the protective mechanisms. As a group, patients with DU have basal and maximal acid outputs in the upper range of normal, but there is such considerable overlap with normal individuals that no definitive conclusions can be drawn. Gastric acid converts pepsinogen molecules into proteolytically active pepsins, and this combination is at the core of the tissue damaging mechanism.[67]

The mucosal defense mechanism is the third factor to be considered. Some reports indicate that patients with DU have lower basal and stimulated bicarbonate output. The cytoprotective effect of prostaglandins seems to be diminished in patients with DU, and is definitely impaired in patients using non-steroidal anti-inflammatory drugs and smokers.[68]

Clinical Presentation

The typical patient is a young adult who has suffered epigastric pain for several weeks to months. The pain is described as burning or as a sensation of hunger that occurs approximately 2 hours after meals and is relieved a few minutes after eating; patients also find relief with antacids. Frequently, the pain awakens the patient in the early hours of the morning. The natural history of untreated DU is characterized by spontaneous healing and subsequent recurrence. Untreated DU has a recurrence rate of 80%-90%.

Evidence of complications of a DU can be gleaned from the clinical presentation. Patients with perforated DU complain of the sudden onset of severe abdominal pain that progressively diffuses throughout the abdomen. The physical examination is characteristic for findings of peritoneal irritation. Patients with a chronic history of bouts of epigastric pain may present with increasing food intolerance, nausea and vomiting, and should be suspected of having a gastric outlet obstruction. Weight loss and findings of nutritional depletion may be present. Physical findings may reveal a distended upper abdomen with a succussion splash. Bleeding is a life-threatening complication of DU, and patients present with hematemesis, melena, and in less significant cases, with anemia from chronic blood loss.

Assessment and Diagnosis

A common initial approach to patients with chronic symptoms, in the absence of any complications or clinical suspicion of malignancy, is a therapeutic trial. Initial evaluation includes symptomatic therapy with proton pump inhibitors, serologic testing for *H pylori*, or a urea breath test and specific antibacterial therapy if either test is positive. Patients who have persistent or recurrent symptoms after an initial trial of 4 weeks of empiric therapy are subjected to diagnostic endoscopy regardless of the presence of *H pylori* on testing. Other indications for upper endoscopy are change in the character of chronic symptoms, uncertainty of diagnosis and clinical suspicion of malignancy.

Characteristics of a typical duodenal ulcer on upper endoscopy are its location in the first portion of the duodenum, sharply defined borders and a clean, smooth ulcer bed. Barium upper GI study is used less frequently, and may also reveal the ulcer crater or a deformity in the first portion of the duodenum. Ulcer location beyond the second portion of the duodenum on endoscopy or on radiographs should raise suspicion for the presence of a gastrinoma.

Patients who present with sudden onset of abdominal pain and peritoneal findings on physical examination require emergency surgery. Initial assessment and management take place simultaneously by rapid rehydration, administration of intravenous antibiotics, and plain chest and abdominal films are made. Likewise, patients who experience an acute upper GI bleed undergo initial resuscitation prior to an emergency endoscopy that is diagnostic of the source of bleeding and therapeutic in the majority of cases.

Patients with clinical evidence of a gastric outlet obstruction undergo initial rehydration and decompression of the stomach with nasogastric suction. Subsequently, an upper GI barium study is performed that reveals a distended stomach, sometimes reaching the pelvis, with a narrowing at the pylorus or at the first portion of the duodenum. Upper endoscopy is indicated to assess the possibility of a malignancy causing obstruction.

Management

Objectives of ulcer therapy are relief of symptoms, facilitation of healing, prevention of complications and prevention of recurrence.

H_2 receptor antagonists (cimetidine, ranitidine, famotidine) are the mainstays of symptomatic therapy and at one time were the standard medications used to heal ulcers. Healing of an ulcer verified by endoscopy is seen in 70% of patients within 4 weeks and in 90% of patients after 8 weeks of therapy.[69] However, the recurrence rate approaches 50% after 1 year and 90% after 2 years if no maintenance therapy is given. Recurrences occur earlier and lead to complications more often in smokers.

PPIs (omeprazole, lanzoprasole) are more effective than H_2 receptor antagonists in providing symptomatic relief and facilitating ulcer healing. Using endoscopic verification, 80% of ulcers are seen to have healed after 2 weeks and 95% after 4 weeks of PPI therapy.[70] Recurrence rates are similar to those seen with H_2 receptor antagonist therapy.[71]

Among less commonly used agents are sucralfate, an agent that coats the ulcer base, alleviating symptoms and promoting healing. Prostaglandin analogs (eg, misoprostol) have cytoprotective and antisecretory effects. Both agents produce similar symptom relief and healing rates as those seen with the use of H_2 receptor antagonists.

Treatment of *H pylori* infection requires combination therapy. Combination regimens are known as triple therapy, and consists of a 2-week course of bismuth subsalycilate, 2 tablets QID, metronidazole, 250 mg TID, and tetracycline hydrochloride, 500 mg QID (or alternatively amoxicillin, 500 mg TID). Triple therapy is successful in eradication of *H pylori* in 90% of cases.[72] The addition of a PPI may raise the efficacy of this regimen to as high as 98% according to one report.[73] Once *H pylori* has been eradicated, the recurrence rate of DU is estimated to be as low as 2% per year.

Surgical treatment of DU was commonplace several decades ago, but the advent of pharmacologic therapy has limited the role of surgery to the management of complications of DU. Indications for surgery are:

- Failure of medical management
- Treatment of a perforated ulcer
- Treatment of a bleeding ulcer
- Treatment of gastric outlet obstruction

Intractability is currently an uncommon indication for surgery with the effectiveness of the currently used regimen of acid suppression therapy and *H pylori* eradication. All operative procedures for DU are based on ablation of the vagal component of acid secretion. The 3 most commonly used procedures are:

- Truncal vagotomy and antrectomy: this is the most effective acid-reduction procedure and it has the lowest recurrence rate, but it carries a higher risk of perioperative complications and long-term functional consequences.[74] The right and left vagus nerves are divided at the esophageal hiatus with careful attention paid to identification and division of branches that separate from the main trunks more proximally. A named branch directed to the fundus of the stomach is the "criminal" nerve of Grassi. Overlooking these small branches may lead to continual acid production and a higher recurrence rate. In addition, resection of the antrum decreases gastrin production and furthers the impact of the vagotomy. The antrectomy must include the mucosal transition zones between the stomach and duodenum distally and between the fundic and antral mucosa proximally. Restoration of gastrointestinal continuity is done in 1 of 2 ways: a Billroth I reconstruction, where an anastomosis is made between the body of the stomach and the duodenum (end-to-end gastroduodenostomy), or a Billroth II reconstruction, where an end-to-side gastrojejunostomy is constructed and the duodenal stump is closed off.

- Truncal vagotomy and drainage (pyloroplasty or gastroenterostomy):[75] a truncal vagotomy is performed in the manner previously described. Approximately one-third of patients will suffer from pyloric dysfunction after a vagotomy, causing a functional gastric outlet obstruction. Therefore, a drainage procedure is routinely added to the vagotomy. A pyloroplasty is most commonly used. Alternatively, in cases where severe scarring at or near the pylorus precludes a safe approach to pyloroplasty, a side-to-side gastroenterostomy can be performed. Disadvantages of gastroenterostomy are continued reflux of gastroduodenal contents into the stomach and the risk of anastomotic ulceration. Important factors in the design of a gastrojejunostomy are that the anastomosis should be long (5-6 cm), placed inframesocolic and retrocolic in the most dependent part of the stomach, and use of a short afferent limb.

- Highly selective vagotomy (parietal cell vagotomy): this procedure is designed to deliberately identify and divide the vagal fibers to the acid-secreting fundic mucosa while preserving the innervation to the antrum and pylorus. This operation is the logical procedure of choice because it decreases the long-term side effects of truncal vagotomy and drainage.[76] In the course of the operation, the vagal trunks are identified and all branches directed to the fundus and body of the stomach are divided with preservation of the antropyloric branches. This entails a thorough dissection in the distal 6 cm of esophagus, with division of the nerve of Grassi and devascularization of the lesser curvature to a distal point where the nerve of Latarget branches into the "crow's foot" located in the distal 5 cm of the antrum.

Early postoperative complications include hemorrhage, duodenal stump leak, anastomotic leak, pancreatitis and gastric outlet obstruction. Long-term side effects are reflux esophagitis, alkaline reflux gastritis, dumping syndrome, postvagotomy diarrhea, anemia, malnutrition and development of gallstones. The indications, relative benefits, risks and long-term morbidity of these procedures are listed in Table 2.

The goals of surgical therapy are management of the complication, to decrease the recurrence rate and to minimize the short- and long-term sequelae of surgery. The operative approach should be tailored to each patient and to the complication being addressed at the time of surgery.

Perforation. Initial management is directed at fluid and electrolyte restoration and administration of intravenous antibiotics. Patients with evidence of acute perforation and peritonitis should undergo surgery as promptly as possible. The primary objectives of surgery are to cleanse the abdomen and to close the perforation to decrease the morbidity from

Table 2

Surgical Procedures in the Management of Complicated Duodenal Ulcer

Operation	Indications	Ulcer recurrence	Complications
Highly selective vagotomy	Intractable DU, type II GU, perforated DU	5%-15%	Mortality <1% Morbidity <1% Postgastrectomy syndrome: very rare
Truncal vagotomy and pyloroplasty	Bleeding or perforated DU	10%-15%	Mortality <1% Morbidity 1%-5% Postgastrectomy syndrome: Dumping 10% Diarrhea 20% Severe symptoms 1%
Truncal vagotomy and antrectomy	Intractable DU or type III GU, perforated or bleeding DU or type I, II, or III GU	1%	Mortality <1% Morbidity 5%-10% Postgastrectomy syndrome: Dumping 15% Diarrhea 20% Severe symptoms 1%-3%
Partial gastrectomy	Intractable type I GU, perforated or bleeding type I, IV GU	2%	Mortality 1% Morbidity 5%-10% Postgastrectomy syndrome: Dumping 15% Diarrhea 5% Severe symptoms 1%-3%

septic complications and ongoing contamination of the peritoneal cavity. Duodenal perforation usually occurs in the anterior wall of the duodenum. The perforation may vary in size from a few millimeters to several centimeters. Omentum has often sealed the perforation at the time of surgery. Several techniques have been used to close the perforation. The edges can be debrided of damaged tissue and the ulcer may be approximated primarily. More commonly, a patch of omentum is sutured over the perforation creating a seal. This is known as a Graham patch. Rarely, very large ulcers with significant necrotic debris may require surgical resection of the antropyloric region. Subsequently the abdomen is irrigated with several liters of warm saline solution. No drainage is required. This procedure can be accomplished through a traditional exploratory laparotomy, but several recent reports support the use of laparoscopic techniques to the same end. Advantages of this technique are reduced postoperative recovery time and decreased morbidity from wound complications.[77]

A secondary consideration is prevention of recurrence in patients with ulcer diathesis. This is a valid concern in patients with a chronic history of symptoms who at presentation are hemodynamically stable and do not have severe contamination of the peritoneum. Several researchers advocate the use of an acid-reduction procedure in these patients. Highly selective vagotomy after closure of the perforation site has emerged as the procedure of choice.[74,78] Enthusiasm for these procedures has significantly decreased with the advent of successful triple therapy for *H pylori* due to the very low ulcer recurrence rate. Furthermore, the performance of acid-reduction surgery requires a longer operative time and specialized skills during laparoscopic surgery.

Nonoperative management of perforated DU has proven to be safe and effective in some subsets of patients.[79,80] Candidates for this approach are those in whom the perforation has spontaneously sealed. Sealing of the perforation and absence of extraluminal contrast must be confirmed by CT with oral thin barium or by an upper gastrointestinal Gastrografin and thin barium study. Patients who present late after the onset of symptoms with localized pain only and without overt signs of sepsis frequently have a sealed perforation. They are treated with nasogastric decompression, intravenous antibiotics and H_2 receptor antagonists.

Bleeding. The patient who presents with acute upper gastrointestinal hemorrhage requires initial fluid and blood volume restoration. Emergency endoscopy should be done as soon as possible as a diagnostic test and to guide therapy. It is also a therapeutic tool in the control of hemorrhage. Indications for surgery are inability to control the bleeding, recurrent bleeding in the same hospitalization and requiring more than 6 units of blood transfusion. Older patients who may not tolerate hemodynamic instability and patients with a visible vessel on endoscopy may benefit from earlier surgery. In addition to the presence of a visible vessel,[81] factors associated with re-bleeding and a higher mortality rate are age older than 60, clinical shock and ulcer crater larger than 1 cm.[82]

The goal of the operative procedure is to control hemorrhage and the prevention of rebleeding. A secondary priority is the decrease of recurrence. Bleeding duodenal ulcers or pyloric channel ulcers can be approached during laparotomy through a gastrotomy that extends through the pylorus into the proximal duodenum. The ulcer bed is usually located in the posterior wall of the duodenum and frequently over the gastroduodenal artery. A suture ligature is applied to the ulcer bed and bleeding vessel. The incision is closed as a pyloroplasty. The operation is completed by a truncal vagotomy. The downside of this operation is a higher rate of rebleeding. Vagotomy and antrectomy with resection of the ulcer has lower rates of recurrent bleeding.

Obstruction. Obstruction occurs in patients with DU in 2 scenarios; as a chronic process where fibrosis is the primary component, or as a consequence of acute inflammation usually complicating a scarred duodenum. Initial management should be directed at restoration of volume status and decompression of the stomach with nasogastric suction. Parenteral nutritional support and intravenous H_2 receptor antagonists are important in the initial management. In the course of the ensuing days, barium studies and upper endoscopy are performed. The role of upper endoscopy is to rule out the presence of a malignancy. Approximately one-third of patients experience significant improvement of the gastric outlet obstruction with medical management. Eventually 75% of patients require surgical intervention for relief of the obstruction.

The primary goal of surgery is to relieve the obstruction and to restore gastrointestinal continuity. An acid reduction procedure is also performed. The status of the pylorus is the primary determinant of the type of surgery to be done. In cases of scarring, a Finney or Jabulay pyloroplasty may be performed in conjunction with a highly selective or a truncal vagotomy. Alternatively, a truncal vagotomy with antrectomy and preferably a Billroth I reconstruction will accomplish the goals of surgery. In cases of very severe scarring and in the presence of a significant inflammatory component, a truncal vagotomy with a gastrojejunostomy is the preferred approach.

Benign Gastric Ulcer (GU)

Gastric ulcers may be of peptic origin or malignant. The most important decision in the care of these patients is to establish whether the lesion is benign or malignant.

Pathophysiology and Clinical Presentation

The pathogenesis of gastric ulcer is not completely understood. Analogous to the pathogenesis of DU, it is multifactorial and the presence of acid is necessary for formation of the ulcer. Again, the formation of an ulcer is a result of an imbalance between aggressors and the mucosal barrier protective mechanism. Nonsteroidal anti-inflammatory drugs play a significant role in as many as one-third of patients. Other factors such as delayed gastric emptying and duodenogastric reflux may also be of significance. *H pylori* is present in approximately 80% of patients with GU and indirect evidence supports its causative role in the genesis of ulcer disease. Patients with GU tend to be older in comparison to patients with DU. GU is a chronic and recurrent disease with symptomatic periods of burning epigastric pain, and symptoms may be exacerbated by meals. Complications of GU are bleeding, obstruction, and perforation. Benign gastric ulcers are classified based on their location and acid secretory status. GU types and their incidence are depicted in Figure 7.

Assessment, Diagnosis and Management

The diagnosis of GU is made by endoscopy. Using endoscopic criteria and biopsy, the benign or malignant nature of the ulcer can be established in approximately 95% of cases.

Figure 7

Types of gastric ulcer (percentages indicate fraction of total cases of GU)

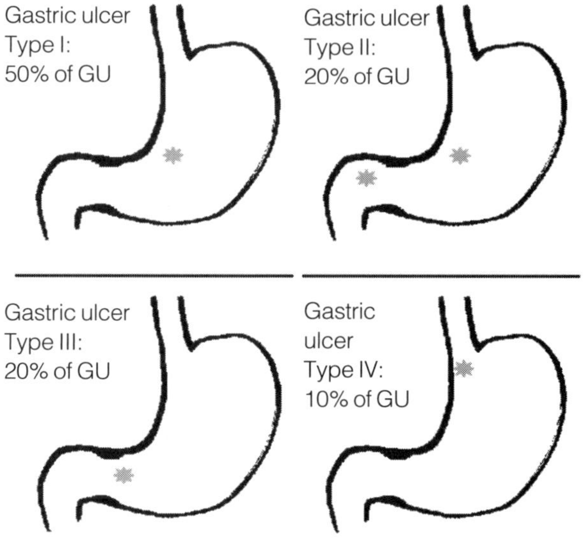

Pharmacologic therapy of GU is similar to that of DU, and the healing rate with pharmacologic acid suppression therapy approaches 80%. Triple therapy for eradication of *H pylori* is the cornerstone of prevention of ulcer recurrence.

Surgery is indicated in patients with GU that does not heal in a 12-week period to exclude the possibility of malignant disease, because the likelihood of healing after that period is low and the complication rate is higher. Surgical excision of the ulcer and acid-reduction surgery is the basis for successful management of these patients. Different surgical approaches for acid-reduction surgery should be tailored based on the indication for surgery (ie, perforation, bleeding, nonhealing, etc.), the physiologic status of the patient, and the type of ulcer. Excision of the gastric ulcer is mandatory for histologic examination. Type I gastric ulcers have a low recurrence rate after gastric resection. There is little proven benefit of adding a vagotomy and it has the added risk of postvagotomy diarrhea. The pathophysiology of type II and type III gastric ulcers, on the other hand, is similar to DU, therefore vagotomy plays an important role in their management, in conjunction with gastric resection.[83,84] In general, highly selective vagotomy is considered to have a higher recurrence rate.[85]

Zollinger-Ellison Syndrome (Z-E)

Definition and Pathobiology

Z-E syndrome is characterized by gastric hypersecretion, intractable peptic disease and a nonbeta islet cell tumor. Gastrinomas occur most commonly in the area known as the "gastrinoma triangle," delineated by the cystic duct, neck of the pancreas and lateral border of the duodenum. The hypersecretory state is caused by production of gastrin by the neuroendocrine tumor. 60% of these tumors are malignant and they frequently have lymph node metastases.

Clinical Presentation and Diagnosis

The presence of ulcer diathesis associated with diarrhea should raise a suspicion of Z-E. It should be suspected in patients who require large doses of antacids, and in patients who fail *H pylori* or surgical therapy for ulcer disease. However, on initial presentation patients with Z-E have clinical characteristics similar to other patients with peptic disease.[86] A familial history is relevant in cases associated with MEN-I syndrome (hyperparathyroidism, pancreatic islet cell tumors and pituitary adenomas).

Once Z-E is suspected, a basal gastrin level should be measured. If it is normal and the gastric pH is high, the diagnosis is excluded. On the other hand, if the level is higher than 1000 pg/mL and the gastric pH is low, there is a high likelihood of Z-E. The diagnosis is confirmed by a secretin stimulation test. In this test, there is a paradoxical elevation of the serum gastrin with the administration of secretin. Patients with gastrin levels less than 1000 pg/mL have a lower incidence of Z-E but should be similarly studied with a secretin test. If positive, it confirms the diagnosis of Z-E.[86]

Management

Initial management requires control of acid hypersecretion with high doses of PPIs or H_2 receptor antagonists. Prior to the use of effective antacid medication, total gastrectomy was used to control symptoms and complications. Total gastrectomy is not necessary with current medical therapy. The focus should be on definitive therapy of the gastrinoma by resection of the primary tumor and lymphatic metastases. In the absence of liver metastases, patients undergo exploration with the aid of intraabdominal ultrasound with a success rate of 85% for identification of the tumor.[87] Postoperatively, normalization of gastrin levels occurs in approximately two-thirds of sporadic cases. Eugastrinemia is rare after surgical resection in patients with MEN-I syndrome, therefore exploration is only considered in patients with a higher likelihood of metastasis, such as patients with tumors larger than 2 cm.[88]

Postgastrectomy Syndromes

These are caused by changes in upper gastrointestinal and small bowel function as a consequence of gastric surgery. The incidence has decreased significantly as a result of a 10-fold decrease in elective gastric surgery. Postgastrectomy syndromes occur in 5%-50% of patients undergoing gastric surgery and their incidence depends on the effect of surgery in disrupting the vagus nerves or bypassing the pylorus.[89]

Dumping Syndrome

This syndrome is caused by the loss of reservoir of the stomach and rapid emptying of osmolar carbohydrate loads into the small intestine. It occurs most commonly after gastrectomy and Billroth II reconstruction.

During ***early dumping*** (within 10-30 minutes of eating), patients complain of gastrointestinal symptoms of fullness, nausea, vomiting and explosive diarrhea. Vasomotor symptoms are diaphoresis, weakness, flushing and palpitations. It is caused by rapid fluid shifts between the intravascular space and the gastrointestinal tract. ***Late dumping*** is caused by the hormonal response to the carbohydrate load, primarily mediated through insulin release. The symptoms are primarily vasomotor. Treatment consists of dietary manipulation, by separating solids from liquids, having smaller, more frequent meals and by taking complex rather than simple carbohydrates.

Postvagotomy Diarrhea

The origin of this disorder is poorly understood, but is likely related to denervation of the gallbladder and small bowel. It occurs in approximately 20% of patients after truncal vagotomy, but in less than 5% of patients after highly selective vagotomy. Treatment consists of dietary changes and use of antidiarrheal agents. In cases of severe diarrhea the use of a 10-cm antiperistaltic jejunal segment has been described with some success.

Afferent Loop Syndrome

This disorder occurs as a consequence of obstruction of the afferent limb of jejunum in a gastrojejunostomy. Major complaints are of severe crampy postprandial abdominal pain and vomiting. The pain is relieved after vomiting of bilious fluid not mixed with the recently ingested food. After evaluation with upper gastrointestinal series and upper endoscopy, surgical correction of the obstructed point is necessary, either by revising the anastomosis to a Roux-en-Y gastrojejunostomy or by creating a side-to-side jejunojejunostomy.

Efferent Loop Syndrome

This is caused by partial or complete obstruction of the gastrojejunostomy. Symptoms consist of postprandial abdominal pain and bilious vomiting. Upper gastrointestinal series and upper endoscopy confirm the diagnosis. Therapy involves a revision of the gastrojejunostomy to a Billroth I anastomosis or to a Roux-en-Y gastrojejunostomy.

7. Benign Tumors of the Esophagus, Stomach and Duodenum

Benign Tumors of the Esophagus

Benign tumors of the esophagus are rare, representing less than 2% of all tumors of the esophagus. Knowledge of these tumors is important because their management is distinctly different than that of malignant tumors of the esophagus. Though there is no uniform classification scheme, classification into polyp lesions and intramural tumors has clinical relevance.

Intramural tumors are tumors that arise in the esophageal wall. Stromal tumors (leiomyomas) account for approximately two-thirds of all benign esophageal tumors. Enterogenous cysts are congenital in origin and contain either esophageal (squamous) or respiratory (ciliated columnar) epithelium. These are also found in the wall of the esophagus.

Clinical Presentation

Benign esophageal tumors tend to occur in a younger age group than malignant lesions. Presenting symptoms are those of a space-occupying lesion of the esophagus. Patients complain of dysphagia of long duration (average, 23 months), but weight loss occurs infrequently.

Assessment, Diagnosis and Management

Initial evaluation in the patient with dysphagia is centered on a barium esophagogram and upper endoscopy. On esophagogram, complete obstruction is very rare. More commonly, a well-defined filling defect with smooth borders is seen in the esophageal lumen. Upper endoscopy allows for direct visualization of the area in question, guided by the esophagogram. The smooth borders and defined limits without ulceration are endoscopic characteristics of benign lesions. The mucosal or intramural nature of these lesions can be defined endoscopically.

Polyps occur more commonly in the cervical region and tend to have normal overlying mucosa. Endoscopic biopsy or polypectomy is obtained for definitive histologic diagnosis. Of course polypectomy is also therapeutic if the diagnosis is benign. A subset of polyps, known as giant fibrovascular polyps, arises in the cervical esophagus and may be very long (several centimeters). These polyps are very vascular and may cause bleeding or airway obstruction. Due to the vascular nature and risk for bleeding and aspiration, these polyps are removed through a cervical or transthoracic esophagotomy.

Management

The management of intramural lesions is dictated by the clinical suspicion of malignancy. The need to biopsy all intramural tumors is controversial. The downside of an endoscopic biopsy is that the mucosa is disrupted and the procedure is likely to cause scarring that may contribute to mucosal injury during enucleation of the tumor.

Symptomatic intramural esophageal tumors that have a benign clinical, radiologic and endoscopic presentation should be resected. The most favored approach is tumor enucleation without esophageal resection, if possible, in order to avoid the morbidity and potential mortality of esophagectomy. The management of incidentally discovered asymptomatic intramural benign lesions is less clear. Tissue diagnosis is difficult to obtain on endoscopic biopsy because these tumors generally do not involve the mucosa. The decision to perform surgery must be individualized and made in conjunction with the patient. Excision of larger lesions in a low-risk patient is reasonable due to the likelihood of growth and of causing symptoms. More recently, endoscopic ultrasound provides a technique for needle-guided biopsy useful in patients who will not undergo surgery.[90]

Gastric Polyps

Epidemiology and Pathophysiology

Benign tumors, in general, represent less than 2% of all tumors of the stomach. Screening in large populations suggests a less than 1% incidence of gastric polyps, with females having a slightly higher incidence than males. The median age of these patients is 65 years.[91]

A number of familial syndromes have a high incidence of gastric polyps. Patients with familial adenomatous polyposis have a 50% incidence of gastric or duodenal polyps with the concomitant risk for cancer. Patients with Peutz-Jeghers syndrome suffer from a 20% incidence of hamartomatous polyps. The incidence of carcinoma transformation is less than for adenomatous polyps, but occurrences have been reported. There is no uniform classification of gastric polyps, but histologic classification assists in the understanding of the origin and consequences of these polyps.

Hyperplastic polyps constitute approximately 75% of all gastric polyps and are regenerative rather than neoplastic. They are also known as inflammatory or hamartomatous polyps. Hyperplastic polyps occur most commonly in association with atrophic gastritis, and they do not undergo malignant transformation.

Adenomatous polyps are the second most common type of gastric polyp. They are neoplastic in origin and represent proliferation of atypical glands. Histologically they are classified into tubular or villous adenomas. They carry a risk of malignant transformation, similar to colorectal adenomatous polyps, and the risk increases with the size of the polyp. Polyps less than 2 cm have a 4% incidence of carcinoma, whereas polyps larger than 2 cm have a 24% incidence of malignancy.

Clinical Presentation, Assessment and Diagnosis

Polyps are commonly found during upper endoscopy, either incidentally or as a result of patients complaining of epigastric pain, upper gastrointestinal bleeding or gastric outlet obstruction. They are diagnosed on upper endoscopy, and polypectomy should be attempted on every polyp seen. Larger, sessile polyps not amenable to endoscopic removal should be extensively biopsied.

Management

Management of gastric polyps is based on 2 factors; first, feasibility of endoscopic removal of the polyp. If feasible, all polyps should be removed endoscopically. Snare polypectomy is commonly applied to pedunculated polyps. The second factor is histologic diagnosis. Adenomatous polyps are premalignant lesions.

In general, smaller sessile polyps can be ablated endoscopically by piecemeal polypectomy or, after obtaining adequate biopsies, by fulguration. Sessile adenomatous polyps not amenable to endoscopic removal, particularly those larger than 2 cm, should be excised to halt the adenoma-carcinoma sequence.

Stromal Tumors of the Stomach

Definition and Epidemiology

These are tumors of mesenchymal origin that arise in the gastric wall, and benign tumors outnumber malignant ones by a margin of 10:1. The majority of benign cases were previously reported as leiomyoma. Stromal tumors occur throughout the gastrointestinal tract, but are most common in the stomach (60%-70%). These tumors represent less than 2% of all gastric tumors.

Pathology

These tumors are grayish-colored nodules arising in the gastric wall with a well-circumscribed pseudocapsule separating tumor from normal smooth muscle. Benign gastrointestinal stromal tumors (GISTs) are small, most specimens being less than 5 cm in size, and have rare or absent mitoses on histology. However, the true benign or malignant nature of these lesions can only be established with certainty by the absence of metastasis and adjacent organ invasion at the time of presentation, and on long-term follow-up.

Clinical Presentation

Erosion of the overlying gastric mucosa can lead to gastrointestinal bleeding presenting as hematemesis, melena or anemia. Infrequently, patients present with mass-effect symptoms and gastric outlet obstruction. Some benign gastrointestinal stromal tumors enlarge extraluminally and reach considerable size, presenting with a palpable abdominal mass that is often freely movable.

Assessment and Diagnosis

Patients usually undergo endoscopic examination as the first means of evaluation. Endoscopy frequently reveals an extraluminal mass with normal overlying mucosa. Umbilication of the mucosa can also be seen. CT scan may show a round mass in the wall of the stomach.

Management

Due to the difficulty in uniformly predicting the benign or malignant potential of gastrointestinal stromal tumors, resection of the lesion with a limited margin of normal tissue is necessary. This can be accomplished with a wedge resection for lesions located in the fundus or body of the stomach, but a formal gastric resection is usually necessary for tumors located in the antrum or near the gastroesophageal junction. Obtaining histologically-negative margins is important in the management of these lesions.[92]

8. References

1. Achar E. Achalasia. *Gastroenterologist*. 1995;3:273-288.

2. Sonnenberg A, Massey B, McCarty D, Jacobsen S. Epidemiology of hospitalization for achalasia in the United States. *Dig Dis Sci*. 1993;38:233-244.

3. Aggestrup S, Uddman R, Sundler F, et al. Lack of vasointestinal polypeptide nerves in esophageal achalasia. *Gastroenterologist*. 1983;84:924-927.

4. Meijsen M, Tilanus H, vanBlankestein M, et al. Achalasia complicated by oesophageal squamous cell carcinoma: a prospective study of 195 patients. *Gut*. 1992;33:155-158.

5. Triadafilopoulos G, Aaronson M, Sackel S, Burakoff R. Medical treatment of esophageal achalasia. *Dig Dis Sci*. 1991;36:260-267.

6. Vaezi MF, Richter JE, Wilcox CM, Schroeder P, et al. Botulinum toxin versus pneumatic dilatation in the treatment of achalasia: a randomised trial. *Gut*. 1999;44:231-239.

7. Singh V, Duseja A, Kumar A, et al. Balloon dilatation in achalasia cardia. *Trop Gastroenterol*. 1999;20:68-69.

8. Katz P, Gilbert J, Castell D. Pneumatic dilatation is effective long-term treatment for achalasia. *Dig Dis Sci*. 1998;43:1973-1977.

9. Schwartz H, Cahow C, Traube M. Outcome after perforation sustained during pneumatic dilatation for achalasia. *Dig Dis Sci*. 1993;38:1409-1413.

10. Vaezi M, Richter J. Current therapies for achalasia: comparison and efficacy. *J Clin Gastroenterol*. 1998;27:21-35.

11. Malthaner R, Todd T, Miller L, Pearson F. Long-term results in surgically managed esophageal achalasia. *Ann Thorac Surg*. 1994;58:1343-1347.

12. Raiser F, Perdikis G, Hinder R. Heller myotomy via minimal access surgery: an evaluation of antireflux procedures. *Arch Surg*. 1996;132:593-598.

13. Patti M, Arcerito M, De Pinto M, et al. Comparison of thoracoscopic and laparoscopic Heller myotomy for achalasia. *J Gastroint Surg*. 1998;2:561-566.

14. Ferguson M. Achalasia: current evaluation and therapy. *Ann Thorac Surg*. 1991;52:336.

15. Patti M, Pellegrini C. Minimally invasive approaches to achalasia. *Semin Gastroint Dis*. 1994;5:108-112.

16. Csendes A, Braghetto I, Henriquez A, Cortes C. Late results of a prospective randomized study comparing forceful dilatation and oesophagomyotomy in patients with achalasia. *Gut*. 1989;30:299.

17. Eypasch E, DeMeester T, Klingman R, et al. Physiologic assessment and surgical management of diffuse esophageal spasm. *J Thorac Cardiovasc Surg*. 1992;104:859-869.

18. Cohen S. The gastrointestinal manifestations of scleroderma: pathogenesis and management. *Gastroenterol*. 1980;79:155-166.

19. Zamost B, Irschberg J, Ippoliti A, et al. Esophagitis in scleroderma. Prevalence and risk factors. *Gastroenterol*. 1987;92:421-428.

20. Poirier N, Taillefer R, Topart P, Duranceau A. Antireflux operations in patients with scleroderma. *Ann Thorac Surg*. 1994;58:66-72.

21. Kahrilas P. Gastroesophageal reflux disease. *JAMA*. 1996;276:983-988.

22. DeMeester T, Wernly J, Bryant G, et al. Clinical and in vitro analysis of determinants of gastroesophageal competence. *Am J Surg*. 1979;137:39.

23. Bonavina L, Evander A, DeMeester TR, et al. Length of the distal esophageal sphincter and competency of the cardia. *Am J Surg*. 1986;151:25.

24. Ott D, Glauser S, Ledbetter S, et al. Association of hiatal hernia and gastroesophageal reflux: Correlation between presence and size of hiatal hernia and 24-hour pH monitoring of the esophagus. *Am J Roentgenol*. 1995;165:557-559.

25. Orlando R. The pathogenesis of gastroesophageal reflux disease: The relationship between epithelial defense, dysmotility, and acid exposure. *Am J Gastroenterol*. 1997;92:3S-7S.

26. Pope C. Acid reflux disorders. *N Engl J Med*. 1994;331:656-660.

27. Johnston B, Troshinsky M, Castel J, Castell D. Comparison of barium radiology with esophageal pH monitoring in the diagnosis of gastroesophageal reflux disease. *Am J Gastroenterol*. 1996;91:1181-1185.

28. Ergun G, Kahrilas P. Clinical applications of esophageal manometry and pH monitoring. *Am J Gastroenterol*. 1996;91:1077-1089.

29. Navarro-Rodriguez T, de Moraes-Filho J, Arakaki E, et al. The screening sensitivity of endoscopy, acid perfusion test and 24-hour pH-monitoring to evaluate esophagitis in patients with heartburn and histological esophagitis. *Arquivos de Gastroenterologia*. 1997;34:148-156.

30. McDougall N, Johnston B, Kee F, et al. Natural history of reflux esophagitis: a 10 year follow up of its effect on patient symptomatology and quality of life. *Gut*. 1996;38:481-486.

31. Harvey R, Gordon P, Hadley N, et al. The effects of sleeping with the bed raised and with ranitidine in patients with severe peptic oesophagitis. *Lancet*. 1987;2:1200-1203.

32. Sontag S. Gastroesophageal reflux disease. *Alimentary Pharmacol Therapeutics*. 1993;7:293-312.

33. DeVault K. Current management of gastroesophageal reflux disease. *Gastroenterologist*. 1996;4:24-32.

34. Galmiche J, Brandsatter G, Evreux M, Hentschel E. Combined therapy with cisapride and cimetidine in severe oesophagitis: a double blind controlled trial. *Gut*. 1988;29:675-681.

35. Kauer W, Peters J, DeMeester T, et al. A tailored approach to antireflux surgery. *J Thorac Cardiovasc Surg*. 1995;110:141-147.

36. Waring J, Hunter J, Oddsdottir M, et al. The preoperative evaluation of patients considered for laparoscopic antireflux surgery. *Am J Gastroenterol*. 1995;90:35-38.

37. Spechler S. Comparison of medical and surgical therapy for complicated gastroesophageal reflux disease in veterans. *N Engl J Med*. 1992;326:786-791.

38. Peters J, Heimbucher J, Kauer W, et al. Clinical and physiologic comparison of laparoscopic and open Nissen fundoplication. *J Am Coll Surg*. 1995;180:385-393.

39. Rice T, Gagner M. Laparoscopic antireflux surgery. *Semin Thorac Cardiovasc Surg*. 1997;9:173-187.

40. Watson A. The role of antireflux surgery combined with fiberoptic endoscopic dilatation in peptic esophageal strictures. *Am J Surg*. 1994;148:346-348.

41. DeMeester S, Campos G, DeMeester T, et al. The impact of an antireflux procedure on intestinal metaplasia of the cardia. *Ann Surg*. 1998;228:547-556.

42. Sampliner R, Effect of up to 3 years of high-dose lansoprazole on Barrett's esophagus. *Am J Gastroenterol*. 1994;89:1844-1849.

43. Bufkin B, Miller J, Mansour K. Esophageal perforation: emphasis on management. *Ann Thorac Surg*. 1996;61:1447-1452.

44. Bjerke H. Boerhaave's syndrome and barogenic injuries of the esophagus. *Chest Surg Clin North Am*. 1994;4:819-825.

45. White R, Morris D. Diagnosis and management of esophageal perforations. *Am Surg*. 1992;58:112.

46. Wilde P, Mullany C. Oesophageal perforation: A review of 37 cases. *Aust NZ J Surg*. 1987;57:743.

47. Cameron JL, Kieffer RF, Hendrix TR, Mehigan DG, Baker RR. Selective non-operative management of contained intrathoracic esophageal disruptions. *Ann Thorac Surg*. 1971;25:346.

48. Schwartz HM, Cahow CE, Traube M. Outcome after perforation sustained during pneumatic dilatation for achalasia. *Dig Dis Sci*. 1993;38:1409.

49. Gouge T, Depan H, Spencer C. Experience with the Grillo pleural wrap procedure in 18 patients with perforation of the thoracic esophagus. *Ann Surg*. 1989;209:612.

50. Whyte R, Iannettoni M, Orringer M. Intrathoracic esophageal perforation: the merit of primary repair. *J Thorac Cardiovasc Surg*. 1995;109:140-146.

51. Eubanks P, Hu E, Nguyen D, et al. Case of Boerhaave's syndrome successfully treated with a self-expandable metallic stent. *Gastroint Endosc*. 1999;49:780-783.

52. Rothstein F. Caustic injuries to the esophagus in children. *Pediatr Clin N Am*. 1986;33:665.

53. Anderson K, Rouse T, Randolph J. A controlled trial of corticosteroids in children with corrosive injury of the esophagus. *N Engl J Med*. 1990;323:637.

54. Peters J, Mason R. The physiopathological basis for Zenker's diverticulum. *Chirurgia*. 1999;70:741-746.

55. Ochando Cerdáan F, Moreno Gonzalez E, Hernandez Garcia D, et al. Diagnosis and treatment of Zenker's diverticulum: review of our series of pharyngo-esophageal diverticula. *Hepatogastroenterol*. 1998;45:447-450.

56. Holinger P, Johnston K. Endoscopic surgery of Zenker's diverticula. Experience with the Dohlman technique. *1961 Ann Otolo, Rhinol Laryngol*. 1995;104:751-757.

57. Allen M. Treatment of epiphrenic diverticula. *Semin Thorac Cardiovasc Surg*. 1999;11:358-362.

58. Chami Z, Fabre J, Navarro F, Domergue J. Abdominal laparoscopic approach for thoracic epiphrenic diverticulum. *Surg Endosc*. 1999;13:164-165.

59. Czaja A, McAlhand C, Pruitt B Jr. Acute gastroduodenal disease after thermal injury. *N Engl J Med*. 1974;291:925.

60. Cheung, L. The pathogenesis, prophylaxis and treatment of stress gastritis. In: Sabiston D, Lyerly H, eds. *Sabiston: Textbook of Surgery. The Biologic Basis of Modern Surgical Practice*. Philadelphia, PA: WB Saunders Co; 1997.

61. Chamberlain C. Acute hemorrhagic gastritis. *Gastroent Clin N Am*. 1993;22:843.

62. Cook D, Fuller H, Guyatt G, et al. Risk factors for gastrointestinal bleeding in critically ill patients. *N Engl J Med*. 1994;330:377.

63. Pemberton LB, Schaefer N, Goehring L, Gaddis M, Arrighi DA. Oral ranitidine as prophylaxis for gastric stress ulcers in intensive care unit patients: Serum concentrations and cost comparisons. *Crit Care Med*. 1992;21:339.

64. Kurata J. Epidemiology: Peptic ulcer risk. *Semin Gastroint Dis*. 1993;4:2-12.

65. Marshall B, Warren J. Unidentified curved bacilli in the stomach of patients with gastritis and peptic ulceration. *Lancet*. 1984;1:1311.

66. Goldschmiedt M, Peterson W. The role of *Helicobacter pylori* in peptic ulcer disease. *Semin Gastrointest Dis*. 1993;4:13-20.

67. Fennerty M. *Helicobacter pylori*. *Arch Int Med*. 1994;154:721-727.

68. Mertz H, Walsch J. Peptic ulcer pathophysiology. *Med Clin N Am*. 1991;75:799-814.

69. McArthur K. Therapy of the uncomplicated ulcer. *Semin Gastrointest Dis*. 1993;4:27-38.

70. Oates J, Wood A. Drug therapy: Omeprazole. *N Engl J Med*. 1991;324:965-975.

71. Graham D, Colon-Pagan J, Morse R, et al. Ulcer recurrence following duodenal ulcer healing with omeprazole, ranitidine or placebo: a double-blind, multicenter 6-month study. *Gastroenterol*. 1992;102:1289-1294.

72. Hentschel E, Brandstatter G, Dragosics B, et al. Effect of ranitidine and amoxicillin plus metronidazole on the eradication of *Helicobacter pylori* and the recurrence of duodenal ulcers. *N Engl J Med*. 1993;328:308-312.

73. Hoskins S, Ling T, Chung S, et al. Duodenal ulcer healing by eradication of *Helicobacter pylori* without anti-acid treatment: randomized controlled trial. *Lancet*. 1994;343:508-510.

74. Jordan P. Surgery for peptic ulcer disease. *Curr Prob Surg*. 1991;28:267-330.

75. Jordan P, Condon R. A prospective evaluation of vagotomy-pyloroplasty and vagotomy-antrectomy for treatment of duodenal ulcer. *Ann Surg*. 1970;172:547-563.

76. Schirmer B. Current status of proximal gastric vagotomy. *Ann Surg*. 1989;209:131-148.

77. Katkhouda N, Mavor E, Mason R, et al. Laparoscopic repair of perforated duodenal ulcers: outcome and efficacy in 30 consecutive patients. *Arch Surg*. 1999;134:845-848.

78. Stabile B, Passaro E Jr. Duodenal ulcer, a disease in evolution. *Curr Prob Surg*. 1984;21:1-79.

79. Crofts T, Park K, Steele R, et al. A randomized trial of nonoperative treatment for perforated peptic ulcer. *N Engl J Med*. 1989;320:970-973.

80. Berne T, Donovan A. Nonoperative treatment of perforated ulcer disease. *Arch Surg*. 1989;124:830-832.

81. Branicki F, Boey J, Fok P, et al. Bleeding duodenal ulcer: A prospective evaluation of risk factors for rebleeding and death. *Ann Surg*. 1990;211:411-418.

82. Hunt P. Bleeding gastroduodenal ulcers: Selection of patients for surgery. *World J Surg*. 1987;11:289-294.

83. Thomas W, Thompson M, Williamson R. The long-term outcome of Billroth I partial gastrectomy for benign gastric ulcers. *Ann Surg*. 1982;189:189.

84. Greenall M, Lehnert T. Vagotomy or gastrectomy for elective treatment of benign gastric ulceration? *Dig Dis Sci*. 1985;30:353-356.

85. Emas S, Grupcev G, Eriksson B. Ten-year follow-up of a prospective, randomized trial of selective proximal vagotomy with ulcer excision and partial gastrectomy with gastroduodenostomy for treating corporal gastric ulcer. *Am J Surg*. 1994;167:596.

86. Weber H, Orbuch M, Jensen R. Diagnosis and management of Zollinger-Ellison syndrome. *Semin Gastro Dis*. 1995;6:79-89.

87. Fraker D, Norton J, Alexander H, et al. Surgery in Zollinger-Ellison syndrome alters the natural history of gastrinoma. *Ann Surg*. 1994;220:320-330.

88. Norton J. Gastrinoma: advances in localization and treatment. *Surg Oncol Clin North Am.* 1998;7:845-862.

89. Eagon J, Miedema B, Kelly K. Postgastrectomy syndromes. *Surg Clin North Am.* 1992;72:445-465.

90. Swisher S, Roth J, Putnam J. Diagnosis and management of benign esophageal tumors. *Cancer Bull*. 1995;47:396-401.

91. Marcial M, Villafaña M, Hernandez-Denton J, Colon-Pagan J. Fundic gland polyps: Prevalence and clinicopathologic features. *Am J Gastroenterol*. 1993;88:10.

92. Morgan B, Compton C, Talbert M, et al. Benign smooth muscle tumors of the gastrointestinal tract. *Ann Surg*. 1990;211:63.

9. Questions

1. The following is ***false*** regarding achalasia:

A. Initial therapy is based on lifestyle changes and medical therapy with calcium channel blockers.

B. Botulinum toxin intersphincteric injection is effective in 60% of patients for less than 6 months.

C. Two-thirds of patients improve after a single balloon dilatation.

D. Surgical esophagomyotomy provides long-term cure in 70%-90% of cases.

2. An otherwise healthy 50-year-old male patient complains of severe retrosternal chest pain during pneumatic dilatation for achalasia. The next step in management should be:

A. Upper endoscopy to rule out an esophageal perforation.

B. Barium esophagogram to rule out an esophageal perforation.

C. Gastrografin esophagogram, and if it does not show extraluminal contrast, then obtain a barium esophagogram.

D. Left thoracotomy with exploration of the mediastinum and repair of the injury, if found.

3. A 72-year-old patient presented with a 2-hour history of severe epigastric, retrosternal pain that radiated to the back. The pain started immediately after several episodes of retching and vomiting. A Gastrografin esophagogram was positive for extraluminal contrast in the distal third of the esophagus and found no other underlying esophageal disease. The best management is:

A. Cervical esophagostomy, gastrotomy and placement of left thoracostomy tubes.

B. Left thoracotomy and distal esophagogastrectomy with intrathoracic esophagogastrostomy.

C. Left thoracotomy, primary repair and serosal patch.

D. Laparotomy, cervical incision and transhiatal esophagectomy with a cervical esophagogastrostomy.

4. A 50-year-old female suffers from a several-year history of reflux symptoms. Chronic use of omeprazole controls the heartburn but she still complains of significant regurgitation and is requesting a definitive solution to her problem. She does not complain of dysphagia. Upper endoscopy revealed esophagitis and a peptic stricture that was easily dilated at 35 cm. Multiple biopsies confirmed the esophagitis and biopsies of the stricture revealed inflammatory changes. There was no columnar metaplasia. Esophageal manometry revealed decreased LES pressure and significantly decreased contraction amplitude in the body of the esophagus. The best operation is:

A. Laparoscopic 270-degree (Toupet, Dor) fundoplication and intraoperative dilatation.

B. Laparoscopic 360-degree (Nissen) fundoplication and intraoperative dilatation.

C. Nissen fundoplication and stricturoplasty.

D. Esophagomyotomy with a 270-degree fundoplication.

5. A 61-year-old female who has no significant complaints underwent an upper endoscopy and colonoscopy for a mild anemia and occult blood in the stool. The bleeding was attributed to a 1.5-cm sigmoid tubular adenoma that was endoscopically removed. Upper endoscopy revealed changes consistent with Barrett's esophagus. Histopathologic diagnosis was Barrett's metaplasia with high-grade dysplasia. The appropriate treatment is:

A. Upper endoscopy as part of a surveillance program for malignancy in 6 months.

B. High-dose therapy with PPIs.

C. Esophageal manometry and laparoscopic fundoplication.

D. Esophagectomy.

6. The following statement about stress gastritis is ***true:***

A. It occurs in 100% of patients who undergo abdominal surgery.

B. It occurs in 10% of patients with sepsis who are ventilator dependent.

C. *Helicobacter pylori* causes stress gastritis.

D. Prophylactic use of H_2 receptor antagonists prevents the development of stress gastritis in ICU patients.

7. The following statement is ***false*** regarding *Helicobacter pylori*:

A. It is found in more than 90% of patients with duodenal ulcer and in 80% of patients with gastric ulcer.

B. The only method of diagnosis of *Helicobacter pylori* infection is by culture of ulcer.

C. Eradication of *Helicobacter pylori* decreases ulcer recurrence to as low as 2% per year.

D. Combination therapy with antibiotics and acid reduction is most effective in eradication of *Helicobacter pylori*.

8. A 45-year-old male patient presented with sudden-onset abdominal pain. The pain started in the epigastrium but became diffuse within a few minutes of its onset. He has a several-year history of recurrent duodenal ulcers that has failed chronic antacid therapy. The patient was tachycardic but normotensive. His abdominal exam was positive for absent bowel sounds, distension, diffuse tenderness and guarding. A chest x-ray revealed free air under the diaphragm. A 3-mm perforation in the anterior wall of the duodenum and significant contamination of the peritoneal cavity was found on exploration. The best surgical treatment is:

A. Truncal vagotomy and antrectomy, including the perforation site.

B. Truncal vagotomy and pyloroplasty.

C. "Graham patch" of the duodenal perforation.

D. "Graham patch" of the duodenal perforation and highly selective vagotomy.

9. The following statement is ***false*** regarding surgical treatment of peptic ulcer disease:

A. Postvagotomy diarrhea is more common after highly selective vagotomy.

B. Ulcer recurrence rate after truncal vagotomy and antrectomy is 1%-2%.

C. Ulcer recurrence rate after highly selective vagotomy is 5%-15%.

D. Dumping occurs more frequently after truncal vagotomy and antrectomy.

10. A 38-year-old obese female had a CT scan of the abdomen after a motor vehicle accident. No significant injuries were seen. However, a 3-cm well-circumscribed mass in the wall of the stomach was seen. There was no evidence of adenopathy and upper endoscopy was normal. The recommended management is:

A. Follow-up CT scan in 6 months.

B. Endoscopic biopsy.

C. CT-guided biopsy.

D. Surgical resection with negative margins

Answers

1. A.
Lifestyle changes are not effective in the therapy of achalasia. Medical therapy with nitrates or calcium channel blockers is used only as a short-term measure in patients with severe symptoms, prior to definitive therapy. Long-term success is dependent on ablation of the sphincter through endoscopic or surgical means.

2. C.
The initial diagnosis of an iatrogenic esophageal perforation is done with Gastrografin esophagogram. Use of this water-soluble contrast does not cause a severe pleural or mediastinal reaction. In approximately 15% of patients, an injury may only be detected by barium contrast. In cases with a large perforation, significant barium contamination of the mediastinum and pleural cavity could occur and lead to significant adherence of bacteria and barium to the tissues.

3. C.
Successful management of barogenic trauma causing esophageal perforation requires prompt recognition and immediate attention. The injury is generally a longitudinal full-thickness tear that can easily be repaired primarily in the early stages of disease. A pleural pedicle flap provides a second layer of coverage. Resection of the esophagus is not necessary in patients without any underlying esophageal pathology, and carries a significant morbidity and mortality risk.

4. A.
Over 80% of patients with easily dilatable peptic strictures do well with an intraoperative dilatation and an antireflux procedure. Patients who do not respond to or require recurrent dilatation are candidates resection. Patients with fibrotic, difficult-to-dilate strictures are also candidates for surgical resection of the stricture. A partial fundoplication is favored because of the decreased contraction amplitude in the esophagus and the risk for postoperative dysphagia with a complete fundic wrap.

5. D.
Patients with high-grade dysplasia in Barrett's esophagus have a risk as high as 40% of having esophageal adenocarcinoma in the Barrett's epithelium. The appropriate conduct is esophagectomy.

6. C.
Overt upper gastrointestinal bleeding can occur in up to 15% of patients in an ICU in the absence of pharmacologic prophylaxis for stress gastritis. ICU patients receiving antacid therapy or H_2 receptor antagonists have a 3% incidence of overt GI bleeding. Therefore, there is an 80% reduction in the risk of bleeding when H_2 receptor antagonists are used for prophylaxis of stress gastritis.

7. B.
A variety of methods are useful in the detection of *H pylori* infection. Histologic examination of the gastric epithelium and urease test allows for the diagnosis on tissue biopsies. Noninvasive methods of determining the presence of *H pylori* are the urease breath test and the measurement of antibodies against *H pylori*.

8. D.
In the individual with no prior dyspeptic symptoms, sealing of the perforation and empiric anti-*H Pylori* therapy should suffice.

9. A.
Postvagotomy diarrhea occurs in approximately 20%-25% of patients after a truncal vagotomy but only 1% of patients suffer from severe or debilitating symptoms. Postvagotomy diarrhea occurs in less than 5% of patients after highly selective vagotomy.

10. D.
Tumors in the wall of the stomach larger than 1-2 cm should be resected in order to establish a definitive diagnosis and to prevent future complications such as bleeding, progressive growth or gastric obstruction. Endoscopic biopsy is notoriously unreliable because the majority of these lesions do not invade the mucosa of the stomach. Fine-needle aspiration EUS is unreliable in predicting the malignant potential of a stromal tumor.

Chapter 10: Barrett's Esophagus and Cancer of the Esophagus, Stomach, Duodenum and Pancreas

Sergio Huerta, MD
Edward H. Livingston, MD

Contents

1. Barrett's Esophagus

The acidic environment from chronic gastroesophageal reflux disease (GERD) causes direct damage to the squamous epithelial lining of the esophagus. The injured lining exposed to acid is progressively replaced by columnar cells as it heals. This metaplastic process is referred to as Barrett's esophagus. Histologically, Barrett's esophagus is characterized by gastric fundic type epithelium, gastric-junctional type epithelium or metaplastic epithelium that contains goblet cells. This process is termed incomplete intestinal metaplasia, specialized columnar epithelium or specialized metaplasia. It is this incomplete intestinal metaplasia that predisposes patients to esophageal cancer. An estimated 14%-20% of American adults are affected by GERD,[1] 10% of patients with GERD will develop Barrett's, and 1% of patients with Barrett's may develop esophageal cancer if prospectively followed in one year.[2]

The clinical prevalence of Barrett's esophagus is less than 10% of that reported by autopsy findings,[3] which reflects the symptomatically silent nature of this condition. Caucasian men are at highest risk and typically present in their mid-50s with symptoms of reflux—heartburn, dysphagia and regurgitation. The severity of symptoms does not correlate with the degree of metaplasia.[4] Any patient with recurrent reflux symptoms following repeated courses of antacid therapy should be evaluated for Barrett's esophagus.

Endoscopy is the diagnostic study of choice for Barrett's esophagus. The diagnosis is made by the presence of specialized metaplasia. The extent of metaplastic lining of the esophagus categorizes Barrett's into long segment (>3 cm) or short segment (<3 cm). The implications and natural history of this classification is unclear and currently these are managed similarly. Identification of the gastroesophageal junction must also be documented. Barium swallow reliably detects complications of Barrett's esophagus (ie, strictures, ulceration), but it has poor sensitivity for identifying mucosal changes. The extent of the disease is measured from the most proximal gastric folds and may contain skip areas. Four-quadrant random biopsies starting at the most proximal gastric fold and continuing to an area just above the squamous epithelial lining of the esophagus prove the diagnosis and exclude the presence of dysplasia or invasive carcinoma. Dysplasia is a histological diagnosis and implies that the epithelial cells have acquired neoplastic genomic abnormalities and potential for malignancy. Thus, metaplasia is the change of the epithelial lining of the esophagus by gastric cells, which is termed Barrett's. Dysplasia, on the other hand, is a pre-malignant abnormality and its risk for cancer is dependent on the degree of dysplasia (ie, low grade vs. high grade). Endoscopy does not identify dysplasia, which is a pathological diagnosis. Thus, random biopsies are taken which have the inherent risk of sampling error. Further, agreement among pathologists for the diagnosis of low grade dysplasia is only around 50%, and circa 85% for high grade dyplasia.[4]

Patients with Barrett's esophagus require lifelong surveillance, regardless of whether the patient is treated medically or surgically for GERD. The treatment of symptomatic Barrett's esophagus is the same as the treatment of GERD. Medical therapy includes elevation of the head of the bed, decreased fat intake, cessation of smoking and discontinuation or change of medications (when possible) that decrease lower esophageal sphincter pressures (nitrates, calcium channel blockers). Histamine-2 (H_2) receptor antagonists and proton pump inhibitors (PPI) are the mainstays of medical therapy. The surgical treatment of Barrett's esophagus without dysplasia consists of a full 360-degree fundoplication (Nissen) or a partial fundoplication (Toupet, Dor, Belsey-Mark IV).

Patients with Barrett's esophagus without dysplasia should undergo surveillance endoscopy every two to three years. Those with low grade dysplasia should be surveyed every 6 and 12 months and annually thereafter if there is no progression of the disease. When high grade dysplasia is identified (and confirmed by expert pathologists), an esophagectomy is the standard treatment option, as 30%-40% of patients with high grade dysplasia harbor invasive cancer. Poor surgical candidates and patients unwilling to undergo surgical intervention require surveillance every 3 months combined with high-dose PPI therapy. Alternatively, these patients can be managed with local ablative strategies. Ablative strategies include endoscopic mucosal resection and photodynamic therapy ablation. Photodynamic therapy ablation uses intravenous sodium porfimer, which is selectively concentrated in dysplastic epithelium. The porfimer is then activated by endoscopic intraesophageal light to chemically ablate dysplastic esophageal mucosa.

Upon healing, ablated areas are replaced with squamous epithelium. Neither medical nor surgical treatment of gastroesophageal reflux disease prevents the development of cancer or can be guaranteed to prevent recurrence of Barrett's esophagus.[3]

2. Esophageal Cancer

Epidemiology

The incidence of esophageal cancer varies according to geographical regions and racial background. Esophageal cancer is common in some areas in China, Puerto Rico and Singapore, but is relatively uncommon in the United States, with 16,470 cases diagnosed in 2008,[5] resulting in 14,280 deaths. Adenocarcinoma and squamous-cell carcinoma (SCC) account for over 90% of esophageal cancers. More than 70% of adenocarcinomas occur in the distal third of the esophagus, whereas SCC is evenly distributed in the upper and middle third of the esophagus. Other uncommon neoplasms of the esophagus include leiomyosarcoma, lymphoma, carcinoid and melanoma. In the United States, the rate of adenocarcinoma of the distal esophagus has risen over the past 20 years,[6] with a parallel decrease in SCC. Adenocarcinoma now accounts for 30%-50% of all esophageal cancers. This striking histological change may be the result of decreased smoking, increased obesity and the increasing use of anti-reflux medications.

SCC is more common in African American men. Risk factors for SCC include tobacco, alcohol, and low income. Several clinical syndromes predispose patients to the development of SCC. Tylosis is an autosomal dominant disease characterized by hyperkeratosis of the skin of the palms and soles and papillomata of the esophagus. SCC may develop in patients with achalasia or caustic burns (lye strictures) at least 15-20 years following the primary diagnosis. The incidence of esophageal cancer in patients with lye stricture is low and does not justify esophagectomy solely for cancer prophylaxis. The incidence of esophageal cancer is also increased in patients with esophageal webs (Plummer-Vinson or Paterson-Kelly syndrome) and to a much lesser degree in patients with esophageal diverticuli.

Adenocarcinoma of the esophagus is more common in Caucasian men. Risk factors for adenocarcinoma include tobacco, obesity and Barrett's esophagus. History of radiation therapy is a predisposing factor for both forms of cancer. Barrett's esophagus can progress from metaplasia to dysplasia and invasive cancer. Patients with Barrett's esophagus have a 1% annual rate of neoplastic transformation into adenocarcinoma. Screening for esophageal cancer is not cost effective and not routinely performed in the United States. However, high-risk patients such as patients with Barrett's esophagus should undergo regular endoscopic surveillance.[7]

Anatomy

The esophagus can be mobilized from the stomach to the level of the aortic arch without risk of devascularization. This is due to the segmental blood supply to the esophagus: the cervical segment of the esophagus is supplied by the inferior thyroid artery; the thoracic esophagus is supplied by the bronchial arteries and aortic branches; and the distal esophagus (the abdominal segment) is supplied by the left gastric and inferior phrenic arteries. Patients with a history of a thyroidectomy with ligation of the inferior thyroid are at great risk of necrosis of the proximal esophagus during mobilization. The esophagus has an extensive lymphatic network. Tumor of any portion of the esophagus may involve lymph nodes from the jugular and supraclavicular region to the celiac basins, including the peritracheal, hilar, subcarinal, para-esophageal, periaortic and pericardial lymph nodes. Esophagectomy for esophageal cancer must encompass at least 10 cm of grossly uninvolved margins to decrease the rate of recurrence. However, submucosal tumor nests may be discontinuous and microscopically negative surgical margins do not obviate local recurrence. Total esophagectomy is required for optimal surgical control.

Clinical Features

History

Most patients with esophageal cancer present during the sixth and seventh decades of life. 75% of patients complain of dysphagia, which is initially experienced with solid foods but in advanced disease may include liquids. Dysphagia generally indicates the presence of a lesion encompassing at least two-thirds of the circumference of the esophagus. Pain on swallowing solids and liquids (odynophagia) is observed in 17% of the patients. Weight loss occurs in 55% of patients. Weight loss more than 10% of normal weight has been associated with decreased survival. GERD is another common finding in these patients, occurring in 21% of the cases.[7] Many patients with esophageal cancers have coexistent cardiopulmonary disease, frequently as a result of tobacco use.

Physical Examination

Early esophageal cancer presents with an unremarkable physical exam. Patients with advanced esophageal cancer may have hepatomegaly, ascites and palpable lymphadenopathy. Supraclavicular adenopathy (Virchow's node) is characteristic, and cervical lymphadenopathy may also be present. Hoarseness (recurrent laryngeal nerve involvement), Horner's syndrome (sympathetic ganglion involvement) and restricted diaphragmatic excursion (phrenic nerve involvement) reflect extensive and typically unresectable disease.

Diagnosis and Staging

The initial screening study consists of a barium-swallow examination (esophagram), which may reveal ulceration or stricture of the esophagus. Upper endoscopy confirms the diagnosis by demonstrating a friable, ulcerated mass. Patients with invasion to the lamina propria or muscularis propria (T1 or T2) and without nodal involvement (N0) are candidates for immediate curative resection (Table 1). The more common patient with T3 or N1 disease may be offered neoadjuvant chemoradiation followed by esophagectomy. The metastatic work-up includes chest radiograph and liver function tests. Tumor markers including CEA, CA 19-9 and CA-125 have poor value in the diagnosis of esophageal cancer. CT scans of the chest, abdomen and pelvis should be obtained for detection of metastatic disease. CT scan is valuable for the recognition of lung and liver metastases, but does not reliably distinguish the characteristics of the tumor or regional lymph node metastases. Magnetic resonance imaging (MRI) may be useful for defining tumor relationship to the thoracic aorta or other vascular structures. 15% of patients who escape identification of metastasis by conventional methods are captured by positron emission tomography (PET) and it is recommended as part of the metastatic work up. Laparoscopic staging has an accuracy of 90%,[8] but its invasive nature makes it less appealing than PET or endoscopic ultrasound (EUS). EUS is the staging procedure of choice. The echo-endoscope allows for accurate staging of tumor size (T1 > 80% and T4 > 95% accurate) as well as nodal involvement (N >70% sensitivity). EUS has the added advantage in that enlarged lymph nodes can be aspirated to distinguish between malignant or inflammatory changes. Patients with upper or middle third esophageal cancers require bronchoscopy to

Table 1

TNM Staging of Esophageal Cancer

T1 Invasion into lamina propria or submucosa
T2 Invasion to muscularis propria
T3 Invasion of adventitia
T4 Invasion of adjacent structures

Stage	**I**	**IIA**	**IIB**	**III**
	T1, N0	T2-3, N0	T1-2, N1	T3, N1 T4, any N
5-year survival	50%-80%	30%-40%	10%-30%	10%-15%

exclude the presence of a tracheo-esophageal fistula, which would preclude surgical resection. Bulging of the posterior membranous trachea or left main stem bronchus or narrowing of the left main stem bronchus indicates an abutting tumor and mandates biopsy and brushing for cytology.

Treatment

Patients with T1 or T2 lesions without lymph node metastases have excellent prognosis and esophagectomy is the mainstay of treatment. Long-term survival in patients with T3 or N1 disease following esophagectomy is unusual. More than 50% of patients with esophageal cancer have metastatic disease or unresectable tumors at the time of presentation. The first aspect to consider determining the form of treatment for esophageal cancer is the histology of the tumor as SCC responds better to ionizing radiation compared to adenocarcioma. The location of the tumor is the next step in determining the form of management. Upper and mid-thoracic tumors may require a thoracotomy, whereas lower esophageal tumors may be resected via the trashiatal approach. The next aspect to consider in terms of management involves the stage of the tumor.

T1 lesions carry a risk of lymph node involvement in less than 50% of the cases. These patients typically do not need neoadjuvant chemoradiation. An esophagectomy is the main stay of treatment and for these patients. It can be performed via more conservative surgical techniques (ie, vagal sparing esophagectomy, transhiatal esphagectomy, minimally invasive procedures). Because of the relatively low risk of lymph node involvement, these patients typically will not benefit from a lyphadenectomy. In these patients, there is no need for adjuvant chemoradiation, unless lymph nodes are positive at the time of resection.[2]

T2 lesions are at risk of a 60% of lymph node involvement. There is a great deal of controversy in the management of these lesions. The aggressive camp advocates: 1.) neoadjuvant chemoradiation, 2.) en-block esophagectomy, 3.) lyphadenectomy, and 4.) ± adjuvant chemoradiation. Conservative advocates suggest: 1.) neoadjuvant chemoradiation, 2.) transhiatal esophagectomy, 3.) no lyphadenectomy, and 4.) definite adjuvant chemoradiation. Advocates for the conservative management argue that chemoradiation addresses positive lymph nodes. Additionally, even with aggressive lymphadenectomy, it is difficult to eradicate all positive disease.

T3 lesions have an 80% risk of lymph node metastasis and require 1.) neoadjuvant chemoradiation, 2.) en-block esophagectomy, 3.) lyphadenectomy, and 4.) adjuvant chemoradiation. A patient with regional local and regional (one lymph node basin away from typical esophageal drainage) lymph node disease might still be considered for resection.[2] **T4** lesions require multimodality therapy. If a lymph node is identified to be more than one basin away from the primary tumor, it is considered a distant lymph node and these patients are considered to have advanced disease. Chemotherapy is the main form of treatment for these patients. Thus, surgery is considered for patients with stage I-III (Table 1) disease, but for patients with stage IV surgical intervention is not curative and these patients are treated with chemotherapy.

Endoscopic mucosal resection (EMR) is being used in Japan for the management of SCC that has not penetrated through the muscularis mucosa (T1a). EMR is beginning to be a treatment modality in Western countries as well.[9,10]

In summary, T1-T3 tumors, even in the presence of local and regional lymph nodes, are considered resectable. T4 tumors without major involvement of adjacent structures might be considered resectable. T4 tumors with involvement of major structures such as great vessels, trachea, liver or pancreas are considered unresectable. Tumor with distant lymph node involvement or systemic metastases are typically considered nonresectable.[11]

Palliation with minimal morbidity is the goal for patients with metastatic disease. Patients with a good performance status do well with esophagectomy. However, the survival of these patients is measured in months, not years. Palliation by nonsurgical means, including radiation with or without endoscopic stenting, should be considered. Patients with malignant tracheoesophageal fistulas present a perplexing treatment dilemma, because they cannot be irradiated. Substernal esophageal bypass to the stomach is an option; however, these patients frequently are not good operative candidates. Endoscopic stenting may palliate these patients.

Chemoradiation

Preoperative administration of radiation therapy or chemotherapy alone followed by surgical resection does not enhance survival in comparison to surgery alone.[7] However, there is a trend towards an improvement in survival when these two modalities are given in combination pre-operatively. Three combined randomized control trial studies suggested that the 3-year survival for patients receiving neoadjuvant chemoratdiation was 37% compared to 28% in patients receiving surgery alone. This was at a cost of a rate of complications of 5% vs. 13%, respectively.[12-14] A recent meta-analysis showed an improved 3-year survival advantage in patients receiving pre-operative chemoradiotherapy and significant downstaging of the tumor.[15] In spite of this evidence neoadjuvant chemoradiation is considered investigational by the National Comprehensive Cancer Network (NCCN).[11] Neoadjuvant chemoradiation typically consisting of induction with paclitaxel and cisplatin followed by 45 Gy and 5-FU/cisplatin/paclitaxel of chemoradiation over 6-7 weeks.[2] Tri-modality therapy (pre-op chemoradiation + surgery with lymphadenectomy) has been recently shown to have a 5-year survival advantage over esophagectomy alone in a small randomized controlled trial study.[16] Esophagectomy is performed 5-6 weeks following the final dose of radiation, which allows local edema to resolve, but is not enough time for fibrous adhesions to form. Patients receiving neoadjuvant therapy are typically restaged prior to surgical intervention. Nutritional support during the preoperative period is essential and can be accomplished with a gastrostomy or jejunostomy feeding tubes, which can be placed endoscopically, percutaneously, laparoscopically or via laparotomy.

Methods of Esophagectomy

Esophagectomy carries a mortality of 4% and substantial postoperative morbidity. Most complications are pulmonary in nature and preoperative evaluation should anticipate respiratory failure especially in patients with an FEV1 less than 50% or a resting elevation of PCO^2.

Transhiatal or blunt esophagectomy (THE) was first described by Denk and popularized by Orringer.[17,18] In this approach, two incisions are required: a midline laparotomy, and a left cervical incision paralleling the medial border of the sternocleidomastoid muscle (Figure 1). Mobilization of the stomach is performed with preservation of the right gastroepiploic arcade. Similarly, mobilization of the duodenum via a generous Kocher maneuver should be performed with preservation of the right gastritic artery. The short and left gastric arteries are then ligated. The vagus nerves

Figure 1

Schematic of transhiatal esophagectomy

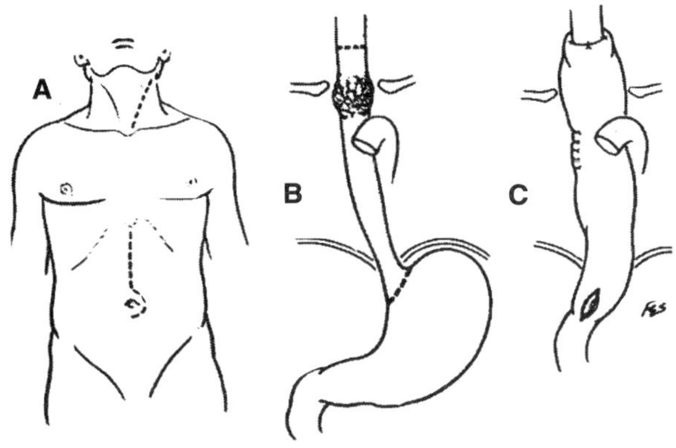

Reprinted from Peters JH, DeMeester TR. Esophagus and diaphragmatic hernia. In: Schwartz SI, Shires GT, Spencer FC, eds. Principles of Surgery. *New York, NY: McGraw-Hill Inc; 1994.*

are divided and the distal esophagus is bluntly dissected from the hiatus to the level of the left mainstem bronchus from within the abdomen. Once the stomach is properly mobilized, the pylorus will reach the hiatus without tension. The cervical esophagus is exposed through a left cervical incision. The esophagus is encircled in the neck with careful preservation of the recurrent laryngeal nerves. The esophagus is bluntly dissected from above until it is entirely freed from mediastinal attachments. Blunt dissection along the esophageal wall prevents accidental tearing of the azygous vein, which could result in uncontrollable hemorrhage. While transhiatal esophagectomy does not allow for the removal of mediastinal lymph nodes other than those visualized through the hiatus, it avoids an intrathoraic anastomosis. Hence, anastomotic leaks are easily managed with the cervical drain without the risk of thoracic empyema or mediastinitis. The avoidance of a thoractomy theoretically improves postoperative pulmonary function. The mortality rate for THE is 4% and the risk of leak is 3%. Injury to the great vessels and stricture rate remain a concern with this type of esophagectomy.

Ivor Lewis Esophagectomy

Ivor Lewis esophagectomy (transthoracic esophagectomy; TEE) requires 2 incisions, a midline laparotomy and a posterior-lateral thoracotomy (Figure 2). The abdominal phase of the operation is similar to that of THE, which consists of complete mobilization of the stomach with preservation of the right gastroepiploic arcade and commonly the right gastric artery. Lymph nodes along the left gastric artery are removed with the specimen. A left thoracotomy is performed in the fourth or fifth intercostal space and the azygous vein is divided. En bloc esophageal resection is undertaken from the hiatus to the apex of the chest. The dissection includes hilar, subcarinal, and periesophageal nodes. A one- or two-layer or stapled anastomosis is done high in the chest and protected with a fundal or pleural wrap. This allows for a 5 cm to 10 cm proximal margin depending on the location of the tumor. Chest tubes are placed for drainage. The theoretical survival benefits of TEE in comparison to transhiatal resection have not been demonstrated.

Limited evidence indicates that pulmonary complications, perioperative morbidity and wound infection rates are lower with the THE approach, but this has not been uniformly observed. THE does increase the risk of recurrent laryngeal nerve injury (occurring in

Figure 2

Schematic of Ivor Lewis esophagectomy

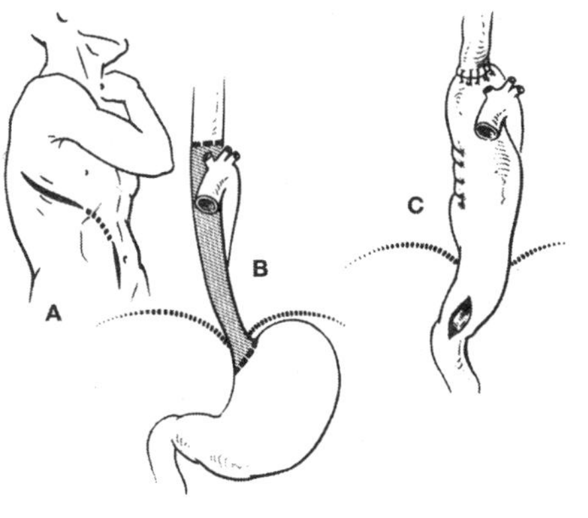

Reprinted from Peters JH, DeMeester TR. Esophagus and diaphragmatic hernia. In: Schwartz SI, Shires GT, Spencer FC, eds. Principles of Surgery. *New York, NY: McGraw-Hill Inc; 1994.*

about 10% of cases) in comparison to TEE. The majority of retrospective studies indicate equivalent survival rates and similar postoperative morbidity and mortality rates between these two surgical techniques.

Radical Esophagectomy

Radical en bloc esophagectomy is a more demanding operation, entailing a cervical incision, laparotomy and thoracotomy. En bloc esophageal dissection proceeds through the chest with complete en bloc mobilization of the esophagus and mediastinal lymph nodes. Following closure of the chest, a midline laparotomy is undertaken with en bloc dissection of perigastric and celiac axis lymph nodes. A left cervical incision allows for mobilization of the esophagus in a manner similar to a THE. A hemigastrectomy with colon interposition is performed from the cervical esophagus to the transected stomach. This technique allows for 10 cm distal and proximal margins and a complete lymphadenectomy. Since the morbidity of this operation is higher than the previously described techniques, patients must be rigorously screened for adequate cardiopulmonary reserve (ejection fraction >40%, FEV1greater than 1.25 L). This operation is indicated in patients with stage IIA and stage IIB disease who are good operative candidates.[19,20] Patients with stage III disease, who are unlikely to be cured regardless of the extent of lymphadenectomy, should not undergo the operative risk of this surgical intervention.

Because these methods of esophagectomy disrupt the vagus nerves, a gastric emptying procedure is required, which can be accomplished via one of three commonly used techniques. Pyloroplasty is an established method of gastric emptying, with almost no incidence of failure. Its main disadvantage is that it requires opening the gastrointestinal tract and also shortens the stomach. A pyloromyotomy has the advantage of disrupting the pylorus without opening the gastrointestinal tract. Finally, the pylorus can be dilated by gently opposing the surgeon's thumb and forefinger through the pyloric channel.

The vagal sparing esophagectomy is similar to the THE, but preserves the vagus nerves. A highly selective vagotomy is required, but no emptying procedure needs to be done. Incomplete resection of the esophagus is a concern with this operation.

Minimally invasive procedures continue to evolve. Esophageal resections can be performed via thoracoscopy to replace the thoracotomy and laparoscopy in place of laparotomy. Currently minimally invasive procedures and the vagal sparing esophagectomy should only be considered for early esophageal cancers.

3. Gastric Adenocarcinoma

Epidemiology

In the year 2008, 21,500 Americans were diagnosed with gastric cancer and 10,880 died from this malignancy.[5] Gastric cancer is the fourteenth most frequent cause of cancer mortality in the United States and the second most common cause of cancer death worldwide. In the United States, there has been a substantial decrease in the incidence of gastric adenocarcinoma in men and women, which is likely the result of improved methods of food storage and changes in diet, including decreased salt intake.[21,22]

Gastric cancer demonstrates a high degree of geographic variability worldwide with the highest incidence in Japan and some South American countries, but remains low in Western Europe and America. First-generation Japanese migrants maintain their native risk for the development of gastric cancer, while their offspring acquire the risk rate of the native country. This reflects the large influence of environmental factors in the development of gastric cancer.[2] Gastric cancer is more common in African American men and typically occurs in the 7th decade of life. Most cases of gastric cancer in the United States occur in the distal stomach (gastric body and antrum).[21] While there has been a plateau and recent decrease in the incidence of distal gastric cancer, a steady increase has been noted in the incidence of proximal and gastroesophageal junction gastric neoplasms.[6]

Figure 3

Lauren intestinal-type gastric cancer characterized by malignant cells that form glandular structures

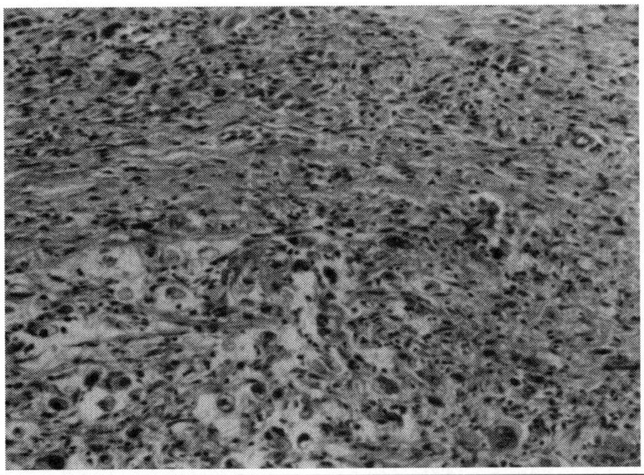

From Dr Charles Theuer's personal collection.

Figure 4

Lauren diffuse-type gastric cancer characterized by malignant cells spread throughout the muscularis propria and lacking glandular structures

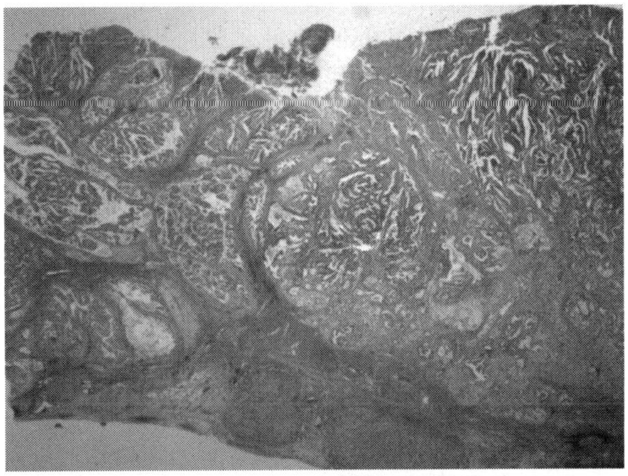

From Dr Charles Theuer's personal collection.

Pathology

Because 95% of all malignant gastric neoplasms are adenocarcinomas, the term *gastric cancer* generally refers to adenocarcinoma of the stomach. The remainder consists of non-Hodgkin's lymphomas and stromal tumors.[23] The stomach is the most common site of gastrointestinal lymphoma. Since treatment options and prognosis are markedly different between lymphoma and adenocarcinoma, early differentiation is crucial. Metastatic spread to the stomach may occur from the liver, pancreas, lung, breast, prostate or melanoma.[24]

Histopathological categorization of gastric cancer involves many classification systems. The two most commonly used are the World Health Organization (WHO) and the Lauren systems. The WHO system histologically categorizes gastric cancer into: adenocarcinoma (intestinal and diffuse), papillary, tubular, mucinous and signet-ring cell. It also assigns grades to adenocarcinoma based on the degree of differentiation from metaplastic intestinal tissue.

More practically, the Lauren system classifies gastric cancer into two histological categories: intestinal and diffuse types.[25] The intestinal-type is characterized by a glandular, solid, intestinal architecture and also displays tubular components (Figure 3). The diffuse-type demonstrates clusters of individually separated cells infiltrating the gastric wall (Figure 4). The Lauren's classification is a useful system for genetic and epidemiological purposes and to assess the natural history of gastric cancer. Intestinal-type gastric cancers are more commonly related to environmental factors (salted fish, meat, smoked foods, cigarette smoking and alcohol) and occur more frequently in the general population. The intestinal type is more common in men and metastatic spread is typically via the hematogenous route. Diffuse-type gastric cancers are more common in women and young patients, have a poorer prognosis, and are likely to have a hereditary etiology. *Helicobacter pylori (H pylori)* infections are associated with both types of gastric cancer.

Risk Factors

5%-10% of gastric cancers show a hereditary component and may develop in families with germ line mutations of p53 (Li-Fraumeni syndrome), BRCA2 and the gene encoding E-cadherin (hereditary diffuse gastric cancer). Gastric cancer may also develop as part of nonpolyposis colon cancer (Lynch II), familial adenomatous polyposis (FAP), Peutz Jeghers and Cowden syndromes. Finally, gastric cancer is more common in patients with blood type A.[21,23,24] Hereditary gastric cancers are histologically of the diffuse type.

Most cases of sporadic gastric cancer occur in the presence of precursor conditions such as chronic atrophic gastritis, intestinal metaplasia or adenomatous polyps. Similarly, patients with pernicious anemia have a 2- to 3-fold increased risk of gastric cancer as a result of the immune type of chronic gastritis affecting the parietal cells of the stomach. Patients with a prior history of partial gastrectomy for benign disease have a 1.5- to 3-fold increased risk of gastric cancer beginning 15 years following their surgery. This risk is probably the result of chronic alkaline duodenal reflux into the remnant stomach. Alternatively, the suppressed acid environment allows for bacterial overgrowth leading to an increased production of carcinogenic nitroso compounds.

Other risks factors include hypertrophic gastropathy (Menetrier's disease) and Barrett's esophagus (particularly gastric cancer in the gastric cardia).[21] *H pylori* infection increases the risk of gastric cancer by 3- to 6-fold. *H pylori* is a fastidious Gram-negative rod that infects the stomach and duodenum following oral ingestion. Once established in the stomach, it may persist for decades in the acidic gastric environment. In most cases, *H pylori* coexists with its host without causing symptoms, but acute or chronic infection may cause atrophic gastritis and ulceration. Patients with gastric cancer not involving the gastroesophageal junction are much more likely to have serologic evidence of prior *H pylori* infection than unaffected controls. *H pylori* is now considered a carcinogenic agent by the International Agency for Research on Cancer, and is estimated to contribute to the development of gastric cancer in 35%-50% of cases worldwide. The role of *H pylori* in the development of gastric cancer is unknown but it is associated with the development of chronic gastritis.[21]

Clinical Features

Gastric cancer is usually fatal in Americans, as 65% of gastric cancers are diagnosed at an advanced stage (T3/T4), with metastasis to lymph nodes in 85% of the cases. This is largely due to the fact that screening is not routinely practiced in the United States. The overall 5-year survival for patients with resectable gastric cancer is 10%-30% with a median survival of 24 months. Patients who undergo palliative surgery have a median survival of 8.1 months and those with advanced metastatic disease 5.4 months.[23,26] The clinical and biological features of gastric cancer in Japan are different than those in the United States. Japanese patients are younger (63 vs. 68 years), more likely to have intestinal-type histology and are much less likely to have cancer of the gastroesophageal junction. Japanese patients with advanced gastric cancer also have superior survival rates compared to Western patients. This stage-stratified survival advantage may reflect higher cure rates and improved staging as a result of more extensive lymphadenectomy, or less aggressive tumor biology in Japanese patients. As a result, the overall 5-year survival rate is above 50% in patients with gastric cancer. This improved survival is, in part, the result of diagnosis at earlier stages of disease in the Japanese population.[23,26]

In America, screening is not cost effective due to the low incidence of the disease and the high costs of upper endoscopy or barium upper gastrointestinal

Table 2

TNM Staging of Gastric Cancer

T1 Invasion of lamina propia or submucosa
T2 Invasion of muscularia propia
T3 Invasion through serosa
T4 Invasion into adjacent structures

N1*[a] Perigastric lymph nodes (3 cm from primary tumor)
N2 Left gastric, common hepatic, or splenic lymph nodes (more than 3 cm from primary)

Stage	**I**	**II**	**III**	**IV**
	T1, N0-1 T2, N0	T1, N2 T2, N1 T3, N0	T2, N1-2 T3, N1-2 T4, N0-1	T4, N2, M0 T4, any N Any T/N, M1
5-year survival				
Japan[31] (1971-1985)	91%	72%	44%	9.0%
United States[32] (1982-1987)	50%	29%	13%	3.0%

*[a] *The most recent classification includes : N1 = 1-6 nodes, N2 = 7-15 nodes, N3 = >15 nodes*[30]

series. Screening has been suggested for high-risk groups in the United States, including the elderly with atrophic gastritis or pernicious anemia, patients more than 20 years post-partial gastrectomy,[23,27] hereditary nonpolyposis colorectal cancer patients, and immigrants of ethnic groups from countries with high rates of gastric carcinoma.

History and Physical Examination

Early gastric cancer produces no symptoms, which delays the diagnosis. Thus, most cases of gastric cancer are diagnosed at the time of locally advanced or metastatic disease. Weight loss and abdominal pain are the most common presenting symptoms of gastric cancer, occurring with a frequency of 62% and 52%, respectively. Gastric outlet obstruction may occur in tumors involving the pylorus, whereas gastric cancers involving the cardia may present with nausea (34%), anorexia (32%) or dysphagia (26%). Gastrointestinal bleeding presenting as melena occurs in 20% of patients with gastric cancer.[21]

Physical examination is generally unyielding in the diagnosis of gastric cancer. An occasional patient will present with a palpable abdominal mass, demonstrating locally advanced disease. There are well described physical exam findings which demonstrate metastatic disease by lymphatic spread such as supraclavicular nodal involvement (Virchow's node), periumbilical implants (Sister Mary Joseph's node), malignant ascites, ovarian masses (Krukenberg tumor) and peritoneal implants in the cul-de-sac (Blumer's shelf). The liver is the most common site of hematogenous spread. Gastric cancer rarely presents with paraneoplastic conditions, including seborrheic keratoses (Leser-Trelat sign), intravascular thrombosis (Trouseau's syndrome), acantosis nigricans (pigmented lesions of mucous membranes and skin folds), nephropathy and hemolytic anemia.[21]

Diagnostic Evaluation

Laboratory exams are typically normal or nonspecific. Anemia, hypoproteinemia, abnormal liver function tests and fecal occult blood may occur in 20%-40% of patients with gastric cancer.[28] Tumor serologic markers such CEA and CA 19-9 are not helpful in the diagnosis of gastric cancer. The diagnosis is generally confirmed with upper GI endoscopy (95% accuracy). Less invasive test such as upper GI barium radiography is not as accurate and also lacks the inability to obtain tissue. Tumor stage and location of the gastric cancer are essential for treatment options and prognosis. TNM staging established by the American Joint Committee on Cancer is the most commonly used system for staging gastric cancer (Table 2). Metastatic work-up consists of chest radiograph, liver function tests, and CT scans of the abdomen and pelvis. Endoscopic ultrasound (EUS) is used by some centers but still not recommended by NCCN guidelines. The accuracy of EUS is best for T3 lesions (90%), but poor for T2 lesions (72%). Nodal staging is only 77% accurate by EUS. Although more invasive, staging laparoscopy is 93% accurate in staging gastric cancer, which can upstage up to 37% of gastric cancers originally deemed resectable and may evade unnecessary surgical intervention.[29] Patients with regional lymph node metastases visible on CT are likely to have advanced gastric cancer, but CT scan is only 25%-80% accurate in the identification of lymph node metastasis, underscoring the utility of diagnostic laparoscopy.[30] Up to 50% of patients identified to have metastatic disease by laparoscopy are successfully palliated with chemotherapy only.[2]

Treatment

Surgical Treatment

The goal for surgical intervention with gastric cancers is to achieve a resection with microscopic negative margins (R0 resection). An R2 resection refers to surgical intervention in which gross tumors was left unresected, while an R1 operation removes all macroscopic disease, but microscopic margins contain disease. Surgical resection with total eradication of the gastric tumor with adequate margins and bordering lymph nodes provides the only option for cure.[31,32]

Two areas in the surgical management of gastric cancer need to be addressed. One is the type of gastrectomy and the second is the degree of lymph node resection to achieve the best chance of cure while minimizing morbidity and motility. The principles for surgical intervention are well established for the former, while the later is under a great deal of current controversy.

The type of gastrectomy (partial vs. total) must address the location of the tumor. Anastomotic recurrence has been noted to occur when the surgical margins are less than 3.5 cm, but is absent when 6.5 cm of negative margins are achieved.[2,32] Thus, frozen sections at the time of gastrectomy have to establish at least 6.0 cm free margins.

Proximal tumors occur in 35%-50% of gastric cancers. These tumors are typically more advanced than distal tumors at the time of surgical exploration. While survival advantage appears to be similar in patients with proximal tumors undergoing a total vs. a proximal gastrectomy,[33,34] morbidity and mortality is substantially superior in patients with proximal tumors undergoing a total gastrectomy. The mortality of patients with proximal partial gastrectomy is up to 16%, compared to 8% in patients treated with a total gastrectomy. Morbidity associated with a partial gastrectomy is substantial and includes dumping syndrome, heartburn and early satiety. Proximal gastric tumors should therefore be treated with a total gastrectomy (Figure 5).[2]

Distal gastric tumors account for nearly 35% of stomach cancers. In contrast to a proximal partial gastrectomy, a distal gastrectomy results in reduced risks of morbidity and mortality compared to a total gastrectomy. Survival is similar in patients with distal tumor treated with a total gastrectomy and distal partial gastrectomy, provided that adequate margins of resection are obtained. Thus, distal gastric tumors can adequately be treated with a distal gastrectomy. Figure 5 depicts the typical extent of dissection based on the location of the tumor.

Patients undergoing subtotal gastrectomy are reconstructed with a Billroth II gastrojejunostomy. A Billroth I gastroduodenostomy is not advocated because the anastomosis lies within the retroperitoneal bed that may contain residual cancer. Recurrence could therefore lead to anastomotic obstruction. Similarly, an antecolic gastrojejunostomy is recommended as it removes the anastomosis from the retroperitoneum. On the other hand, a retrocolic gastrojejunostomy has the theoretical advantage of superior dependent

Figure 5

Extent of resection required for R1 and R2 lymphadenectomy based on the site of the primary gastric cancer

R = scope of lymphadenectomy (broken line). To qualify as an R2, all R1-designated nodes must be removed and most of R2-designated nodes must be removed.

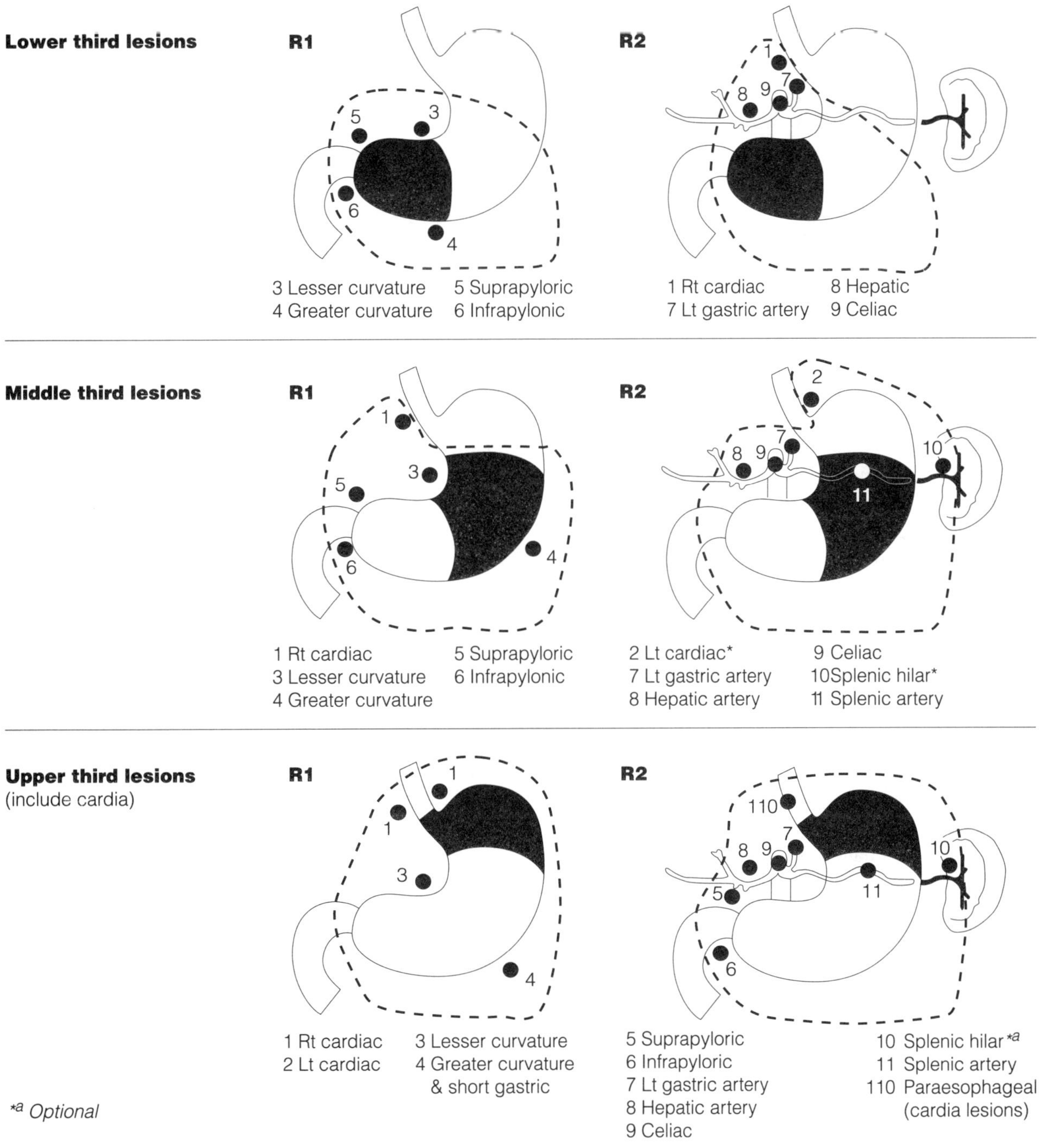

*a Optional

Reprinted from Smith J, Shiu MH, Kelsey L, et al. Morbidity of radical lymphadenectomy in the curative resection of gastric carcinoma. Arch Surg. *1991;126:1469-1473.*

gastric emptying. Randomized comparisons of antecolic and retrocolic reconstructions are unavailable. Patients undergoing a total gastrectomy should undergo a Roux-en Y esophagojenunostomy. A feeding jejunostomy is routinely placed in patients undergoing total gastrectomy.

Nearly one-fourth of patients with gastric cancers present with stage IV disease at the time of diagnosis. Patients with pathologically proven peritoneal implants, liver metastases or paraaortic lymphadenopathy are not curable. A palliative gastrectomy (including omentectomy) should be undertaken in these patients (without liver metastases or malignant ascites).[35] A palliative bypass is the operation of choice for unresectable gastric cancer causing gastric outlet obstruction. Endoscopic dilation with stent placement is another modality of choice available for patient with obstructive symptoms.

There is substantial controversy concerning the degree of extent for lymph node dissection (LND). Japanese data assert that extended LND prolongs survival and allows for more appropriate staging. Roughly, group 1 nodes are nodes located in the perigastric area (D1). Group 2 nodes (D2) are nodes located along the celiac axis distribution (hepatic proper, right gastric and splenic). An extended LND includes resection of D2 nodes. Finally, group 3 nodes (D3) are nodes in the para-aortic area.

In Eastern Asia, gastrectomy with D2 lymphadenectomy is the standard treatment for curable gastric cancer.[36] This practice emanates from repeated studies in Japan that confirmed the original finding by Kodama demonstrating a survival advantage in patients with gastic cancer receiving a D2 (39%) vs. a D1 (18%) lymphadenectomy.[37] However, these findings have not been supported by Western studies. For instance, well randomized studies (the Dutch and the British Randomized trials)[23,31] assessing the effect of D1 vs. D2 lymphadenectomy have demonstrated increased morbidity and mortality in patients undergoing D2 LND with equivalent survival rates to those receiving a D1 LND.[23,31] Current guidelines by the National Comprehensive Cancer Network (NCCN) recommend a D1 resection with assessment of at least 15 lymph nodes. A D2 resection in the United States remains investigational and should be performed in specialized centers. Splenectomy and distal pancreatectomy increase operative morbidity and mortality and are not employed unless required for en bloc resection of the primary tumor.[23,31] The need for more aggressive lymph node dissection has been recently resolved by a Japanese study which demonstrated no survival advantage in patients submitting to D2 LND vs. a D2 LND + para-aortic nodal dissection (D3 LND).[36]

Technical Considerations

The best exposure to the stomach can be achieved either via a Chevron or upper midline incision. After thorough inspection of the peritoneal surfaces and the liver, the greater omentum is divided at its colonic attachment and the lesser omentum is divided at its hepatic attachment. These maneuvers allow palpation of the para-aortic lymph nodes. Peritoneal, hepatic and omental implants are sampled. Metastases to these structures or the para-aortic nodes indicate incurable gastric cancer, and a palliative resection, including omentectomy, is performed. The chest should not be opened for the purpose of achieving a negative margin during palliative gastrectomy. Thoracotomy increases postoperative morbidity and is not justified unless a curative gastrectomy is entertained.

In cases where abdominal exploration indicates that a curative gastrectomy is possible, dissection continues in the lesser sac. Posterior gastric attachments are divided. The right gastroepiploic arcade is identified and branching veins between this arcade and the middle colic vein are divided. The arcade is completely dissected to the origin of the gastroepiploic artery from the gastroduodenal artery. Ligation of the arcade at the origin ensures removal of the infrapyloric nodes. The common hepatic artery is identified in the retroperitoneum. It is dissected to the origin of the right gastric artery. Ligation of the right gastric artery at its origin allows for the removal of suprapyloric nodes. The duodenum is divided and the closure may be reinforced with Lembert sutures. Attention is then directed to the origin of the left gastric artery. This artery and the coronary vein are best approached through the lesser sac. The vein and artery are ligated at the superior border of the pancreas after careful mobilization of the left gastric and celiac lymph nodes so they are included in the surgical specimen. The lesser and greater curves of the stomach are exposed at least 6 cm above the tumor and the stomach is divided with a linear stapler.

Radiation and Chemotherapy

Preoperative and postoperative radiation, chemotherapy and chemoradiation all have been employed with moderate reported success. A few well randomized studies continue to accumulate to support this practice. The current recommendations from the National Comprehensive Cancer Network advocate for the use of chemoradiation (5-FU based) for patients with T3/4 or node positive tumors in whom an R0 resection was undertaken. Patients with R1 resections might also be considered candidates for postoperative (adjuvant) chemoradiation.

Chemoradiation (5-FU and leucovorin + 45 Gy of radiation) has been shown to increase survival by nine months in patients treated with this modality vs. surgery alone. Additionally, recurrence rates were 10% higher in patients who did not receive chemoradiation therapy. The medical adjuvant gastric infusional chemotherapy (MAGIC) trial showed a significant improvement in overall survival as well as progression disease survival in patients with operable cancers of the stomach and lower esophagus receiving neoadjuvant and adjuvant chemotherapy. Chemotherapy consisted of three pre-operative and three post-operative cycles of epirubicin, cisplatin and 5-FU.[38]

In patients with metastatic disease, chemotherapy is the only modality available (epirubicin, cisplatin, 5FU, etoposide). Chemotherapy increases survival by up to 9 months. Symptomatic patients with metastatic disease should undergo palliation therapy with chemotherapy, radiation therapy or surgical intervention. In spite of aggressive chemotherapy or palliative interventions, the median survival for patients with metastatic disease is less than 10 months.

4. Gastric Lymphoma

Primary gastric lymphomas are non-Hodgkin's lymphomas (NHL). Although non-Hodgkin's lymphoma of the stomach accounts for less than 5% of gastric malignancies, the stomach is the most common site of extranodal NHL. Gastric NHL is categorized into low grade (indolent) and high grade (aggressive). Forty percent of gastric NHLs are low grade and the vast majority arise from mucosa-associated lymphoid tissue (MALT). MALT is a specialized form of lymphoid tissue such as that found in Peyer's patches. The stomach typically lacks lymphoid tissue. Chronic Helicobacter pylori (*H pylori*) infection results in interleukin-2 production and other cytokines inducing proliferation of B cells in the gastric mucosa and formation of MALT.[39] Thus, *H pylori* infection is the primary risk factor for low grade NHL of the stomach and its eradication is paramount in the treatment of this lesion. Other risk factors include inflammatory bowel disease, celiac disease, immunosuppresion (particularly following organ transplantation) and HIV infection. Low grade gastric NHL may progress to the high grade type. However, high grade NHL may also occur *de novo* and spread locally or distally via lymphatics. Patients are typically in their sixties and there is no gender predilection. Gastric NHL usually presents with a clinical history similar to gastric adenocarcinoma, with pain being the most common symptom. Vomiting occurs with gastric outlet obstruction whereas bleeding may accompany ulceration and peritonitis due to perforation. One-eighth of patients have systemic symptoms including weight loss, night sweats and fever (B-symptoms).

Signs of diffuse lymphoma, including splenomegaly or peripheral lymphadenopathy, may be present in advanced disease. Fifteen percent of patients with low grade NHL have lymph node involvement, whereas nearly all cases of high grade NHL present with lymph node metastasis. The diagnosis of gastric lymphoma is usually made with upper endoscopy and biopsy. Further diagnostic evaluation should focus on whether the stomach is the primary or secondary site of lymphoma and staging of the disease. This evaluation includes CT scans of the chest, abdomen, and pelvis, biopsy of enlarged peripheral lymph nodes and bone marrow biopsy. EUS is helpful in determining the depth of tumor invasion and perigastric lymphadenopathy. PET is also a useful modality in staging of this lesion.

Patients with low grade MALT localized to the stomach and perigastric lymph nodes (stage I and stage II disease) have a good prognosis with 5-year survival rates of 80%-90%. The initial treatment for all types of gastric NHL should consist of *H pylori* eradication. Three regimens of *H pylori* eradication have shown 80%-95% response rate, these consist of 14 days of: a.) proton pump inhibitor (lansoprazole/omeprazole), clarithromycin, and metronidazole; b.) proton pump inhibitor (lansoprazole/omeprazole), bismuth, metronidazole, and tetracycline, or c.) H_2 blocker, bismuth, metronidazole and tetracycline. *H pylori* eradication and close endoscopic surveillance should suffice for patients with stage I gastric NHL. A small percentage of patients with stage I low grade gastric lymphoma who do not respond to *H pylori* eradication within a few months should be suspected of having non-MALT gastric lymphoma or an *H pylori* translocated strain [translocation t(911:18)]. These patients as well as those with stage II disease should be treated with radiation therapy (30 Gy) and/or chemotherapy in addition to *H pylori* eradication. Radiation and/or chemotherapy are the mainstay of treatment in patients with stage III and IV low grade lesions. Patients with disseminated disease are best treated with chemotherapy without radiation. Currently, surgical intervention is indicated for patients with residual disease after aggressive medical management or patients with perforation or bleeding.[40] Chemotherapy consists of cyclophosphamide, vincristine, nitrogen mustard, procarbazine and prednisone (CMOPP) or cyclophosphamide, doxorubicin, vincristine and prednisone (CHOP). The monoclonal antibody rituximab has also been used, in addition to chemotherapy.

5. Ampullary Adenocarcinoma

Periampullary tumors are defined as neoplasms within 2 cm of the ampulla in the duodenum. These cancers include tumors of the duodenum, head of the pancreas, ampulla and lower common bile duct. These lesions present with similar clinical symptomatology, but their outcome depends on the site of origin of the primary tumor. Periampullary cancers are staged based on the depth of invasion into the duodenum or pancreas rather than the size of the tumor.[41]

Ampullary cancers have the most favorable prognosis of all periampullary neoplasms. 80% of ampullary tumors are benign. Additionally, because of their location, ampullary tumors generally become symptomatic when they are small (less than 2 cm), and therefore lymphatic metastases are less frequent. Although the symptoms are not specific, consisting of vague abdominal pain, upper GI bleeding or obstruction, increased liver function tests, jaundice or recurrent pancreatitis, these symptoms usually mandate further work-up, resulting in the discovery of the tumor. The diagnostic modality of choice is ERCP. CT scan is useful to exclude metastases, but does not reliably reveal the primary tumor due to its small size and location. Treatment with pancreaticoduodenectomy results in 5-year survival rates of nearly 50% for nodenegative disease, and 20%-30% for node-positive disease. Local resection should be performed for villous adenomas of the ampulla or for invasive cancer in patients who are unable to tolerate pancreaticoduodenectomy. Local resection of suspected benign lesions that prove to be invasive on final pathology should be treated with pancreaticoduodenectomy in good operative candidates. Ampullary tumors should be considered premalignant lesions if discovered in the setting of familial polyposis syndromes.[42]

6. Duodenal Adenocarcinoma

Primary adenocarcinoma of the duodenum is a rare neoplasm accounting for less than 0.4% of all gastrointestinal neoplasms.[43,44] Its surgical management and prognosis is highly dependent on the location of the tumor along the duodenum. Tumors located in the first and second portions of the duodenum mimic pancreatic head cancer in terms of clinical presentation and surgical management. The diagnosis is usually delayed because the symptoms are nonspecific. Patients may present with jaundice or gastric outlet obstruction. The preoperative evaluation and treatment are identical to that of cancer of the head of the pancreas. The tumor is frequently inaccessible by standard endoscopy. However, EUS is very useful in these patients to identify and sample the mass. Pancreaticoduodenectomy is the standard curative procedure. Survival after pancreaticoduodenectomy in the absence of local lymph node invasion is 68% at 5 years, but nearly zero at 3 years when there is regional invasion of the lymph nodes.[43] Survival rate after palliative excisions is 15 months, which is still superior to the cure rate for resected pancreatic cancer.

Patients with carcinoma of the third and fourth portions of the duodenum have much better prognosis. The predominant symptoms of tumors in this part of duodenum are related to upper intestinal obstruction. The diagnostic modality of choice is endoscopy. Although segmental duodenectomy limits the extent of lymphadenectomy, it is the preferred treatment for resectable duodenal cancers in these segments of the duodenum.[45]

7. Pancreatic Adenocarcinoma

Epidemiology

Cancer of the exocrine pancreas was diagnosed in 37,680 patients in the United States in 2008 and accounted for 91% of deaths (34,290) from this malignancy, making it the fourth-leading cause of cancer death.[5] The similar incidence and death rates emphasize that most pancreatic cancers are fatal as a result of the late development of clinical symptoms. Eighty percent of patients with pancreatic cancers have metastatic disease at the time of diagnosis and treatment options for advanced disease are ineffective. The vast majority of malignancies of the pancreas are infiltrating ductal adenocarcinomas and the term *pancreatic cancer* generally refers to adenocarcinoma of the pancreas. The average age at diagnosis is 65 years. Pancreatic cancer is more common in men than women (relative risk 1.35) and occurs 30%-40% more frequently in African Americans.[46] Cigarette smoking is the most firmly recognized risk factor (2- to 3-fold increase risk) for pancreatic cancer. Tobacco smoking contributes to nearly 30% of pancreatic cancers. Obesity and reduced physical activity have an increased pancreatic cancer risk.[47] In contrast, diets low in fat and high in vegetables, citrus fruits, fiber and vitamin C are associated with lower pancreatic cancer rates.[40] Coffee and alcohol consumption have not been associated with the development of this disease. Host risk factors associated with pancreatic cancer include chronic and hereditary pancreatitis. Non-insulin-dependent diabetes mellitus (relative risk 2.0) may be a risk factor but this association is controversial.

Familial pancreatic cancer accounts for less than 10% of all pancreatic cancers. Data from the National Familial Tumor Registry demonstrates that the risk of cancer of the pancreas is 18-fold higher if two first degree relatives are involved and 57-fold higher if three first-degree family members are affected.[48] Included among these are six recognized genetic syndromes caused by germline mutations which have demonstrated a substantial increase in pancreatic cancer risk. For instance, patients with *Peutz-Jeghers* syndrome have a 130-fold increased risk for pancreatic cancer. Familial breast cancer patients with germline mutations of the BRCA2 gene have a 3.5- to 10-fold increased risk for development of pancreatic cancer. Familial atypical multiple mole melanoma syndrome with germline mutation in the *p*16 gene have a 12- to 20-fold increased risk for the development of pancreatic cancer. Patients with Hereditary Pancreatitis (mutation in the PRSS1 gene) have a 50-fold increased risk for pancreatic cancer. Finally, patients with Lynch II syndrome (mutation in the mismatch repair genes *hMLH1 and hMSH2*) and ataxiate-langiectasia have also shown an increased risk for pancreatic cancer.[46]

The molecular genetics of pancreatic cancer are complex. Nearly all cancers involve mutations of multiple genes. Mutant oncogenes *K-ras* and epidermal growth factor receptor expression are seen in almost all cases. Loss of heterozygosity at loci of tumor suppressor genes, including *p16, p53*, is also usually present in patients with pancreatic cancers.

Pathology

During pancreatic development, undifferentiated precursor cells are responsible for generating mature ductal, acinar and islet cell types. Each mature cell has the potential to become malignant. Pancreatic cancer generally refers to carcinomas arising from the exocrine pancreas. Virtually all these cancers begin with ductal epithelium. The acinar cells give origin to less than 1% of malignant tumors. Endocrine tumors arise from the pancreatic islets and comprise less that 2% of all pancreatic neoplasms. 5% of all pancreatic tumors are cystic neoplasms. Metastatic spread to the pancreas is extraordinarily rare, but it has been reported from renal cell carcinoma, non-small cell lung cancer, sarcoma, melanoma and bladder cancers.[49] Two-thirds of pancreatic ductal adenocarcinomas occur in the head of the pancreas.

Clinical Features

History

There are no established screening tests for pancreatic cancer. The vague and nonspecific symptoms in pancreatic cancer contribute to its delay in diagnosis. Patients with lesions of the head of the pancreas present with painless jaundice and weight loss. Accompanying the jaundice may be dark urine, light stools and pruritus, and accompanying weight loss, anorexia and weakness. A subset of these patients present with epigastric and/or back pain as a result of distension of the pancreatic capsule, obstruction of the pancreatic duct or perineural invasion. Patients with lesions of the body and tail present primarily with pain and weight loss (these tumors are typically larger and diagnosed at a more advanced stage). Constant pain is attributed to tumor invasion of the celiac and mesenteric plexuses and occurs with advanced disease. Patients present with a mean duration of symptoms of eight weeks. New-onset diabetes mellitus may be an initial presenting symptom in 10% of patients with pancreatic cancer. Some degree of glucose intolerance occurs in 15%-20% of patients with pancreatic cancer, and the development of diabetes in a patient with chronic pancreatitis may be suggestive of a neoplastic process of the pancreas. A small percentage of pancreatic cancer patients (10%) will have had symptoms attributed to cholelithiasis and will have undergone recent cholecystectomy prior to the diagnosis of pancreatic cancer.[46,50]

Physical Examination

Physical examination is usually unrewarding. Since two-thirds of pancreatic adenocarcinomas occur in the head of the pancreas, the most common presenting physical finding is jaundice. Hepatomegaly, ascites or a palpable gallbladder (Courvoisier's sign) may be present in some patients with advanced cancers. Courvoisier's sign, in the absence of cholangitis, is present in one-fourth of patients and is indicative of malignant obstruction of the common bile duct until proven otherwise. Physical findings in patients with disseminated disease include supraclavicular lymphadenopathy (Virchow's node) or peritoneal seeding (Sister Mary Joseph's nodule or Blumer's shelf). Migratory thrombophlebitis (Trousseau's sign), which is evidence of intravascular thrombosis, may occur in patients with advanced pancreatic cancer as well as other advanced cancers resulting from a hypercoagulable state from malignant disease.

Diagnostic Evaluation and Staging

Routine laboratory analyses are rarely abnormal and if abnormal they lack specificity. Evidence of extrahepatic obstruction may be revealed by increased levels of serum alkaline phophatase and bilirubin with mild elevation of gamma-glutamyl transferase and hepatic aminotransferases. Hypoalbuminemia and anemia may be present in patients with advanced disease. Mild coagulopathy may also be observed. Hyperamylasemia and/or hyperlipasemia are atypical.

There are no accurate or reliable serum markers to aid in the diagnosis of pancreatic cancer. Low sensitivity and cross-reactivity with other tumors have prevented the clinical use of carcinoembryonic antigen (CEA), fetoprotein and pancreatic oncofetal antigen in the diagnosis of pancreatic cancer. Carbohydrate antigen 19-9 levels (normal <37 units/mL) has been the most useful commercially available test. CA 19-9 is a Lewis blood group-related mucin clinically used in the diagnosis, prognosis and monitoring of pancreatic cancer. However, the accuracy of CA 19-9 is only 80% and does not identify early curable tumors. The accuracy of CA 19-9 in the diagnosis of pancreatic cancer is excellent when combined with ERCP, abdominal CT or abdominal US.[51] Higher levels of CA 19-9 indicate poor prognosis and tumor unresectability. CA 19-9 is also useful to monitor therapeutic intervention response.

Imaging studies are essential in the management of pancreatic cancer. The most important goal of imaging is to determine tumor resectability. Involvement of superior mesenteric/portal venous structures and nodal involvement are paramount in selecting treatment options. The investigation of most patients with pancreatic cancer generally begins with a right upper quadrant ultrasound to evaluate jaundice. Abdominal ultrasound (US) examination reliably detects extrahepatic ductal dilatation (greater than 7 mm). However, accurate identification of a pancreatic mass may be compromised by operator experience, bowel gas interference or obesity, and is successful in half of cases and does not provide information regarding tumor involvement of the mesenteric/portal venous structures or lymph node involvement. In advanced disease, ascites and liver metastases (>1 cm) may be seen by abdominal US.

Computed tomography (CT) performed with oral and intravenous contrast with 3 mm cuts through the pancreas remains the initial procedure of choice for diagnosis and staging of pancreatic cancer. The sensitivity for lesions greater than 1 cm is 95%.[52] The false positive rate is low, but can occur as a result of focal pancreatitis or anatomic variability. High resolution CT with thin cuts provides excellent visualization of the relationship of the tumor to the major vessels of interest (ie, the superior mesenteric vein and artery). Involvement of the superior mesenteric artery indicates that the tumor is unresectable (T4 - lesions). Invasion of the superior mesenteric vein or portal vein (T-3 lesions) may be considered by some surgeons to be an indication of unresectability. Some centers, however, advocate en bloc excision of the superior mesenteric vein (SMV) or portal vein in cases without evidence of nodal metastases.[53] The SMV can be primarily repaired, or interposition grafting can be done with internal jugular vein or PTFE. Patients who undergo vein reconstruction have generally poor survival, and resectability in patients with portal/SM vein involvement must include careful decision making. Thus, stage I/II patients are considered for surgical resection, whereas stage III and IV cancers are typically deemed unresectable.[2] The overall accuracy of CT for determination of tumor resectalbity is 95%. However, about one-third of patients who appear resectable on CT will prove to be unresectable at operation. Additionally, CT is unreliable in predicting nodal involvement.[54] MRI has no advantage over CT in assessing tumor resectability.[55]

Endoscopic retrograde cholangiopancreatography (ERCP) is a sensitive test for the diagnosis of pancreatic cancer. ERCP allows direct visualization of the duodenum and ampulla, delineation of the biliary and pancreatic ductal systems, and tissue sampling. ERCP may disclose the classic "double duct" sign of biliary and pancreatic ductal obstruction. ERCP may also be used to obtain "brush" samples for cytology, thus providing the most accurate diagnosis and making it the gold standard test for the diagnosis of pancreatic cancer. However, regardless of the ERCP findings, if a patient is suspected to have pancreatic cancer, resection is indicated regardless of the results of ERCP.[2] Additionally, ERCP is a valuable means of palliating patients with obstructive jaundice from pancreatic cancer with metastatic or locally advanced disease who are not candidates for resection. These patients benefit from sphincterotomy and/or stent placement. Routine stenting of patients with resectable pancreatic cancer, however, has not been shown to lower the morbidity of subsequent resection.

Endoscopic ultrasound (EUS) combined with fine needle aspiration (EUS-FNA) has rapidly become a common staging test for pancreatic cancer (Table 3). The accuracy of EUS is operator dependent and it is not yet available at many community hospitals. At experienced centers, EUS has been shown to have a similar sensitivity and specificity for the diagnosis of pancreatic cancer to that of thin section CT.[55] EUS has the advantage of allowing sampling of the tumor mass, regional nodes, liver lesions and ascites during the diagnostic evaluation. EUS-FNA has a diagnostic accuracy of 92% with a sensitivity, specificity and positive predictive value of 91%, 100% and 100%, respectively. However, the negative predictive value is only 44%, emphasizing that a negative cytologic examination does not exclude cancer. No mortalities have been reported with EUS-FNA and morbidity is only 2%.[56]

Centers without personnel experienced with EUS FNA rely on percutaneous fine-needle aspiration (FNA) of pancreatic masses to establish a diagnosis. CT-guided percutaneous FNA is the diagnostic procedure of choice in patients with unresectable disease. FNA is rarely associated with complications. Seeding of the needle tract is a theoretical possibility, but no data has shown this conclusively. Biopsy for tissue diagnosis is more important for patients with unresectable tumor than patients whose tumor and overall status indicate surgical intervention. For the non-operative candidate, tissue diagnosis is required for chemo-radiotherapeutic interventions. Negative results on tissue diagnosis with a suspicious mass by CT does not preclude surgical intervention.

20-40% of patients staged by CT, MRI, ERCP or EUS will have undetected disseminated disease by laparoscopic exploration.[2] Laparoscopic exploration for patients with pancreatic lesions is best used selectively and may have a larger role in resectable tumors of the body and tail of the pancreas.[29,57]

Neoadjuvant Therapy

Only a few studies have been undertaken to determine the role of radiation/chemotherapy in the management of pancreatic cancer. These studies demonstrate a modest role for neoadjuvant therapy in both downstaging of tumors and improving overall survival.[58-60]

Surgical Treatment

Removal of all evaluable disease offers the patient the only chance of long-term survival. Less than 10% of patients diagnosed with pancreatic cancer are considered resectable. Those who undergo surgical resection have a disappointing 20% 5-year survival (Table 3).

The general exploration of the abdomen includes careful inspection of the peritoneal surfaces and liver for metastases, which can be more accurately determined by intra operative liver ultrasonography. Suspicious lymph nodes are submitted for frozen section histology to evaluate for metastatic disease. The presence of peritoneal implants and liver metastases render the patient incurable. Similarly, histologically proven metastases in lymph nodes accessible during the initial abdominal exploration makes the chance of cure highly remote. Resectability is best determined preoperatively rather than intraoperatively. Only those patients without extrapancreatic disease (ie, a patent superior mesenteric vein-portal vein confluence, and no direct tumor extension to the celiac axis or superior mesenteric artery) are candidates for curative resection. If there is no evidence of disease outside the anticipated margins of resection, formal resection is undertaken. Pancreaticodudenectomy with or without preservation of the pylorus and proximal duodenum (Whipple procedure) is currently the procedure of choice for ductal adenocarcinoma of the head of the pancreas.

Figure 6

Schematic diagram showing the proposed lines of resection for pancreaticoduodenectomy (Whipple procedure)

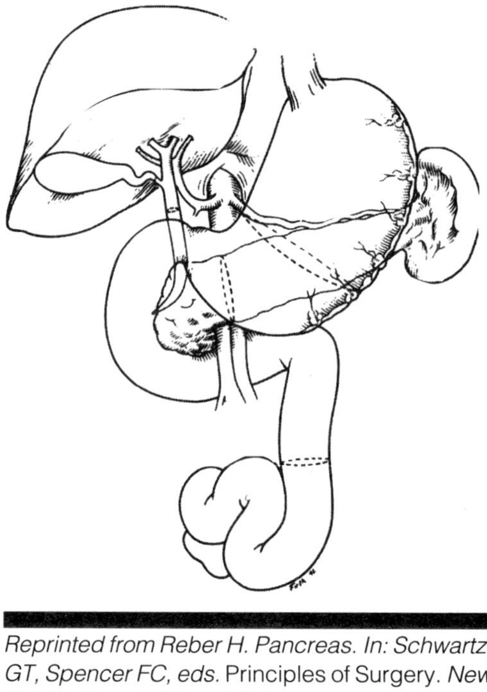

Reprinted from Reber H. Pancreas. In: Schwartz SI, Shires GT, Spencer FC, eds. Principles of Surgery. *New York, NY: McGraw-Hill Inc; 1994.*

Table 3

TNM Staging of Pancreatic Cancer

T1 Tumor limited to pancreas <2cm
T2 Tumor limited to pancreas >2cm
T3 Tumor extends beyond pancreas but does not involve celiac axis or SMA
T4 Tumor invades celiac axis and SMA

N1 Regional lymph node metastasis

Stage	**I**	**II**	**III**	**IV**
	T1, N0 T2, N0	T3, N0 T1-3, N1	T2, N1-2 T3, N1-2	Any T/N, M1
5-year survival	20%-40%	10%-25%	10%-15%	0%-8%

Technical considerations for standard pancreaticoduodenectomy (PD) have been reviewed extensively.[53] The proposed lines of resection are shown in Figure 6. Following abdominal exploration, the right colon is mobilized and retracted inferiorly. The lesser sac is entered and posterior attachments of the stomach are divided. The superior mesenteric vein is identified by tracing the middle colic vein proximally, or after Kocherization by following the sweep of the duodenum medially. The gallbladder is mobilized and the common hepatic duct and gastroduodenal arteries are divided. These maneuvers allow exposure of the anterior surface of the portal vein. The portal vein and superior mesenteric vein are carefully separated from the overlying pancreas. The stomach (or duodenum in cases of pylorus-preserving pancreaticoduodenectomy [PPPD]), small bowel and pancreas are then divided sequentially. The uncinate process is liberated from its retroperitoneal attachments to complete the dissection (Figure 7). Gastrointestinal continuity is re-established by a pancraticojejunostomy (or pancreaticogastrostomy), choledocojejunostomy and gastrojejunostomy (or duodenojejunostomy in the case of PPPD). Anastomoses are done in sequence: pancreas, then bile duct then stomach (or duodenum in the case of PPPD) (Figure 8, Figure 9).

Figure 7

Schematic showing the proposed anastomoses following specimen removal during pancreaticoduodenectomy

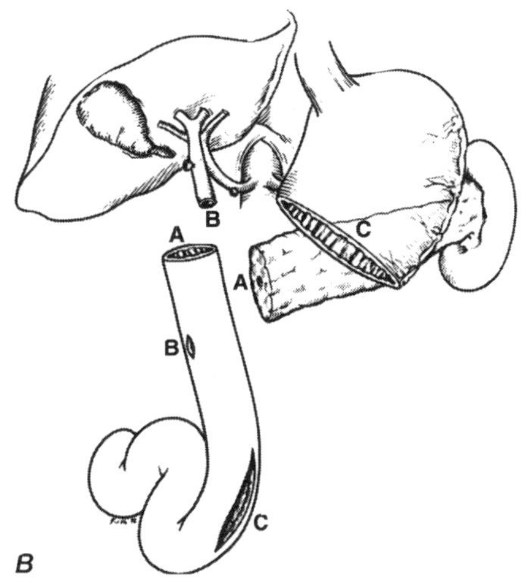

Reprinted from Reber H. Pancreas. In: Schwartz SI, Shires GT, Spencer FC, eds. Principles of Surgery. *New York, NY: McGraw-Hill Inc; 1994.*

Pancreatojejunostomy may be performed as an end-to-end "dunking" procedure, an end-to-side anastomosis between pancreas and jejunum, or an end-to-side duct-to-mucosa anastomosis. A duct-to-mucosa anastomosis may be performed over a stent. Pancreaticogastrostomy is performed in an end-to-side fashion. The primary theoretical advantage of duct-to-mucosa pancreaticojejunostomy is long-term patency. There is no evidence that the type of pancreatic-enteric anastomosis affects the rate of pancreatic fistula.

The biliary and pancreatic anastomoses are drained and jejunostomy (for feeding) and gastrostomy (for decompression) tubes are placed prior to closure. Routine placement of feeding and decompression tubes is paramount in the postoperative management of patients following a pancreatico-dudodenectomy.

PPPD is a modification of the standard Whipple procedure in which the entire stomach, including the pylorus, and 2 cm to 3 cm of the duodenal cuff, are preserved. This modification retains the entire stomach as a reservoir and may prevent the development of postgastrectomy syndromes, marginal ulceration and enterogastric reflux. PPPD is touted to result in shorter operative times, less blood loss and fewer transfusions. It appears to be associated with better long-term gastric function and patient well-being. The disadvantage of PPPD is the inability to obtain clear wide margins and potential increase in recurrence. A small survival advantage has been noted in patients undergoing standard Whipple procedure versus PPPD,[61] although randomized studies of PPPD vs. standard pancreaticodudenectomy have not been done.

Total pancreatectomy for pancreatic cancer is rarely performed. Total pancreatectomy had been proposed to obtain superior tumor margins and provide a more extensive lymph node dissection. In practice, total pancreatectomy is associated with increased postoperative mortality and no change in survival compared to standard pancreaticodu-denectomy. Postoperative diabetes is extremely difficult to manage in patients undergoing total pancreatectomy.

Figure 8

Intraoperative photograph following specimen removal during pancreaticoduodenectomy

A plastic stent has been placed in the pancreatic duct. The bile duct is occluded by a noncrushing clamp. The portal-mesenteric venous confluence is clearly seen.

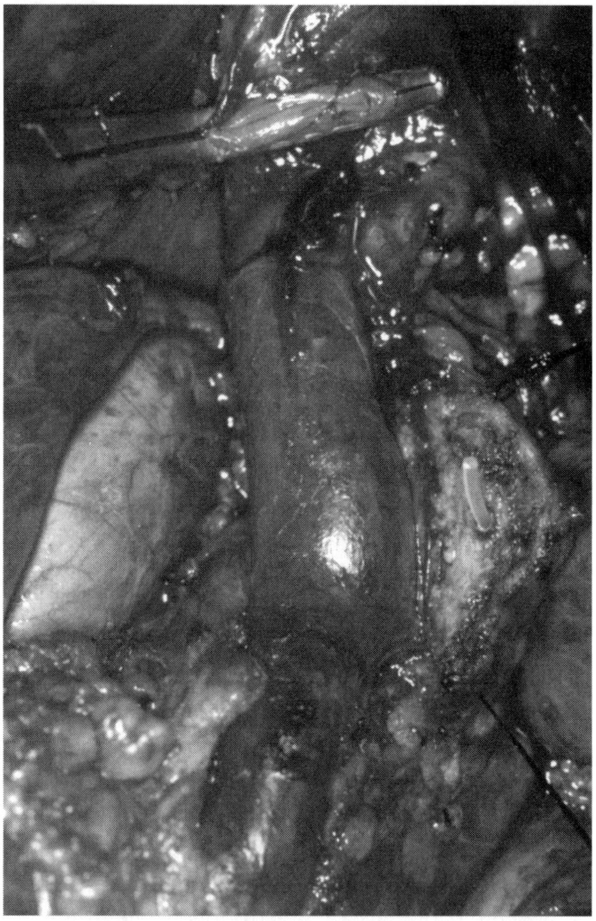

From Dr Charles Theuer's personal collection.

Figure 9

Schematic showing completed anastomoses during pancreaticoduodenectomy

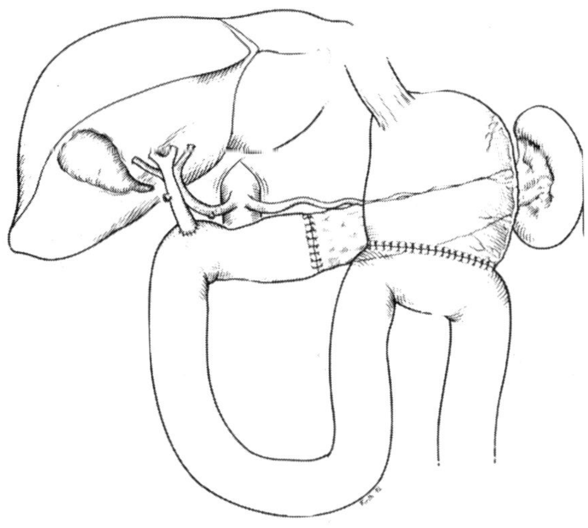

Reprinted from Reber H. Pancreas. In: Schwartz SI, Shires GT, Spencer FC, eds. Principles of Surgery. *New York, NY: McGraw-Hill Inc; 1994.*

15% of pancreatic adenocarcinomas occur in the body and the tail of the pancreas. Because these tumors typically do not cause biliary obstruction, its diagnosis is not made until the disease is very advanced and unresectable. Distal pancreatectomy with splenectomy is reserved for rare instances when the tumor located in the body or the tail of the pancreas is resectable.

Palliation

Palliation of pancreatic cancer patients may be the goal of operative exploration or may result from operative findings indicating unresectablility. Palliation can be performed operatively and nonoperatively and this decision should be individualized depending on the overall status of the patient. Whether palliation is accomplished operatively or nonoperatively, relief of obstructive jaundice, duodenal obstruction and back pain are the primary goals.

Internal drainage of obstructive jaundice from pancreatic cancer can be accomplished with choledochojejunostomy, choledochoduodenostomy or cholecystojejunostomy. The gallbladder is a useful conduit if the cystic duct is patent and more than 2 cm away from the tumor mass. Gallstones, if present, should be removed. Late bypass failure may occur in cases where progressive tumor growth obstructs the cystic duct. Choledochojejunostomy has the advantage of avoiding this problem because the anastomosis is created at the common hepatic duct. Choledochoenteric bypass is associated with shorter operating times and less blood loss, but has increased postoperative morbidity and late bypass failure.[62] A choledochojejunostomy can be constructed either via a loop jejunostomy or Roux-en-Y limb. A defunctionalized limb of the Roux-en Y requires an extra anastomosis, but has the advantage of preventing leaks mixed with enteric contents. The risk of cholangitis is not different with either of these two biliary drainage procedures.[63] Choledochoduodenostomy is yet another alternative to relieve biliary obstructive symptoms with reported excellent long-term palliation.

Duodenal obstruction occurs in 15%-30% of patients with unresectable pancreatic cancer and these patients should undergo a gastrojejunostomy. It is less clear whether patients without gastric outlet obstruction benefit from prophylactic gastrojejunostomy at the time of internal biliary bypass. Approximately 20% of patients who undergo biliary bypass alone develop symptoms of gastric outlet obstruction.[63,64] A gastrojejunostomy does not increase operative mortality and will obviate the need for further operative intervention. Since these patients have very advanced pancreatic cancer, reoperative surgery is accompanied by a significant morbidity and mortality. Thus, a prophylactic gastrojejunostomy in patients undergoing internal biliary bypass is the favored practice by some surgeons. Others argue that a gastrojejunostomy may be accompanied by long-term delayed gastric emptying in patients who have a limited survival and care must be individualized. The theoretical advantage of an antecolic gastrojejunostomy away from the tumor bed may be offset by delayed postoperative gastric emptying that may accompany antecolic rather than retrocolic gastrojejunostomy. Vagotomy serves to further inhibit gastric emptying and should not be performed; patients are at risk for marginal ulceration since biliary flow does not traverse the gastrojejunostomy in most cases. Proton pump inhibitors are used postoperatively to prevent this potential complication.

Pain associated with pancreatic cancer may be relieved with chemical splanchnicectomy. Alcohol injected at the time of palliative operation into the celiac ganglia on either side of the aorta decreases cancer-associated pain without an increase in complications.[65]

For the patient with severely advanced disease and who are poor surgical candidates, palliation can be accomplished nonoperatively. ERCP with stent placement may alleviate biliary obstructive symptoms, a percutaneus gastrostomy tube (PEG) may relieve gastric outlet obstruction and chemical sphanchnicectomy can be accomplished with CT or EUS guidance. The role of laparoscopy in palliation for patients with pancreatic cancer is still controversial.

Complications

The mortality rate in high volume centers performing pancreatiocoduodenectomies is 2%-4%. Postoperative complications occur in 25%-40% of patients following this operation. Delayed gastric emptying occurs in 15%-40% of these patients (either by standard PD or PPPD).[2] Mechanical obstruction should be excluded by upper endoscopy or upper gastrointestinal series. Upper GI series also serves to qualify the degree of gastroparesis. Patients are treated with decompression via nasogastric or gastrostomy tube. Erythromycin or metoclopramide may reduce the incidence of gastric emptying by only 37%.[66] Thus, a jejunostomy tube for prolonged postoperative feeding as well as a gastrostomy tube for postoperative venting should be routinely employed during pancreaticoduodenectomy.

Pancreatic fistula (defined as the output of more than 50 cc of amylase-rich fluid) accompanies 10%-20% of cases and is directly responsible for 20% of postoperative deaths, which constitutes the most serious complication of pancreaticoduodenectomy. Pancreatic fistula indicates disruption of the pancreatic-enteric anastomosis and occurs at the same rate regardless of anastomosis (ie, pancreaticogastrostomy vs. pancreaticojejunostomy). Disruption of biliary and gastric anastomoses are rare and less serious.

Patients with pancreatic fistula may be completely asymptomatic if it is a controlled fistula and the output is well captured by the drain. These patients do well with a clear liquid diet, enteral nutrition through a jejunostomy tube or parenteral nutrition. A CT scan should be performed to exclude abdominal fluid collections. The benefits of somatostatin in this setting are unclear. Drains may be progressively advanced as output decreases. 80% of patients can be managed conservatively. An additional 10%-15% of patients with this complication respond well to percutaneous drainage.

Patients with sepsis or hemorrhage related to pancreaticoenteric anastomotic disruption necessitate immediate and aggressive intervention. Abscesses may be drained percutaneously. Septic patients who do not respond to aggressive medical management within 48 hours should be explored. Operative intervention has the goals of decontaminating the source of sepsis and eliminating the need for further pancreaticoenteric anastomosis. More than half of these critically ill patients can be salvaged with completion pancreatectomy. Hemorrhage associated with pancreatic fistula can be managed with angiographic embolization. Patients who require operative exploration and have diffuse retroperitoneal hemorrhage and necrosis require completion pancreatectomy. The rare cases of hemobilia and hemopancreaticus are best diagnosed and treated angiographically.

Endocrine pancreatic function is rarely impaired and diabetes is unusual following pancreaticoduodenectomy. Exocrine pancreatic function, on the other hand, is affected to various degrees and in severe cases may require lifelong exogenous enzyme supplementation.

Adjuvant Therapy

The management of patients with pancreatic cancer is based on the stage of the tumor (Table 3). Generally, four groups of patients required various forms of treatment: patients with resectable tumors; patients with locally advanced disease; patients with unresectable tumors, and; patients with metastatic disease. Adjuvant therapy (5-fluorouracil and +/- radiation) improves survival in patients with resected adenocarcinomas. At the present time, the standard of care for patients with locally advanced disease is continuous infusion of 5-FU with radiation therapy.[67] However, the role of radiation therapy is still questionable. Current chemotherapeutic agents include gemcitabine and other growth-factor and cell-signal inhibitors.[68]

Gemcitabine is the cornerstone for the treatment of metastatic disease. The 1-year survival of patients treated with gemcitabine versus 5-FU is 18% and 2%, respectively. The median survival remains disappointingly low at 5.7% vs. 4.4% months, respectively.[68]

Acinar Cell Carcinoma

Acinar tumors are malignant tumors with acinar differentiation and account for less than 1% of all pancreatic malignant cancers. 50% of these lesions present with metastatic disease. These lesions are evenly distributed throughout the pancreas. Clinically, these tumors may present with subcutaneous fat necrosis, rash, peripheral eosinophilia or polyarthralgias. In general, patients with acinar cell carcinoma of the pancreas have slightly better survival (19 months) compared to ductal adenocarcinomas.[46]

Solid-Pseudopapillary Tumor of the Pancreas

Solid-pseudopapllilary tumors of the pancreas (SPTP) are rare, benign or low grade malignant epithelial tumors. The low 1%-2% frequency of SPTP amongst exocrine tumors appears to be increasing in recent years. The signs and symptoms of SPTPs are related to their mass effect and consist of abdominal discomfort or pain. When these tumors present with symptoms, physical examination demonstrates an easily palpable, well-demarcated mass in the abdomen. These are generally large tumors with an average size of 8 cm to 10 cm. Serologic tumor markers and laboratory values are usually within normal limits. Computed tomography is the test of choice and demonstrates a well-defined, solid and cystic mass. Prognosis for patients with SPTP is excellent. Surgical resection is the mainstay of treatment.[69,70]

8. Cystic Pancreatic Neoplasms

The vast majority of cystic lesions of the pancreas are pancreatic pseudocysts. A pancreatic pseudocyst is a fluid collection of pancreatic juices that arise from pancreatitis. There is no true lining, but a fibrous capsule around the fluid collection. During the formation of the fibrous wall, there is exchange of pancreatic enzymes between the fluid collection and the plasma. This decreases as the fibrous wall matures at around 4-6 weeks following the initial attack of pancreatitis. Pancreatic pseudocysts lack a true epithelial lining. This is to be contrasted with true pancreatic cysts such as cystic neoplasms and congenital pancreatic cysts or cystic neoplasms. 15% of cystic lesions of the pancreas are cystic neoplasms and one half of these are malignant. The most common cystic neoplasms of the pancreas encountered are serous cystadenomas (35%), mucinous cystic neoplasms (10%-40%) and intraductal papillary mucinous tumors (IPMTs ([20%-30%]). Serous cystadenomas have very low malignant potential, but may grow to very large sizes. These lesions typically contain glycogen rather than mucin and are usually multilocular. Mucinous cystadenomas have the potential to turn into mucinous cystadenocarcinoma. They contain mucin and are commonly unilocular. The histological characteristics of IPMTs are similar to mucinous cystadenomas. Unlike mucinous cystadenomas, IPMTs communicate with the pancreatic ductal system.[71,72]

History and a physical exam may aid in differentiating a cystic neoplasm from pancreatic pseudocyts. Prior history of pancreatitis preceding a fluid collection should point to pancreatic pseduocyst. A young female with a pancreatic cystic lesion without history of pancreatitis should be treated as a patient with a cystic neoplasm until proven otherwise. Incidental pancreatic cystic masses present with symptoms in 63% of the cases and the most common complaint is abdominal pain (70%). Weight loss, pancreatitis, back pain, and jaundice occur less frequently. CT scan is the initial test of choice for evaluation of a pancreatic cystic mass. Serum levels of CA 19-9 and CEA may occasionally be elevated in pancreatic malignancies. Endoscopic ultrasound with fine-needle aspiration (EUS-FNA) provides cytologic information in addition to a more accurate location and size of the tumor. EUS-FNA may also provide information on cystic fluid CEA levels which can be useful in the diagnosis of pancreatic neoplasms. Similarly high levels of amylase and lipase in the pancreatic cyst are suggestive of pancreatic pseudocysts.

Surgical resection is indicated in most patients with pancreatic cysts that are symptomatic. Serous cystadenomas are equally distributed throughout the pancreas, and its surgical management depends on the location of the tumor (ie, body/tail may be treated with a distal pancreatectomy, whereas pancreatic head neoplasms may require a pancreaticoduodenectomy). Mucinous cystadenomas are more commonly found in the body and tail of the pancreas, and distal pancreatectomy should be the procedure of choice for premalignant lesions. IPMTs are commonly located in the head of the pancreas and require a pancreaticoduodenectomy for appropriate management. Up to 19% of patients require a total pancreatectomy due to the characteristic growth of the tumor along the pancreatic duct, making attainable free margins difficult. The 5-year survival for patients with complete resection of mucious tumors is nearly 100% and over 50% for patients with complete excision of IPMTs.[71,72]

9. Islet Cell Tumors

Islet cell tumors arise from neuroendocrine stem cells within the pancreatic duct epithelium. These pluripotent cells give rise to five distinct clinical islet cell tumor syndromes: insulinoma, gastrinoma, glucagonoma, VIPoma and somatostatinoma. These tumors are much more uncommon than adenocarcinoma of the pancreas. The relative frequency of these tumors and their metastatic potential is depicted in Table 4. The most important features regarding islet cell tumors are: 1.) to establish the diagnosis; 2.) to localize the tumor; and 3.) and to determine whether the tumor is a component of the multiple endocrine neoplasia syndrome type-1 (MEN-1).

The diagnosis of islet cell tumors is made on biochemical grounds rather than radiologic imaging. For instance, the diagnosis of insulinoma is established by an inappropriately high level of insulin relative to serum glucose levels during an episode of severe hypoglycemia. Gastrinomas are diagnosed by a high basal acid output and hypergastrinemia. The rest of islet cell tumors are diagnosed by clinical suspicion and confirmed by measurement of the respective serum level of the hormonal component of the tumor (Table 4).

Once the diagnosis of an islet cell tumor has been established, it must be localized before proceeding with further management. CT and MRI studies are of little value in localizing these tumors as the sensitivity is only 40%-60%. However, they may be obtained as part of the metastatic work up. Though invasive and technically challenging, suprahepatic vein measurement following secretagoge injection is an excellent test to localize these tumors as this relays on the good vasculature of islet neoplasms. Endoscopic ultrasound with fine-needle aspiration (EUS-FNA) and octreotide scans are currently the preferred tests to localize these tumors.[73]

Up to one-fourth of the pancreatic endocrine tumors are a part of MEN-1 syndrome.[73] The components of MEN-1 include parathyroid hyperplasia, pancreatic islet tumors and pituitary tumors. An islet tumor concomitant with hyperparathyroidism is diagnostic of MEN-1. Calcium levels should be measured on all patients with pancreatic endocrine tumors. Diagnosis of MEN-1 mandates attention to the management of the parathyroid gland prior to proceeding with resection of the pancreatic tumor. Thus, recognition of MEN-1 is essential in the management of pancreatic endocrine tumors.

Insulinoma

Insulinomas are the most common, yet the least malignant islet cell tumors. These are typically solitary and less than 2 cm in size, but may be multiple, especially in cases associated with MEN-1. They are uniformly distributed throughout the pancreas. Patients with insulinomas manifest may present with neuropsychiatric symptoms as a result of hypoglycemia. Whipple's triad, consisting of symptoms of hypoglycemia at fasting, blood glucose levels of less than 45 mg/dL and relief of symptoms following the administration of glucose, is typically seen. The diagnosis is confirmed by severe hypoglycemia during supervised fasting, in which symptoms are typically seen within 24 hours. At the time of hypoglycemia, serum levels of glucose, insulin and C-peptide should be determined. Elevated C-peptide levels confirms endogenous insulin production rather than exogenous administration. Serum glucose less than 45 mg/dL in

Table 4

Pancreatic Islet Cell Tumors

Islet Cell Tumor	Incidence	Malignancy Rate	Component of MEN-1	Clinical Presentation	Diagnosis
Insulinoma	42%	13%	16%	Neuroglycopenia, Whipple's triad = symptoms of hypoglycemia, resolution of symptoms with glucose administration and glucose level <45 mg/dL	Fasting glucose to insulin ratio >0.3
Gastrinoma	35%	60%	40%	Peptic ulcer disease refractory to medical treatment, ZES	Gastrin level, basal acid output, secretin test for ZES
Glucagonoma	6%	80%	58%	Glucose intolerance, diabetes mellitus, weight loss, anemia, necrolytic migratory erythema	Glucagon level
PPoma	3%	65%	50%	Silent	PP level
VIPoma	3%	50%	50%	WDHA = watery diarrhea, hypokalemia, and achlorhydria	VIP level
Somatostatinoma	1%	90%	Rare	Dyspepsia, steatorrhea, gallstones, mild diabetes mellitus	Somatostatin level
Nonfunctioning	10%	Rare	5%	None	None

the presence of a serum insulin level of greater than 6 mU/mL establishes the diagnosis of insulinoma. Medical treatment of hypoglycemia consists of diet modification, avoidance of exercise, as well as diazoxide and somatostatin administration to control hypoglycemia.

The preferred test to localize insulinomas is EUS (sensitivity 88%, specificity 100%). Unlike the rest of pancreatic islet tumors, octreotide scan has poor sensitivity for localizing insulinomas (60%) due to the fact that these tumors lack sufficient somatostatin receptors compared to the rest of pancreatic neuroendocrine tumors. If EUS fails to disclose the tumor, selective arteriography with calcium infusion while measuring hepatic venous insulin is useful in delineating the major arterial supply to the tumor, and surgical resection can be performed. Intraoperative ultrasound (IOUS) combined with manual palpation, after thoroughly exposing the pancreas, can localize insulinomas in 91% of the cases. IOUS has the added advantage of allowing for identification of the pancreatic ducts. Small benign tumors can be treated with enucleation. Pancreatic resection is reserved for malignant tumors or tumors whose proximity to the CBD does not allow for simple removal of the lesion because of inability to develop a proper plane. Tumors in the body or the tail of the pancreas are treated with a distal pancreatectomy, with splenic preservation if possible. Large rare tumors of the head of the pancreas may require a pancreaticoduodenectomy. In cases where the tumor can not be localized intraoperatively, a blind pancreatectomy should not be performed. When associated with MEN-1, insulinomas of the head of the pancreas should undergo enucleation, and those in the body and tail, a distal pancreatectomy.[74] Metastatic disease should be resected, if possible, by formal resection. Debulking is undertaken for palliation.

Gastrinoma

Gastrinoma is the second most common pancreatic islet cell tumor. These tumors are usually malignant and more typically associated with MEN-1. In fact, gastrinomas are the most frequently found pancreatic tumors in patients with MEN-1. Gastrinomas may cause the Zollinger-Ellison Syndrome (ZES). The diagnosis of gastrinoma is established by demonstrating basal acid output over 15 mEq/hr with fasting gastrin levels above 500 pg/mL. A paradoxical rise in serum gastrin levels of more than 200 pg/mL above baseline in response to intravenous secretin administration is diagnostic for ZES. The ulcer diathesis of ZES can be controlled with proton pump inhibitor therapy. Total gastrectomy is rarely required even if the gastrinoma cannot be completely excised.

Since most gastrinomas metastasize to regional lymph nodes and liver (15%-50%), common staging tests include CT, MRI and octreotide scan. CT and MRI are useful for excluding hepatic metastases, but frequently do not visualize the primary tumor. Octreotide scan is the most useful modality to localize the tumor as well as metastases. EUS is also employed to aid in the localization of this tumor, but nearly half of patients undergo operative exploration without successful preoperative localization. Since half of gastrinomas are palpable, the intraoperative use of ultrasound, endoscopy and duodenotomy successfully localizes the majority of these tumors. The vast majority of gastrinomas lie within the gastrinoma triangle formed by the junctions of the cystic and common bile duct, the body and neck of the pancreas, and the second and third portions of the duodenum.[75] Gastrinomas most commonly occur in the duodenal wall, but may occur as primary tumors in periduodenal or peripancreatic lymph nodes. Intraoperative ultrasound is helpful in defining the relationship of the tumor to vascular structures and aids in the planning of resection. When the tumor is in the duodenum, it is resected by a full thickness duodenotomy and the duodenum is subsequently repaired longitudinally. Small tumors are treated by enucleation. Involved lymph nodes are resected and unilobar liver metastases should be treated with wedge resection or lobectomy. Aggressive medical management is recommended for patients with multiple gastrinomas associated with MEN-1, as these tend to be less malignant.

Glucagonoma

In contrast to insulinomas and gastrinomas, glucagonomas are large tumors (>3 cm) and usually occur in the body and tail of the pancreas (80%). Most of these tumors are malignant and liver metastases are commonly found at the time of diagnosis. Patients present with symptoms of glucose intolerance, weight loss, and a characteristic rash called necrolytic migratory erythema. Patients may have anemia, glossitis and diarrhea, and stomatitis and thromboembolism occurs in a third of patients. A serum glucagon level in excess of 1000 pg/mL is diagnostic. Tumors are usually visualized by CT and/or octeotride scan. Resection of the tumor is successfully achieved by distal pancreatectomy and splenectomy. Metastatic disease in lymph nodes and the liver should be resected. Unresectable disease may be treated with chemotherapy. Octreotide improves skin rash and diarrhea, but does not affect diabetes.

VIPoma

Most VIPomas are solitary lesions greater than 3 cm in size commonly localized in the tail of the pancreas. VIPomas secrete vasoactive intestinal peptide, causing a profuse watery diarrhea (10 L/d) leading to profound metabolic disturbances. This syndrome is typically characterized by an acronym for watery diarrhea, hypokalemia and metabolic acidosis (WDHA). Fasting VIP levels greater than 200 pg/mL establish the diagnosis.[76] CT and/or octreotide scans generally localize this lesion. 50% of all VIPomas are malignant. While small tumors may be enucleated, larger ones should be formally resected, along with any involved lymph nodes and hepatic metastases. Debulking unresectable disease ameliorates symptoms, and such tumors can be treated with chemotherapy. Somatostatin is the cornerstone in amelioration of symptoms.

Somatostatinoma

Somatostatinomas are very rare tumors of the endocrine pancreas. They are typically large and frequently malignant. Most of these neoplasms are located in the head of the pancreas, but some occur in the duodenum. Symptoms are nonspecific and include biliary colic from gallstones, steatorrhea and diarrhea. Surgical management generally requires pancreaticoduodenectomy and survival rates are poor.

10. References

1. Kahrilas PJ. Clinical practice. Gastroesophageal reflux disease. *N Engl J Med*. 2008; 359:1700-1707.

2. Townsend Jr CM, Beauchamp RD, Evers BM, et al. *Townsend: Sabiston Textbook of Surgery*. 18th Ed. Philadelphia, PA: Saunders Elsevier; 2008.

3. Cameron AJ, Lomboy CT. Barrett's esophagus: age, prevalence, and extent of columnar epithelium. *Gastroenterology*. 1992; 103:1241-1245.

4. Spechler SJ. Clinical practice. Barrett's Esophagus. *N Engl J Med*. 2002; 346:836-842.

5. Jemal A, Siegel R, Ward E, et al. Cancer statistics, 2008. *CA Cancer J Clin*. 2008; 58:71-96.

6. Blot WJ, Devesa SS, Kneller RW, et al. Rising incidence of adenocarcinoma of the esophagus and gastric cardia. *JAMA*. 1991; 265:1287-1289.

7. Enzinger PC, Mayer RJ. Esophageal cancer. *N Engl J Med*. 2003; 349:2241-2252.

8. Krasna MJ, Flowers JL, Attar S, et al. Combined thoracoscopic/laparoscopic staging of esophageal cancer. *J Thorac Cardiovasc Surg*. 1996; 111:800-806.

9. Maish MS, DeMeester SR. Endoscopic mucosal resection as a staging technique to determine the depth of invasion of esophageal adenocarcinoma. *Ann Thorac Surg*. 2004; 78:1777-1782.

10. Soetikno R, Kaltenbach T, Yeh R, et al. Endoscopic mucosal resection for early cancers of the upper gastrointestinal tract. *J Clin Oncol*. 2005; 23:4490-4498.

11. Ajani JA, Barthel JS, Bekaii-Saab T, et al. Esophageal cancer. *J Natl Compr Canc Netw*. 2008; 6:818-849.

12. Bosset JF, Gignoux M, Triboulet JP, et al. Chemoradiotherapy followed by surgery compared with surgery alone in squamous-cell cancer of the esophagus. *N Engl J Med*. 1997; 337:161-167.

13. Nygaard K, Hagen S, Hansen HS, et al. Pre-operative radiotherapy prolongs survival in operable esophageal carcinoma: a randomized, multicenter study of pre-operative radiotherapy and chemotherapy. The second Scandinavian trial in esophageal cancer. *World J Surg*. 1992; 16:1104-1109.

14. Walsh TN, Noonan N, Hollywood D, et al. A comparison of multimodal therapy and surgery for esophageal adenocarcinoma. *N Engl J Med*. 1996; 335:462-467.

15. Urschel JD, Vasan H. A meta-analysis of randomized controlled trials that compared neoadjuvant chemoradiation and surgery to surgery alone for resectable esophageal cancer. *Am J Surg*. 2003; 185:538-543.

16. Tepper J, Krasna MJ, Niedzwiecki D, et al. Phase III trial of trimodality therapy with cisplatin, fluorouracil, radiotherapy, and surgery compared with surgery alone for esophageal cancer: CALGB 9781. *J Clin Oncol*. 2008; 26:1086-1092.

17. Orringer MB. Transhiatal esophagectomy without thoracotomy for carcinoma of the thoracic esophagus. *Ann Surg*. 1984; 200:282-288.

18. Orringer MB, Marshall B, Stirling MC. Transhiatal esophagectomy for benign and malignant disease. *J Thorac Cardiovasc Surg*. 1993; 105:265-276.

19. Skinner DB, Dowlatshahi KD, DeMeester TR. Potentially curable cancer of the esophagus. *Cancer*. 1982; 50:2571-2575.

20. Skinner DB, Little AG, Ferguson MK, et al. Selection of operation for esophageal cancer based on staging. *Ann Surg*. 1986; 204:391-401.

21. Fuchs CS, Mayer RJ. Gastric carcinoma. *N Engl J Med*. 1995; 333:32-41.

22. Tsugane S. Salt, salted food intake, and risk of gastric cancer: epidemiologic evidence. *Cancer Sci*. 2005; 96:1-6.

23. Dicken BJ, Bigam DL, Cass C, et al. Gastric adenocarcinoma: review and considerations for future directions. *Ann Surg*. 2005; 241:27-39.

24. Master SS. Gastric carcinoma. *Dis Mon*. 2004; 50:532-539.

25. Lauren P. The two histological main types of gastric carcinoma: diffuse and so called intestinal-type carcinoma. An attempt at histo-clinical classification. *Acta Pathol Microbiol Scand*. 1965; 64:31-49.

26. Hundahl SA, Phillips JL, Menck HR. The National Cancer Data Base Report on poor survival of U.S. gastric carcinoma patients treated with gastrectomy: Fifth Edition American Joint Committee on Cancer staging, proximal disease, and the "different disease" hypothesis. *Cancer.* 2000; 88:921-932.

27. Greene FL. Management of gastric remnant carcinoma based on the results of a 15-year endoscopic screening program. *Ann Surg*. 1996; 223:701-706.

28. Weed TE, Nuessle W, Ochsner A. Carcinoma of the stomach. Why are we falling to improve survival? *Ann Surg*. 1981; 193:407-413.

29. Lowy AM, Mansfield PF, Leach SD, et al. Laparoscopic staging for gastric cancer. *Surgery*. 1996; 119:611-614.

30. Mani NB, Suri S, Gupta S, et al. Two-phase dynamic contrast-enhanced computed tomography with water-filling method for staging of gastric carcinoma. *Clin Imaging*. 2001; 25:38-43.

31. Kodera Y, Schwarz RE, Nakao A. Extended lymph node dissection in gastric carcinoma: where do we stand after the Dutch and British randomized trials? *J Am Coll Surg*. 2002; 195:855-864.

32. Willis S, Truong S, Gribnitz S, et al. Endoscopic ultrasonography in the preoperative staging of gastric cancer: accuracy and impact on surgical therapy. *Surg Endosc*. 2000; 14:951-954.

33. Bozzetti F, Bonfanti G, Bufalino R, et al. Adequacy of margins of resection in gastrectomy for cancer. *Ann Surg*. 1982; 196:685-690.

34. Bozzetti F, Marubini E, Bonfanti G, et al. Subtotal versus total gastrectomy for gastric cancer: five-year survival rates in a multicenter randomized Italian trial. Italian Gastrointestinal Tumor Study Group. *Ann Surg*. 1999; 230:170-178.

35. Butler JA, Dubrow TJ, Trezona T, et al. Total gastrectomy in the treatment of advanced gastric cancer. *Am J Surg*. 1989; 158:602-604.

36. Sasako M, Sano T, Yamamoto S, et al. D2 lymphadenectomy alone or with para-aortic nodal dissection for gastric cancer. *N Engl J Med*. 2008; 359:453-462.

37. Kodama Y, Sugimachi K, Soejima K, et al. Evaluation of extensive lymph node dissection for carcinoma of the stomach. *World J Surg*. 1981; 5:241-248.

38. Cunningham D, Allum WH, Stenning SP, et al. Perioperative chemotherapy versus surgery alone for resectable gastroesophageal cancer. *N Engl J Med*. 2006; 355:11-20.

39. Hussell T, Isaacson PG, Crabtree JE, et al. The response of cells from low grade B-cell gastric lymphomas of mucosa-associated lymphoid tissue to Helicobacter pylori. *Lancet*. 1993; 342:571-574.

40. Yoon SS, Coit DG, Portlock CS, et al. The diminishing role of surgery in the treatment of gastric lymphoma. *Ann Surg*. 2004; 240:28-37.

41. Chan C, Herrera MF, de la GL, et al. Clinical behavior and prognostic factors of periampullary adenocarcinoma. *Ann Surg*. 1995; 222:632-637.

42. Ross WA, Bismar MM. Evaluation and management of periampullary tumors. *Curr Gastroenterol Rep*. 2004; 6:362-370.

43. Rudan N, Nola P, Popovic S. Primary adenocarcinoma of the duodenum. Report of two cases. *Cancer*. 1984; 54:1105-1109.

44. Sarma DP, Weilbaecher TG. Adenocarcinoma of the duodenum. *J Surg Oncol*. 1987; 34:262-263.

45. Lowell JA, Rossi RL, Munson JL, et al. Primary adenocarcinoma of third and fourth portions of duodenum. Favorable prognosis after resection. *Arch Surg*. 1992; 127:557-560.

46. Yeo TP, Hruban RH, Leach SD, et al. Pancreatic cancer. *Curr Probl Cancer*. 2002; 26:176-275.

47. Michaud DS, Giovannucci E, Willett WC, et al. Physical activity, obesity, height, and the risk of pancreatic cancer. *JAMA*. 2001; 286:921-929.

48. Tersmette AC, Petersen GM, Offerhaus GJ, et al. Increased risk of incident pancreatic cancer among first-degree relatives of patients with familial pancreatic cancer. *Clin Cancer Res*. 2001; 7:738-744.

49. Hiotis SP, Klimstra DS, Conlon KC, et al. Results after pancreatic resection for metastatic lesions. *Ann Surg Oncol*. 2002; 9:675-679.

50. Murr MM, Sarr MG, Oishi AJ, et al. Pancreatic cancer. *CA Cancer J Clin*. 1994; 44:304-318.

51. Ritts RE, Jr., Nagorney DM, Jacobsen DJ, et al. Comparison of preoperative serum CA19-9 levels with results of diagnostic imaging modalities in patients undergoing laparotomy for suspected pancreatic or gallbladder disease. *Pancreas*. 1994; 9:707-716.

52. Freeny PC, Traverso LW, Ryan JA. Diagnosis and staging of pancreatic adenocarcinoma with dynamic computed tomography. *Am J Surg*. 1993; 165:600-606.

53. Tyler DS, Evans DB. Reoperative pancreaticoduodenectomy. *Ann Surg*. 1994; 219:211-221.

54. Roche CJ, Hughes ML, Garvey CJ, et al. CT and pathologic assessment of prospective nodal staging in patients with ductal adenocarcinoma of the head of the pancreas. *AJR Am J Roentgenol*. 2003; 180:475-480.

55. Soriano A, Castells A, Ayuso C, et al. Preoperative staging and tumor resectability assessment of pancreatic cancer: prospective study comparing endoscopic ultrasonography, helical computed tomography, magnetic resonance imaging, and angiography. *Am J Gastroenterol*. 2004; 99:492-501.

56. Raut CP, Grau AM, Staerkel GA, et al. Diagnostic accuracy of endoscopic ultrasound-guided fine-needle aspiration in patients with presumed pancreatic cancer. *J Gastrointest Surg*. 2003; 7:118-126.

57. Nieveen van Dijkum EJ, Romijn MG, Terwee CB, et al. Laparoscopic staging and subsequent palliation in patients with peripancreatic carcinoma. *Ann Surg*. 2003; 237:66-73.

58. Ammori JB, Colletti LM, Zalupski MM, et al. Surgical resection following radiation therapy with concurrent gemcitabine in patients with previously unresectable adenocarcinoma of the pancreas. *J Gastrointest Surg*. 2003; 7:766-772.

59. Kalser MH, Ellenberg SS. Pancreatic cancer. Adjuvant combined radiation and chemotherapy following curative resection. *Arch Surg*. 1985; 120:899-903.

60. Magnin V, Moutardier V, Giovannini MH, et al. Neoadjuvant preoperative chemoradiation in patients with pancreatic cancer. *Int J Radiat Oncol Biol Phys*. 2003; 55:1300-1304.

61. Roder JD, Stein HJ, Huttl W, et al. Pylorus-preserving versus standard pancreatico-duodenectomy: an analysis of 110 pancreatic and periampullary carcinomas. *Br J Surg*. 1992; 79:152-155.

62. Sarfeh IJ, Rypins EB, Jakowatz JG, et al. A prospective, randomized clinical investigation of cholecystoenterostomy and choledochoenterostomy. *Am J Surg*. 1988; 155:411-414.

63. Sarr MG, Cameron JL. Surgical management of unresectable carcinoma of the pancreas. *Surgery*. 1982; 91:123-133.

64. Singh SM, Reber HA. Surgical palliation for pancreatic cancer. *Surg Clin North Am*. 1989; 69:599-611.

65. Lillemoe KD, Cameron JL, Kaufman HS, et al. Chemical splanchnicectomy in patients with unresectable pancreatic cancer. A prospective randomized trial. *Ann Surg*. 1993; 217:447-455.

66. Yeo CJ, Barry MK, Sauter PK, et al. Erythromycin accelerates gastric emptying after pancreaticoduodenectomy. A prospective, randomized, placebo-controlled trial. *Ann Surg*. 1993; 218:229-237.

67. Whittington R, Neuberg D, Tester WJ, et al. Protracted intravenous fluorouracil infusion with radiation therapy in the management of localized pancreaticobiliary carcinoma: a phase I Eastern Cooperative Oncology Group Trial. *J Clin Oncol*. 1995; 13:227-232.

68. Lockhart AC, Rothenberg ML, Berlin JD. Treatment for pancreatic cancer: current therapy and continued progress. *Gastroenterology*. 2005; 128:1642-1654.

69. Huerta S, Janssen M, Marcus DR. Solid pseudopapillary tumor of the pancreas diagnosed postpartum. *Surgery*. 2005; 137:480-481.

70. Pettinato G, Di Vizio D, Manivel JC, et al. Solid-pseudopapillary tumor of the pancreas: a neoplasm with distinct and highly characteristic cytological features. Diagn Cytopathol. 2002; 27:325-334.

71. Brugge WR, Lauwers GY, Sahani D, et al. Cystic neoplasms of the pancreas. *N Engl J Med*. 2004; 351:1218-1226.

72. Fernandez-del Castillo C, Targarona J, Thayer SP, et al. Incidental pancreatic cysts: clinicopathologic characteristics and comparison with symptomatic patients. *Arch Surg*. 2003; 138:427-423.

73. Proye CA, Lokey JS. Current concepts in functioning endocrine tumors of the pancreas. *World J Surg*. 2004; 28:1231-1238.

74. Thompson NW, Pasieka J, Fukuuchi A. Duodenal gastrinomas, duodenotomy, and duodenal exploration in the surgical management of Zollinger-Ellison syndrome. *World J Surg*. 1993; 17:455-462.

75. Passaro E Jr, Howard TJ, Sawicki MP, et al. The origin of sporadic gastrinomas within the gastrinoma triangle: a theory. *Arch Surg*. 1998; 133:13-16.

76. Ghaferi AA, Chojnacki KA, Long WD, et al. Pancreatic VIPomas: subject review and one institutional experience. *J Gastrointest Surg*. 2008; 12:382-393.

11. Questions

1. All the following factors increase the risk of developing gastric cancer except:

A. History of peptic ulcer disease

B. A father who died of diffuse-type gastric cancer

C. History of gastrectomy for the treatment of peptic ulcer disease

D. Low consumption of fruits and vegetables

E. Pernicious anemia

2. A pancreaticoduodenectomy for a mass in the head of the pancreas:

A. Has worse prognosis if performed for the management of an ampullary tumor

B. Should be done only after a biopsy proves the diagnosis of malignancy

C. Results in better functional outcome with a pylorus-sparing procedure

D. Results in reduced operative mortality when performed in centers which average at least one Whipple procedure per month

3. With regards to the surgical management of pancreatic cancer:

A. Total pancreatectomy offers the best chance of survival

B. Pylorus-sparing procedure results is less rate of recurrence than the standard Whipple procedure

C. Gastrostomy and jejunostomy tube placement should be avoided during a pancreaticoduedenectomy as this adds to the operative time and may increase the rate of complications

D. Pancreatico-enteric fistula occurs at the same rate regardless of the type of anastomosis (ie, pancreaticogastrostomy vs. pancreaticojejunostomy)

4. In cystic neoplasms of the pancreas:

A. Serum levels of CA-19-9 are typically elevated

B. The 5-year survival following surgical excision is similar to acinar cell carcinoma of the pancreas

C. CT scan reliably distinguishes pancreatic cystic neoplasms from pancreatic pseudocysts

D. EUS with FNA can sample fluid from the cystic lesion and aid in the diagnosis

5. A patient diagnosed with gastrinoma should have the following test:

A. CT of the head

B. Measurement of urinary pH to establish the diagnosis

C. Serum calcium levels

D. Secretin level

6. All of the following statements are true regarding Barrett's esophagus except:

A. Aggressive medical management or surgical intervention for gastroesophageal reflux disease effectively prevents the development of cancer from Barrett's esophagus

B. Patients with symptomatic Barrett's esophagus without dysplasia should be treated as patients with gastroesophageal reflux disease

C. Patients with Barrett's esophagus with low-grade dysplasia require endoscopic surveillance at least once a year

D. The treatment for Barrett's esophagus with high grade dysplasia requires an esophagectomy

7. Which upper gastrointestinal malignancy requires the widest resection margins for optimal local control?

A. Solid-pseudo papillary tumor of the pancreas

B. Pancreas

C. Esophagus

D. Duodenum

8. Which periampullary adenocarcinoma has the best 5-year survival?

A. Ampullary

B. Pancreas

C. Duodenum

D. Cholangiocarcinoma

9. Which is the most accurate preoperative staging test for the diagnosis of T and N stage in esophageal cancer?

A. Computed tomography

B. Endoscopic ultrasound

C. Barium swallow

D. Upper endoscopy with biopsy

10. Which upper gastrointestinal malignancy has the highest 5-year survival rate following curative resection?

A. Gastric lymphoma

B. Gastric adenocarcinoma

C. Pancreatic adenocarcinoma

D. Duodenal adenocarcinoma

11. Which method of esophageal resection has the shortest operating time and is associated with the lowest blood loss?

A. Transhiatal esophagectomy

B. Ivor Lewis esophagectomy

C. Radical en bloc esophagectomy

D. Thoracoabdominal esophagectomy

12. A 65-year-old man develops increased drain output and fever seven days following pancreaticoduodenectomy. Oliguria responds to a fluid challenge. Appropriate initial diagnostic evaluation would include all of the following except:

A. Computed tomography

B. Determination of drain fluid amylase content

C. Serum electrolytes

D. Fistulogram

13. *Helicobacter pylori* infection is associated with all of the following malignancies except:

A. Gastric lymphoma

B. Distal gastric adenocarcinoma

C. Gastroesophageal junction adenocarcinoma

D. Intestinal-type gastric adenocarcinoma

14. All of the following obviate curative resection for pancreatic cancer except:

A. Superior mesenteric artery involvement

B. Superior mesenteric vein involvement

C. Thrombosis of portal-mesenteric vein confluence

D. Liver metastases

15. A patient presenting with watery diarrhea, hypokalemia, and acidosis should be screened for which type of tumor?

A. Insulinoma

B. Gastrinoma

C. Glucagonoma

D. VIPoma

E. Somatostatinoma

16. Barrett's esophagus

A. Is a disease of Caucasian men that predisposes those without dysplasia to a 1.0 % risk of squamous cell carcinoma per year

B. Patients with low grade dysplasia should be considered candidates for an esophagectomy

C. A fundoplication substantially reduces the risk of cancer for these patients

D. Agreement among pathologists regarding the diagnosis of high grade dysplasia is higher than that for low grade dysplasia

E. It is defined when the esophageal squamous epithelium undergoes dysplasia as a result of the constant exposure of acid from GERD

Answers

1. A.

Risk factors for gastric cancer include chronic atrophic gastritis, intestinal metaplasia or adenomatous polyps. Patients with pernicious anemia have a 2-to-3-fold increased risk of gastric cancer. Patients with a prior history of partial gastrectomy for benign disease have a 1.5- to 3-fold increased risk of gastric cancer beginning 20 years following their surgery. Other risks factors include hypertrophic gastropathy (Menetrier's disease) and Barrett's esophagus (particularly gastric cancer in the gastric cardia). *H pylori* infection increases the risk of gastric cancer by 3- to 6-fold. Peptic ulcer disease is not a recognized risk factor for gastric cancer.

2. D.

Complete removal of all disease offers the only chance for cure in patients with pancreatic cancer. Patients with a mass in the head of the pancreas should undergo a Whipple procedure. Typically, biopsy is not needed to proceed with surgical management, as this will not alter treatment options. Ampullary tumors have the best prognosis of all periampullary cancers. The pylorus-sparing procedure has not demonstrated functional advantage over the standard Whipple procedure. Centers which average at least one Whipple procedure per month have the least number of complications.

3. D.

Postoperative complications following a Whipple procedure occur in 25% of patients. Delayed gastric emptying occurs in one-third of these patients and these patients should have routine placement of gastrostomy and jujunostomy tubes for decompression and feeding, respectively. Pancreatic fistula is the most serious complication of pancreaticoduodenectomy. Pancreatic fistula indicates disruption of the pancreatic-enteric anastomosis and occurs at the same rate regardless of anastomosis (ie, pancreaticogastrostomy vs. pancreaticojejunostomy). Total pancreatectomy does not offer survival advantage over a standard Whipple procedure.

4. D.

The most common cystic neoplasms of the pancreas encountered are serous cystadenomas (35%), mucinous cystic neoplasms (10%-40%), and intraductal papillary mucinous neoplasms (IPMT [20%-30%]). Serous cystadenomas have very low malignant potential, but may grow to very large sizes. These lesions typically contain glycogen rather than mucin and are usually multilocular. Mucinous cystadenomas have the potential to turn into mucinous cystadenocarcinoma. They contain mucin and are commonly unilocular. The histological characteristics of IPMTs are similar to mucinous cystadenomas. Unlike mucinous cystadenomas, IPMTs communicate with the pancreatic ductal system. Once excised, these tumors have an excellent prognosis. It is typically difficult to distinguish between a pancreatic pseudocyst and cystic neoplasms of the pancreas. EUS-FNA may aid in the diagnosis by sampling the fluid and assessing whether the fluid is rich in amylase and lipase, which would point towards a pseudocyst, whereas elevated levels of CEA should suggest cystic neoplasms. Serum levels of CA-19-9 may be elevated in pancreatic adenocarcinoma but are typically normal in patients with cystic neoplasms.

5. C.

It is important to recognize that up to one-fourth of pancreatic endocrine tumors are part of the MEN-1 syndrome. Elevated calcium levels suggesting hyperparathyroidism concomitant with a pancreatic endocrine tumor establishes the diagnosis of MEN-1.

6. A.

Neither medical nor surgical treatment of gastroesophageal reflux disease prevents the development of cancer or can be guaranteed to prevent recurrence of Barrett's esophagus, and lifelong surveillance is mandatory. Patients with Barrett's esophagus without dysplasia should undergo surveillance endoscopy every two to three years. Those with low grade dysplasia should be surveyed after 6 and 12 months, and annually thereafter if there is no progression of the disease. When high grade dysplasia is identified, an esophagectomy is the standard treatment option, as 30%-40% of patients with high grade dysplasia harbor invasive cancer.

7. C.
The esophagus has an extensive submucosal lymphatic network. Submucosal tumor nests may be discontinuous and microscopically negative margins do not obviate local recurrence. Esophagectomy should encompass the entire esophagus to ensure optimal local control.

8. A.
Patients with ampullary carcinoma present with smaller tumors than patients with the other tumors listed. 5-year survival rates near 50% for nodenegative patients and 30% for node-positive patients have been reported.

9. B.
Endoscopic ultrasound has become the diagnostic staging tool of choice for esophageal cancer. The echo-endoscope reliably assesses T stage (95% sensitivity) and also N stage (70% sensitivity). Fine-needle aspiration can be done to obtain a tissue diagnosis. The echo-endoscope also reliably detects liver masses and ascites, both of which may be sampled by FNA.

10. A.
Gastric lymphoma has the best 5-year survival. Currently, surgical intervention is indicated for patients with residual disease after aggressive medical management or patients with perforation or bleeding.

11. A.
Transhiatal esophagectomy has been clearly shown to be associated with lower blood loss and shorter operating times than other types of esophagectomy. Data indicating that transhiatal esophagectomy is associated with fewer postoperative complications is inconsistent.

12. D.
The patient in question likely has a pancreatic fistula. The diagnosis can be confirmed by assessing the amylase content of the drain fluid. An amylase concentration greater than the serum amylase establishes the diagnosis. The fistula may be completely captured by the drain. However, CT scan is indicated to assess for undrained fluid collections. These may be drained using CT guidance. Fistulograms seldom yield useful information in the early postoperative course. Exploratory laparotomy is reserved for patients with sepsis or those who do not respond to conservative management.

13. C.
Helicobacter pylori is a Gram-negative rod that selectively infects the stomach and duodenum. It is associated with intestinal-type distal gastric cancer and gastric lymphoma, but not with cancer of the gastroesophageal junction.

14. B.
Pancreatic cancer should be thoroughly staged preoperatively. Distant metastases preclude curative resection. Involvement of the superior mesenteric artery requires interposition grafting for en bloc resection. This maneuver is associated with unacceptable perioperative morbidity and mortality. Thrombosis of the portal vein-superior mesenteric vein confluence as a result of tumor infiltration makes curative resection impossible. Isolated superior mesenteric vein involvement by tumor can be treated by experienced pancreatic surgeons with local vein resection and primary repair or interposition grafting with internal jugular vein or PTFE.

15. D.
VIPomas secrete vasoactive intestinal peptide, causing a profuse watery diarrhea (10 L/d) leading to profound metabolic disturbances. This syndrome is typically characterized by an acronym for watery diarrhea, hypokalemia and achlorhydria (WDHA).

16. D.
Barrett's esophagus is indeed a disease of Caucasian older men, but the risk is for adenocarcinoma of the esophagus and not SCC. An esophagectomy is a treatment option for patients with high grade dysplasia and *not* low grade dysplasia. No anti-acid modality medical or surgical has been shown to actually reduce the rate of cancer in patients with Barrett's. Barrett's is defined when the esophageal lining undergoes metaplasia not dysplasia. Agreement regarding high grade dyplasia is around 85% among two expert pathologists. This inter-agreement is only 50% for cases of low grade dysplasia.

Chapter 11: Hepatobiliary and Pancreas Surgery

Maki Yamamoto, MD
David K. Imagawa, MD, PhD

Contents

1. Liver

Infections of the Liver

Pyogenic abscesses. Although rare, pyogenic abscesses of the liver are increasing in incidence over the last 3 decades and are usually secondary to perihepatic or remote infections.[1] Malignant and benign obstruction of the biliary tree can lead to abscesses caused by ascending cholangitis. Hematogenous seeding can occur through the portal vein (eg, appendicitis or diverticulitis) or hepatic artery (eg, bacterial endocarditis). Other less common etiologies include trauma, direct extension from surrounding disease processes and cryptogenic etiologies.[2] Organisms usually found in pyogenic liver abscesses are those of enteric flora including Gram-negative rods, streptococci and anaerobes.[3] Males and females appear to be equally affected, and abscesses most commonly occur in the elderly.

The most common clinical manifestations of pyogenic liver abscesses are non-specific and include fevers, chills and abdominal pain. Jaundice occurs in a minority of patients and suggests biliary tract involvement. Laboratory studies usually reveal leukocytosis, elevated alkaline phosphatase and elevated transaminases. Imaging by ultrasound or CT scan will reveal solitary or multiple abscesses with or without loculations.

Treatment of pyogenic abscesses is directed against the primary infection and the secondary hepatic abscess. Pyogenic hepatic abscesses are drained by percutaneous methods under CT or ultrasound guidance, and intravenous antibiotics to cover enteric organisms (eg, carbapenems, second and third generation cephalosporins) are initiated. The appropriate length of intravenous antibiotic treatment is still undefined, and conversion to oral antibiotics after an intravenous antibiotic course for a total of six weeks has been described.[4,5] Operative drainage is for patients who do not respond to conservative therapies for large loculated collections or for patients who need abdominal surgery for other indications.

Amebic abscess. Entamoeba histolytica is an ameba transmitted by the fecal-oral route that can cause amebic colitis and hepatic amebic abscesses in humans. Amebic infections predominantly occur in areas with poor sanitation. Patients with recent travel to endemic areas (eg, tropical climates) and those with immunodeficiencies are at increased risk for amebic liver infection.[6]

Clinical and laboratory manifestations of amebic liver abscesses are similar to those caused by pyogenic abscesses. Differentiation from pyogenic abscesses can be achieved by a serologic testing for *Entamoeba antigens*. Ultrasound and CT scan imaging will reveal abscesses that are indistinguishable from pyogenic abscesses. Unlike hydatid cysts, amebic abscesses do not calcify. Diagnosis of amebic liver abscess is thus more likely in a patient with the appropriate risk factors, presence of abscesses on imaging studies, and a positive serum ELISA for Entamoeba antigens. Some experts have even proposed the initiation of medical treatment prior to serologic diagnosis.[7]

Treatment of amebic liver abscesses is a two-week course of intravenous or oral metronidazole. Percutaneous aspiration is indicated in cases that lack response to medical treatment. Surgery is indicated for amebic abscesses that rupture.

Hydatid disease. The echinococcal tapeworms *E granulosis* and *E multilocularis* are rare causes of liver infection in the United States. Dogs are the definitive hosts. Humans, as intermediate hosts, can acquire this infection by ingesting echinococcal eggs in contaminated food.

Although infection can occur anywhere in the human body, the liver is the most frequently involved. Echinococcal embryos enter via the portal blood stream and lodge in the liver. Embryos that survive host defenses then develop into hydatid cysts.

Clinical manifestations of hydatid cysts include abdominal pain, biliary obstruction, and portal hypertension, although most patients are asymptomatic. These manifestations are secondary to the size of the slow-growing hydatid cyst. Occasionally as a complication these cysts may undergo rupture into the abdominal cavity causing anaphylaxis. Laboratory tests may reveal nonspecific elevations in liver transaminases and bilirubin. Eosinophilia may be present. ELISAs for echinococcal specific antigens may help establish the diagnosis of hydatid infection. CT scan is the preferred imaging modality and will demonstrate a solitary cyst with a calcific rim. Occasionally surrounding daughter cysts may be present.

The treatment of choice for hydatid cysts is surgical removal or obliteration. Nonoperative management with albendazole therapy may be attempted in patients with inaccessible, small fluid-filled cysts with thin walls located deep within the liver. Surgical removal and obliteration of hydatid cysts may be through the open or laparoscopic approach. Cysts are first injected with a scolicidal agent such as hypertonic saline if cyst aspirates are nonbilious. Cyst removal may be accomplished by careful pericystic dissection or partial hepatic resection. Recently, a new technique in percutaneous drainage with injection of scolicidal agent (eg, hypertonic saline or alcohol) and subsequent reaspiration has been shown to be a treatment option in select groups of patients. Regardless of the operative treatment, the fundamental rule that applies to any treatment is the prevention of scoleces dissemination.[8]

Benign Tumors of the Liver

Hepatic adenoma. Hepatic adenomas are benign lesions characterized histologically by a collection of well-circumscribed hepatocytes without defined bile duct architecture. The association of oral contraceptives and hepatic adenomas is well documented and the lesions have been shown to decrease in size when the contraceptives are stopped. Over 90% of cases occur in women between the ages of 20 and 40 years. Hepatic adenomas are not considered to be premalignant. The complications of hepatic adenomas are related to its risk for rupture and hemorrhage. Hepatic adenoma rupture and hemorrhage occur in up to 50% of patients with a mortality approaching 10%.[9]

Clinical manifestations of hepatic adenomas include abdominal pain related to adenoma rupture or bleeding and hepatomegaly. Laboratory tests are usually normal unless rupture and bleeding has occurred. Imaging of hepatic adenomas can be performed adequately with CT scan and ultrasound, although there are no pathognomic radiological findings.

Hepatic adenoma rupture and hemorrhage requires emergent operation. Asymptomatic patients or those who are hemodynamically stable are also best managed with operative resection. Discontinuation of hormones/oral contraceptives may decrease the risk of adenoma growth and complication, but adenoma resolution is unpredictable.

Focal nodular hyperplasia. Focal nodular hyperplasia is a benign liver tumor that occurs mostly in women of childbearing age, with only about 10%-20% of cases occurring in men.[10] This benign lesion's association with oral contraceptives is controversial. As its name implies, this lesion results from a hyperplastic process that, unlike hepatic adenomas, involves all liver parenchymal cell types. It has a central fibrous lesion that may contain arteries or rarely, portal vessels.

Patients with focal nodular hyperplasia are usually asymptomatic, although the rare symptomatic patient may complain of abdominal discomfort and have hepatomegaly on physical exam. CT scan or ultrasound may demonstrate a lesion with a characteristic central, stellate scar. Secondary to Kupffer cell activity, a nuclear medicine scan (^{99m}Tc sulfur colloid) will demonstrate an isodense lesion with the surrounding parenchyma in focal nodular hyperplasia; whereas a hepatic adenoma will show decreased uptake. Asymptomatic patients do not require any treatment; whereas surgical management is reserved for symptomatic patients or those with unclear diagnoses.[11]

Hemangioma. Cavernous hemangioma is a benign vascular lesion of the liver. It is the most common benign tumor of the liver and is most often found in females. Cavernous hemangiomas are characterized by large endothelial cell-lined vascular cavities within the liver. Complications of this tumor are fortunately rare and include biliary obstruction, rupture and high-output congestive heart failure. Another rare complication of hepatic hemangiomas that deserves mention here is the Kasabach-Merrit syndrome, which is characterized by coagulopathy due to trapping of platelets within the hemangioma.

Clinical manifestations of cavernous hemangiomas include abdominal pain, early satiety, nausea or vomiting. Laboratory values are usually normal unless complication is present. Imaging by CT scan, MRI, and nuclear medicine tagged red cell scan aid in the diagnosis. Hemangiomas less than 4 cm are usually observed and large, symptomatic ones may be surgically resected.[11]

Polycystic liver disease. Polycystic liver disease is usually found in association with polycystic kidney disease, although hepatic and renal components of the disease may vary in severity. Infantile polycystic disease is an autosomal recessive disorder characterized by a more severe hepatic component in those children who survive renal failure caused by renal cysts. Adult polycystic disease is an autosomal dominant disorder characterized by dominance of either hepatic or renal components. About 4% of patients with adult polycystic disease may have intracranial aneurysms.[12]

Clinical manifestations depend on the severity of disease. The infantile form may be found incidentally or as a cause of congenital hepatic fibrosis. The adult form is usually symptomatic, and patients with large hepatic cysts may present with abdominal pain, early satiety, and nausea with vomiting. Treatment of hepatic cysts includes excision or liver transplantation in suitable candidates.

Malignant Lesions of the Liver

Hepatocellular carcinoma. Hepatocellular carcinoma (HCC) is the most common solid tumor worldwide and is increasing in prevalence. The U.S. is no exception, where incidence and mortality rates of have steadily increased over the past 20 years. The incidence of liver cancer is highest in Asian Americans, due to the prevalence of hepatitis B and C in that population. Other risk factors for liver cancer include alcohol abuse, aflatoxins, cirrhosis, hematochromatosis and other metabolic disorders. Roughly 80% of primary liver tumors are hepatocellular carcinoma (HCC), where tumor cells resemble hepatocytes. It is an aggressive form of liver cancer, the third leading cause of cancer death worldwide with a dismal 5-year survival rate of 9%.

Unfortunately, there is often a long delay between the occurrence of HCC and diagnosis. The disease is relatively asymptomatic until it progresses to a state where patients experience abdominal pain, weight loss, jaundice or gastrointestinal hemorrhage. However, there are methods that promote the early detection of HCC in groups that are at risk. The most widely used tools are ultrasound and monitoring of alpha-fetoprotein (AFP). Studies have shown that when used in combination, ultrasound and AFP have a sensitivity approaching 100%.[13] Nonspecific laboratory abnormalities include elevated liver transaminases and bilirubin. CT scan with intravenous contrast is the imaging test of choice. Percutaneous core biopsy or fine needle aspiration can be used to establish tissue diagnosis in ambiguous cases, but such procedures carry the risk of tumor implantation into biopsy needle tracts and in most cases are unnecessary.

HCC can be classified as well-differentiated, moderately differentiated or poorly differentiated lesions. Well-differentiated HCC may be difficult to distinguish from normal liver or adenomas. Poorly differentiated HCC may have a varied cellular appearance. A fibrolamellar variant of HCC deserves mention because of its better prognosis and its prevalence in young Caucasian patients.[14]

Due to the advanced stage of the disease at the time of presentation, curative treatment (transplant or surgical resection) can be offered only in a small proportion of patients with HCC. Surgical approaches include anatomic or nonanatomic resections as well as orthotopic liver transplantation. HCC is amenable to resection if the remaining hepatic mass has adequate functional reserve, the operation is technically feasible and there is no evidence of extrahepatic spread. The lack of suitable donors for transplant also limits the ability to effectively treat patients with HCC. Indications for liver transplantation in the HCC patient vary from center to center but generally include unresectable tumors (due to inadequate functional reserve or technical feasibility of resection) less than 5 cm, minimal intrahepatic tumor dissemination (<3 tumors, largest <3 cm) and absence of extrahepatic spread. Although there are multiple palliative modalities of treatment, including embolization (TAE), chemoembolization (TACE), alcohol ablation and radiofrequency ablation, the effectiveness of these modalities are illustrated with the dismal 5-year survival rate.[15]

Cholangiocarcinoma. Cholangiocarcinoma is a rare malignancy that originates from the biliary epithelium. It is more common in males with an average age of over 50 years. Patients with gallstones seem to be at increased risk, although this association is not as strong as that seen in gallbladder cancer. Although the exact etiology is unknown, the following risk factors are well established: primary sclerosing cholangitis, choledochal cysts and congenital hepatic fibrosis.[16]

Clinical symptoms are those of biliary obstruction, jaundice, abdominal pain and cholangitis. Weight loss, anorexia and pruritis are seen in patients who present with advanced disease. Laboratory evaluation can show an elevated alkaline phosphatase, bilirubin and CA 19-9. Ultrasound or CT scan may reveal dilated bile ducts but usually does not reveal the tumor. Imaging by endoscopic retrograde cholangiopancreatography (ERCP), percutaneous transhepatic cholangiography (PTC), or endoscopic ultrasound (EUS) may be required to identify bile duct tumors. ERCP has the additional advantage of providing brushings for cytological diagnosis of proximal bile duct tumors. EUS-guided needle biopsy is an important tool in staging for lymph node metastases.

Surgical resection or liver transplantation remain the only options for curative intent. Cholangiocarcinoma of the proximal and middle portions of the extrahepatic bile ducts are best treated with resection and reconstruction with a biliary-enteric anastomosis may be required (choledochojejunostomy or hepaticojejunostomy). Cholangiocarcinoma of the bifurcation or more distal extra/intra-hepatic ducts (Klatskin tumor) are usually unresectable, although addition of hepatic resection may result in complete tumor removal in a few patients. Prognosis for hilar cholangiocarcinoma is poor with a 5-year survival rate of less than 20%. With microscopic negative margins in surgical resection, 5-year survival improves up to 45%.

Patients with metastatic disease, vascular invasion, or bilateral intrahepatic spread are considered unresectable. Palliative treatments of these patients to relieve biliary obstruction include surgically created biliary-enteric anastomosis, external stenting or endoprosthesis placement.[17]

Metastatic liver disease. Metastatic cancer to the liver is the most common type of hepatic tumor.[18] The most common types of cancers that metastasize to the liver include colorectal, breast, melanoma, lung and pancreatic islet tumors. Patients with colorectal cancer who undergo primary tumor resection have a recurrence rate of approximately 40%. 20% of recurrent colorectal cancer occurs as isolated hepatic metastasis, and these patients are potentially curable with surgery.

Patients with colorectal metastasis are considered resectable if there is no extrahepatic metastasis, a 1 cm margin around the tumor is obtainable, and there are less than 5 metastases. Patients who meet these criteria and undergo adequate surgical resection may achieve a 5-year survival of up to 40%, although the average 5-year survival rate is approximately 25%.[19] Addition of a hepatic artery infusion pump for chemotherapy may increase the two-year survival up to 86%.[20] For patients who are initially deemed unresectable due to extent of intrahepatic lesions, underlying liver dysfunction (eg, chemotherapy-induced steatosis), and proximity to portal confluence, other modalities can be utilized, such as portal vein embolization, staged hepatectomies or resection combined with ablative techniques.

Cirrhosis and Portal Hypertension. Cirrhosis results from chronic liver damage and regeneration that result in the diffuse loss of hepatic architecture and deposition of connective tissue.[21] Cirrhosis can be classified as macronodular, micronodular or mixed according to morphological characteristics. Micronodular cirrhosis is seen in alcoholic cirrhosis; macronodular is seen in hepatitis-induced cirrhosis. As mentioned earlier, cirrhosis has a multitude of etiologies including alcohol, chronic hepatitis B and C infection, hemochromatosis, alpha 1-antitrypsin deficiency, biliary obstruction and Wilson disease. The pathophysiological mechanism

Table 1

Causes of Portal Hypertension

Posthepatic	
Hepatic vein thrombosis (Budd-Chiari syndrome)	
Severe right sided heart failure	
Constrictive pericarditis	
Hepatic veno-occlusive disease	
Intrahepatic	
Cirrhosis	
Schistosomiasis	
Massive fatty change	
Diffuse fibrosing granulomatous disease (tuberculosis and sarcoidosis)	
Idiopathic	
Prehepatic	
Portal vein thrombosis	
Splenic vein thrombosis	
Arteriovenous fistula	

underlying the various etiologies of cirrhosis is the cycle of parenchymal damage and necrosis followed by regeneration that increasingly becomes more disorganized and fibrotic with each cycle of injury.

The causes of portal hypertension can be classified according to where the lesion or obstruction of portal venous flow is located (Table 1). Posthepatic portal hypertension results from obstruction of hepatic vein outflow. A classic but rare example of this type of portal hypertension is Budd-Chiari syndrome. Budd-Chiari syndrome is characterized by thrombosis of the hepatic veins, which may be caused by hypercoagulability, congenital venous webs, tumors or infections. Intrahepatic portal hypertension is caused by intrahepatic lesions or diseases that obstruct portal venous flow. Cirrhosis is an example of an intrahepatic disease that promotes portal venous obstruction or increased resistance to portal venous flow. Prehepatic portal hypertension is caused by lesions or diseases that promote the obstruction of portal venous flow proximal to where the portal vein enters the liver. Pancreatitis may result in splenic vein thrombosis that impedes venous outflow from the proximal stomach. This left-sided portal hypertension, also known as sinistral portal hypertension, is an important cause of gastroesophogeal varices and is usually treated with splenectomy.

Complications of cirrhosis include portal hypertension and HCC (see Table 1). Approximately one-third of patients with cirrhosis will develop portal

Table 2

Location of Portosystemic Venous Shunts

Gastroesophageal region	Esophageal tributaries of the left gastric vein anastomose with the esophageal veins, which empty into the azygous vein.
Anorectal region	Superior rectal vein anastomoses with the middle and inferior rectal veins.
Paraumbilical region	Paraumbilical veins in the falciform ligament anastomose with subcutaneous veins in the anterior abdominal wall.
Retroperitoneal region	Tributaries of the splenic and pancreatic veins anastomose with the left renal vein. Short veins also connect the splenic and colic veins to the lumbar veins of the posterior abdominal wall.

Figure 1

Surgical vascular shunts used in portal hypertension

Normal portal venous anatomy (A)
Selective distal splenorenal shunt (B)
Partial Sarfeh shunt (C)
Nonselective end-to-side portacaval shunt (D)

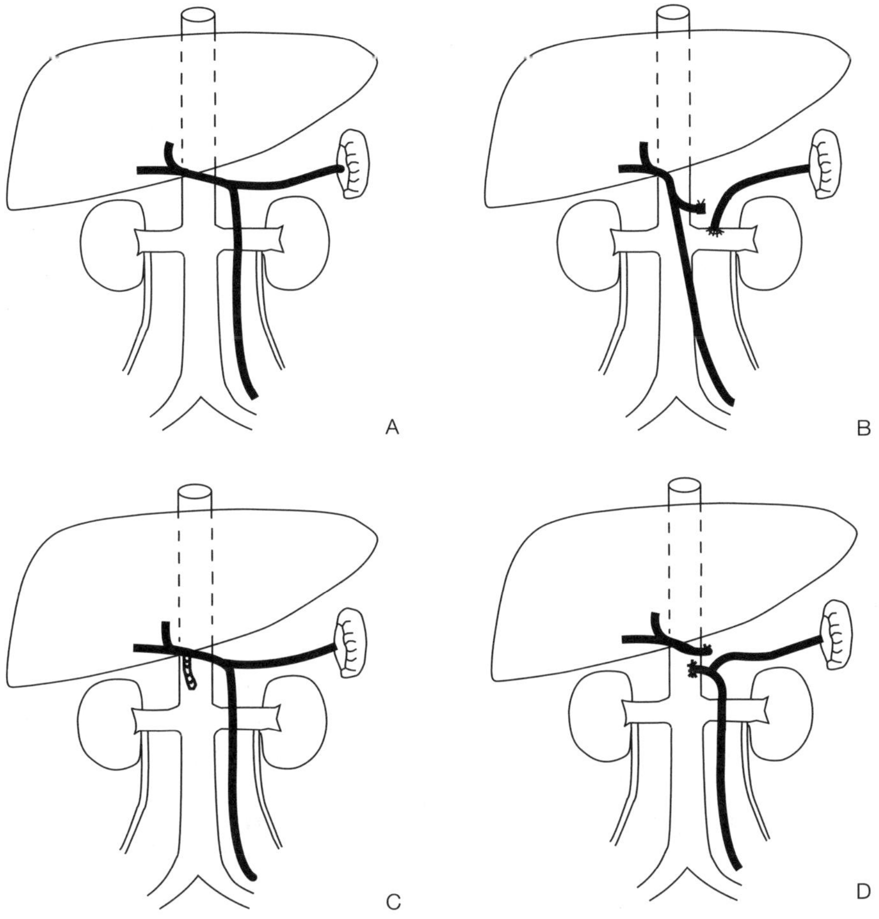

hypertension. Normal portal venous pressure is 6-8 mm Hg and portal hypertension results when portal pressure is greater than 12 mm Hg. Portal hypertension is due to an increased resistance to portal venous flow. Chronic portal hypertension results in the development of portal systemic collaterals, plasma volume expansion, increased cardiac output and splanchnic vasodilatation.

Patients with portal hypertension may present with hepatosplenomegaly, variceal bleeding, ascites or hepatic encephalopathy. Ascites is a collection of fluid within the peritoneal cavity that has low protein and cellular concentrations. Portosystemic venous shunts may arise in several regions and are summarized in Table 2. These shunts are sites of variceal bleeding due to rupture of these distended, thin-walled veins. Patients with varices are at significant risk of bleeding and over two-thirds of patients who have bled from varices will rebleed within 18 to 24 months. Mortality from acute variceal bleeding is up to 50% per occurrence.

Acute variceal bleeding is controlled by endoscopic sclerotherapy and IV vasopressin or octreotide. Currently, octreotide is preferred as vasopressin may cause intestinal and myocardial ischemia by selective vasoconstriction. For refractory bleeding, a Sengstaken-Blakemore tube may be used to tamponade bleeding as a temporizing measure. Medical treatment with nitrates and β-blockers may help prevent variceal bleeding by lowering portal venous pressure but their impact on survival in this set of patients is unclear.

Surgical treatment with decompressive shunts is the most efficacious way of stopping and preventing bleeding, but it is limited to patients who have favorable operative risk. Portal venous decompressive shunts can be divided into: 1.) nonselective portal systemic shunts and 2.) selective variceal decompressive shunts.

Nonselective portal systemic shunts divert portal venous blood flow into the systemic venous system by way of the inferior vena cava (IVC). This type of shunt includes the end-to-side portocaval shunt (Eck) and side-to-side total portocaval shunts. Due to the complete diversion of portal flow into the systemic circulation, it is an extremely effective treatment for medically refractory variceal bleeding and ascites, with the resultant high incidence of hepatic failure and encephalopathy. A third type of nonselective shunt is a transjugular intrahepatic portosystemic shunt (TIPS). Since it is performed by interventional radiology, it has almost completely replaced surgically created nonselective shunts.

Selective variceal decompression may be achieved with a distal splenorenal (Warren) shunt or a selective portocaval shunt. A distal splenorenal shunt is effective at preventing variceal hemorrhage, but it may be associated with increased ascites. A partial portal decompression may be achieved by a small diameter (8 mm) shunt between the portal vein and IVC (Sarfeh shunt).[22] Sarfeh shunts are able to control variceal bleeding with a decreased risk of encephalopathy.[23]

2. Gallbladder and Biliary Tree

Benign Gallbladder Disease

Cholelithiasis. Gallstones can be divided into cholesterol, pigmented, and mixed types. In the Western World, cholesterol gallstones make up the majority of gallstones and are associated with advanced age, obesity, female sex, and a Western diet. Pigmented and mixed stones are associated with hemolytic anemia, ileal resection, biliary stasis or infection. Most patients with gallstones are asymptomatic and should not receive surgical treatment unless there is an increased risk for gallbladder cancer. Porcelain gallbladder (calcified gallbladder walls) and gallstones in a patient with American Indian descent are significant risk factors for gallbladder cancer.

Symptomatic and uncomplicated gallstones manifest as biliary colic. Biliary colic is characterized by severe epigastric or RUQ that occurs hours after a meal. Physical exam may reveal a tender RUQ. An abdominal ultrasound will demonstrate gallstones but not gallbladder wall thickening or pericholecystic fluid. Initial treatment of biliary colic is analgesia and avoidance of fatty meals. Laparoscopic cholecystectomy may be performed for patients with uncomplicated gallstone disease if their biliary colic is recurrent despite dietary changes. Complications of cholelithiasis include acute cholecystitis, cholangitis, gallstone ileus and gallstone pancreatitis.

Acute cholecystitis. Acute cholecystitis results from gallstones that obstruct the gallbladder outflow track (gallbladder neck or cystic duct). Acute cholecystitis may result in wall inflammation, wall perforation and abdominal abscess formation. The pain that patients with acute cholecystitis experience is similar to that of biliary colic but more severe. Patients may also complain of nausea, vomiting, fevers and chills. Clinical findings may include fever, RUQ tenderness, and a Murphy's sign (inspiratory arrest upon deep palpation of the RUQ region). Laboratory studies may show a mild leukocytosis, but in severe cases such as emphysematous cholecystitis (presence of gas in the gallbladder wall) the WBC may be over 20,000 μL^{-1}. LFTs and bilirubin may also be elevated and suggests choledocholithiasis (stone in the common bile duct). Ultrasound is the imaging modality of choice to diagnose cholecystitis. The presence of gallstones, pericholecystic fluid and thickened gallbladder wall are all suggestive of acute cholecystitis. In cases where ultrasound investigation is not definitive, radionuclide cholescintigraphy can be performed (eg, HIDA scan). Initial treatment of cholecystitis includes making the patient NPO and giving IV hydration and IV antibiotics that cover enteric flora (eg, 2nd or 3rd generation cephalosporins). Early cholecystectomy is usually performed if the acute cholecystitis has been present for no more than 4 days. Delayed cholecystectomy is performed in those who have symptoms for more than 4 days or those who recover with systemic antibiotic treatment.

Acute cholangitis. Acute cholangitis is a life-threatening infection and complication of cholelithiasis. It is an ascending biliary infection that results from obstruction of the biliary tree. Choledocholithiasis is the most common cause of biliary obstruction. Cholangitis may also be caused by bile duct stricture (benign or malignant) and parasites. Charcot's triad describes the symptoms of cholangitis: fever, jaundice and RUQ pain. Toxic cholangitis can be described by Reynold's pentad: Charcot's triad plus hypotension and mental status change. Laboratory studies will reveal a prominent leukocytosis, elevated bilirubin and elevated LFTs. Ultrasound and CT scan may reveal biliary duct dilatation from the obstructing choledocholithiasis. Definitive diagnosis is performed with ERCP or PTC (percutaneous transhepatic cholangiography). Initial treatments are making the patient NPO and giving IV hydration and systemic antibiotics for enteric flora. ERCP or PTC should be able to diagnose as well as decompress the biliary tree. Later removal of the stones by ERCP or operative technique should be performed in the stabilized patient.

Gallstone ileus. Gallstone ileus is a small bowel obstruction caused by a large gallstone. The obstructing gallstone first erodes through the gallbladder into the duodenum and travels to the ileum where it usually causes obstruction. The patient presents with a small bowel obstruction and pneumobilia from the cholecystoduodenal fistula that allowed the gallstone to pass from the gallbladder to the duodenum. Treatment is surgical removal of the impacted stone. It is still controversial whether or not it is prudent to divide the cholecystoduodenal fistula.

Gallbladder Cancer. Gallbladder carcinoma is a very rare (incidence 1-15 per 100,000) disease with a poor prognosis. Five-year survival is 5% with long-term survivors limited to those with early stage disease. It is more common in females in the seventh decade of life.[24] Risk factors are related to cholelithiasis and porcelain gallbladder. The clinical presentation is non-specific, including abdominal pain, nausea and vomiting, jaundice, and weight loss, causing the delayed presentation of this disease. Ultrasound, EUS, ERCP and CT scan are useful adjuncts for diagnosis and staging of disease. Early diagnosis is usually found incidentally during routine laparoscopic cholecystectomies. Tis or T1 (confined to lamina propria) lesions can be treated successfully with simple cholecystectomies. More advanced stages of the disease may require a more radical resection, including resection of segment V and IVB with regional lymph node dissection. Treatment is resection for those without disseminated disease or biliary diversion for palliation in those with unresectable disease. Prognosis is very poor with a near 100% one=-year mortality after diagnosis.[25]

3. Pancreas

Benign Disease of the Pancreas

Acute pancreatitis. Alcohol abuse and gallstone disease are the major causes of acute pancreatitis.[6] Less common etiologies of acute pancreatitis are idiopathic, familial, drug-induced (thiazides, corticosteroids, azathioprine and tetracyclines), iatrogenic or are due to hypercalcemia, hyperlipidemia or infections. A rare cause of acute pancreatitis is a scorpion sting.[7] The patient with acute pancreatitis usually presents with epigastric pain, which may radiate to the back, and nausea and vomiting. Patients with severe pancreatitis may present with symptoms of hypovolemia because of fluid sequestration in and around the inflamed pancreas; therefore, tachycardia, orthostatic hypotension and even shock may be present.

Physical examination reveals decreased bowel sounds and epigastric tenderness. In hemorrhagic pancreatitis, blood may dissect through retroperitoneal planes and present as ecchymotic-appearing skin findings in the flank (Grey Turner's sign) or periumbilical area (Cullen's sign). Laboratory findings include a small increase in the WBC count (in noninfected cases), an extreme elevation in serum and urine amylase, and an elevation in lipase. Abdominal radiographs may show a segment of dilated small bowel or transverse colon adjacent to the pancreas called the sentinel loop. Abdominal CT scan may reveal a phlegmon (mass of inflamed tissues), pseudocyst, necrosis or abscess.

Initial treatment is supportive, including bowel rest, nasogastric suction, fluid resuscitation, electrolyte disturbance correction and oxygen supplementation. If the pancreatitis is secondary to choledocholithiasis, then ERCP can be performed to remove the obstructing biliary duct stone. Surgical management is reserved only for severe necrotizing pancreatitis.

Complications of acute pancreatitis are rare and include pseudocyst and abscess. Pseudocysts are fluid-filled structures devoid of epithelial lining that may become infected, bleed, and rupture. Intervention for pseudocysts is indicated if they are chronic (>6 weeks), large (>5 cm diameter), infected, ruptured or bleeding. Percutaneous drainage can be performed on the severely ill patient who will not tolerate a laparotomy; however, internal drainage methods such as a cystojejunostomy, cystogastrostomy and cystoduodenostomy are preferred and have better long-term results. For pancreatic abscesses, management includes intravenous antibiotics with broad spectrum coverage and drainage. Percutaneous drainage is less invasive, but if peripancreatic areas are infected, surgical debridement is necessary.

Prognosis of acute pancreatitis can be gauged by the Ranson's criteria. Ranson's initial presentation criteria include: age >55 years; blood glucose >200 mg/dL; WBC >16,000 μL^{-1}; LDH >350 IU/L, and AST >250 IU/dL. Ranson's criteria for the first 24 hours are: BUN rise >8 mg/dL; Ca^{2+} <8 mg/dL; PaO_2 <60 mm Hg; base deficit >4 mEq/L; estimated fluid sequestration >600 mL, and hematocrit fall >10%. Mortality for 0-2 criteria is 2%; for 3-4, 15%; for 5-6, 40%; and for 7-8, 100%. Necrotizing pancreatitis has a very poor prognosis.

Chronic pancreatitis. Chronic alcoholism is the main cause of chronic pancreatitis. Gallstones, hyperlipidemia, hypercalcemia and pancreatic ductal strictures are less common causes of chronic pancreatitis. Clinical manifestations of chronic pancreatitis include abdominal pain, malabsorption and diabetes mellitus. The pain is epigastric and may radiate to the back. The pain can be intermittent at first but eventually becomes constant and severe in intensity. The malabsorption and diabetes mellitus are results of pancreatic insufficiency caused by the chronic pancreatitis. Malabsorption is a sign of significant loss of exocrine pancreatic function. Steatorrhea is caused by a deficiency in pancreatic lipase secretion and results in oily bowel movements and abdominal bloating. Weight loss is common and fat-soluble vitamin deficiencies (vitamins A, D, E, and K) may also occur. Physical exam may reveal splenomegaly from splenic congestion secondary to splenic vein thrombosis. Laboratory investigation may reveal a normal amylase level, hyperglycemia and hyperbilirubinemia secondary to biliary duct obstruction. Abdominal plain film usually reveals calcification of the pancreas. ERCP is also helpful in making the diagnosis.

Complications of chronic pancreatitis include pseudocyst formation, pancreatic insufficiency, biliary obstruction duodenal obstruction and pancreatic cancer.[28,29] Obstruction of adjacent biliary ducts and duodenum arises from peripancreatic inflammation and fibrosis. Splenic vein thrombosis may also occur, leading to the formation of gastroesophageal varices and sinistral (left-sided, prehepatic) portal hypertension.

Treatment includes complete cessation of alcohol intake, insulin administration for diabetes and pancreatic enzyme supplementation with meals. Surgical drainage or resection is indicated for intractable pain. The Puestow procedure involves a Roux-en-Y with longitudinal pancreaticojejunostomy. This procedure improves pain in most patients. For patients with small ducts in which the Puestow procedure would not benefit, a pancreaticoduodenectomy (Whipple's procedure) is indicated and results are favorable in the majority of patients.[30,31,32] In select cases, total pancreatectomy with islet autotransplantation can be considered.[33]

Pancreatic Cancer

Pancreatic cancer is more commonly seen in the elderly, African Americans, males and diabetics. Smoking, a diet consisting of fried meat and fat, and previous gastrectomy are also risk factors. Most of the primary tumors arise in the head of the gland and most have ductal adenocarcinoma histology. The tumor spreads quickly to surrounding structures and metastasizes to regional lymph nodes and the liver. Distant spread occurs later in the course of the disease.

Symptoms of pancreatic cancer located in the head of the gland include weight loss, jaundice and abdominal pain. A mass palpable on physical exam usually signifies an advanced stage that is not amenable to surgical management. A palpable, nontender gallbladder in a jaundiced patient suggests an occult neoplasm obstructing the biliary tree (Courvoisier's law). On the other hand, pancreatic cancer that arises in the body or tail of the pancreas will not cause biliary obstruction and thus may only present late with weight loss and abdominal pain.

Laboratory findings include hyperbilirubinemia with biliary duct obstruction or elevated LFTs with hepatic metastases. The tumor marker CA 19-9 can be used to follow response to treatment but is usually not sensitive enough for a screening tool. Imaging is best performed with a CT scan to define the boundaries of the tumor and identify any metastatic spread. ERCP and EUS may also be useful diagnostic tools. Percutaneous biopsy is helpful in establishing the diagnosis of presumptive nonresectable pancreatic cancer. Percutaneous biopsy is contraindicated in cases where resection is plausible.

The treatment of pancreatic cancer is still limited in most cases. Surgical resection and cure is possible if the tumor has not spread locally and distantly and if there is no arterial involvement. Most patients do not meet these criteria for surgical resection. The surgical resection used for head of the pancreas lesions is pancreaticoduodenectomy (Whipple's procedure).[34] For lesions in the tail of the pancreas, surgery would involve a distal pancreatectomy. With the advent of laparoscopy, this procedure can be performed with minimally invasive techniques.[35] For the remainder of unresectable cases, palliative procedures such as cholecystojejunostomy or choledochojejunostomy are performed to relieve biliary obstruction. Chemotherapy and radiation therapy have not been shown to be efficacious in pancreatic cancer, although there are a number of ongoing clinical trials that evaluate new chemotherapeutic agents for pancreatic cancer.[36,37,38]

4. References

1. Huang C-J, Pitt HA, Lipsett PA, et al. Pyogenic hepatic abscess: changing trends over 42 years. *Ann Surg*. 1996; 223:600-609.

2. Pitt HA. Surgical management of hepatic abscesses. *World J Surg*. 1990; 498-504.

3. Frey CF, Zhu Y, Suzuki M, Isaji S. Liver abscesses. *Surg Clin North Am*.1989; 69:259-271.

4. Donovan AJ, Yellin AE, Ralls PW. Hepatic abscess. *World J Surg*.1991;15:162-169.

5. Ng FH, Wong WM, Wong BC, et al. Sequential intravenous/oral antibiotic vs. continuous intravenous antibiotic in the treatment of pyogenic liver abscess. *Aliment Pharmacol Ther*. 2002;16:1083-1090.

6. Seeto RK, Rockey DC. Amebic liver abscess: epidemiology, clinical features, and outcome. *West J Med*. 1999;170:104-109.

7. Goessling W, Chung RT. Amebic liver abscess. *Curr Treat Options Gastroenterol*. 2002;5:443-449.

8. Sayek U, Tirnaksiz MB, Dogan R. Cystic hyatid disease: current trends in diagnosis and management. *Surg Today*. 2004;34:987–996.

9. Shortell CK, Schwartz SI. Hepatic adenoma and focal nodular hyperplasia. *Surg Gynecol Obstet*. 1991;173:426-431.

10. Bioulac-Sage P, Balabaud C, Wanless IR. Diagnosis of focal nodular hyperplasia: not so easy. *Am J Surg Pathol*.2001;25:1322-1325.

11. Choi BY, Nguyen MH. The diagnosis and management of benign hepatic tumors. *J Clin Gastroenterol*. 2005;39:401–412.

12. Chapman AB, Rubinstein D, Hughes R, et al. Intracranial aneurysms in autosomal dominant polycystic kidney disease. *N Engl J Med*. 1992;327:916-920.

13. Daniele B, Bencivenga A, Megna AS, Tinessa V. Alpha-fetoprotein and ultrasonography screening for hepatocellular carcinoma. *Gastroenterology*. 2004;127(5 suppl 1): S108-S112.

14. Saab S, Yao F. Fibrolamellar hepatocellular carcinoma. Case reports and a review of the literature. *Dig Dis Sci*.1996;41:1981-1985.

15. Rocken C, Carl-McGrath S. Pathology and pathogenesis of hepatocellular carcinoma. *Dig Dis Sci*. 2001;19:269-278.

16. Chapman RW. Risk factors for biliary tract carcinogenesis. Ann Oncol. 1999;(suppl 10)4:308-311.

17. Ustundag Y, Bayraktar Y. Cholangiocarcinoma: A compact review of the literature. *World J Gastroenterol*. 2008;14:6458-6466.

18. Vogl TJ, Muller PK, Mack MG, Straub R, Engelmann K, Neuhaus P. Liver metastases: interventional therapeutic techniques and results, state of the art. *Eur Radiol*. 1999;9:675-684.

19. Sasson AR, Sigurdson ER. Surgical treatment of liver metastases. *Semin Oncol*. 2002;29:107-118.

20. Heslin MJ, Medina-Franco H, Parker M, Vickers SM, Aldrete J, Urist MM. Colorectal hepatic metastases: resection, local ablation, and hepatic artery infusion pump are associated with prolonged survival. *Arch Surg*. 2001;136:318-323.

21. Wright AS, Rikkers LF. Current management of portal hypertension. *J Gastrointest Surg*. 2005;9:992-1005.

22. Collins JC, Ong MJ, Rypins EB, Sarfeh IJ. Partial portacaval shunt for variceal hemorrhage: longitudinal analysis of effectiveness. *Arch Surg*. 1998;133:590-592.

23. Capussotti L, Vergara V, Polastri R, Marucci MM, Bouzari H, Fava C. A critical appraisal of the small-diameter portacaval H-graft. *Am J Surg*. 1995;170:10-14.

24. Lazcano-Ponce EC, Miquel JF, Munoz N, et al. Epidemiology and molecular pathology of gallbladder cancer. *CA Cancer J Clin*. 2001;51:349-364.

25. Reid KM, Ramos-De la Medina A, Donohue JH. Diagnosis and surgical management of gallbladder cancer:a review. *J Gastrointest Surg*. 2007;11:671–681.

26. Bank S, Indaram A. Causes of acute and recurrent pancreatitis. Clinical considerations and clues to diagnosis. *Gastroenterol Clin North Am*. 1999;28:571-589, viii.

27. George Angus LD, Salzman S, Fritz K, Ramirez J, Yaman M, Gintautas J. Chronic relapsing pancreatitis from a scorpion sting in Trinidad. *Ann Trop Paediatr*. 1995;15:285-289.

28. Ho HS, Frey CF. Current approach to the surgical management of chronic pancreatitis. *Gastroenterologist*. 1997;5:128-136.

29. Malka D, Hammel P, Maire F, et al. Risk of pancreatic adenocarcinoma in chronic pancreatitis. *Gut*. 2002;51:849-852.

30. Jordan PH, Jr, Pikoulis M. Operative treatment for chronic pancreatitis pain. *J Am Coll Surg*. 2001;192:498-509.

31. Sakorafas GH, Sarr MG. Changing trends in operations for chronic pancreatitis: a 22-year experience. *Eur J Surg*.2000;166:633-637.

32. Sakorafas GH, Farnell MB, Nagorney DM, Sarr MG. Surgical management of chronic pancreatitis at the Mayo Clinic. *Surg Clin North Am*. 2001;81:457-465.

33. Blondet JJ, Carlson AM, Kobayashi T, et al. The role of total pancreatectomy and islet autotransplantation for chronic pancreatitis. *Surg Clin N Am*. 2007; 87:1477–1501.

34. Lillemoe KD, Yeo CJ, Cameron JL. Pancreatic cancer: state-of-the-art care. CA Cancer J Clin. 2000;50:241-268.

35. Yamamoto M, Hayashi MS, Jones BU, et al. Laparoscopic distal pancreatectomy and splenectomy for insulinoma. Presented at: American Hepato-Pancreato-Biliary Association Congress; April 19-22, 2007; Las Vegas, NV.

36. Bramhall SR, Rosemurgy A, Brown PD, Bowry C, Buckels JA. Marimastat as first-line therapy for patients with unresectable pancreatic cancer: a randomized trial. *J Clin Oncol*. 2001;19:3447-3455.

37. Lima CM, Leong SS, Sherman CA, et al. Irinotecan and gemcitabine in patients with solid tumors: phase I trial. *Oncology*. 2002;16:19-24.

38. Yamamoto M, Imagawa DK, Katz MH. Multidisciplinary management of resectable adenocarcinoma of the pancreatic head. *Expert Review of Anticancer Therapy*. 2008;8:1611-1621.

5. Questions

1. A 78-year-old bedridden male with dementia was transferred from a nursing home with a four day history of abdominal pain and fevers. Physical exam and diagnostic evaluation revealed a perforated appendicitis for which he underwent appendectomy. Seven days postoperatively he developed a fever and abdominal pain. Physical exam reveals mild diffuse abdominal tenderness. Laboratory studies reveal a mild leukocytosis. The *least* likely diagnosis that may explain this patient's clinical and diagnostic findings is:

   A. Wound infection

   B. Urinary tract infection

   C. Pneumonia

   D. Deep venous thrombosis

   E. Intra-abdominal abscess

   F. Hepatic pyogenic abscess

2. The above patient's wound was inspected and was found to be without erythema, drainage, fluctuance or tenderness. Urinalysis revealed no WBCs and no leukocyte esterase. A chest radiograph did not show any infiltrate. There were minimal D-dimers and fibrin split products on laboratory investigation. What is the next most useful step in this patient's management?

   A. Broaden antibiotic coverage

   B. Initiate antifungal coverage

   C. Abdominal pelvis CT scan with contrast

   D. Do nothing

3. A 45-year-old obese female with a family history of "kidney disease" presents with chronic, progressive abdominal pain. Physical exam reveals hepatomegaly and right upper quadrant tenderness. Laboratory studies are significant for a WBC 12,000; sodium 138; potassium 4.3; chloride 100; BUN 30; and creatinine 1.9. Transaminases are mildly elevated. Which *one* of the following imaging studies is most appropriate for this patient:

   A. CT scan of the abdomen and pelvis with PO and IV contrast

   B. Noncontrast CT scan of the abdomen and pelvis

   C. Abdominal ultrasound

   D. Abdominal plain films

4. The above patient receives the appropriate imaging study, which reveals cysts in both the liver and kidney. Which of the following are reasonable in the clinical management of this patient:

   A. Evaluate for kidney and liver transplantation

   B. CT scan of the head

   C. Family/genetic screening

   D. None of the above

5. A 65-year-old male with chronic hepatitis C and alcoholic liver cirrhosis is referred by his primary care provider for evaluation of a 2 cm right lobe liver mass diagnosed by ultrasound. The most likely diagnosis is:

   A. Hepatic adenoma

   B. Hemangioma

   C. Metastatic cancer

D. Simple hepatic cyst

E. Hepatocellular carcinoma

6. Reasonable treatment options for this patient include:

A. Chemotherapy

B. Radiation therapy

C. Implantation of hepatic artery chemotherapy infusion pump

D. Chemoembolization

E. Liver transplantation

F. Anatomical resection

7. A 43-year-old obese female presents to the emergency room with severe nausea, vomiting and epigastric pain. This is her first episode of these symptoms, and it started after she ate dinner. Physical exam is pertinent for a temperature of 37.7 and a mildly tender abdomen in the epigastric and right upper quadrant regions. What are reasonable diagnostic studies that would aid in the management of this patient:

A. Nothing

B. WBC

C. AST, ALT, alkaline phosphatase, total bilirubin

D. Amylase

E. Right upper quadrant ultrasound

F. Contrast CT scan of the abdomen

8. The appropriate imaging study reveals a gallbladder with gallstones, no wall thickening and no pericholecystic fluid. The common bile duct is not dilated. The patient is still complaining of pain and nausea. The next steps in this patient's care should include which of the following:

A. Admit for bowel rest, IV antibiotics and cholecystectomy

B. Administration of analgesics and antiemetics

C. Diet education

D. PO trial

9. The above patient presents to the emergency room five weeks later with similar symptoms. In addition, she has fever, icterus and some right upper quadrant pain. What is the most important initial consideration in this patient?

A. Gallstone pancreatitis

B. Acute cholecystitis

C. Acute hepatitis

D. Ascending cholangitis

10. The above patient is found to be hypotensive. What immediate steps should be taken?

A. Emergent laparoscopic cholecystectomy

B. Emergent open cholecystectomy

C. Fluid resuscitation

D. Broad spectrum IV antibiotics

E. Emergent ERCP or PTC to remove common duct stone

F. Emergent cholecystostomy tube placement

Answers

1. F.
Hepatic pyogenic abscesses used to be common in the preantibiotic era. Now with the use of intravenous antibiotics the incidence of hepatic pyogenic abscesses has become minimal. Common causes of postoperative fever such as wound infection, urinary tract infection, pneumonia, atelectasis or deep venous thrombosis should be considered.

2. C.
The risk of intra-abdominal and pyogenic abscess formation is increased in perforated appendicitis. These abscesses are best diagnosed by a CT scan with contrast. In addition, percutaneous drains may be placed in these abscesses during a CT scan. Broadening antibiotic coverage or initiating antifungals are not appropriate without evaluating for the presence of intra-abdominal abscesses.

3. C.
Hepatomegaly, abdominal pain, renal insufficiency and family history make polycystic liver/kidney disease likely in this patient. Abdominal ultrasound can accurately identify liver and renal cysts. CT scan with IV contrast should be done with caution in this patient because of her renal insufficiency. A CT scan without IV contrast may be an alternative if ultrasound is not available.

4. A., B., and C.
Polycystic liver/kidney disease is an indication for kidney and/or liver transplantation. CT scan of the head is reasonable to identify individuals with intracranial aneurysms. Adult polycystic liver disease has an autosomal dominant inheritance pattern, and thus family screening is warranted.

5. E.
In the setting of hepatitis B or C and cirrhosis, a new liver mass is treated as a hepatocellular carcinoma until proven otherwise.

6. D., E., and F.
Hepatocellular carcinoma may be resected if surgically feasible and if the patient has enough remaining liver reserve. Otherwise, chemoembolization may be used to control or even shrink hepatocellular carcinoma lesions for eventual liver transplantation.

7. B., C., D., and E.
This patient has symptoms of biliary colic. Complications of cholelithiasis, such as acute cholecystitis and choledocholithiasis, must be ruled out. A right upper quadrant ultrasound can be used to diagnose cholelithiasis and rule out cholecystitis and choledocholithiasis in this patient. Laboratory studies will also aid in the diagnosis of cholecystitis, pancreatitis or bile duct obstruction.

8. B., C., and D.
Biliary colic should be treated with analgesics, antiemetics and diet restriction (complete fat avoidance). This patient should be given a PO trial before discharge from the ER to ensure ability to hydrate herself via the oral route.

9. D.
Ascending cholangitis is a complication of choledocholithiasis. This is a life-threatening infection that must be diagnosed and treated immediately.

10. C. and D.
This patient has acute cholangitis. Although ERCP and PTC will remove the obstruction causing the cholangitis, the patient should be first fluid resuscitated and started on IV antibiotics in the setting sepsis. Once hemodynamic stability is achieved, the patient should have the bile duct obstruction resolved.

Chapter 12: Benign and Malignant Diseases of the Small and Large Intestine

Russell A. Williams, MD

Contents

1. Diseases of the Small Intestine

Physiology

Water and Electrolytes

Volume of fluid entering the small bowel each day: From the pancreas: 1-2 L, clear, pH alkaline (7-8.3), containing the enzymes for digestion of protein, fat and starch. From the biliary system: 0.5-1.5 L, containing the bile salts which are reabsorbed in the last 200 cm of the ileum. From the stomach: 2.5 L (about 1 L of this is saliva). About 1 L of fluid passes from the terminal ileum into the colon and all but 200 mL are absorbed in the colon.

Bile salts participate in micelle formation and then pass through the lumen of the small bowel to the terminal ileum for reabsorption via the enterohepatic circulation. Loss of the terminal ileum (eg, in Crohn's disease, surgical resection, or with short bowel syndrome) decreases the absorption of bile salts and increases the likelihood of gallstone formation. The increased passage of bile salts into the colon may produce diarrhea.

Endocrine and ***immunologic functions*** occur in the small bowel mucosa. In particular, the mucosal cells produce regulatory peptide hormones, such as secretin, cholecystokinin, and vasoactive intestinal polypeptide. IgA antibodies originate in the plasma cells of the lamina propria. These antibody molecules protect the individual by binding with bacteria, viruses and toxins in the mucus of the intestinal lumen.

Motility of the small bowel is either segmental, mixing the food and enzymes and increasing contact with the intestinal absorptive surface, or peristaltic, moving the contents through the lumen of the small bowel. If the motility is deficient, it can result in luminal contents not passing through the nonmotile segment of small bowel, a condition known as nonmechanical bowel obstruction, present when patients are diagnosed with paralytic ileus or the much rarer condition idiopathic intestinal pseudo-obstruction.

Neoplasms of the Small Intestine

Neoplasms of the small intestine can develop in any of the cell types in each layer of the small bowel. Furthermore, the cells lining the small bowel divide with great rapidity. Yet, despite this and the large amount of small intestinal tissues with potential for neoplasia, small bowel tumors are extremely uncommon, accounting for less than 5% of all tumors in the gastrointestinal tract.

Benign Tumors of the Small Bowel[1]

Benign tumors develop in the small intestine about 10 times more frequently than their malignant counterparts. *Leiomyomas, lipomas and adenomas* are the most common benign tumors and occur with about equal frequency (15%-20%). Other less common tumors are hemangiomas, neurofibromas and fibromas. Endometriosis may also occur in the small bowel and be an unusual cause of bleeding coinciding with menstruation. Tumors such as these may all be precursors to intussusception, and in the adult patient are the commonest cause of this condition.

The leiomyoma may outgrow its blood supply, ulcerate, and expose the underlying artery, resulting in bleeding which can be massive. Hemangiomas can occur in isolation or may be multiple and part of the autosomal dominant inherited disease hereditary hemorrhagic telangiectasia (Osler-Rendu-Weber syndrome).

The benign tumors are mostly asymptomatic, but they do account for about one-quarter of bowel neoplasms that become symptomatic. The most common presentation of this type of tumor is with obstruction, which may be due to intussusception. Other benign tumors, particularly the hemangiomas and leiomyosarcomas, present with bleeding typically chronic in nature, leading to iron deficiency anemia.

These benign tumors may be diagnosed on contrast or CT studies of the small bowel, and if small bowel endoscopy is available, it will demonstrate the tumor. In patients in whom the tumor is the source of major hemorrhage, it will be seen on angiography of the mesenteric arteries and may be approximately localized to the small bowel with a radionuclide-tagged red cell scan (bleeding scan).

At operation, the segment of small bowel harboring the tumor is resected, with reanastomosis of the divided ends. A careful search of the remainder of the small bowel is always carried out, to look for other benign tumors that are known to occur in association with the symptomatic lesion.

Malignant Tumors of the Small Bowel

The most common primary malignancy of the small bowel is ***lymphoma***, which develops most often in the lymphoid-rich tissue of the ileum. The increase in non-Hodgkin's B-cell lymphoma, one manifestation of HIV infection, accounts for lymphoma now being the most common malignancy of the small bowel. In patients with celiac disease, lymphoma can develop in the proximal small bowel.

Adenocarcinoma is the next most frequent malignant tumor of the small bowel and is more likely to develop in the proximal jejunum. Crohn's disease of the small bowel increases the likelihood of development of small bowel adenocarcinoma, and in these patients the cancer develops in the terminal ileum that may have been surgically bypassed in an operation once done to treat Crohn's disease. The next most common tumor is carcinoid, and even less common are tumors of the mesenchymal tissues, particularly leiomyosarcoma.

Lymphoma developing in a segment of bowel may cause a marked thickening of the circumference of a length of intestine, and this distinctive diagnostic appearance may be seen on CT examination of the abdomen. The patient may have intestinal malabsorption, if there is extensive involvement of thesmall bowel mucosa.

The intestine is the most common site for development of extranodal lymphoma. A lymphoma that originates primarily in the small bowel will not have peripheral or mediastinal lymphadenopathy, the tumor will not spread beyond the bowel and regional lymph nodes, and there will be no tumor involvement of the liver or spleen. In addition, the white cell count will be normal and have a normal distribution.

Primary small intestinal lymphomas of the Western type arise focally and may be polypoid or ulcerated. They present with obstruction, bleeding and perforation. Operation is done to establish the diagnosis and remove the tumor if it is confined to a resectable field of the small bowel.

Adenocarcinoma is often asymptomatic, or the patient may complain of vague abdominal symptoms. Since the tumor advances to involve most of the small bowel circumference or may form a large mass in the lumen of the bowel, the diagnosis becomes easier as specific obstructive symptoms emerge. The patient loses weight and may have anemia or a positive test for blood in the stool.

At the time of operation the majority of patients with adenocarcinoma of the small bowel have lymph node metastatic spread, and this is associated with a poor prognosis. Metastatic involvement of the nodes adjacent to the superior mesenteric artery may make resection of the involved tissues unsafe. Operation resects the segment of small intestine and the involved adjacent mesentery and lymph nodes. The 5-year survival in patients who have had resection of a small bowel adenocarcinoma is 25%.

Carcinoid tumors arise from the neuroendocrine cells, known as the enterochromaffin or Kulchitsky cells in the crypts of Lieberkuhn.[2] They most commonly (about 50% of cases) develop in the appendix, with about 25% occurring in the small bowel, particularly the terminal ileum, and are multiple in about 40% of patients. The other major site of carcinoid occurrence is the rectum.

Carcinoid tumors develop in patients at a younger age than adenocarcinoma, typically between 25 and 45 years of age. The carcinoids that develop in the ileum are malignant in about one-third of cases, with a high likelihood, if over 2 cm in diameter, of having spread to the local lymph nodes and the liver. The tumors arising from the rectum and the appendix are rarely malignant. Up to 15% of patients with carcinoid tumor will have another noncarcinoid tumor elsewhere in the body, particularly the stomach, breast, colon or lung.

On gross appearance the carcinoid tumor is a yellow, firm, submucosal mass. Characteristically, the serotonin produced by the carcinoid tumor stimulates the growth of surrounding fibrous tissue, so that the bowel and the adjacent mesentery are narrowed and kinked and bound in place by the densely sclerotic tissues. Bowel obstruction is a common presentation due to fibrotic contracture and stricture of the small bowel, rather than growth of the tumor mass to occlude the lumen of the ileum. The primary carcinoid tumor is at times remarkably much smaller than the metastases that evolve from it.

The carcinoid syndrome develops with carcinoid of the small bowel only when liver metastases are present. Normally, the serotonin produced by the carcinoid tumor and released into the portal circulation is metabolized by the hepatocytes into 5-hydroxyindoleacetic acid (5-HIAA) and is excreted in the urine. With hepatic metastases, the serotonin and other vasoactive substances secreted by the tumor escape hepatic degradation and enter the systemic circulation directly. About 10% of patients with small intestinal carcinoid tumor develop the carcinoid syndrome. This syndrome can also develop in association with carcinoid tumors in the testis, ovary and bronchus, and the serotonin is secreted directly into the systemic circulation, with resultant symptoms.

The carcinoid syndrome is characterized by:

- ***Cutaneous flushing*** (about 80% of patients) mediated by the vasoactive peptides secreted by the tumor. The flushing can occur spontaneously, or may be triggered by excitement, exercise and some foods or alcohol.

- ***Diarrhea*** (about 80% of patients) is caused by the raised levels of serotonin that increase intestinal peristaltic activity and fluid secretion.

- ***Bronchospasm*** (about 25% of patients) is the result of serotonin, bradykinin and histamine elaborated by the carcinoid tumor.

- ***Right heart valve fibrosis*** (about 50% of patients) is due to fibrosis of the endocardium under stimulation from serotonin. The tricuspid and pulmonary valves become sclerotic, resulting in valvular stenosis and incompetence. The serotonin is inactivated by enzymes in the lungs, accounting for the fact that the valves in the left side of the heart are not similarly sclerosed.

Diagnosis of Carcinoid Tumors and the Carcinoid Syndrome

Barium studies and CT with contrast are useful radiological tests for demonstrating intrinsic and extrinsic masses in the small bowel. In addition, these studies may identify kinking or fixation of the loops of intestine due to the associated fibrotic reaction in carcinoid tumors. If the tumor is in a segment of the small bowel accessible by endoscopy it will be seen as a yellow submucosal mass, reminiscent of a lipoma. Biopsy will confirm its carcinoid nature.

In addition, the serotonin metabolite 5-HIAA, that is secreted in the urine in large amounts, can be measured to detect and confirm the presence of a carcinoid tumor. About half the patients with carcinoid tumors have elevated levels of 5-HIAA in their urine, regardless of whether the carcinoid syndrome has developed. If more than 20 mg of urinary 5-HIAA is excreted over 24 hours, a carcinoid tumor is present. Hepatic metastases are detected on CT scan, and can be biopsied to make the diagnosis.

The management of carcinoid tumors and the carcinoid syndrome is both operative and pharmacologic. All tumors over 1 cm in diameter are resected en bloc with the associated mesentery and lymph nodes. This is also recommended for multiple tumors. The overall 5-year survival after resection of a small intestinal carcinoid is 70%.

If unresectable metastases are found by the surgeon at the time of operation, reduction of tumor bulk has been shown to be of benefit, increasing survival and reducing symptoms. It also preempts another operation to treat the bowel obstruction that will likely develop if the primary tumor is left in place. About 20% of patients with hepatic metastases and 40% of patients with inoperable metastatic disease survive 5 years or more.

Hepatic metastases may be quite massive and replace much of the liver. Resection of localized tumor masses in the liver is recommended because this aids in the control of symptoms.

Carcinoid tumors grow very slowly, hence the practice of resecting all tumor tissue that can be safely removed, even in the face of disseminated carcinoid tumor. The median survival for patients from the time of histological diagnosis of carcinoid is about 14 years. After the onset of the carcinoid syndrome the survival is about 8 years.

Furthermore, many of the symptoms that develop in patients with carcinoid are attributable to the pronounced sclerosis that occurs in conjunction with the carcinoid tumor, and lysis of this tissue will often ameliorate the associated complaints.

Other treatments for the control of metastatic disease and the symptoms include:

- The use of serotonin antagonists to control diarrhea
- Interferon therapy for the control of flushing
- Alpha-adrenergic blocking agents to control the effect of kallikrein and reduce flushing
- Somatostatin and its analog octreotide have been most effective in controlling the carcinoid syndrome in patients whose symptoms are aggravated by exposure to stress
- Hepatic artery ligation or embolization for control of symptoms where resection of metastases is not possible
- Heart valve replacement
- Orthotopic liver transplant

Simple appendectomy and no further surgery is needed for carcinoid tumors less than 1 cm in diameter that are asymptomatic and found in the appendix on histological examination. However, if the tumor is 2 cm or more in diameter, a right hemicolectomy is recommended. Table 1 summarizes the features of gastrointestinal carcinoid tumors.

Leiomyosarcoma may occur in the smooth muscle of any segment of the small bowel, but is most often found in the jejunum. This tumor develops in the submucosa, and as it enlarges it outgrows its blood supply and ulcerates into the lumen of the small bowel. The tumor is usually large, but it bleeds rather than produces bowel obstruction, and patients usually present with melena. The bleeding can be massive as the ulcer erodes into the arterial supply of the tumor.

Metastatic tumors are more common than primary malignancies of the small bowel. The most common metastases are from melanoma and breast cancer primaries. These cause bowel obstruction and may be the presentation of the disease, the true nature of which is identified after the histology of the small bowel metastasis is elucidated.

Gastrointestinal Stromal Tumors (GIST)[17]

GIST tumors are rare, mesenchymal neoplasms (sarcomas), composed of spindle-shaped cells in 70%-80% and epithlioid type cells in 20%-30%, which account for less than 3% of gastrointestinal (GI) malignancies, but are the most common GI tract sarcoma. The majority (70%) occurs in the stomach, 20% in the small intestine and the rest in the esophagus. About one-third are malignant when diagnosed. Small tumors are usually benign but large tumors metastasized to the liver and sites within the abdomen, including the mesentery, peritoneum and omentum. GIST tumors are thought to arise from the interstitial cells of Cajal, which are the pacemakers for peristaltic function. Although the neoplasm develops because of a mutation in the c-kit gene, most cases are sporadic rather than familial.

The GIST tumor grows outward from the bowel wall and upon outstripping its blood supply, develops necrosis and ulceration. When the ulceration communicates with the intestinal lumen, gastrointestinal bleeding, the most common symptom, ensues. Small tumors will not be visible on upper GI series, but are readily recognized on upper endoscopy. Biopsy and immunochemistry identification of c-kit will provide definitive diagnosis.

Surgical excision, either by open laparotomy or laparoscopy, is the recommended treatment. Small tumors (<2 cm) are usually benign, do not require wide resection, lymph node dissection or adjuvant therapy. Large tumors (>5 cm) may disseminate or recur. The tyrosine kinase inhibitor, imatinib

Table 1

Carcinoid Tumors of the Gastrointestinal Tract

	Gastric	**Small Bowel**	**Appendiceal**	**Colonic**	**Rectal**
Classification	CAG-A[b],[a] ZE,[b] Sporadic				Glucagon peptide rather than serotonin
Incidence	<1% of gastric tumors 75% with CAG-A Women > Men	33% of small bowel tumors	Most common cancer of appendix Women > Men	<1% of colonic tumors	1%-2% of rectal tumors
Age	6th-7th decade	6th-7th decade	4th-5th decade	7th decade	6th decade
Site	Multifocal in body or fundus	Distal ileum, multicentric		66% Rt. colon, mostly cecum	
Symptoms & Signs	Abdominal pain, pernicious anemia, hypochlorhydria, hypergastrinemia	Vague abdominal symptoms, pain, obstruction	90% asymptomatic because 75% are in distal third causing no obstruction	Pain, anorexia, weight loss	50% asymptomatic; rectal bleeding, pain, constipation
Syndrome[a]		5-7% of cases	If liver metastases present	<5% of cases	Rare
Metastases	<10% of cases	Majority of patients at presentation	Rare if <2 cm 30% of ≥2 cm	66% of patients at presentation	
Site of Metastases		Nodes and/or liver	Nodes, distant, liver	Nodal or distant	Local nodes, liver; rarely lung, bone
Medical Treatment		Somatostatin analogue Interferon alpha			
Surgical Treatment	<1 cm = Endoscopy, resection >1 cm = Antrectomy Sporadic type = radical gastrectomy	Small bowel resection with associated mesentery	<2 cm = Appendectomy >2 cm = Rt. hemicolectomy	Radical colectomy	<1 cm = local excision ≥2 cm = local anterior resection, abdominoperineal resection
Prognosis and 5-Year Recurrence Rate	No deaths in treated patients; sporadic carcinoid of stomach is often fatal	65% if localized; 36% if distant metastases	94% for local disease 85% if regional metastases 34% if distant metastases	70% if local 44% if regional metastases 20% if distant metastases	81% if local disease 47% if regular metastases 18% if distant metastases

[a] *carcinoid syndrome: caused by release of hormones from tumorous neuroendocrine cells; episodic flushing, wheezing, diarrhea, right-sided valvular heart disease and failure.*

[b] *chronic atrophic gastritis type A, Zollinger-Ellison associated.*

Adapted from Kulke MH, Mayer RJ. N Engl J Med. *1999; 18:858-868.*

(Gleevec®) elicits an approximately 50% response in advanced neoplasms with unresectability (eg, invasion of the mesenteric root) or metastasis.

Meckel's Diverticulum

A Meckel's diverticulum is a congenital or true diverticulum, involving all 3 layers of the intestinal wall. It is a remnant of the vitellointestinal duct, found on the antimesenteric border of the ileum in about 2% of the population, and is situated up to 2 feet from the ileocecal junction.

The diverticulum varies greatly in size, ranging from an outpouching of the ileum with a lumen of the same diameter as the ileum, to a small finger-like attachment to the ileum with a lumen that is nearly obliterated. In some cases, the vitellointestinal duct remains patent and forms a congenital fistula between the ileum and the umbilicus. In other cases, there is a fibrous remnant of the vitellointestinal duct extending from the ileum to the anterior abdominal wall which tethers the ileal loop, and thus may predispose to volvulus of the small bowel or small bowel entrapment by the band, causing bowel obstruction. A Meckel's diverticulum commonly contains heterotopic intestinal tissue, particularly gastric mucosa with acid-secreting parietal cells.

Rare complications that may develop in a Meckel's diverticulum are:

- ***Bleeding***, due to acid production by the parietal cells. The acid causes ulceration of the ileal mucosa adjacent to the neck of the diverticulum. This is the commonest cause of massive lower gastrointestinal bleeding in children and teenaged patients. The Meckel's may be identified by a contrast enema or small bowel study. The presence of gastric mucosa is confirmed with a technetium scan that shows lower right quadrant abdominal concentration of the radionuclide as the result of the technetium being taken up by the parietal cells in the Meckel's diverticulum.

- ***Infection***, which develops similarly to appendicitis. Meckel's diverticulitis is always considered in patients operated on for the clinical diagnosis of appendicitis, but who at exploration are found to have a normal appendix.

- ***Intussusception*** with the Meckel's diverticulum, as the lead point develops when the Meckel's invaginates into the lumen of the ileum and is then propelled further along the bowel by peristalsis.

Management of the bleeding or infected Meckel's diverticulum is removal of the diverticulum. This is usually achieved by removing a short segment of the ileum bearing the diverticulum and reanastomosing the two ends of the ileum.

If a Meckel's diverticulum is found incidentally at laparotomy and is not the site of a complication it is usually not removed. Some authorities recommend removing a narrow-necked diverticulum, which is believed more likely to become the site of diverticulitis.

Short Bowel Syndrome

In the normal condition, humans have small intestinal absorptive ability far in excess of what is needed to sustain them in a healthy condition. However, the surgical treatment of some diseases, such as acute mesenteric infarction, trauma, volvulus of the midgut with gangrene, and some patients who have had repeated small bowel resection for conditions such as multiple small bowel fistulas or Crohn's disease can sustain loss of large lengths of small intestine.

Normally, a patient will survive and maintain their nutrition and body mass with 3 or more meters of small intestine. With lesser lengths this becomes more problematic, and the patient may need nutritional supplements and parenteral nutrition. With marginal absorptive capacity, he or she will almost certainly need nutritional support for a time while the remaining small bowel hypertrophies.

Patients with short bowel syndrome have diarrhea which is debilitating. This is a more marked problem in patients who have also had part or all of their entire colon resected. In addition to malabsorption of nutrients, patients with short bowel syndrome have *hypersecretion of gastric acid* and this may further damage the mucosa of the remaining small bowel. To prevent this, patients are treated with agents that block the secretion of acid by the parietal cells of the stomach. Patients with extensive loss of their ileum and an intact colon form *oxalate kidney stones*. Unabsorbed fatty acids combine with calcium, decreasing the formation of calcium oxalate, and the excess oxalate is absorbed in the colon, a condition known as enteric hyperoxaluria.

The ileocecal valve functions to prevent reflux of bacteria into the small bowel and also controls the delivery of small bowel contents to the colon. Bacterial overgrowth in the small bowel leads to enteritis and increases the diarrhea.

Surgical procedures, such as reversal of a segment of small intestine to impede passage of a coordinated peristaltic wave along the intestinal length, thus slowing intestinal transit, and construction of intestinal valves in an attempt to mimic the ileocecal valve, have not been generally adopted because they do not have a reliable outcome. Furthermore, these operations may be troublesome because they utilize or may destroy even more of the small bowel, exacerbating the original problem.

Blind Loop Syndrome

Changes in the normal flora of the small intestine can result in the blind loop syndrome, clinically characterized by malabsorption, steatorrhea and vitamin B_{12} deficiency.

The small bowel in healthy individuals contains less than 105 bacteria/mL, primarily streptococci, staphylococci, lactobacilli and fungi. Anaerobes are not present in the upper small bowel but do occur along with coliforms in the distal ileum. Patients with blind loop syndrome have a small bowel concentration of between 106 and 1011 organisms with multiple species, coliforms and anaerobes.

The bacterial population characteristics of the small bowel are in part maintained because of the acidity of the stomach. The concentration of gastric organisms increases as the pH is increased to neutral. This is changed with gastric surgery, vagotomy, atrophic gastritis and in patients on acid-reducing medications, such as H_2-receptor antagonists.

In addition, the normal aboral, peristaltic, propulsive activity of the small bowel is essential for the maintenance of normal intestinal flora, and in conditions of altered motility such as intestinal pseudo-obstruction, bacterial overgrowth may further complicate the patient's symptoms.

Blind loops are frequently created in certain operations, including the Billroth II anastomosis, gastric bypass and biliary pancreatic diversion, in the formation of some side-to-side and end-to-side anastomoses, and in diseases in which bowel strictures develop, such as radiation enteritis or Crohn's disease.

The cause of the steatorrhea is most likely deconjugation of the bile acids in the gut, resulting in their early reabsorption, lowering their concentration below the level critical for micellar formation necessary for fat digestion. Unconjugated bile salts irritate mucosal cells and impair the transport of electrolytes and water in the colon and small bowel with resultant diarrhea. Bacteria, particularly anaerobes, sequestrate the vitamin B_{12} and the intrinsic factor-cobalamin complex. Hypoalbuminemia and protein deficiency are aggravated by the intraluminal deamination of protein by bacteria in addition to diarrheal loss.

The syndrome is diagnosed by bacterial culture of the jejunal aspirate with attention focused on any increase in the variety and number of organisms, including *Bacteroides* and the coliforms. Alternately, an overgrowth of organisms can be correlated with measured changes in the concentration in the breath of substances normally absorbed intact, but that may be metabolized by abnormal bacteria in the small bowel to produce a volatile metabolite that is absorbed into the blood and exhaled in the breath.

The patient's underlying medical condition may obscure the symptoms of the blind loop syndrome, hence the importance of considering its presence in patients at risk. Their principal complaint is diarrhea and further study will reveal malabsorption.

The treatment is 2-fold: any surgical problem thought to underlie the overgrowth of the bacteria is corrected. If there is none, the patient is treated with antibiotics on a rotating schedule to lower the likelihood of resistant strains emerging.

2. Appendicitis

Appendicitis is the most common acute surgical disease of the abdomen and affects 1 in 700 members of the population. It affects men about 1.5 times more frequently than women, and patients are most often under age 30. Children under the age of 3 and adults over the age of 50 years are rarely affected.

Infection of the appendix, or *appendicitis*, is established when the appendix lumen becomes obstructed at its base, most often by a fecolith—a semisolid, inspissated, aggregation of fecal material. In some patients, the lumen is obstructed by hypertrophied lymphoid tissue, stimulated to enlarge by an intercurrent viral infection, such as measles. There is abundant bacterial flora of makeup identical to that of the adjacent colon.

The inflammation is accompanied by an outpouring of purulent fluid, with increased pressure in the lumen of the appendix and consequent venous, then arterial, obstruction of the blood supply to the appendix. Gangrene resulting from pressure necrosis then ensues at the base and in the appendix wall overlying the fecolith. Gangrene may also develop at the tip of the appendix, which is most remote from the origin of the arterial supply. The gangrenous region of the appendix ruptures, with spillage of the pus and fecal material from the lumen of the appendix into the adjacent space, which is usually walled off by the patient's omentum, or freely into the general peritoneal cavity with consequent generalized peritonitis.

If the appendicitis is not treated—a rare occurrence—the infection will invade the portal venous system with resultant portal pyemia and multiple abscess formation in the liver. In about 10% of patients, the inflammation in the appendix resolves spontaneously, an observation based on patients reporting a previous similar illness at the time they had an appendectomy. In about 4%, they had this on more than 1 occasion.

The bacterial flora of an inflamed appendix is polymicrobial, consisting mostly of anaerobic organisms, particularly *Bacteroides* species, *Escherichia coli*, and *Streptococcus*. The fluid around an inflamed appendix grows bacteria in about half of patients. *Bacteroides* is found in about 80% of cases and the likelihood of isolating organisms is greatest in patients who have perforated appendicitis. Abscesses and infection can complicate appendicitis, developing in sites remote from the appendicitis, and much more likely to appear in patients with perforation of the appendix.

The clinical manifestations of appendicitis are pain, nausea, or vomiting, abdominal tenderness and fever, which usually evolve in that sequence. Pain is a complaint in nearly 100% of patients. It starts in the peri umbilical area or epigastrium, is colicky, and after about 6 hours moves to the right lower abdominal quadrant, and is then of a constant quality. At this time, the inflammation has spread through the wall of the appendix and there is involvement of the parietal wall peritoneum, explaining the transition of symptoms from the poorly localized visceral colic to the pain of local peritonitis. The latter is accompanied by local tenderness.

Constipation is most often reported, but at times patients will have diarrhea. This is a symptom with retroileal appendicitis, in which the inflamed appendix produces local enteritis. Later in the course of appendicitis, mucoid diarrhea heralds the development of a pelvic abscess. The purulent collection adjacent to the rectum stimulates secretion of large amounts of mucus by the rectum.

With the appendix located retrocecally, it may be cushioned from the examiner's finger and the patient does not complain of tenderness. Other maneuvers performed during the physical examination disturb the posterior abdominal wall parietal peritoneum, and if it is inflamed, produce the obturator sign psoas sign and Rovsing's sign.

In some patients with a longer history of symptoms, a mass may be felt in the lower quadrant of the abdomen. In most patients this is an amassing of the omentum and inflammatory changes of tissues adjacent to the inflamed appendix. At times, however, there is also a collection of purulent material. Usually this mass is tender and not appreciated because of abdominal guarding, and only becomes evident when the abdomen is relaxed under anesthesia in preparation for appendectomy.

If the patient neglects the abscess, it will enlarge and point onto the skin of the loin, flank or the abdominal wall. At times, it enlarges down into the pelvis and will be felt on rectal examination.If the appendix has perforated, the degree and region of abdominal tenderness is dependent on the extent of peritoneal cavity involvement in the inflammation that tracks outward from the ruptured appendix.

The diagnosis of appendicitis is usually clinical. It is more accurate in men because women may have inflammatory conditions of the pelvic reproductive organs that mimic appendicitis. The appendix is found to be normal (a negative finding of appendicitis) at appendectomy in 10% and 15% of patients, respectively, for men and women. If surgery is performed less frequently, more patients will have complications of appendicitis, such as perforation or abscess formation. If the negative appendectomy rate is raised to 23%, as has been suggested, an increased number of unnecessary operations will be done, but fewer patients will have the diagnosis missed. For this to be acceptable, the mortality for a negative appendectomy must be practically zero, as is now the case.

Variations in the clinical course of appendicitis in the elderly, pregnant, and younger patient are well known. In the elderly and younger patients, the appendix is more likely to be ruptured when the patient has surgery. This is observed in about 40% and 70% of patients under 10 and over 50 years of age, respectively.

Older patients with intraabdominal sepsis are known to manifest fewer symptoms and signs, leading to delay in seeking treatment, or delay in the appreciation by the physician of the true nature of the patient's problem. In infants, the incidence of perforation is particularly high, around 85%, and this may be because children frequently cannot give a detailed history, and straining and crying make the abdominal examination particularly difficult to interpret. Often the only clue is the mother noticing that something is wrong.

Appendicitis is the most frequent extrauterine surgical complication in the pregnant woman. Pain in the tight lower quadrant is the most reliable complaint of appendicitis during pregnancy. However, this is often interpreted as change associated with the pregnancy itself or attributed to a urinary infection, which often complicates pregnancy. Fetal loss is increased with appendicitis to about 9% with simple appendicitis, and rises to 36% in patients with peritonitis.

Patients with HIV/AIDS infection have the customary presentation with appendicitis, but they will usually not have an increase in the white cell count. In some, the apparently normal white cell count found when they present with appendicitis may actually be elevated above their baseline in a patient with neutropenia. In some patients with AIDS, cytomegalovirus infection, which can cause colitis that primarily involves the right colon, can cause inflammation of the appendix. In others, the appendix can be the site of involvement with Kaposi's sarcoma.

If there is uncertainty about the diagnosis in a patient suspected of having appendicitis, they are admitted to hospital for observation for 12-24 hours. An ultrasound study may help to clarify the picture, showing a noncompressible, tender structure in the region of the abdomen. The inflamed concentric layers of the appendix wall and enlarged lumen produce a bull's-eye target appearance. The appendix is not always seen on this study, and in this situation no conclusion about the diagnosis is possible.

CT examination of the abdomen is most helpful in making the diagnosis, and this is the best study to perform when the diagnosis is in question, and it ultimately may prove to be the most efficient means to rule out appendicitis. Further, if there is an abscess identified on the study, it can be drained under radiologic guidance.

Laparoscopy is also very effective for diagnosing appendicitis, particularly in those with early symptoms. In addition, the appendix can be removed using this technique. Laparoscopy also readily allows the surgeon to diagnose other conditions within the abdomen, particularly those involving the female reproductive organs.

Acute appendicitis is treated with appendectomy. Antimicrobial agents are given in the perioperative period for simple appendicitis. With perforation, these agents are continued until the clinical evidence shows resolution of the infection.

A periappendiceal abscess is drained, usually at operation, and if the appendix can be safely removed during the same procedure, this is done. However, it frequently is very difficult, and may result in accidental enterotomies and a surgical situation requiring a much more extensive procedure, such as right hemicolectomy or a stoma formation. Prudence would dictate leaving the appendix to be removed another time, before becoming entrapped in such a dangerous course.

If an appendiceal mass is palpable and the patient is not septic, a trial of nonoperative antimicrobial therapy is recommended. During the 24-48 hours of treatment, the patient is observed for untoward changes in vital signs, and the mass is regularly palpated and its size recorded to determine progress, with the expectation it will decrease in size and the patient will not become toxic. No change or enlargement of the mass or spread of infection indicates need for operative treatment.

3. Diseases Affecting Both the Small and Large Intestine

Obstruction

Mechanical Obstruction

Definition. Total or partial physical obstruction of the lumen of the small or large bowel, resulting in failure of the intestinal contents to pass distally beyond the point of obstruction. The agent that physically obstructs the bowel may be within its lumen, in the wall of the bowel, or outside the bowel. The term ileus means bowel obstruction, and strictly used includes mechanical causes of obstruction. However, ileus in common parlance refers to paralytic or adynamic ileus or obstruction of the bowel. Table 2 summarizes the causes of mechanical bowel obstruction.

Adhesions cause about two-thirds of the episodes of small bowel obstruction, followed by hernia (about 20%) and tumor (eg, cancer of the cecum, about 15%). Adhesions are the result of previous abdominal surgery in an adult, but in children may be congenital. Adhesions are not a cause of obstruction of the large intestine, probably because the colon lumen is much larger than that of the small bowel, and is less likely to be compromised when anchored to an adjacent structure with a resultant twist, such as is caused by an adhesion.

Volvulus, or twisting of the bowel, is more likely to occur when the bowel is redundant and attached to the posterior abdominal wall with a short-based mesentery. The redundant loop twists on the mesenteric root, and it becomes a closed loop, which rapidly becomes distended and tense as secretions accumulate inside. The twist of the loop at its base occludes the blood supply to the bowel and ischemia occurs early.

Volvulus can involve the entire small bowel, especially in individuals who have an abnormal mesenteric attachment as typically occurs with intestinal malrotation. If surgical intervention is delayed, the patient with volvulus of the small bowel may be found to have gangrene of the entire midgut, requiring resection and leaving the patient with a serious permanent intestinal deficit because of short or absent small bowel.

Table 2

Causes of Small and Large Bowel Mechanical Obstruction

Intraluminal	
	Foreign body
	Bezoar
	Tumor
	Gallstone
	Intussusception
	Meconium
	Inspissated stool
Intramural	
	Tumor
	Inflammation
	Fibrosis
	Hematoma
	Intussusception
Extramural	
	Hernia
	Volvulus
	Adhesion

Volvulus can also involve the sigmoid colon and the cecum. In sigmoid volvulus, the massively distended sigmoid loop is seen filling the right side of the patient's abdomen on a plain radiograph. There is a characteristic bird's-beak appearance at the site of torsion on contrast enema. When recognized early, sigmoid volvulus may be reduced by using a sigmoidoscope or colonoscope to induce untwisting of the base of the colon. If operative intervention is needed because the bowel is thought to be ischemic, then resection with a colostomy is the procedure of choice. Cecal volvulus occurs in patients with a large, flexible, mobile cecum. In patients with cecal volvulus, the massively distended cecum fills the left upper quadrant of the abdomen. This condition requires operative correction and fixation of the cecum.

Intussusception in the young child usually begins with hypertrophied lymphoid tissue. It can be safely treated early, before bowel ischemia supervenes, with hydrostatic radiologically-guided reduction, and no resection of the bowel is needed.[3] In adults, however, the origin of the intussusception is very often a tumor of the small bowel, therefore the recommended treatment in adults is to resect the segment of the bowel involved in the intussusception, thus relieving the obstruction and removing any tumor that is present.

Patients with bowel obstruction complain of *pain, vomiting, constipation* and *abdominal distention*. The pain is colicky in nature and located in the central, periumbilical region of the abdomen in patients with small bowel (midgut) obstruction. In patients with more distal, colonic (hindgut) obstruction, the pain is lower in the abdomen, in the hypogastrium.

Vomiting occurs early, starting with the onset of the colicky pain when the small bowel is obstructed in the more proximal jejunum. This results in decompression of the obstructed segment of bowel, minimizing the distention of the abdomen that would otherwise be present. In distal obstruction, the vomiting is feculent in character. With the stasis of the obstructed bowel contents, the bacteria multiply and take on the characteristics of colonic flora, and these organisms account for the feculent nature of the vomitus.

Distention is a pronounced clinical finding in patients with the obstructing lesion located more distally in the bowel. With distal obstruction, the onset of vomiting is late, 24-48 hours after the onset of abdominal pain. Obvious swelling of the abdomen helps the physician to clinically localize the obstructing lesion to the distal bowel.

Constipation becomes obstipation (total constipation) when the contents of the bowel beyond the point of obstruction have passed and there is no further passage of flatus or feces. In the early stage of high bowel obstruction, the increased peristaltic activity both proximal and distal to the obstruction results in rapid emptying of the distal bowel and may produce a misleading impression that the bowel is not obstructed.

Bowel ischemia and *gangrene* can complicate all types of intestinal obstruction and interventions should be timed to prevent this. With volvulus, the vessels in the twist at the base supply the bowel beyond the point of torsion and are obstructed early. Ischemic necrosis of the intestinal loops or segment of bowel beyond the twist sets in early.

The onset of severe and unrelenting abdominal pain more constant than colicky in character, with complaints of pain on palpation of the abdomen out of proportion to the physical findings, are indications of ischemia, and regular and frequent examination of the patient is necessary to detect it. If symptoms of ischemia are noted early in the course of intestinal obstruction, volvulus is likely and urgent treatment is indicated. In addition, a rise in the white cell count and elevation of body temperature are other signs of ischemia. The aforementioned are all indications for immediate surgical intervention to avoid the loss of any intestine because of infarction.

Strangulation because of trapping of the mesenteric vessels is more likely in patients with a band adhesion or hernia, where the sharp fascial margins of the herniating ring, particularly the femoral ring, occlude the blood supply to the trapped bowel segment. In other cases of obstruction, dilation of the bowel and increased intraluminal pressure results in venous obstruction, and there is a slower progression to arterial obstruction and gangrene of the intestinal wall.

The diagnosis of intestinal obstruction can usually be made on the basis of the clinical history and physical examination. A plain radiograph of the abdomen shows characteristic findings confirming the diagnosis. The obstructed, dilated, gas- and fluid-filled bowel loops have the features summarized in Table 3, which details plain-film findings related to the site of obstruction and the pathological condition of the bowel.

Radiological studies using contrast medium will more precisely localize the obstruction site and can demonstrate its cause. A contrast enema using barium or Gastrografin or a CT scan with contrast will outline an obstructing tumor of the distal bowel, as well as a sigmoid or cecal volvulus, and allow for the planning of surgery and discussion with the patient on the likelihood of the need to perform a colostomy. A Gastrografin study of the upper intestinal tract will similarly diagnose cancer, intussusception or a simple stricture, or may show adhesions to be the cause of the obstruction.

The plain x-ray appearance of gallstone ileus is diagnostic. Gas outlines the biliary tree, and a mass with rims of partial calcification is often present in the right lower quadrant, lodged in the terminal ileum, and the small bowel is obstructed proximal to the region of the stone.

The management of bowel obstruction may be entirely nonsurgical, particularly in a patient who has adhesions as the cause. The treatment is simply intravenous fluids and electrolytes to replace those that are lost into the bowel. In addition, nasogastric suction decompresses the stomach and a short length of the proximal bowel and makes the patient comfortable because it prevents vomiting. However, a patient with adhesions managed in this manner must attain certain milestones within a predefined time frame in order to continue with nonsurgical management. Failure to progress on the predetermined course is usually an indication for operation.

To minimize the chance of problems with this treatment, the patient should be frequently reexamined by the same surgeon to ensure the most reliable interpretation is made of any change in the patient's status. The management regimen includes monitoring of body temperature and vital signs, supplemented with plain x-ray and blood studies to detect and correct any change in the electrolytes and to note any change in the white cell count. Vomiting and the net loss of fluid from the circulation into the bowel lumen may lead to hypovolemia and shock.

Table 3

Features of Obstructed Bowel Seen on Plain X-Ray

Pathology/Site of Obstruction	Findings on Plain X-Ray
Jejunum	Prominent mucosal folds, (valvulae connivente) traversing the width of the jejunum; upper abdominal location
Ileum	Parallel walls, producing a featureless, tube-like appearance; located in lower right abdominal quadrant
Colon	"Picture frame" appearance around the perimeter of the abdomen; haustra protruding partly across the colon lumen; stool in lumen with a competent ileocecal valve, only the colon is distended (a closed-loop type of obstruction)
Obstruction	Air-fluid levels, in step-like pattern; these are best seen when the film is taken with the patient standing and may not be seen when the patient is lying flat
Ischemia	Gas slivers, bubbles, or small gas pockets in the thickened bowel wall; gas in the portal venous system or liver; gas in the peritoneal cavity

Early evidence of this is manifested by decreased urinary output, uremia and hemoconcentration.

A change in the abdominal examination, such as increasing pain, and an alteration in the pain from colic to constant with abdominal tenderness, may indicate the presence of underlying bowel ischemia, and the need for urgent operation. An elevation in body temperature, white cell count, and pulse may accompany intestinal ischemia. If the obstruction is not resolved after a period of 24-48 hours, in the absence of any of the foregoing signs of ischemia, operation is indicated, because the process is unlikely to resolve with further nonoperative treatment. If the cause of the intestinal obstruction has been identified by preoperative studies to be primarily treatable with surgery, such as a tumor or stricture, and not adhesions, the patient is rehydrated and resuscitated and operation should be scheduled immediately.

The operation may be difficult because of the dilated bowel obscuring view and access to the peritoneal cavity, and it may also complicate closure of the surgical incision. Milking the contents into the stomach and aspirating them through the nasogastric tube is a safe method to decompress the bowel and avoids an enterotomy to aspirate the bowel contents.

Untwisting a volvulus releases the stagnant contents of the closed loop into the adjacent normal segments of bowel. The loop contents typically contain bacterial toxins, which may be absorbed into the systemic circulation and produce shock, so this should be anticipated to minimize this complication.

The obstructing lesion can be found by tracing the collapsed distal bowel back to the point it becomes dilated. The obstruction is relieved by dividing an adhesion, reducing a hernia and resection of gangrenous bowel.

The segment of bowel containing the obstructing pathology is usually resected and the small intestine reanastomosed. Anastomosis of dilated colon is not usually advised, since it is more likely to break down and lead to abscess or fistula formation. Instead, a temporary colostomy is recommended. In some patients with obstructing tumors of the distal transverse or descending colon, performing an extended intestinal resection, removing the dilated colon, and anastomosing the terminal ileum to the distal colonic segment may avoid this.

In complicated obstruction ("hostile abdomen"), in which the peritoneal cavity is obscured by multiple adhesions or disseminated peritoneal metastases, the obstruction is most expeditiously relieved by an intestinal bypass of the obstructed bowel. The operation may simply consist of anastomosis of proximal distended bowel to collapsed distal bowel, because safe dissection and localization of the obstruction is not possible, and if attempted would surely result in multiple enterotomies and postoperative fistulas.

Reoperation is delayed in patients who have bowel obstruction postoperatively, or in those with obstruction due to Crohn's disease or radiation treatment. A fibrinous adhesion causing obstruction will likely undergo postoperative natural fibrinolysis, and time should be allowed for this to take place. Patients with radiation-induced strictures often suffer from repeated bowel obstructions, operations and inadequate healing of the anastomosis with fistula formation. Crohn's disease has a well-defined management regimen, which is followed in patients believed to have an inflammatory rather than a fibrous stricture obstructing the bowel.

Paralytic Ileus

The intestine is almost always paralyzed and nonmotile after abdominal surgery, due to a neurogenic failure of intestinal contraction, preventing the contents from being propelled distally. The pathogenesis is only partially understood, but probably is related to inflammatory mediators released at the time of surgery, along with activation of inhibitory neurogenic stimuli. It also is related to the magnitude of the surgical procedure because postoperative ileus is less pronounced after laparoscopic surgical procedures than after traditional open procedures.

The bowel is dilated, but the involved segment, which may encompass the entire small bowel, does not show peristaltic activity. Nonmotility may also involve only a segment of the intestine adjacent to an area of inflammation due to diverticulitis or appendicitis. In this situation, particularly if there is a considerable length of paralyzed small bowel, the proximal bowel will dilate and show increased peristaltic activity, experienced by the patient as colic, and the segment of paralyzed bowel may act as a mechanical obstruction. The colon and the stomach may be similarly paralyzed, and the earliest region of the intestinal tract to recover is the small bowel, followed by the stomach and then the colon. Signs that activity has returned to the different regions of the gut are summarized in Table 4.

Table 4

Indications of Return of Bowel Function in the Stomach, Small Bowel and Colon

Stomach	Decreasing volume of gastric aspirate measured over a 4-hour period. If persistently high volumes of gastric fluid are aspirated after a prolonged period, the tube may be malpositioned and aspirating fluid that would otherwise pass distally. Cease aspiration for 4 hours and record the residual volume of nasogastric aspiration, or place the tube to gravity
Small Bowel	Return of bowel sounds and decreasing abdominal distention
Colon	Passage of flatus and stool

Paralytic ileus also occurs in generalized or localized peritonitis, bowel ischemia and trauma. Its course is protracted by the use of the narcotics frequently necessary for management of postoperative pain, and also by electrolyte imbalance, particularly hypokalemia. The extent of the paralysis of the bowel is related to the amount of operative trauma to which it has been subjected. For example, it would be anticipated that the entire bowel would remain paralyzed for a much longer period (up to 5-6 days) after an extended resection of the pancreas and lymph nodes to remove a tumor, but no ileus may appear after a laparoscopic cholecystectomy.

Paralytic ileus may also be a response by the bowel to an injury or to the presence of a noxious agent, and as such has survival value to the organism. Lack of motility allows the injured or anastomosed bowel to heal and regain tensile strength. Inactivity of the bowel also diminishes the spread throughout the peritoneal cavity of toxins produced by bacterial multiplication, and prevents the spread of the inflammatory response that develops with peritonitis. Paralytic ileus is treated with nasogastric suction, fluid and electrolyte replacement, and withdrawal or substitution of narcotic analgesics. In some cases, this disorder has a prolonged course and the patient may need intravenous hyperalimentation until bowel function returns. It has been a longstanding belief that the best way to prevent ileus was with a nasogastric tube into the stomach, which extracts air, thereby reducing the amount of swallowed air entering the intestines. This has been increasingly questioned, especially since the publication of a recent Cochrane systematic review based on 4194 patients from 28 studies where patients were randomly assigned to routine vs. selective or no use of a nasogastric tube.[14] Patients without a tube had a highly significant earlier return of bowel function ($P < .00001$). There were no complications reported when tubes were not used.

Patients who had postoperative ileus differ in several ways from patients without ileus: they are almost a decade older, have greater illness severity, longer operations and require more opiate medications. Mortality rate is higher in patients with postoperative illness: 3.7% compared with 2.3% for nonileus patients ($P \leq .05$). The mean length of hospital stay for patients with ileus is reported to be 10.6 days compared with 5.4 days for patients without ileus; the total cost for the treatment of patients with ileus is approximately $16,000 compared with $10,000 for patients without ileus.

Drugs in the Treatment of Postoperative Ileus

Pharmacologic agents have been used with limited success to stimulate the paralyzed bowel and prevent ileus, but this has not been widely adopted in clinical practice.

Alvimopan

Until recently, effective drug therapy to prevent or reduce the severity of ileus did not exist. Since opioids are known to increase postoperative ileus, a new agent, alvimopan, that blocks the gastrointestinal effect of opioids but does not interfere with the analgesic effect, has been studied. A total of 1594 patients randomly received either 6 or 12 mg alvimopan or placebo. Alvimopan at either dosage level significantly reduced the need for nasogastric tube insertion, decreased the frequency of postoperative ileus, shortened hospital stay, and reduced the frequency of hospital readmission. There were no adverse effects on the integrity of the intestinal anastomosis.

Cox-2 Inhibitory Drugs

Any drug that reduces the need for postoperative opioids should reduce the frequency of postoperative ileus. In a randomized trial of valdecoxib, a Cox-2 inhibitor in patients undergoing elective colorectal resection, it was found that recovery of bowel function was shorter in the treated group. This corresponded to a reduced need for opioid pain medication. Although this drug appears to be effective, it is unlikely to be used for the control of ileus, since the FDA, responding to reports of drug-related cardiovascular side effects, has asked that the agent be withdrawn from the market.

Paralytic ileus is differentiated from mechanical obstruction based on clinical and radiological findings. The patient usually does not complain of colic, has an underlying predisposing cause for the paralytic ileus, and a Gastrografin study will reveal slow transit of the contrast medium through the paralyzed bowel and no mechanical obstruction.

Intestinal Pseudo-Obstruction

Chronic intestinal pseudo-obstruction is a condition in which the patient has recurrent symptoms and signs of intestinal obstruction without detectable mechanical obstruction. It is caused by markedly abnormal intestinal motility resulting from either smooth muscle dysfunction or uncoordinated motility. Esophageal dysfunction with dysphagia, gastroparesis and colonic dysmotility may accompany the small intestinal dysmotility.

Patients present with recurrent symptoms and signs of intestinal obstruction. The severity of the dysmotility and accompanying symptoms varies among patients. In some, the episodes may be separated by long periods of time while in other patients the symptoms may be nearly continuous. Patients are malnourished and consequently have a large weight loss because of malabsorption due to intestinal bacterial overgrowth. The abdomen is distended, and at times some patients will have nausea and vomiting.

There are many causes of intestinal pseudo-obstruction, including familial visceral myopathies, collagen disease such as scleroderma and systemic lupus erythematosus, neurological diseases and pharmacological agents, and the diagnosis is made by ruling out mechanical causes. The symptoms usually appear after meals and treatment generally involves changing the eating pattern to minimize the occurrence of symptoms. To ensure adequate caloric intake, some patients need to take supplementary diet formulas. Occasionally, obstructive symptoms will require alleviation through nasogastric suction. Parenteral nutrition is required in a small subset of patients with persistent symptoms. The prognosis for the patient with generalized involvement of the small bowel is poor.

In some patients, the dysmotility is limited to a short segment of the intestine, which may be drained using a side-to-side anastomosis or resection. Megaduodenum is seen in patients with scleroderma and systemic lupus erythematosus.

Diverticular Disease

Diverticular Disease of the Small Bowel

Diverticula of the jejunum and the ileum are uncommon and are rarely the sites of disease. They are acquired or false diverticula because their walls have no well-developed outer muscular coat, and are composed only of intestinal mucosa covered by an attenuated layer representing the submucosa. The diverticula pouch out through the sites of least resistance around the circumference of the bowel wall. These sites of relative weakness in the bowel wall integrity—*the locus minoris resistentiae*—are adjacent to the blood vessels that penetrate the muscular layers of the bowel on the mesenteric aspect of the small intestine. It is not understood why these diverticula develop, but presumably it relates to an abnormality of increased intraluminal pressure in the small bowel. Localized hyperperistalsis and smooth muscle hypertrophy are seen in the intestinal wall at the sites diverticula occur, but whether these are the cause or an effect of them is not known.

Diverticula of the small intestine are most often found in the jejunum and are usually multiple, involving a contiguous length of bowel, but on rare occasions clusters of diverticula are separated by segments of normal bowel of considerable length. The diverticula are diagnosed at laparotomy or with a barium study of the upper gastrointestinal tract. They are usually wide-mouthed and the barium passes into and out of them freely. The barium study sometimes detects abnormalities of the intestinal movement that siphons the barium back and forth from the intestinal lumen into the diverticulum. This abnormal motility is called jejunal dyskinesia. In some cases the proximal jejunum is dilated with hypertrophy of its walls.

Barium may not enter the diverticula, thus they may not be seen. If the diagnosis is under serious consideration, a repeat film of the abdomen 24 hours later may show barium retained in the diverticula, a likely indicator of stagnation.

Complications Attributable to Diverticula of the Small Intestine

Small bowel obstruction, which may be mild and nonmechanical, is part of the syndrome of jejunal dyskinesia. Alternatively, the obstruction may be mechanical and require surgical treatment. Adhesions develop at the site of repeated low-grade diverticulitis. Patients with jejunal dyskinesia have been relieved of their symptoms through resection of the abnormally hypertrophied intestine bearing the diverticula.

Inflammation with perforation of the diverticulum is the next most frequent complication. The contents of the diverticulum spread into the adjacent mesentery or freely into the peritoneal cavity. Only a single diverticulum is seen to be involved in the inflammatory process when the segment of bowel containing the perforated diverticulum that has been resected is examined microscopically. Presumably the inflammation was initiated by obstruction of the drainage of the diverticulum.

Preoperatively, it will not be clear to the surgeon that the disease is in the small bowel. Patients present with peritonitis, which may be localized to the epigastrium or more generalized. Local resection of the inflamed mass of tissue and the adjacent small bowel is effective treatment. At operation it may not be apparent that the patient has diverticulosis of the small bowel, because the fat of the mesentery in which they reside obscures the diverticula.

Bleeding is another well-documented complication of diverticula, and it may be massive due to erosion into one of the arteries adjacent to the diverticulum. Many patients give a history of previous bleeding from the bowel. The bleeding diverticulum may be demonstrated on a mesenteric angiogram.

Malabsorption may be the result of jejunal diverticula becoming colonized with colonic bacteria. These organisms rapidly multiply within the stagnant confines of the small intestinal diverticula. It is thought that they either absorb or destroy ingested nutrients, especially vitamin B_{12}. Alternatively, the organisms may produce toxic materials that interfere with absorption by the mucosal cells. This better explains the malabsorption seen of materials other than vitamin B_{12}, such as fat, carbohydrate and vitamin A, which are found in large quantities in the normal diet and would not be totally assimilated by the overgrowth of bacteria in the diverticula.

The syndrome is diagnosed by radiologic demonstration of jejunal diverticula and the laboratory demonstration of malabsorption, especially of vitamin B_{12}.

Further investigation will reveal bacterial growth in the *duodenal* fluid and the return to normal of radioactive vitamin B_{12} absorption following antibiotic treatment.

Diverticular Disease of the Colon

Diverticula of the colon are common in the elderly population and many physicians accept the condition as part of the aging process. The majority of people will remain without symptoms from the diverticula.[4]

The characteristic saccular diverticula occur in 2 rows on either side of the colonic mesentery between the mesenteric and antemesenteric teniae. They may be difficult to see at operation with the naked eye, because they occur in association with the appendicae epiploicae and are obscured from view by the surrounding fat.

Colonic diverticula are generally pseudodiverticula-their walls do not contain muscle, apart from that located at the neck where the diverticulum penetrates the circular layer of colonic wall muscle. The neck is also intimately related to the colonic arterial blood vessels as they enter the colon wall, and this anatomical juxtaposition accounts for the arterial quality of bleeding that may occur as a complication of the diverticula.

Giant diverticula of the colon are occasionally demonstrated on barium enema; however, these usually represent areas of localized perforation which have been walled off, and are chronic abscess cavities rather than mucosal-lined pockets.

In Western societies, the diverticula occur predominantly in the left colon. About 65% of people will have involvement of the sigmoid colon, and only 30% will have the sigmoid and another segment, typically the descending colon, affected. Occasionally right-sided diverticula occur in association with the sigmoid diverticula and rarely (in about 5%), diverticula are found only in the right colon.

The incidence increases with age, and 30% of people over 50, 50% over 70, and 65% over 80 years of age will develop diverticulosis. Once established, the extent of colonic involvement usually does not extend to include the more proximal colon. New diverticula usually form within the same involved segment. People of Asian origin who adopt a Western diet are increasingly developing diverticulosis, typically affecting the right colon.

It is believed that abnormal motility of the colon causing increased intraluminal pressure plays a role in the development of colonic diverticula. This is very likely related to the decreased amount of nonabsorbable fiber in the current western diet. Low-fiber diets have been shown to increase the colonic intraluminal pressure, though corresponding studies on high-fiber ingestion produce variable results.

Symptoms attributable to colonic diverticulosis include intermittent lower abdominal or left iliac fossa pain, altered bowel habits including either constipation or diarrhea, abdominal bloating and the passage of clear mucus. These are all symptoms of nonspecific colonic dysfunction and may be reported in other colonic conditions such as irritable bowel syndrome.

Acute diverticulitis develops in about 10%-20% of patients with diverticular disease. These patients present with left iliac fossa abdominal pain, which is initially colicky but after some hours becomes constant and is then associated with tenderness in the abdominal left lower quadrant. Most often, the sigmoid colon is the site of involvement and clinical findings are seen in the left lower quadrant of the abdomen. However, because this part of the colon is mobile and at times resides in the right lower abdominal quadrant, sigmoid diverticulitis will occasionally present with findings on the right side of the abdomen, mimicking appendicitis. A tender mass may be present in the left lower quadrant, which contains the adjacent small bowel and the inflamed sigmoid and omentum. Occasionally this inflammatory phlegmon is in the pelvis and may be felt as an extrinsic, tender mass on rectal examination.

A significant proportion of patients with acute diverticulitis also have urinary frequency and dysuria because the phlegmon lays adjacent to the bladder, producing a sympathetic cystitis. As the inflammation advances, a series of complications ensue. These are *peridiverticular abscess*, fistulization into adjacent structures, and occasionally, generalized fecal peritonitis.

Most patients with acute diverticulitis have an elevated temperature and leukocytosis, and about one-half also have occult blood in the stool. If there is an iron deficiency anemia, however, this suggests another diagnosis, such as cecal cancer, rather than diverticulitis.

Most patients with symptoms suggesting colonic disease will be investigated with either a barium enema or colonoscopy. The barium enema gives useful information about the number and distribution of the diverticula, although it has been suggested that colonoscopy is more sensitive at diagnosing coexisting colonic neoplasia. A 35% error rate has been shown in the barium enema diagnosis of coexistent colonic neoplasia in patients with sigmoid diverticulosis. Colonic neoplasia and diverticulosis occur in the same age group, and in view of this high error rate, the authors concluded all patients with sigmoid diverticulosis shown on contrast enema should also have a colonoscopy. However, there are many other studies showing a comparable rate of diagnostic accuracy between the 2 methods for diagnosing colonic neoplasia, and the choice ultimately depends on the equipment and expertise available. Economically, the investigation of colonic dysfunction symptoms with both studies is not justified, with the exception of the patient who has a chronic stricture.

Acute diverticulitis is usually diagnosed clinically and treatment started without special investigations. The high pressures generated within the colon with properly-performed barium enema or colonoscopy may aggravate an existing colon perforation. In those who require assessment of extraluminal complications of diverticulitis, the CT scan has excellent diagnostic accuracy.

Ultrasonography may have diminished accuracy in the diagnosis of interloop abscesses and abscesses filled with gas, and will not detect underlying malignancy. Diverticulitis may be confused with acute appendicitis, inflammatory bowel disease, ischemic colitis, foreign body perforation of the colon and pseudomembranous colitis. Crohn's disease with its characteristic transmural inflammation and local complications is a special consideration because it may have findings similar to those of diverticulitis.

Inflammatory Complications

Acute diverticulitis results from perforation of a single diverticulum, and with incomplete resolution of the peridiverticulitis the walled-off inflammation will result in a peridiverticular abscess. Patients with this complication usually have a 3-4 day history of lower abdominal pain and high fever. A tender mass is often felt in the left lower quadrant of the abdomen if it is not obscured by involuntary guarding. The diagnosis is confirmed with a CT scan of the abdomen that demonstrates the abscess. An abscess should be suspected in patients treated for diverticulitis but who fail to improve after 48-72 hours.

Once identified, the abscess is drained with CT or ultrasound guidance. This permits control of the initial sepsis and a single-stage resection with anastomosis at a later date. About 75% of peridiverticular abscesses can be drained in this manner. This may fail if the abscess is multilocular and may be complicated by the formation of a fecal fistula. The latter may be an indication of underlying cancer of the sigmoid.

Fistulas form as the result of rupture of a peridiverticular abscess into an adjacent organ, such as the bladder, small bowel, vagina or the anterior abdominal wall. A colovesical fistula forms in about 2% of patients with diverticulitis. The patient complains of fecaluria or pneumaturia, and about one-third of patients develop symptoms of systemic infection. Most colovesical fistulas occur in men or in women who have had a hysterectomy. In women, the uterus normally intercedes between the bladder and the inflammation in the colon.

The colovesical fistula is diagnosed on the basis of the history. It may be demonstrated on barium enema, cystography or cystoscopy, or CT scan. However, the fistula may not appear on any of these studies. This complication is treated once the urinary sepsis is controlled with antimicrobial therapy. After adequate bowel preparation, the bowel is excised with the fistula, and a primary colonic anastomosis is done, closing the fistulous opening in the bladder, rather than resecting a part of the bladder wall. In a patient who is a poor operative risk, a diverting colostomy is done to control the urinary infection, and the sigmoid resection is performed once their health has improved.

A colovaginal fistula is a rarer complication of peridiverticular abscess, and the region of the bowel from which it originates may be demonstrated with a barium enema or a vaginogram. This fistula requires surgical correction and the procedure is usually done in one stage. Again, if the patient is frail, a diverting colostomy will alleviate the symptoms.

Fistulas occasionally develop between the colon and small bowel and bacterial overgrowth in the small bowel will produce marked diarrhea. This will also exclude a length of the small bowel, and if of considerable length, this exclusion will produce malabsorption and the blind loop syndrome.

Colocutaneous fistula is a rare spontaneous complication that most often follows a surgical procedure or abscess drainage.

Free perforation is particularly likely when there is a large perforation of the colon or of a peridiverticular abscess. The patient has florid, fecal peritonitis, and initially complains of lower abdominal pain and the desire to urinate; this is quickly followed by severe generalized abdominal pain and septic shock. The treatment is resuscitation and operation to resect the perforated colon and clean the peritoneal cavity. A colostomy is done rather than a primary anastomosis.

Diverticular stricture, small bowel obstruction, and ureteric obstruction may all require operation for correction, particularly if the result of inflammatory fibrosis. External compression due to peridiverticular inflammation will regress when the inflammation resolves.

About 15%-20% of patients with diverticula will have at least one episode of rectal bleeding, and about 5% will bleed massively and require transfusion. The hemorrhage is characteristically of sudden onset, brisk and arterial. Despite the fact that diverticula are predominantly on the left side of the colon, the bleeding is usually from the colon proximal to the splenic flexure and originates from a single diverticulum. The bleeding often stops spontaneously, but about one-quarter of the patients will rebleed. Those who do so will require aggressive investigation and treatment based on the localization of the bleeding point.

The majority of episodes of acute diverticulitis are mild or moderate in severity and respond to conservative medical treatment. Antimicrobials are administered to control the overgrowth of colonic aerobic and anaerobic flora. Recovery should be clearly in progress after 48-72 hours. Operation is indicated in patients who fail conservative treatment, after recurrent (2 attacks) of diverticulitis, and if malignancy cannot be excluded.

In the recent past, nonresolving diverticulitis was treated surgically with a 3-stage procedure. Today there is increased use of a 1-stage or at most 2-stage procedure, depending on the degree of inflammation at the site of the original operation. Fecal or generalized peritonitis dictates the need for a protecting colostomy (two-staged) to minimize complications of anastomosis healing and reduce mortality. Most surgeons excise the inflamed colon at the first operation rather than leave a site of ongoing infection in the abdomen.

The majority of patients will only have 1 attack of acute diverticulitis. About one-quarter, however, will have a second episode, and it is these patients who are considered for operation. The colon resection in these patients is done in one stage. Colonic resection is generally not recommended for refractory symptomatic diverticulosis. In patients under 40 years of age, acute diverticulitis is a more aggressive disease than in older age groups. Over two-thirds of patients under age 40 with acute diverticulitis may require operation early because of persistent symptoms after 72 hours of treatment.

It has been reported that over half the patients under 40 years of age who were medically managed after their first presentation were readmitted with symptoms within about 2 years, and a significant proportion had serious complications. Because of these findings, there is now a consensus among surgeons that colonic resection after resolution of the first attack of acute diverticulitis is the best management of the patient under age 40.

Fistulas

A ***fistula*** is an abnormal communication between 2 epithelial surfaces, and can form at any site in the intestinal tract. The most common type of fistula develops between the bowel and the skin—an enterocutaneous fistula or a colocutaneous fistula—and the majority of these are a complication of an abdominal or bowel operation. A *postoperative fistula* is more likely to be a complication of an operation in which there are extensive adhesions, or may appear if the bowel itself is diseased (eg, Crohn's disease or radiation enteritis), compromising its normal healing.

Fistulas may also form spontaneously, and these are usually the result of a localized abscess that may have developed following the perforation of a diseased segment of bowel or another abdominal organ, such as the gallbladder, bile duct or urinary tract. The abscess is walled off from the peritoneal cavity by fibrous tissue and it erodes into an adjacent structure, such as the bladder, vagina, uterus, another segment of small bowel, the colon or onto the skin. The result is that the 2 parts of the anatomy communicate and the bowel or other organ may discharge contents to the other structure, with varying consequences. The fistula may form between the end or the side of the bowel and the location of output of the fistula will vary greatly. The larger the diameter of the communicating track, the greater the output. Fistulas that discharge more than 500 mL/day are known as *high-output fistulas*, and they pose serious problems with management if they discharge onto the patient's skin.[5]

The loss of the bowel contents through the fistula may have a wide range of consequences, depending on the make-up of the material and its volume. If the fistula is from the proximal small bowel, it has the potential to discharge high volumes, perhaps liters of fluid daily. This fluid contains electrolytes, acid, bile, activated digestive enzymes and nutrients ingested by the patient. The result is the patient will very rapidly become hypovolemic and develop marked abnormalities of electrolytes, and will become severely malnourished. If the enzyme-rich fistula fluid makes contact with the patient's skin, it causes a very pronounced chemical irritation that interferes with healing. With more distal bowel fistulas, the volume of fluid lost is much lower and its composition is more fecal in character. These fistulas are much less of a problem in terms of development of fluid and electrolyte abnormalities and malnutrition.[6]

The following factors have an influence on the likelihood of a fistula healing:

- *The segment of bowel in which the fistula develops*: a fistula from the proximal small bowel or an end fistula, in contrast to a lateral or side fistula, usually results in much greater losses of nutrients and fluids, and if untreated the malnutrition results in greatly compromised healing of the bowel and fistula track. A colocutaneous fistula will heal spontaneously with predictable regularity, unlike a fistula from the jejunum to the skin. With the latter the patient requires intensive nursing care and parenteral or elemental nutrition, depending on the output volume of the fistula. In a colonic or fecal fistula, less nursing care is required and the patient usually continues to eat a normal diet, which has little influence on the output of the fistula.

- *The disease that underlies the development of the fistula*: otherwise healthy bowel can be expected to heal, provided the nutrition of the patient is maintained. If the bowel is the site of an unusual infection, such as tuberculosis or actinomycosis, or is the site of unusual inflammation, such as that caused by radiation enteritis, Crohn's disease or a malignancy, the fistula is extremely unlikely to heal.

- *The presence of a foreign body adjacent to the bowel or in the fistula track*: the best example of a foreign body is a drain tube placed by the surgeon at operation. It may occasionally erode into the bowel anastomosis. If a fistula arises in the presence of a drain, the drain should be partially removed to disengage it from contact with the anastomosis. On rare occasions, an unsuspected foreign body such as a swab or laparotomy sponge will cause fistula formation. This is easily seen on imaging and should always be excluded as a cause for fistula.

- *The length of the fistula track*: short tracks between the bowel and the skin or an adjacent organ are lined with epithelium, which prevents fibrosis and closure of the track. An example is a bowel stoma, such as a colostomy, in which the skin and the bowel epithelium are directly anastomosed so the stoma remains patent. A fistula between the vagina and the rectum, or a fistula between the colon or the bladder and an adherent segment of bowel typically has a very short track that is epithelialized, accounting for persistence of these fistulas.

- *The presence of obstruction in the bowel distal to the fistula*: this is an obvious explanation for persistence of a fistula. The bowel contents discharge through the path of least resistance, a pattern that continues until the distal obstruction is removed. Radiologic studies are obtained to examine the bowel beyond the fistula, and may include barium enema or upper gastrointestinal contrast imaging, or a study obtained through the fistula itself (a fistulagram). Contrast agent is injected through the fistula, allowing visualization of the state of the bowel and any distal obstruction. A barium enema is routinely obtained to exclude distal obstruction before the closure of a stoma. If distal obstruction is present and not corrected before closing the stoma, the repair of the bowel wall breaks down and forms a persistent fistula.

Management of a Bowel Fistula[7]

Maintain the nutrition of the patient to facilitate healing. The ideal means for the patient to obtain adequate nutrition is for them to continue eating; however, this may only be an option with distally situated fistulas with a low output that can be captured in a dressing or a stoma appliance. Feeding the patient an elemental diet or providing nutrition with total parenteral nutrition may reduce the output through the fistula and be the only means to provide adequate calories and nutrients.

Prevent damage to the skin adjacent to the fistula. This requires expert management, usually with the assistance of a stomal therapist. If the output cannot be captured in a dressing, a stomal appliance attached to the abdominal skin around the margins of the fistula can usually be fashioned to protect the skin from injury by the chemicals in the fistula fluid.

Control any infection in the region of the fistula. This is particularly important if an abscess has formed. Drainage is often possible using radiologic guidance. At times when percutaneous drainage is not possible, an operation is needed, particularly with recurrent abscess formation.

Study the fistula to exclude reasons for its persistence. These are outlined in the foregoing section and they may be scrutinized using radiological, histological and microbiological studies.

Operation to close the fistula. This is done once it is established that the fistula is unlikely to heal. Surgery may be performed after a 4-6 week course of the treatment outlined above. Fistula closure is a semi-elective operation, and proper preoperative patient care will ensure he or she is in a good state of nutrition and fluid balance.

Fistulas that have formed high in the small bowel are more likely to require operative closure than those located more distally. A fistula with a short track, such as a colovaginal or enterovesical fistula, needs surgery for correction, because it will not heal spontaneously. This should be acknowledged early in its course to avoid unnecessary and futile treatment and delay.

Vascular Diseases

Acute and chronic visceral ischemia are manifestations of peripheral vascular disease, although they do not occur with the great frequency of ischemic disease in the heart, brain or legs. The specific ischemic disorders of the intestine are acute mesenteric ischemia, ischemic colon disease, chronic mesenteric ischemia, mesenteric venous occlusion, the celiac axis syndrome and portal or mesenteric venous thrombosis. The most common are acute mesenteric ischemia and ischemic colon disease; chronic mesenteric ischemia and portal venous thrombosis are rare.[8]

Acute mesenteric ischemia evolves in the region of supply of the superior mesenteric artery. The potentially abundant collaterals between the midgut and the fore- and hindgut are not sufficiently developed to prevent infarction of the bowel in the face of an acute reduction in blood flow from the superior mesenteric artery. The disorder results from low flow or occlusion in the superior mesenteric artery. Patients who develop low flow do so after an episode of hemodynamic instability that produces shock. The shock has usually been treated adequately at the time the intestinal ischemia manifests itself. Myocardial infarction, severe heart failure, cardiac arrhythmias or sepsis are common antecedents of the shock and low flow in the mesenteric circulation. Improvement in cardiac function and repletion of the intravascular volume does not always reverse the vasospasm. The longer the tissues of the gut have been ischemic, the lower the likelihood of correction of a hemodynamic abnormality and improved blood flow in the intestinal circulation. After an unknown period the vasospasm is irreversible. At an early point in the progression of the disease, it may be possible to restore normal hemodynamics through the infusion of vasodilators such as papaverine, and this treatment may be useful to clinically overcome what would otherwise be persistent mesenteric vasoconstriction.

Occlusive acute mesenteric ischemia follows thrombosis, which is preceded by formation of atherosclerotic plaques that frequently develop at the origin of the superior mesenteric artery. Thus thrombotic occlusion is followed by extensive bowel ischemia. Emboli lodge more distally in the superior mesenteric arterial tree at narrowed branch points and produce less extensive ischemia the further distally they occlude.

In its purest form, where there is no atherosclerotic disease in the celiac and inferior mesenteric arteries, gangrene is limited to the midgut, involving the small bowel from several inches beyond the duodenojejunal flexure to a point on the transverse colon which may be on either side of the middle colic artery. Such extensive loss of bowel leaves the patient with a serious lifetime intestinal deficit.

The typical patient with acute mesenteric ischemia is elderly and often hospitalized with cardiac disease or other conditions predisposing to hemodynamic instability. The patient develops sudden, severe abdominal pain at the time of onset of the acute ischemia. The pain is constant and usually in the center of the abdomen. Palpation by the surgeon surprisingly reveals a lack of physical signs such as guarding accompanying the patient's complaint of unrelenting intense abdominal pain. This marked disparity between the abdominal physical examination findings and the patient's complaints of pain is the best and only clinical indication of early intestinal ischemia. Unfortunately, this syndrome may be ignored and the complaints dismissed, missing the opportunity for early diagnosis and cure of the disease. At this time the ischemia is limited to the intestinal mucosa, but after 24 hours or more it progresses to become transmural, and at that time the customary finding of peritonitis is detected. Unfortunately, the only effective treatment at this stage is resection of the gangrenous bowel.

Initial plain radiographs of the abdomen are usually normal. However, if they can be compared with films of the abdomen taken when the intestinal blood flow was normal, the gas in the ischemic bowel will appear to be reduced. The acutely ischemic bowel goes into spasm and expels its gaseous contents. With the progression of the ischemia to full-thickness necrosis, bacteria multiply in the tissues of the bowel wall and invade the portal vein, establishing infection in the parenchyma of the liver. Gas is seen in the intestinal wall dissecting linearly between its layers on plain film or CT of the abdomen. With advancing septicemia, bowel organisms may be grown from cultures of the peripheral blood.

Angiography shows whether the patient has occlusive intestinal ischemia and may differentiate embolus from thrombosis. Definitive operative treatment is likely to salvage these patients early in the disease's course. Alternatively, thrombolytic therapy may be considered, but this may waste vital time and should it fail to remove the occlusion, it will increase the likelihood of gut necrosis. If the angiogram shows nonocclusive acute mesenteric ischemia, the angiogram catheter is left in the mesenteric artery and can be used for infusion of papaverine.

At operation, the surgeon must decide on the location of the transition point between ischemic and viable bowel; this can be of critical importance in cases where there is a massive amount of infarcted bowel, and each centimeter preserved becomes significant. In patients in whom there is uncertainty it is wise to use a second-look procedure, reexamining the bowel 24-48 hours following the initial operation. Sometimes, however, the patient is dramatically improved when reassessed postoperatively and the decision to reoperate may wrongly be deferred. Any remaining portion of ischemic bowel will not produce symptoms early, but will manifest its presence a week or more later, when it perforates and there is resultant peritonitis.

Ischemic colon disease produces an entire range of tissue damage, from disease limited to the mucosa to that involving the full thickness of the colon wall. Colonic ischemia characteristically involves a short segment of the colon rather than the entire hindgut, and very often it affects the splenic flexure or descending colon. Ischemia may develop in all segments of the colon, including the rectum.

Ischemia of the colon follows arterial occlusion or low blood flow. Of interest to the vascular surgeon is colon ischemia that follows ligation of the inferior mesenteric artery at the time of aortic aneurysm or colon resection. With ligation, full thickness, rather than mucosal, ischemia follows. At operation, attention should be paid to the back flow in the divided inferior mesenteric artery, or its stump pressure can be measured to determine if it should be reimplanted. Low flow ischemia of the colon may occur after any of the previously described antecedent conditions that produce hemodynamic instability and shock.

Patients with ischemia of the colon usually complain of sudden severe left-sided abdominal pain, and they often report the onset of dark, bloody diarrhea coincident with the pain, but the bleeding is usually not excessive. There is tenderness and guarding in the left lower quadrant of the abdomen. Definite signs of peritonitis are noted if the colon is infarcted, but these are less pronounced if the ischemia is limited to the mucosa and submucosa. This condition needs to be distinguished from Crohn's disease and ulcerative colitis.

The ischemic mucosa can be seen on colonoscopy or sigmoidoscopy. It appears as black to maroon-colored hemorrhagic blebs that progress to ulceration before healing. Results of stool cultures are negative. A contrast enema shows the characteristic thumbprint-like appearance of ischemic colitis. A repeat of this study 1 week later will show marked resolution of this appearance, an event considered to be confirmation of the diagnosis. In some patients, the ischemic segment of colon will heal with stricture formation.

Abdominal angina is the well-known term describing the pain occurring after meals in patients who have chronic mesenteric ischemia. In about half the patients who present with intestinal angina, this complaint is an antecedent to acute mesenteric ischemia.

Although the presence of atherosclerosis is almost universal in the older patient, it is uncommonly associated with intestinal angina. With the evolution of chronic obstruction of the mesenteric vessels, there is an accompanying hypertrophy of the normal and other collateral vessels, such as the meandering artery of Riolan, to compensate for the decrease in blood flow. A plaque adjacent to their origin in the aorta nearly always partially or totally occludes the major vessels, and there is nearly always advanced disease in the aorta. However, it is difficult to correlate the degree of atherosclerosis with the development of intestinal angina, due to the variable development of collaterals.

In order to make the diagnosis of chronic intestinal ischemia, all 3 intestinal vessels must be involved with significant atherosclerosis, and 1 of the 3 must be occluded, accompanied by severe atherosclerotic narrowing of 1 or both of the other remaining arteries. The celiac axis is most often occluded and the superior mesenteric artery is usually most markedly narrowed by atherosclerosis.

The chief complaint is pain following meals, beginning within 15 minutes to 1 hour of eating, and rising to a plateau over the succeeding several hours. Patients may develop a fear of eating and lose a large amount of weight, and may appear as if they have a malignancy. In some cases, the tips of the intestinal villi necrose, and the patient develops malabsorption and steatorrhea or a motility disorder of the intestine.

Chronic intestinal ischemia is confirmed with an angiogram showing the previously described extent and location of atherosclerosis. Markedly enlarged collateral vessels such as those seen connecting the celiac axis and the superior mesenteric artery are an indication of chronic intestinal ischemia. Patients must also be investigated for more common causes of these gastrointestinal symptoms, particularly a neoplasm. The diagnosis of chronic intestinal ischemia is one of exclusion.

Simple mesenteric bypass or transaortic thromboendarterectomy are done to treat chronic mesenteric ischemia. The bypass is usually constructed between the superior mesenteric artery and the aorta or the iliac arteries. Some 70% of patients treated for symptoms of chronic mesenteric ischemia have relief following revascularization. This likely also protects the patient from the future development of acute intestinal ischemia.

Mesenteric venous thrombosis usually occurs spontaneously. However, in some patients it may be associated with underlying abnormalities, such as hypercoaguable states; or in some patients there may be restriction of the outflow of the mesenteric venous system at the portal vein by a lesion such as a pancreatic neoplasm. The extent of ischemic damage that follows mesenteric venous occlusion depends on how widely the thrombosis has spread through the intestinal veins.

Patients with mesenteric venous thrombosis complain of poorly localized abdominal discomfort, loss of appetite and a change in bowel habits, usually with bloody diarrhea. With venous obstruction, the intestinal wall becomes thickened and edematous, accompanied by the formation of ascites, so abdominal swelling is seen. The disease may evolve over a week or more as the clot propagates throughout the venous ramifications.

The venous phase of the mesenteric angiogram or CT with contrast shows the clot in the portal, splenic, and larger mesenteric veins. Treatment includes observation with the expectation of resolution with opening of alternate venous pathways in the abdomen, thrombolytic therapy and, rarely, operation to resect gangrenous bowel.

The celiac axis compression syndrome presents in patients younger than the typical patient with atherosclerotic disease. Patients are usually women, and the diagnosis is made after exclusion of more common abdominal conditions. Often the patient has had surgery to remove their appendix, uterus and ovaries, or gallbladder, and the symptoms persist.

Compression of the celiac axis is found as an isolated abnormality of the visceral arteries, and could be the result of entrapment by the fibers of the celiac ganglion or within the fibers of the median arcuate ligament. A bruit is commonly heard in the upper abdomen.

Operation to treat celiac axis compression syndrome involves division of the median arcuate ligament together with ganglionectomy if there is neural compression of the celiac axis. Some patients who are treated with operation have permanent resolution of their symptoms, but many do not. The ability of the mesenteric circulation to compensate for reduced blood flow in one or another region through function of collateral vessels makes it seem unlikely that the syndrome has a vascular origin.

4. Diseases of the Large Intestine

Physiology

The colon absorbs water and electrolytes, but this function is not essential for maintenance of health, because patients without a colon may live a normal life. The colon receives about 1-2 L of fluid from the ileum daily and all but about 200 mL of the water contained therein is absorbed. The absorption is greater in the right than in the left colon. Short chain fatty acids are the end product of bacterial metabolism of starch, and these are required for the maintenance of healthy colon mucosa.

Malignant Tumors of the Colon

Colorectal cancer is now the third most common cancer affecting males (after lung and prostate) and females (after lung and breast) in the United States, according to the Centers for Disease Control. Overall, colorectal cancer is the second most common malignancy after lung cancer in the developed world, and this very likely relates to the increased amount of calories and fat in the Western diet. The cancer is usually solitary, although in about 5% of patients with a tumor in their colon, a second cancer is also present, hence preoperative investigation with colonoscopy or barium enema is needed to examine the entire length of the colon.[9]

There are nearly 150,000 new cases of colorectal cancer diagnosed in the United States each year, and of these cases, approximately 30% originate in the rectum.

Although most patients will require surgery, additional drug therapy along with radiotherapy is often beneficial. Over the past 25 years, survival from colorectal cancer has improved for all patients groups, probably because of earlier diagnosis and better therapy.

The factors that increase the likelihood of developing cancer of the colon are:

- ***Previous cancer:*** those patients who have had a cancer are more likely to develop a second cancer, and these appear in up to one-third of patients who are followed for 40 years.

- ***Genetic predisposition (Hereditary polyposis syndromes)***

Figure 1

5-year relative survival (all ages) from colorectal cancer in the United States during various time periods

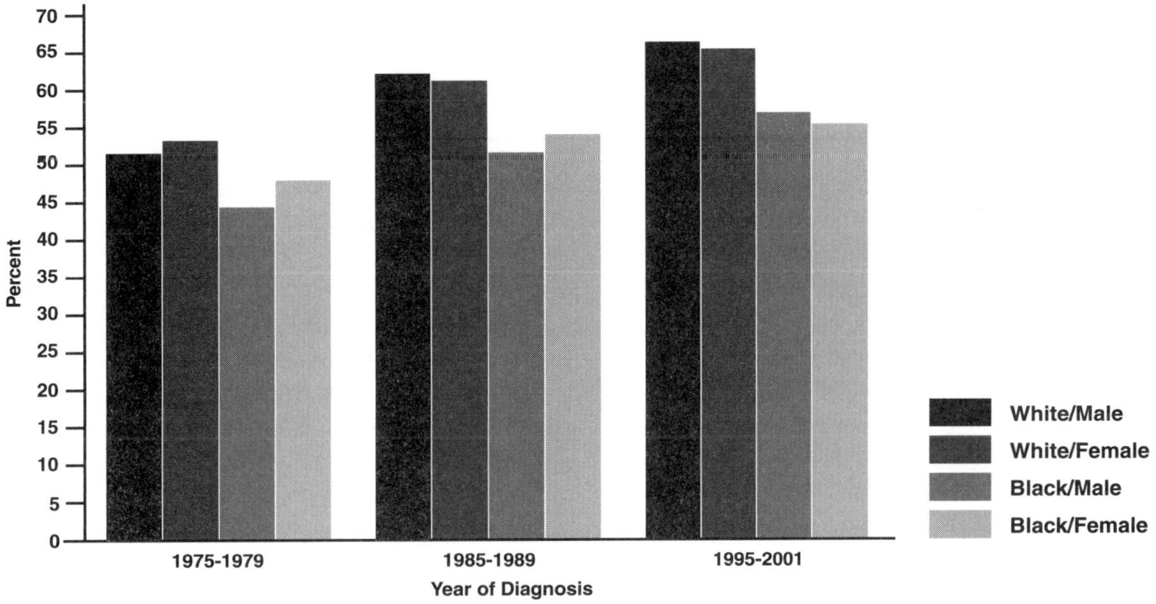

Ries LA, Eisner MP, Kosary CL, et al, eds. SEER Cancer Statistics Review, 1975-2002. *Bethesda, MD: National Cancer Institute; 2005.*

Hereditary Nonpolyposis Colorectal Cancer (HNPCC)

(HNPCC-Lynch Syndrome) is the commonest form of inherited colorectal cancer. This syndrome is an autosomal dominant disease, with a population incidence of approximately 1:1000, and is responsible for up to 5% of all cases of colorectal cancer. Patients with HNPCC have up to an 80% lifetime risk of developing colorectal cancer, and a 60% lifetime risk of developing endometrial carcinoma. Affected individuals are also at an increased risk for other cancers, such as stomach, ovarian, small bowel, biliary and kidney cancers.

In contrast to familial adenomatous polyposis, patients with HNPCC develop adenomas at a normal rate but progress more rapidly through the stages of carcinogenesis. Relative to sporadic colorectal cancer, adenomas and carcinomas in HNPCC occur predominantly in the proximal colon due to an increased rate of transformation.

Diagnosis of HNPCC is primarily based on clinical criteria. The Amsterdam Criteria were the first diagnostic guidelines to be developed, but they can only identify approximately 60% of the patients with HNPCC. The latter led to the development of the revised criteria (Amsterdam II Criteria, which take into consideration the presence of extracolonic cancer and have a sensitivity of detection of approximately 80%). New guidelines (The Bethesda Guidelines) were also developed to aid in the decision process regarding whether patients who do not fulfill Amsterdam Criteria should undergo gene testing for HNPCC, and this further increased the sensitivity of detection to 94%.

The pathogenesis of HNPCC is typified by the presence of widespread alterations in short, repeated DNA sequences in tumor cells—a phenomenon called microsatellite instability (MSI). This indicates that numerous replication errors occur during the formation of tumors. Indeed, subsequent genetic analysis identified their existence in HNPCC as a group of Tumor Suppressor Genes that encode proteins involved in repairing mismatched DNA sequences (MMR genes). The genes identified to date include *MSH2*, *MLH1*, *PMS2*, *MSH6* and *PMS1*. Among these, approximately 85% of the mutations involve *MSH2* and *MLH1*.

An important consequence of mutations in the MMR genes is the subsequent inactivation of other genes due to the presence of microsatellite sequences in their coding regions. Some of these targeted genes are involved in important aspects of regulation of cell proliferation. Examples include the type II receptor for transforming growth factor beta; the type II receptor for the insulin-like growth factor 2; and BAX, which is involved in the control of apoptosis. Inactivation of these genes leads to derangement of cell proliferation and subsequent tumor formation.

Routine molecular screening for Lynch syndrome, or hereditary nonpolyposis colorectal cancer, is possible and useful in patients with colorectal adenocarcinoma, according to the results of a study. Germ-line mutations in the mismatch-repair genes *MLH1*, *MSH2*, *MSH6* and *PMS2* lead to the development of the Lynch syndrome (hereditary nonpolyposis colorectal cancer), conferring a strong susceptibility to cancer.

Because genotyping analysis in screening for Lynch syndrome is expensive and not always conclusive, this method was compared with screening for tumor microsatellite instability among a cohort of patients with colon cancer.

Of the 1066 participants with a new diagnosis of colorectal adenocarcinoma, 208 (19.5%) had microsatellite instability, and 23 (2.2%) had a mutation causing Lynch syndrome. Of these 23 probands with Lynch syndrome, 10 were older than 50 years, and 5 met neither the Amsterdam criteria nor the Bethesda guidelines for the diagnosis of hereditary nonpolyposis colorectal cancer, including age and family history as markers to identify patients at high risk for Lynch syndrome.

Routine molecular screening of patients with colorectal adenocarcinoma for the Lynch syndrome identified mutations in patients and their family members that otherwise would not have been detected. These data suggest that the effectiveness of screening with immunohistochemical analysis of the mismatch-repair proteins would be similar to that of the more complex strategy of genotyping for microsatellite instability.

Whether insurers will be persuaded that the screening using this technique is cost effective remains to be seen.

Familial Adenomatous Polyposis (FAP)

FAP is an autosomal dominant disorder in which patients typically develop colorectal cancer in early adult life, secondary to extensive adenomatous polyp formation in the colon. Polyps also develop in the upper gastrointestinal tract, and malignancies may occur in other sites, including the brain and the thyroid.

A phenotypic variant of FAP—the Gardner syndrome—is characterized by colonic polyposis with extraintestinal tumors, especially osteomas, and a rather characteristic retinal lesion known as congenital hypertrophy of the retinal pigment. The onset of polyposis in affected individuals often coincides with puberty, and untreated patients invariably develop colorectal cancer, with a median age at diagnosis of 40 years. Prophylactic colectomy is the treatment of choice once colonic polyposis is manifested.

The Hamartomatous Polyposis Syndromes

Hamartoma refers to an excessive but focal overgrowth of cells and tissues native to the organ in which it occurs. Although the cellular elements are mature and identical to those found in the remainder of the organ, they do not reproduce the normal architecture of the surrounding tissue. In the intestinal tract, several discrete familial syndromes characterized by multiple hamartomatous polyps have been described—these include the Peutz-Jeghers syndrome, juvenile polyposis syndrome and related syndromes, such as Cowden's syndrome and Bannayan-Ruvalcaba-Riley syndrome. The hamartomatous polyps in these diseases are derived from the epithelial, stromal or from both components of the intestine. Affected patients are at risk for developing cancer of the intestinal tract.

Peutz-Jeghers Syndrome

This syndrome is an autosomal dominant disorder first described by Peutz in 1921, followed by Jeghers in 1949. Characteristics of this disease include the presence of pigmentation on the lips, buccal mucosa, hands and feet; hamartomatous polyps throughout the gastrointestinal tract; and increased risk for gastrointestinal, breast, ovarian and testicular cancers. The cumulative risk of colon cancer is 39%, with similar rates for gastric and pancreatic cancer.

Juvenile Polyposis Syndrome

Juvenile polyps are distinctive hamartomas that have a smooth surface and are covered by normal colonic epithelium. Juvenile polyposis syndrome is defined by any one of the following criteria: 10 or more colonic juvenile polyps; juvenile polyps throughout the gastrointestinal tract; or any number of juvenile polyps, with a family history of juvenile polyposis.

The risk of colon cancer is increased in familial juvenile polyposis, with cancer occurring at an average age of 34 years. Although the juvenile polyps per se are not considered neoplastic, the synchronous adenomatous polyps and mixed juvenile-adenomatous polyps of these patients may give rise to concern.

The APC I1307K Mutation

Most of the APC mutations found in hereditary and sporadic colorectal cancer are nonsense mutations (ie, they lead to the formation of a truncated protein). In contrast, the *APC* I1307K mutation is a missense point mutation in nucleotide position 3920, causing a T to A transversion and, consequently, the substitution of lysine (K) for isoleucine (I) in amino acid position 1307 of the *APC* protein. This mutation is predominantly seen in Ashkenazi Hebrews and carries a predisposition to colorectal cancer. The increased risk for CRC is about 2-fold, indicating that the mutation has a low penetrance despite a relatively high prevalence of about 6.1% in American Hebrews of European origin.

MYH-Associated Polyposis

Although the majority of FAP is attributed to germline mutations in the *APC* gene, a small number of familial cases of polyposis have no identified *APC* mutations. Recent studies of these *APC*-negative probands identified germline mutations in the *MYH* gene, which functions in base excision repair. Somatic mutations in the *APC* gene can be found in tumors from carriers with biallelic mutations that are either missense or nonsense. Hereditary polyposis due to *MYH* mutations has been termed *MYH*-associated polyposis and follows a distinct genetic pathway. It has been estimated that *MYH*-associated polyposis contributes to approximately 1% of unselected CRC.

- *Close relatives with colon cancer*: first degree relatives of patients who have had colon cancer have an up to 3-fold increased risk for development of colon cancer.

- *History of ulcerative colitis and Crohn's disease*: patients with a history of ulcerative colitis and Crohn's disease of the colon have an increased risk for development of cancer that starts about 10-15 years after diagnosis, and risk is also increased with pancolitis and onset of ulcerative colitis before the age of 15 years.

- *History of polyps*: colorectal polyps of the adenomatous type are found in about 40% of the population at age 60 years, and 50% have them at age 70. Over half the polyps occur in the rectum or the sigmoid colon. Adenomas are felt to be premalignant, and malignant change is found in 10% of polyps between 1 and 2 cm in diameter, and in 45% of polyps greater than 2 cm in size.

Adenomas and cancer increase with age and both have a similar distribution throughout the colon. Patients with a cancer have adenomas in the resected specimen in about one-third of cases. With an increase in the number of adenomas there is increased likelihood of a coexistent cancer. (If 5 or more adenomas are found on colonoscopy, about one-quarter of patients will also have a cancer).

The American Cancer Society recommends screening as follows: an annual rectal examination from the age of 40 years onwards, fecal testing for occult blood each year after age 50 years and flexible sigmoidoscopy every 3-5 years from 50 years on. For those who are at high risk for colon cancer development, colonoscopy is the best study. In those with hereditary predispositions this is begun early in life.

Fecal Blood Testing in Colorectal Cancer Screening

The use of a fecal occult blood test (FOBT) by high-risk patients participating in a colonoscopy-based colorectal cancer screening program may increase the rate of discovery of a number of neoplastic lesions. Screening colonoscopy may not detect some significant lesions. By adding FOBT between colonoscopies, this miss rate can be reduced.

The use of an FOBT between colonoscopy screening can detect significant pathology in individuals already enrolled in a screening program because of a personal or family history of colorectal neoplasias. In total, 785 (47.8%) of 1641 subjects invited by mail participated in immunochemical FOBT screening. A positive result was obtained for 57, and 52 underwent colonoscopy. 14 of the patients (1.8%) had significant neoplastic lesions. These consisted of 6 colorectal cancers and 8 significant adenomas.

This approach may be feasible, should there be a nearly 50% participation rate. At least one FOBT should be considered in the interval between surveillance colonoscopies, particularly in those patients who have a past history of colorectal neoplasia.

The diagnosis of colon cancer is suspected in any patient who reports a change in bowel habits, be it a change from constipation to loose bowel movements or diarrhea, or the emergence of constipation. It is likely that tumors are present for 2 or more years, increasing in size without symptoms. Tumors on the right side of the colon tend to be exophytic, growing into the lumen of the colon, which is of greater diameter than the left. Because of this, right-sided tumors do not obstruct the bowel until late in their course (unless the cancer is adjacent to the ileocecal junction, in which case the terminal ileum becomes obstructed relatively early in the course of its growth). Cancers in the right colon ulcerate and bleed slowly so that the patient will have blood detectable in their stool and develop an iron deficiency anemia. Patients may also complain of vague discomfort in the right lower quadrant of the abdomen with no change in bowel habit.

Cancers on the left side of the colon where the lumen of the bowel is smaller and the stool is less liquid are more likely to obstruct the lumen of the bowel and produce changes in bowel habits. Bleeding may be noticed by the patient as dark streaks in the stool, and sometimes dark blood and mucus with clots are also reported. It is important to note that rectal bleeding and hemorrhoids are common, but in the older patient cancer of the colon must be excluded before it is concluded that hemorrhoids are the cause of the bleeding. In younger patients, diagnostic or therapeutic treatment of the hemorrhoids should stop the bleeding, and if this does not occur, then a cancer of the colon should be sought and excluded.

Diagnostic studies include colonoscopy, barium enema and CT scan of the abdomen with contrast medium. Colonoscopy is the study used most often to detect and biopsy suspected cancers of the colon. Barium enema is used less often, but one should be obtained to examine the portion of the colon proximal to the viewing limit of the flexible sigmoidoscope. In some patients the cancer may have narrowed the colon lumen so that the colonoscope will not pass, in which case the remainder of the colon is studied with a barium enema. Barium enema will miss small tumors that may be seen with colonoscopy (about 20% of tumors are less than 0.5 cm in diameter). Many cancers in the bowel are seen on CT examination and this study is used to assess the extent of cancer, demonstrate the lymph nodes in the retroperitoneum and the liver, and a CT study of the chest will detect pulmonary metastases.

Blood tests are done to assess the degree and type of the patient's anemia, the liver functions (which may be abnormal with liver metastases) and the presence of the tumor marker carcinoembryonic antigen (CEA). CEA is helpful in detecting recurrent cancer and this antigen is elevated in about 70% of patients with colon cancer. If the CEA level does not fall after resection, the implication is that cancer cells are still present and it bodes for a poor prognosis. If there is a fall to normal in the level of CEA after operation and it subsequently rises, recurrent cancer is present and investigations are done to locate the metastasis, with a view to reoperation and resection. A test for radiolabeled monoclonal antibodies to CEA is one of the tests used to characterize possible metastases as originating from a cancer of the colon.

The *surgical treatment* is resection of the tumor and the regional lymph nodes with primary anastomosis of the bowel.[10] If metastases are present and the patient's condition is good, it is generally recommended that the primary tumor be resected to prevent future obstruction and bleeding. If the tumor is obstructing the colon, primary resection is done as an extended procedure, anastomosing the ileum to the distal colon. Alternately, a limited colon resection with reanastomosis and proximal protecting colostomy is a prudent choice of operation. If the tumor is perforated, the resection and reanastomosis is protected with a proximal stoma. In those patients with local spread of the tumor, resection of the primary tumor in continuity with the involved organ or tissue en bloc is the recommended management. Obstruction, perforation, and local spread decrease the curability of the colon cancer.

The patient is followed after the operation with CEA, liver function tests, CT of the abdomen and colonoscopy. If there is no recurrence at 12 months, the frequency of the follow-up is decreased. If recurrent disease is found, then an assessment is made as to whether it can successfully be resected with a secondary operation.

The mainstay of treatment for colorectal cancer remains adequate surgical resection. In recent years survival has improved considerably because of earlier diagnosis and improved efficacy of chemotherapy and radiotherapy. Potential benefits of using laparoscopic-assisted surgery compared with conventional surgery for colorectal cancer include less pain, quicker return of GI tract function, shorter hospital stay, fewer wound complications, quicker recovery and less need for immunosuppression.

Laparoscopy-assisted Colectomy

Between July 1996 and July 2002, 794 patients with colorectal cancer who were enrolled from 27 U.K. centers were randomized to receive laparoscopic-assisted (n = 526) or open surgery (n = 268) as part of the UK Medical Research Council trial of conventional vs. laparoscopic-assisted surgery in a colorectal cancer (CLASICC) trial.[11]

29% of patients underwent conversion. In this group, hospital stay was extended. The most common reasons for conversion were excessive tumor fixity, uncertainty of tumor clearance and obesity. Mortality was higher in patients who underwent conversion (9% vs. 5% in the open and 4% in the laparoscopic group).

In the laparoscopic group, length of incision was shorter, duration of surgery was longer and mean hospital stay was 2 days shorter. Time to resumption of bowel movement and normal diet was similar. For patients with colon cancer, hospital stay was similar for both procedures.

For patients with rectal cancer, hospital stay was 2 days shorter for laparoscopic than for open surgery, and 3 days shorter than for patients who underwent surgery conversion.

The rate of abdominoperineal resection for rectal cancer was 27% in the open and 25% in the laparoscopic group, and most resections were undertaken because the tumor location was too low. The proportions of Duke's C2 tumors were similar between open and laparoscopic procedures.

Positive circumferential resection margins (CRM) rates were similar, with 5% for the open and 6% for the laparoscopic group. CRM rates did not vary when per protocol analysis was applied. The rate of positive CRMs was higher in patients with rectal cancer. Distance of tumor from mesenteric resection margin was similar in open and in laparoscopic surgery (9 cm for open vs. 8 cm for laparoscopic). Intraoperative complications were similar. The transfusion rates were similar (15% and 20%).

30-day postoperative complication rates were similar at 32%. The laparoscopic patients had more pneumonias. The rates of 3-month complications were similar at 7%. There were no significant differences in quality-of-life measures up to 3 months. The proportions of Duke's C2 tumors were similar between open and laparoscopic procedures.

In the United States, ***the Clinical Outcomes of Surgical Therapy Study Group*** published the results of a similar study.[12] This trial was conducted at 48 institutions which randomly assigned 872 patients with adenocarcinoma of the colon to undergo open or laparoscopically-assisted colectomy performed by credentialed surgeons. The median follow-up was 4.4 years. The primary end point was the time to tumor recurrence.

At 3 years, the rates of recurrence were similar in the 2 groups—16% among patients in the group that underwent laparoscopically-assisted surgery and 18% among patients in the open-colectomy group. Recurrence rates in surgical wounds were less than 1% in both groups.

The overall survival rate at 3 years was also very similar in the 2 groups (86% in the laparoscopic-surgery group and 85% in the open-colectomy group; hazard ratio for death in the laparoscopic-surgery group, 0.91; 95% confidence interval, 0.68 to 1.21).

There was no significant difference between groups in the time to recurrence or overall survival for patients with any stage of cancer.

Perioperative recovery was faster in the laparoscopic-surgery group than in the open-colectomy group, as reflected by a shorter median hospital stay (5 days vs. 6 days), and briefer use of parenteral narcotics (3 days vs. 4 days), and oral analgesics (1 day vs. 2 days).

The rates of intraoperative complications, 30-day postoperative mortality, complications at discharge and 60 days, hospital readmission, and reoperation were very similar between groups.

In this multi-institutional study, the rates of recurrent cancer were similar after laparoscopically-assisted colectomy and open colectomy, suggesting that the laparoscopic approach is an acceptable alternative to open surgery for colon cancer.

Preparation for Laparoscopic Colectomy

Patients who are being considered for laparoscopic bowel surgery should have a definitive diagnosis. The distance from the tumor to the anal verge is readily measured in the course of colonoscopy, but this measurement does not always happen to be the true distance from the anal verge found at the operation.

The ileocecal valve (which remains a constant and easily identifiable landmark) is reliably identified at laparoscopy; however, the anatomy of other parts of the colon can be quite indistinct. A useful maneuver to avoid errors in identifying the location of the tumor at laparoscopy is to use preoperative India ink tattooing to mark lesions located in segments of the bowel outside the area of the ileocecal valve, thus facilitating intraoperative localization of the tumor.

Bowel Preparation Prior to Colorectal Surgery

There has been a long tradition of preparing the colon to reduce bacterial numbers before colectomy. Because of the many regimens, surgeons may have concern about which therapeutic regimen should be used. R.L. Nelson, from the University of Illinois, in collaboration with the Cochrane group, reviewed 197 published studies covering 49 different antibiotics. Of particular note, there were 10 randomized studies comparing any antibiotic vs. no antibiotic (placebo); as would be anticipated, antibiotics markedly reduced the risk of infection: relative risk = 0.3, 95% confidence interval = 0.22-0.41.

Both aerobic and anaerobic coverage should be included, and a combination of oral plus a single intravenous (IV) dose provides excellent protection. These investigators concluded that any antibiotic or combination of antibiotics works well, and that a combination of IV and oral routes is particularly efficacious.

Another component of bowel preparation has traditionally included mechanical cleansing of the bowel. A recent report suggests, however, that with antibiotic use and current surgical techniques, mechanical bowel cleansing may no longer be required.

Benign Tumors of the Colon

The most common benign tumors are polyps of various types. These are of importance because of their varying potential for malignant change. A number of syndromes described in more detail in the section on Genetic Predisposition to Malignant Tumors of the colon, including polyps of the large and small bowel, are of importance to the surgeon.[13]

Familial adenomatous polyposis is an autosomal dominant disease in which the patient develops adenomatous polyps in the colon and rectum from puberty onwards. The treatment is proctocolectomy with ileal pouch anal anastomosis or ileorectal anastomosis, with close endoscopic follow-up of the rectal pouch and endoscopic removal of polyps. *Gardener's syndrome* (polyposis, desmoid tumors, osteomas of the skull and mandible, and sebaceous cysts) and *Turcot's syndrome* (polyposis and glioma or medulloblastoma) are variants of familial adenomatous polyposis with extracolonic manifestations. Juvenile polyps are hamartomas and of low malignant potential. These syndromes, *juvenile polyposis* coli, and generalized juvenile gastrointestinal polyposis are inherited autosomal dominant conditions.

The *Cronkhite-Canada syndrome* is juvenile polyposis with ectodermal lesions. *Peutz-Jeghers syndrome* is also a rare autosomal dominant condition with multiple hamartomatous polyps throughout the entire bowel and melanotic pigmentation of the skin and mucous membranes. The polyps are only removed if large and symptomatic, although there is an increase in development of cancer from the polyps in the stomach, duodenum, and pancreas, as well as in the small bowel and breast.

Colonic Dysmotility[14]

Constipation as a symptom is difficult to define, because it is based on the patient's perception of what a normal pattern of defecation is. This is usually a complaint of women of reproductive age and will typically develop by about age 20. Bowel movements occur several times a week, and are accompanied by straining and incomplete rectal evacuation, in addition to nausea, abdominal distention and pain. The patient will often complain of the need to assist defecation by manual extraction of the stool from the rectum or digital pressure in the vagina. Patients are incapacitated by the constipation and become fixated on their abdominal symptoms and aberrant defecatory pattern.

Constipation is measured by recording the colonic transit time of radiopaque markers using daily radiographs of the abdomen. This measures the mean transit time of a bolus of markers and is not reproducible from day to day. To be reproducible, a longer period of ingestion and establishment of a steady state are needed. On the basis of these studies, 3 groups are identified. The first has a propulsion defect in the colon and there is colonic delay. In the second, the stool passes normally through the colon until it reaches either the left colon or the rectum, where its passage is abnormally prolonged (known as hindgut and outlet obstruction, respectively). In the third group of patients with constipation the transit time is normal.

Delayed transit in the ascending colon is known as *colonic inertia* and is seldom an isolated finding, but is associated with overall slowed colorectal transit. *Anismus* is an abnormal condition in which the voluntary muscle of the pelvic floor contracts rather than relaxes during straining. Patients with anismus may have normal transit time, but complain of incomplete evacuation of stool and excessive straining and bloating. There is no abnormality on anal manometry of the recorded resting or contracting anal pressures in patients with either anismus or slow-transit constipation. On defecography, patients with anismus have a significantly higher degree of acute anorectal anterior angulation and less descent of the perineum. Slow transit constipation and colonic inertia account for the most severe constipation.

In the patient complaining of constipation, a trial of a high-fiber diet is given before any diagnostic studies are done. It will usually not improve symptoms in patients with slow transit constipation or colonic inertia, and will often make the complaints worse.

Biofeedback to control any recorded objective change in abnormal anorectal manometric studies has been useful in treating some patients with constipation. Anismus disappears and constipation eases during and after biofeedback therapy in such patients. The patient with severely symptomatic colonic dysmotility is managed with intense but relatively simple medical therapy, including administration of enemas and oral laxatives such as milk of magnesia, and mineral oil, although these agents tend to lose their effectiveness over time. Other treatment includes lactulose and daily oral polyethylene glycol solution. The promotility agents cisapride, erythromycin and prostigmine are also used.

In patients debilitated by constipation, operation may be recommended. These patients should have been investigated extensively, should not have diffuse abnormalities involving parts of the bowel other than the colon, and should have no psychiatric abnormalities. Total abdominal colectomy with ileorectal anastomosis is the procedure recommended. Segmental resection of the right or left side of the colon usually does not improve the symptoms, and may require additional, more extensive resection for symptom control.

Massive Lower Gastrointestinal Bleeding

Massive bleeding in the lower gastrointestinal tract can develop without any warning in an older patient, and if untreated, the patient may develop hypovolemic shock. The management is focused on localizing the bleeding site, which in about 70% of patients is in the colon. The remainder are divided between the small intestine, stomach and duodenum.[15]

The patient will frequently give a history of the painless passage of bloody stools. Abnormalities of clotting are excluded, and in patients with bleeding diverticulosis, reversing the effects of an anticoagulant such as warfarin will control the bleeding. Physical examination may give an indication to the surgeon of the likely lesion, such as in patients found to have a cirrhotic liver or telangiectatic lesions on the lips as a manifestation of Osler-Rendu-Weber syndrome.

Sigmoidoscopy or *colonoscopy* will show the abnormal mucosa of Crohn's disease, ulcerative colitis or ischemic colitis. Internal hemorrhoids are rarely the source of massive bleeding. Rapidly accumulating blood and clots may make it technically difficult for the colonoscopist to clearly view colonic pathology, and if this examination is done while bleeding is profuse, it is usually of low diagnostic yield. However, if performed after bleeding has stopped and the colon is cleared, colonoscopy may be the only study that will reveal the nature of a bleeding site, such as a locally adherent clot at the orifice of a diverticulum. The colonoscope may also be introduced into the bowel at the time of operation to localize a mucosal lesion which may not be palpable and evident to the surgeon.

It is critically important in the surgical management of patients with massive rectal bleeding to exclude a bleeding site in the stomach, duodenum, esophagus, small bowel and rectum. A nasogastric tube is used to aspirate fluid from the upper tract, and if the fluid sample contains bile and is negative for blood on testing, a rapidly bleeding upper intestinal site is unlikely. If there is any doubt, an upper tract endoscopy will identify the site of bleeding.

Mesenteric angiography is recommended for identification of the bleeding site in patients who are bleeding relatively rapidly; in patients in whom colonoscopy would be obscured by the large amount of blood in the colon; or in patients whose view of the colon was adequate at colonoscopy, but no bleeding site was found and the bleeding persists. Angiography demonstrates the anatomy of the various vascular malformations in the small and large intestines. These include angiodysplastic lesions of the colon and arteriovenous malformations, which are more likely in the small bowel. Pooled or extravasated contrast medium is seen in the bowel adjacent to the bleeding site, and this finding establishes the fact that the patient is bleeding at a rate of more than 0.5 mL/minute. The mesenteric angiogram studies the 3 mesenteric vessels, selectively cannulating each one. If no site of bleeding is seen at the time of angiography and no lesion is present, a repeat angiogram may be obtained via the angiogram catheter, which should be left in place in anticipation of recurrent bleeding.

Barium contrast studies can be obtained in a patient in whom the bleeding appears to have either stopped or markedly diminished in rate. It is important to remember that angiographic findings are obscured by residual barium in the bowel, so if angiography is planned it should be performed before proceeding with the barium study. A contrast enema will only show contour abnormalities such as diverticula, neoplasms, or colonic mucosal ulcerations or swelling. When there are no clues to the site of bleeding and both the small and large bowel are to be studied with contrast examinations, the small bowel study precedes the barium enema, since no bowel preparation is necessary, and the small bowel anatomy will not be obscured by residual barium in the colon.

Radionuclide-labeled red blood cell scans may be useful for demonstrating the region of the bowel from which blood is originating, particularly if the rate of bleeding is relatively slow and it is felt that angiography would very likely not reveal the site of bleeding.

In patients with no site for gastrointestinal bleeding located, the likelihood of negative or indeterminate findings at diagnostic laparotomy is as high as 70%, so surgery is not recommended without rigorous preoperative investigation.

Diffuse colonic diverticulosis is the cause of massive hemorrhage in over two-thirds of patients. In the elderly there is a high incidence of associated disease, especially of the cardiovascular system. The bleeding site is in the right colon in three-quarters of cases, and is thought not to be a complication of a localized episode of diverticulitis. A mesenteric angiogram, a tagged red cell bleeding scan or a colonoscopy will localize the site of the bleeding diverticulum. Diverticula will only be shown on colonoscopy, CT with contrast or a barium enema.

Angiodysplasia accounts for a significant number of cases of lower gastrointestinal bleeding and is second only to diverticulosis as its cause. Angiodysplasia includes telangiectasias, hamartomas and hemangiomas. These are probably acquired, since patients with bleeding from these vascular lesions are nearly always elderly. The majority of these lesions occur in the right colon and are identified on colonoscopy or angiography. They are submucosal lesions and will not be seen on barium enema or when the surgeon examines the unopened bowel at operation. On angiography, these lesions appear as dilated, tortuous intramural veins that empty late, as a small vascular tuft in the arterial phase or as an early-filling vein indicating arteriovenous shunting.

Ischemic colitis and inflammatory bowel disease are very uncommon sources of massive rectal bleeding. Intestinal varices are also a very uncommon source of massive rectal bleeding in patients with cirrhosis and portal hypertension. These are seen as mucosal imprints on barium contrast study or when visualized by sigmoidoscopy or colonoscopy. The venous phase of a mesenteric angiogram will outline intestinal varices. Other less-common causes of massive bleeding are benign or malignant tumors, intussusception, Meckel's diverticulum and aortoenteric fistula.

If the bleeding is uncontrolled and its origin is known, then a segmental resection of the bowel to remove the bleeding lesion is the recommended treatment. If the bleeding site has not been identified and sites in the upper intestinal tract and the rectum are excluded, it is recommended that a subtotal colectomy be done. This more extensive operation removes the length of colon which harbors the majority of the lesions responsible for massive lower gastrointestinal bleeding. A partial colectomy without previous localization of the bleeding point in patients with diverticulosis requires a second operation in about half the patients, and the performance of a second operation to treat continued bleeding is associated with greatly increased mortality.

Inflammatory Bowel Disease[16]

Ulcerative colitis and *Crohn's disease* are both defined empirically, on the basis of clinical features, pathological, radiological and endoscopic findings, and laboratory results. There are other variant forms of colitis known as *lymphocytic colitis*, visible on microscopy, and *collagenous colitis*, indicated by response to the administration of sulfasalazine and normal appearance of the bowel mucosa on inspection with the naked eye. Inflammation also develops in segments of the bowel after surgery in 2 conditions:

- ***Diversion colitis***, in which the abnormalities are the result of a deficiency of short chain fatty acids required for the maintenance of the colonic epithelium, and which are normally produced by luminal bacteria. Topical administration of butyric acid reverses the changes. This disorder occurs in a segment of colon disconnected from the fecal stream (eg, the rectum) following Hartman's procedure.

- ***Pouchitis***, an inflammation that may arise in the ileal pouch in some patients after surgical treatment of ulcerative colitis. The cause of pouchitis is not known; however, administration of antimicrobials effective against anaerobes usually cures the inflammation.

There has been an increase in the prevalence of Crohn's disease in the United States and Western Europe, whereas the ulcerative colitis rate remains stable. The prevalence of the 2 diseases is now equal. Ulcerative colitis involves the mucosa and the superficial submucosa; the inflammation rarely spares the rectum and extends in a contiguous fashion proximally. It is characterized by the formation of ulcers, mucopurulent exudates, pseudopolyps and bloody diarrhea. The severity of the illness relates to the extent and activity of the inflammation. The inflammation is most severe in patients with pancolitis.

Within 3 years of establishing the diagnosis of ulcerative colitis, about one-third of patients who have pancolitis will have a colectomy due to the severity of symptoms. In the same period, about 10% of patients with less extensive colitis and 2% of those with ulcerative proctitis will have a colectomy. Recurrence is characteristic of ulcerative colitis and about half the patients in any cohort will have symptoms at any time.

Crohn's disease is characterized by transmural inflammation of the bowel wall, and ulceration which is aphthoid in the early stages, and later becomes linear or fissure-like, with the inner aspect of the bowel mucosa taking on a cobblestone appearance on gross inspection. Noncaseating granulomas are found in the inflammatory tissue on microscopic examination in about 50% of patients.

The terminal ileum is the most common site for development of Crohn's disease; however, it also occurs elsewhere and is limited to the colon in 30% of cases, occurs in both the colon and the small bowel in about 30% of cases, and in the remaining 40% of patients is limited to the small bowel. Unlike ulcerative colitis, Crohn's disease spares the rectum, and involves scattered segments of the bowel rather than extending contiguously, leaving lengths of bowel free of disease, creating an overall appearance known as "skip areas." Patients with Crohn's disease often have perianal suppuration as a complication. In Crohn's disease, the sites of inflammation, fibrosis and scarring are diverse, the illness is dominated by pain and diarrhea, and there is retardation of growth in children. Crohn's disease is indolent; patients usually seek medical care 3 years after the onset of symptoms, and the disease is diagnosed 9 months after that. About one-third of patients need operation in the first year after diagnosis, and 5% per year after that. About 5% of patients need reoperation each year.

The complications of inflammatory bowel disease include toxic megacolon in both ulcerative colitis and Crohn's disease; fistula formation in Crohn's disease; and perianal disease, which occurs much more frequently in Crohn's disease. The extraintestinal manifestations of arthritis, uveitis and skin inflammation occur during the active phase of these disorders, and spondylitis and cholangitis may develop and progress while the diseases are inactive or cured. Conditions that sometimes complicate Crohn's disease include gallstones, thromboembolic disease, nutritional deficiency, renal colic and oxalate stones, and ureteric obstruction.

The drug therapy for Crohn's disease and ulcerative colitis includes *sulfasalazine*, which reduces the frequency and severity of attacks in ulcerative colitis and controls the acute process in Crohn's disease, but has no prophylactic activity. Only 20% of patients can tolerate this drug. The active component of the drug is 5-aminosalicylic acid (ASA) and the sulfapyridine causes the side effects. The 5-ASA is delivered to the small bowel or colon in high concentration in the newer formulations of the drug.

Steroids are very useful for the treatment of patients with moderate to severe ulcerative colitis and Crohn's disease of the small bowel, and are used in Crohn's disease of the colon. The newer topical steroids are metabolized in large part on first passage through the liver. The *antimetabolites* 6-mercaptopurine, azathioprine and methotrexate are all used late in the treatment of these diseases in patients unresponsive to ASA and steroids, often in conjunction with these agents. Metronidazole is used for the treatment of perianal fistula disease.

In patients with ulcerative colitis there is an increased risk of developing cancer of the colon that starts about 10-15 years after the diagnosis is made. After 10-15 years the risk is 0.5%-1% with pancolitis and rises to 30% 35 years after the diagnosis. This figure increases to 49% if the diagnosis is made before the patient reaches the age of 15 years. With less extensive disease, the risk is lower. The cancer has the same prognosis as that associated with sporadic colon cancer. Symptoms associated with the underlying colitis do not change when the cancer is present and are of no use in making the diagnosis of cancer. Endoscopic biopsy of the mucosa showing high-grade dysplasia is an indicator of high likelihood of cancer developing imminently, or already existent in the colon.

In patients with Crohn's colitis there is a 6-fold increase in the likelihood of developing cancer of the colon. There is also an increased chance of developing cancer of the small bowel or in a bypassed ileum, which at one time was an operation done for the treatment of Crohn's disease. Patients with ulcerative colitis are at an increased risk for development of cholangiocarcinoma in addition to adenocarcinoma of the colon.

In Crohn's disease, surgery is reserved for the management of complications, used in conjunction with medical therapy. It is not curative, although it can bring great improvement in the patient's quality of life. The major indication for surgery, accounting for 50% of operations, is obstruction due to a chronic sclerotic stricture. Other complications treated surgically are internal and external fistulas and abscesses, and perianal fistulas and infections. In each of these conditions, resection of the involved segment of bowel is performed with the aim of minimizing the length of excised bowel, because of the recurrent nature of Crohn's disease and the likely need for additional operations. This philosophy minimizes the chance of the patient completely losing all of the small bowel and sustaining permanent digestive impairment. Many chronic fibrous strictures are managed with stricturoplasty, which is a side-to-side enterostomy of the strictured length of bowel. With multiple strictures, this is appealing as a means of retaining bowel length.

Some patients with ulcerative colitis require an urgent operation to treat toxic megacolon, severe hemorrhage, or fulminant colitis, after a failed course of intense medical therapy. The decision to operate in each of these conditions is made early, when the patient fails to meet objective clinical improvement criteria. Surgery is performed if there is no improvement after 24-36 hours with toxic megacolon, and after 3-4 days of intense medical management in fulminant colitis. This practice minimizes the chance of colonic perforation.

With chronic ulcerative colitis, operation is recommended if exacerbations are frequent, if the patient is unable to work or has low quality of life, has frequent readmissions to hospital, or a high-maintenance steroid dose is needed to maintain remission. In some patients the risk of developing or the actual presence of a colon cancer is the reason for the operation.

Ulcerative colitis is cured with a total proctocolectomy. In past years this was coupled with a permanent ileostomy, but today the standard reconstruction is ileal pouch anal anastomosis. This operation is usually done in conjunction with a protecting temporary ileostomy, especially in patients who are at increased risk for complications of healing. This group of patients includes those on high doses of steroids, malnourished individuals, and those needing an emergency operation for severe colitis. Variants of this surgery include the use of a J or S pouch, rectal mucosectomy or a very low resection of the rectum with anastomosis of the pouch to the stump of the rectum, leaving a small ring of mucosa. About 5% of patients having this operation need conversion to a permanent ileostomy because of complications, including uncontrollable pouchitis, poor control with overflow onto the perianal skin and severe excoriation of the perianal skin. The typical patient has good rectal sensation, is continent, can hold their stool until convenient to empty the pouch and has about 6 bowel movements daily, varying with the diet.

5. References

1. Rossini FP, Risio M, Pennazio M. Small bowel tumors and polyposis syndromes. *Gastrointest Endosc Clin N Am.* 1999 ;9(1):93-114.

2. Oberg K. Neuroendocrine gastrointestinal tumors-a condensed overview of diagnosis and treatment. *Ann Oncol.* 1999;10(suppl 2):S3-S8.

3. Eisen LK, Cunningham JD, Aufses AH Jr. Intussusception in adults: institutional review. *Am Coll Surg.* 1999 ;188(4):390-395.

4. Stollman NH, Raskin JB. Diverticular disease of the colon. *J Clin Gastroenterol.* 1999 ;29(3):241-252.

5. Foster CE III, Lefor AT. General management of gastrointestinal fistulas. Recognition, stabilization, and correction of fluid and electrolyte imbalances. *Surg Clin North Am.* 1996;76(5): 1019-1033.

6. Berry SM, Fischer JE. Classification and pathophysiology of enterocutaneous fistulas. *Surg Clin North Am.* 1996;76(5):1009-1018.

7. Tassiopoulos AK, Baum G, Halverson JD. Small bowel fistulas. *Surg Clin North Am.* 1996t;76(5):1175-1181.

8. Haglund U, Bergqvist D. Intestinal ischemia–the basics. *Langenbecks Arch Surg.* 1999;384(3):233-238.

9. Potter JD. Colorectal cancer: molecules and populations. *J Natl Cancer Inst.* 1999; 91(11):916-932.

10. Muto T, Watanabe T. Colorectal carcinoma: recent advances in its biology and treatment. *J Cancer Res Clin Oncol.* 1999;125(3-4):245-253.

11. Guillou PJ, Quirke P, Thorpe H. MRC CLASICC trial group Short-term endpoints of conventional versus laparoscopic-assisted surgery in patients with colorectal cancer (MRC CLASICC trial): multicentre, randomised controlled trial. *Lancet.* 2005;365:1666-1668,1718-1726.

12. The Clinical Outcomes of Surgical Therapy Study Group. A comparison of laparoscopically assisted and open colectomy for colon cancer. *N Engl J Med.* 2004;350:2050.

13. Guillem JG, Smith AJ, Calle JP, Ruo L. Gastrointestinal polyposis syndromes. *Curr Probl Surg.* 1999 ;36(4):217-323.

14. Spiller RC. Disturbances in large bowel motility. *Bailliere's Best Pract Res Clin Gastroenterol.* 1999;13(3):397-413.

15. Billingham RP. The conundrum of lower gastrointestinal bleeding (Review). *Surg Clin North Am.* 1997;77(1):241-252.

16. Becker JM. Surgical therapy for ulcerative colitis and Crohn's disease. *Gastroenterol Clin North Am.* 1999;28(2):371-390, vi.

17. Kingham TP, Dematteo RP. Multidisciplinary treatment of gastrointestinal stromal tumors. *Surg Clin North Am.* 2009;89 (1):217-233.

6. Questions

1. A 50-year-old man presents with recent onset of rectal bleeding. His hemoglobin is 10.5 g/dL and he has been taking a moderate dosage of aspirin to treat pain from a knee injury. He otherwise feels well and said he had some bleeding similar to this episode that resolved when he added fiber to his diet when he was 35 years old. Examination of his abdomen reveals no abnormal findings and on proctoscopy he has large hemorrhoids that bleed on contact with the sigmoidoscope. Your next step in his management is:

   A. Place rubber bands on the hemorrhoids and investigate for other sites of origin of the bleeding only if he continues to bleed.

   B. Advise that he restart the fiber in his diet.

   C. Perform a flexible sigmoidoscopy, and if this is normal, treat the hemorrhoids.

   D. Perform a sigmoidoscopy and barium enema to examine the proximal colon.

   E. Arrange for him to have a barium enema examination of the colon.

2. A 76-year-old woman admitted to the medical intensive care unit with an acute myocardial infarction and cardiogenic shock complains of severe and unremitting central abdominal pain that came on suddenly 5 days after her admission to hospital for treatment of the infarction. On examination her temperature is normal, pulse is 110 beats/min and irregular in rhythm, and her abdomen is soft with no guarding, although she complains of pain. The next step in management of the pain is:

   A. Administer an intravenous dose of morphine and continue to monitor her symptoms.

   B. Obtain a plain radiograph of her abdomen and if this shows no abnormality prescribe analgesic medication.

   C. Have a mesenteric angiogram done urgently.

   D. Return in 4 hours and reexamine her abdomen for signs of peritonitis should they develop.

   E. Obtain an echocardiogram to determine if there are clots on the valves of the heart or attached to the endocardium.

3. A 25-year-old man admitted with symptoms of appendicitis for the preceding 6 days is found to have an 8-cm diameter mass that is moderately tender in his right lower abdominal quadrant. His temperature is 37.5°C, pulse is 75 beats/ min and an ultrasound study is reported as appendicitis. Your management of this man is:

   A. Urgent operation to remove the appendix.

   B. Operation done through a midline incision and removal of the appendix.

   C. Observe the patient for change in the mass and start him on antimicrobial therapy.

   D. Investigate the mass further with colonoscopy, to exclude carcinoma.

   E. Needle biopsy of the mass with radiological guidance to exclude malignancy.

4. A 45-year-old man presents to the emergency room having passed large amounts of bright red blood per rectum. His hemoglobin is 7 g/dL and his pulse is 130 beats/min. He is resuscitated and given 2 units of blood. There is no blood in the gastroduodenal aspirate. A colonoscopy done 24 hours after admission showed diverticula of the descending and sigmoid colon. On the third day postadmission he suddenly develops massive rectal bleeding and shock. The best plan for management of this patient is:

   A. Resuscitate, and when stabilized, perform a left hemicolectomy, removing all colon involved with diverticula.

   B. Resuscitate and arrange for an urgent mesenteric angiogram.

C. Resuscitate, and when stabilized, arrange for a tagged red cell bleeding scan.

D. Resuscitate, and when stabilized, perform a total colectomy.

E. Resuscitate and then perform an endoscopic exam of the upper gastrointestinal tract; if this is normal, perform a total colectomy.

5. A 29-year-old man presents with perforation of a transverse colon carcinoma, which was treated with a right hemicolectomy and placement of an ileostomy. The segment of colon that was removed contained multiple polyps and had metastases to 2 of 20 lymph nodes in the mesentery. He had 2 brothers who also had their colons removed when they were in their twenties. Which of the following statements is true of this patient?

A. This patient will require a residual colectomy and proctectomy with rectal mucosectomy and ileal pouch anal anastomosis.

B. The remainder of his colon will be normal.

C. The patient will not require chemotherapy.

D. The polyps in the colon specimen are juvenile polyps.

E. The bowel can be reanastomosed once he has recovered.

6. A 35-year-old man is admitted with severe pain in the left lower quadrant of his abdomen, loose bowel movements and abdominal distention. His abdomen is tender and a mass is palpable in the left lower quadrant. His temperature is 39°C and his white cell count is 25,000. A plain x-ray of his abdomen shows air-fluid levels in the left lower quadrant. Based on these data, which of the following statements is correct?

A. He has small bowel obstruction and needs an urgent laparotomy.

B. Once he has recovered from this acute illness he should have a sigmoid colectomy.

C. This patient has inflammatory bowel disease.

D. If he develops an abscess it should be drained operatively.

E. Urgent sigmoidoscopy is required to make a diagnosis.

7. Each of the following statements is true ***except***:

A. A colonic fistula will heal without operation.

B. A jejunocutaneous fistula will heal more quickly than a colonic fistula.

C. A jejunal fistula can result in hypovolemic shock.

D. Obstruction of the bowel beyond the fistula decreases the likelihood of the fistula healing.

E. A colovaginal fistula will not heal spontaneously.

8. A 35-year-old woman is seen in consultation complaining of colicky abdominal pain, nausea and vomiting. For the last 6 months she has noticed facial flushing and diarrhea when she drinks alcohol. On examination of her abdomen she has an enlarged, firm liver. What information is needed to confirm the diagnosis?

A. A CT scan of the abdomen and liver showing liver metastases.

B. A 5-hydroxyindole acetic acid level of more than 20 mg in the urine measured daily.

C. A barium study of the small bowel that shows ileal obstruction.

D. Metastases in the lymph nodes of the small bowel adjacent to the site of obstruction.

E. An 0.5-cm diameter carcinoid tumor at the base of the appendix.

9. A 56-year-old woman recently noted fecal material discharging from her vagina. Examination of her abdomen and pelvis is normal. A barium enema shows colonic diverticula, but no communication of the colon with the vagina, and a contrast study of the small bowel is normal. How would you manage this patient?

A. Perform a proximal diverting colostomy with the expectation that the fistula into the vagina will heal.

B. Study the colon with endoscopy to determine if there is a communication with the vagina.

C. Perform a laparotomy and resect the colon containing the fistula to the vagina, and protect the anastomosis with a proximal colostomy.

D. Resect the colon containing the fistula to the vagina, and primarily reanastomose the colon.

E. Place the patient on nothing but mouth and parenteral nutrition with the expectation the fistula will heal.

10. A 45-year-old patient presents with colicky abdominal pain, distention, vomiting and constipation. On barium enema there is obstruction of the colon at the splenic flexure and the proximal colon is massively distended. The next step in management of this patient is:

A. Colonoscopy.

B. A period of nasogastric suction and intravenous fluids with the expectation that the obstruction will resolve.

C. Resection of the splenic flexure with primary anastomosis of the colon.

D. Resection of the proximal colon to a point beyond the obstruction and reanastomose this to the ileum.

E. Passage of a rectal tube to open the obstruction in the splenic flexure.

Sesap 14

If colonoscopy is +ve for polyp - what is the surveillance ~~patte~~ recommendations.
(1) Small Rectal hyperplastic polyps → ∅ (Regular Colonoscopy)
(2) 1-2 small tubular adenomas (5-10 yrs)
(3) 3-10 adenomas; or any adenoma ≥ 1cm; or adenoma with villous features or high grade dysplasia - 3yrs
(4) > 10 adenomas → ≤ 3yrs.
(5) sessile adenoma removed in piecemeal fashion (2-6 mo).

Answers

1. D.

The concern in a patient of this age with recent onset of rectal bleeding is potential for carcinoma of the colon. In a younger patient, the hemorrhoids could be treated and investigation done only if the bleeding persisted. The best method to examine the colon is colonoscopy; however, that is not a choice in this question. Sigmoidoscopy with barium enema is another method for examining the entire length of the colon, as is barium enema alone. The enema study may miss small tumors of the colon.

2. C.

This is the typical patient who is at risk for the development of acute mesenteric ischemia. Her pain is very likely to be caused by an embolus either from the mural thrombus that may be associated with the infarcted area of the heart, or alternately from the atrium, since her irregular pulse suggests she has atrial fibrillation. There are no peritoneal signs in the early stage of mesenteric ischemia when the infarction of the bowel is limited to the mucosa. An angiogram will demonstrate occlusion of the mesenteric vessels and treatment is started immediately, usually operative.

3. C.

This man has an appendix phlegmon and when he came to the hospital he did have abnormal vital signs indicating he was septic, indicating that his immune mechanisms had detected the appendicitis, and that with more time he would likely resolve the acute problem without treatment. Operating on a phlegmon can be difficult and dangerous for the patient. The recently formed adhesions are often numerous and dense and dissection is fraught with the risk of enterotomies that may lead to extensive bowel resection and the need for a stoma. The phlegmon will likely resolve and antimicrobials can be expected to hasten that process. The margins of the underlying appendix mass are marked on the abdomen skin, and repeat clinical examinations are done to determine that the mass is not enlarging or becoming tender, and the patient's vital signs checked regularly to make sure they are normal. If the mass should enlarge or the vitals were to change radically, operation would then be indicated, or radiographically-guided drainage of an abscess could be performed if one is visualized on CT scan of the abdomen. An interval appendectomy may be done.

4. B.

It is likely that the bleeding is from a colonic site since no blood was found in the nasogastric aspirate, which was tested at the time of admission. The source could be the diverticula, although no clot was seen at the mouth of any of the diverticula to suggest this, and left-sided diverticula are less likely to be the source of major bleeding than right-sided diverticula. Angiodysplasia may not have been visible on the endoscopy, particularly if the patient was not fully resuscitated, and this could well be the source of his bleeding. The angiogram is done to demonstrate this lesion, and also to detect any vascular malformations in the small bowel, which could also be the source of the bleeding. A tagged red cell scan is used for the study of patients bleeding more slowly or if the angiogram is normal, along with the other studies. This study will only roughly localize the bleeding site and does not yield information about the pathology. A total colectomy is only done when the colon is the site of persistent massive bleeding, and in this patient a site in the colon has not been localized, and there is no bleeding from the rectum or proximal to the ileocecal valve. Ideally a limited resection is done, removing only the lesion that has been shown to be bleeding.

5. A.

This patient has hereditary polyposis of the colon. Colonoscopy will show multiple adenomatous polyps in the colon and rectum. He will require chemotherapy for complete treatment of the Duke's B cancer to improve survival. After this is completed the best operation to restore bowel continuity is the ileal pouch anal anastomosis. He should have a mucosectomy to remove all mucosa at risk for development of cancer.

6. B.

The symptoms and signs are those of acute colonic diverticulitis, which may be complicated by abscess formation. An abscess is treated with CT-guided drainage rather than operation, and once the patient has recovered from the first episode of diverticulitis he should be advised to have a sigmoid colectomy. Diverticulitis in patients under age 40 is more aggressive than in older patients. This age group is more likely to have a repeat attack within 2 years and it will likely be associated with severe complications. In older patients, operation is recommended after the second episode.

7. B.

These are all well-known facts about fistulas. A high small bowel fistula, with voluminous output, is unlikely to heal without operation.

8. B.

These statements all relate to the carcinoid syndrome. For this to be manifest in patients with a carcinoid tumor, liver metastases must be present. The primary tumor is usually located in the terminal ileum. The metastases replace normal liver tissue, and the liver no longer has the capacity to remove serotonin, which enters the systemic circulation and produces the syndrome. The primary tumor is often small and may produce bowel obstruction through the marked sclerotic reaction well known to accompany it. Tumors less than 2 cm in diameter are very rarely malignant. The diagnosis is confirmed by finding elevated levels of 5-hydroxyindole acetic acid in the urine. This is a product of serotonin metabolism, from the serotonin produced by the carcinoid tumor.

9. D.

Colovaginal fistulas will not heal without an operation to resect the colon containing the fistula. The track of the fistula is short and epithelialized. It may be difficult to demonstrate the communication of the fistula with the bowel, regardless of the study used. In this patient, the symptoms clearly indicate vaginal communication with the colon. With proper bowel preparation the resection can be done in one stage, without the need for a protecting colostomy. At operation, care is taken to separate the site of the colon anastomosis from the repaired communication with the vagina by placing omentum between them. This lessens the likelihood of a recurrence.

10. D.

The patient very likely has a cancer obstructing the colon. It is rare that colonic obstruction is due to adhesions. The treatment for this is resection of the tumor. Primary anastomosis of the colon to proximal distended colon is unsafe and likely to be complicated by breakdown of the anastomosis. To avoid this an extended resection of the proximal colon is done, the terminal ileum is anastomosed to the distal colon, and no protecting stoma is made.

Chapter 13: Anorectal Disorders

Tracey Arnell, MD
Michael J. Stamos, MD

Contents

1. Anatomy

Anus

The definition of the anal canal has some variation. Surgically it extends inferiorly from above at the top of the puborectalis to the anal verge, which is the caudal extent of the internal sphincter at the intersphincteric groove. The physiologic anal canal extends from the anal verge proximally to the dentate line. The dentate line is the point at which the endoderm meets the ectoderm, with columnar epithelium proximal and squamous epithelium (skin) distal. Anal glands originate from the anal crypts located at the dentate line. The area 1-2 cm proximal to the dentate line is the anal transitional zone (ATZ) or cloacogenic area, and is composed of transitional epithelium. The innervation, venous, and lymphatic drainage above and below the transitional area are different. Cephalad, innervation is autonomic and drainage is to the hypogastric vessels and lymphatics, whereas caudad the innervation is somatic and drainage is to the inferior hemorrhoidal and inguinal vessels and lymph nodes.

The internal anal sphincter is composed of smooth (involuntary) muscle that is a continuation of the inner circular muscle of the rectum. The external sphincter is contiguous with the puborectalis and is striated (voluntary) muscle. At the superior extent of the surgical anal canal, the levators form the pelvic floor. They are composed of (medial to lateral) the puborectalis, pubococcygeus and iliococcygeus muscles. The levators originate from the pubis and form a sling around the anorectal junction. The mechanisms of continence are described later.

Rectum

The rectum begins where the taeniae coli fuse to form the longitudinal muscle layer at the sacral promontory, and ends at the levators. It is 13-15 cm in length and lies in the concavity of the sacrum, ending just beyond the tip of the coccyx. Anteriorly, the rectum is approximately equally divided into a proximal intraperitoneal and a distal extraperitoneal portion. Posteriorly, the rectum is entirely extraperitoneal. The rectum is lined by columnar epithelium identical to that of the colon, but differs in that it lacks taeniae, a complete serosa, haustra, and epiploic appendices. There are three mucosal folds known as the valves of Houston, 2 on the left and 1 on the right. The middle valve corresponds to the peritoneal reflection anteriorly. Venous drainage is dual, through the inferior mesenteric and hypogastric vessels. Lymphatic drainage is via the mesorectum which lies posterior and lateral to the rectum contained within its fascia propria. The mesorectum is penetrated by the terminal branches of the sacral nerve roots and branches of the middle rectal vessels.

Blood Supply

The anorectum is supplied by the superior, middle and inferior rectal vessels, which originate from the inferior mesenteric, hypogastric and pudendal arteries, respectively. The middle rectal artery is variable and often small, entering the rectum anterolaterally at the level of the levators. There is an extensive submucosal plexus of vessels contributing to the excellent vascularity of the anorectum.[1,2]

2. Benign Anorectal Conditions

Anorectal Abscess and *Fistula in Ano*

Definition

An *anorectal abscess* is a perianal or ischiorectal infection most commonly originating from the anal canal. These perianal infections originating from the crypts of the anus are the initial event in the formation of a *fistula in ano,* which is a connection between the anal canal and the skin.

Epidemiology

There are few studies documenting the incidence of anorectal sepsis and fistula. In a 10-year study of one population, the incidence in men was 12 per 100,000 compared to 5.6 per 100,000 in women. Several other studies have confirmed this male predominance. The second and third decade is the most common age of presentation, accounting for 65% of cases.[3] Patients with hematologic abnormalities are especially prone to anorectal infections. When the neutrophil count is less than 500/mm^3, up to 11% of patients may develop perianal sepsis.[4]

Etiology

The cryptoglandular theory is the generally accepted explanation for the etiology of over 90% of perianal abscesses and fistulae. Based on anatomic studies dating to 1878 by Chiari, and expanded upon by Parks and others, anal glands are found to drain into the anal crypts at the dentate line. There are an average of 6 glands per individual (more in men) and the majority are posterior. The depth of penetration of the glands is variable; 80% are submucosal, 10% penetrate the internal sphincter (IS), 2% enter the intersphincteric space and only 1% penetrate the external sphincter (ES). These individual differences in number and depth of glands may explain the variability in individual susceptibility and subsequent location of infection. The remaining 10% of anorectal abscesses not due to cryptoglandular disease occur for a variety of reasons are listed in Table 1.[4-8]

Table 1

Alternate Causes of Perianal Abscesses

Cryptoglandular infection
Hidradenitis
Trauma
Obstetrical
Foreign body
Surgical (anorectal procedures)
Neoplasms
Anal canal
Anal margin
Hematologic malignancies

A thorough understanding of the anatomy of the perianal area is imperative in evaluating patients with perianal sepsis and fistulae. There are several important spaces that may become involved in the disease process (see Figure 1). The most common site is perianal (55%), followed by ischiorectal (35%), submucosal and intersphincteric. Least common and often most challenging are supralevator abscesses. Infections of the deep postanal space deserve separate consideration because of the frequency of missed diagnosis. Figure 2 demonstrates the location of the deep postanal space. An infection in this area may spread to the surrounding lateral spaces, resulting in a horseshoe abscess.

The location of the initial perianal infection determines the type of fistula that develops. Park's classification identifies intersphincteric, transsphincteric, suprasphincteric and extrasphincteric fistulas, and is the most commonly used system.[6,9,10]

Clinical Presentation

Based on the cryptoglandular theory of perianal sepsis, the inciting event leading to a fistula is a perianal infection. The usual presenting symptoms are pain (90%), swelling (50%), discharge, bleeding and occasionally fever. The pain is often of a throbbing nature, continuous and worse with bowel movements. It may result in fecal impaction and urinary retention.

The incidence of subsequent *fistula in ano* in patients treated for abscesses has been reported to be 50%-75%. Additionally, some patients will present initially with a fistula, likely from an episode of

Figure 1

Locations of perirectal and perianal spaces

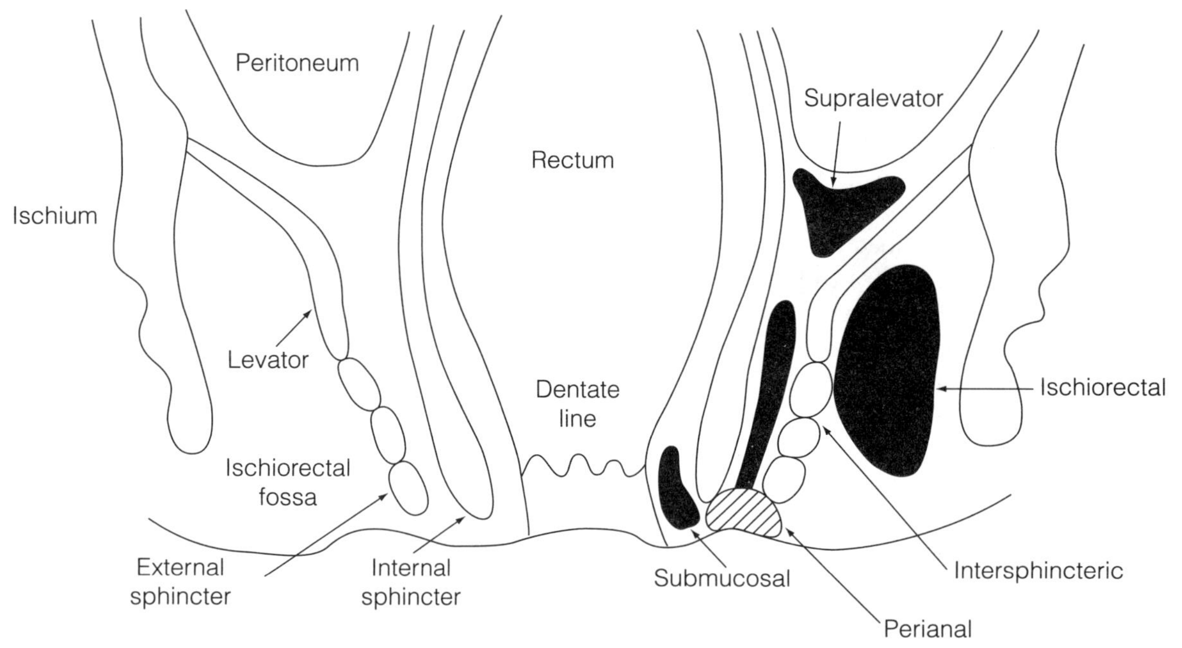

Figure 2

Potential postanal and rectal spaces

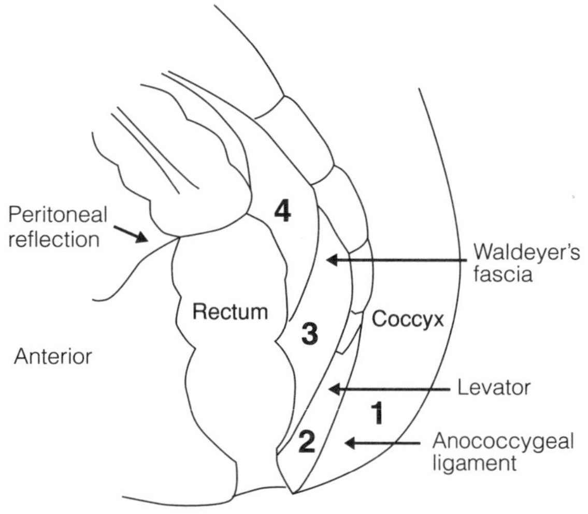

1, superficial postanal space; 2, deep postanal space; 3, supralevator space; 4, retrorectal space

perianal infection that spontaneously drained/decompressed. The most common complaint is that of drainage and discharge, but recurrent episodes of perianal infections may also occur.[11-13]

Evaluation

On physical examination, fever and tachycardia may occur with moderate to severe perianal infection. Externally, an area of erythema and induration is often evident. Fluctuance may not be present and is not to be awaited before incision and drainage. Digital rectal examination (DRE) may reveal a fluctuant area in the anal canal. In patients with an intersphincteric, supralevator, or deep postanal space infection or who are immunosuppressed, findings may be limited to this or asymmetric tenderness externally. Upon visual anoscopic inspection of the anal canal, a crypt draining purulent fluid is occasionally seen. If tenderness precludes a complete examination, an examination under anesthesia should be performed. Extensive laboratory examination is unnecessary, but an elevation in the white blood cell count may occur. Hyperglycemia and diabetic ketoacidosis can occur in diabetics. Patients who are immunosup pressed may not manifest any of these signs, and if typical symptoms are present (ie, pain, fever, tenderness), anorectal sepsis should be suspected. In selected patients, a computed tomographic examination may disclose the presence and extent of a perirectal abscess but should not be done routinely.

Fistula in Ano

Patients presenting with symptoms of *fistula in ano* will usually have one or more external openings which appear as punctate, granulating elevations. An internal opening should be sought and can be expected to be located at the level of the dentate line. The location of the external opening can predict the location of the internal opening according to Goodsall's rule (see Figure 3). Goodsall's rule has been found to be more than 90% accurate in predicting posterior fistulas, but less than 75% correct in cases of anterior external openings.[12] A useful technique is to perform a DRE and feel for a cord or knot in the anal canal. Palpation of the area between the external opening and the anal canal with a lubricated index finger may also identify a cord that corresponds to the fistula tract. Direct examination of the anal canal using an anal retractor may reveal a hypertrophied papilla or discharge from a crypt. If the opening is not identified, gentle probing with a crypt or lacrimal probe through the external or internal opening can be performed. If these techniques fail, injection of a liquid into the external opening with observation of the anal canal can locate the internal opening. Commonly used liq uids include hydrogen peroxide, milk and methylene blue. Methylene blue has the disadvantage of staining the surrounding area. If an internal opening is still not found, more involved investigations such as endoanal ultrasound, magnetic resonance imaging (MRI) and/or fistulograms may be necessary.

Figure 3

Goodsall's rule of fistula tract direction

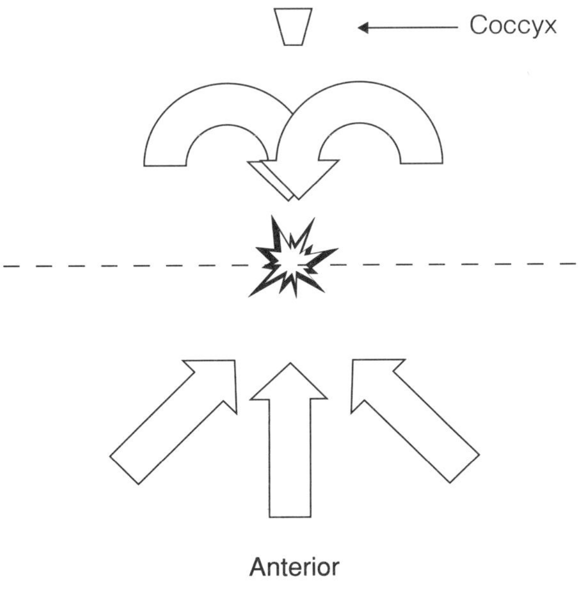

Up to one-third of patients with Crohn's disease may develop perianal infections and fistulas, and in 10% they may be the presenting symptom. Patients with multiple external openings and/or fistulas, complex fistulas, associated bowel symptoms or other atypical signs and symptoms should undergo investigation of the colon and terminal ileum. The treatment of these patients is often quite different and directed at control of the inflammatory bowel disease.[14,15]

Treatment

The most important principle in the treatment of patients with perianal infections and fistulas is for surgeons to perform only the techniques they are familiar and comfortable with. Overzealous debridement, probing and fistulotomies may result in recurrence, increasingly complex fistulas and alterations in continence.

The treatment of most perianal abscesses is straightforward after identification of the area of infection. For perianal and ischiorectal abscesses, a simple oval or cruciate incision over the fluctuant area, often done under local anesthesia, may be performed. The wound does not need to be aggressively curetted or deeply packed. After irrigation, a wick may be placed and removed the following day. Intersphincteric abscesses may be more complicated. The optimal treatment is to divide the internal sphincter overlying the abscess to the dentate line. Because of the difficulty in identifying intersphincteric abscesses and the need to divide the internal sphincter, these abscesses are more appropriately drained in the operating room. If a horseshoe ischiorectal abscess is identified, a deep postanal space infection should be sought. The deep postanal space is drained through an incision between the tip of the coccyx and the anal canal. Using a Kelly clamp, the fibers of the anococcygeal ligament are spread to allow entry into the deep postanal space. It is important not to divide the anococcygeal ligament because this may lead to incontinence. Failure to identify and drain a deep postanal space infection will often lead to recurrence or persistence of the abscess. Supralevator abscesses are the most unusual and potentially difficult to treat correctly. They occur either as an upward extension of an intersphincteric or ischiorectal abscess, or a downward extension from an intra-abdominal process (ie, diverticulitis, appendicitis). Those arising from abdominal sources require treatment of the primary process. Supralevator abscesses resulting from intersphincteric infections should be drained through the rectum because drainage through the ischiorectal fossa may result in a supralevator fistula. Those that result from an ischiorectal abscess should be drained through the ischiorectal fossa or an extrasphincteric fistula may result (see Figure 4).

In experienced hands, performing a fistulotomy at the time of drainage of a perianal abscess is safe in a patient with normal continence. The decision whether or not to do this should be influenced by the knowledge that up to 50% of patients will not develop a fistula, and also be based on the individual surgeon's experience.[16]

The use of antibiotics is not always necessary. In an immunocompetent patient without systemic signs of infection or severe induration and erythema, drainage is sufficient. Immunocompromised patients, and those with evidence of sepsis or severe cellulitic skin changes should receive antibiotics. The spectrum of the antibiotic should cover the common bowel organisms and include adequate anaerobic coverage.

Figure 4

Correct drainage of a supralevator abscess

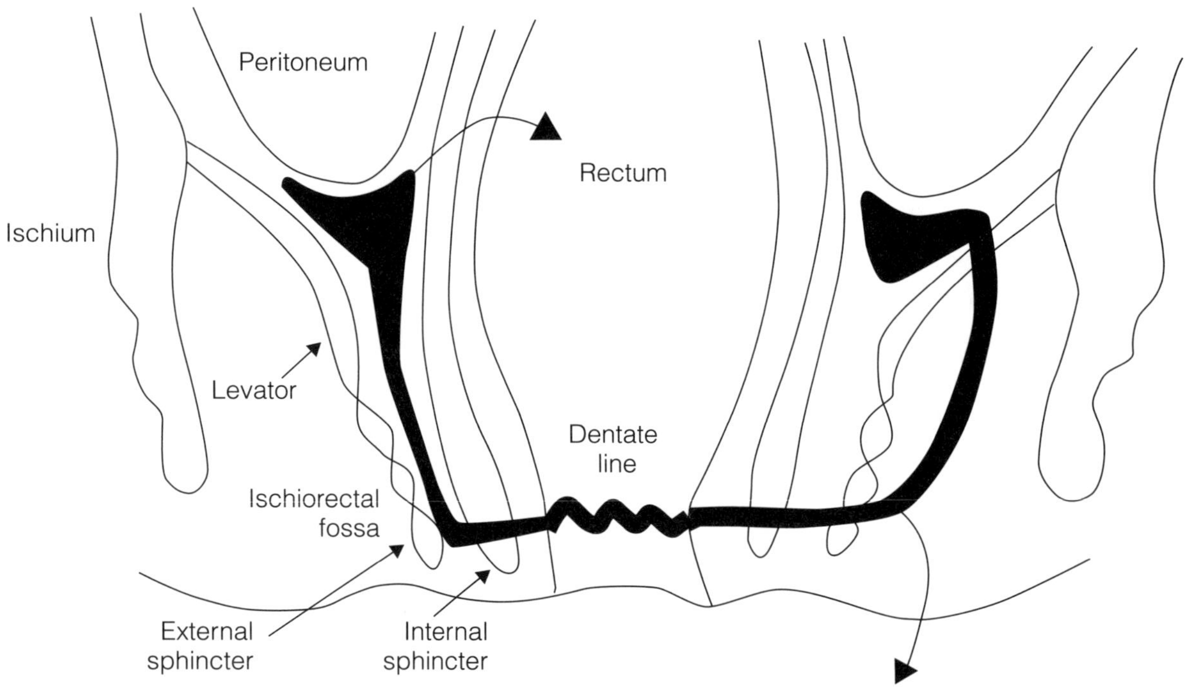

If severe perineal sepsis (Fournier's gangrene) with skin changes consistent with necrotizing infection is present, wide surgical debridement must be carried out urgently. This is often performed in conjunction with a urologist because of the frequent involvement of the scrotum. The need for a colostomy is dependent on the extent of debridement and involvement of the sphincter, but is rarely indicated at the time of the initial debridement. Surgical debridement may also be necessary in the neutropenic patient.

If a fistula is not identified and treated at the primary abscess drainage, fistula treatment may be necessary if patency persists. The evaluation is as previously described, and rarely are more extensive tests required. If the internal opening is not correctly identified at operation, recurrence is the rule. Once the fistula tract has been identified, the question is how to eradicate it: how much sphincter can be divided? The previous rule had been that the internal and external sphincter below the puborectalis can be divided without interfering with continence, but this has to be tailored to the individual patient based on a detailed continence history including trauma and childbirth injuries. Elderly patients, women (especially those with multiple vaginal deliveries), patients with alterations in continence preoperatively and those with fistulas in the anterior quadrants are at higher risk for developing incontinence. In these patients, more conservative treatment is warranted. In all patients, division of the puborectalis will result in gross fecal incontinence. With these factors in mind, treatment of the fistula should be decided on an individual basis.

Providing that the patient will tolerate division of the involved sphincter, a primary fistulotomy can be performed; the tract is gently curetted and left open. If a horseshoe fistula is present, counterincisions or laying open of the horseshoe tracts to the posterior midline followed by a fistulotomy in the posterior midline is carried out (see Figure 5).

For management of fistulas in which the primary fistulotomy may compromise continence, a cutting seton may be used. Setons are nonabsorbable materials such as silk, Silastic catheters, Penrose drains and vascular loops, that are threaded through the intact fistula tract after curetting. The skin bridge and subcutaneous tissue between the internal and external opening is divided, leaving the underlying muscle intact. The seton is sequentially tightened over a period of weeks to slowly divide the sphincter, allowing the divided sphincter to scar rather than splay open. Whether this preserves continence more safely than primary fistulotomy is controversial and generally should not be performed in patients with preexisting incontinence of any degree.[17]

The other use of a seton is as a drain. This is most commonly used in fistulas associated with Crohn's disease. The duration of the seton is based on the activity of the underlying Crohn's disease, and its function is to prevent and treat perianal sepsis.

More advanced techniques may be necessary in patients with any degree of incontinence or concern for same, recurrent fistulas, high fistulas and those associated with a large degree of sphincter involvement. Options include fibrin glue, anal fistula plug and mucosal or skin flaps to obliterate the internal opening. For any technique, the most important factors in successful resolution of the fistula are knowledge of the anatomy of the anal canal and fistulas, and identification of the internal opening. The most common cause for fistulotomy failure and recurrence of abscess or fistula is incorrect or inadequate identification of the internal opening.

Fissure

Definition

A *fissure in ano* is a tear in the anoderm. Fissures with symptoms lasting less than 3 months and without chronic changes are considered acute. If symptoms are of longer duration or associated with chronic skin changes, they are defined as chronic.

Epidemiology

Fissure in ano has been estimated to be responsible for up to 15% of visits to colon and rectal surgery clinics. It occurs at all ages, but is most common in young and middle-aged adults. Most studies find an equal incidence in men and women although the distribution of fissure location may differ.[18] As with perianal infections and fistulas, they may occur in patients with Crohn's disease as well.

Figure 5

Drainage of a postanal space abscess

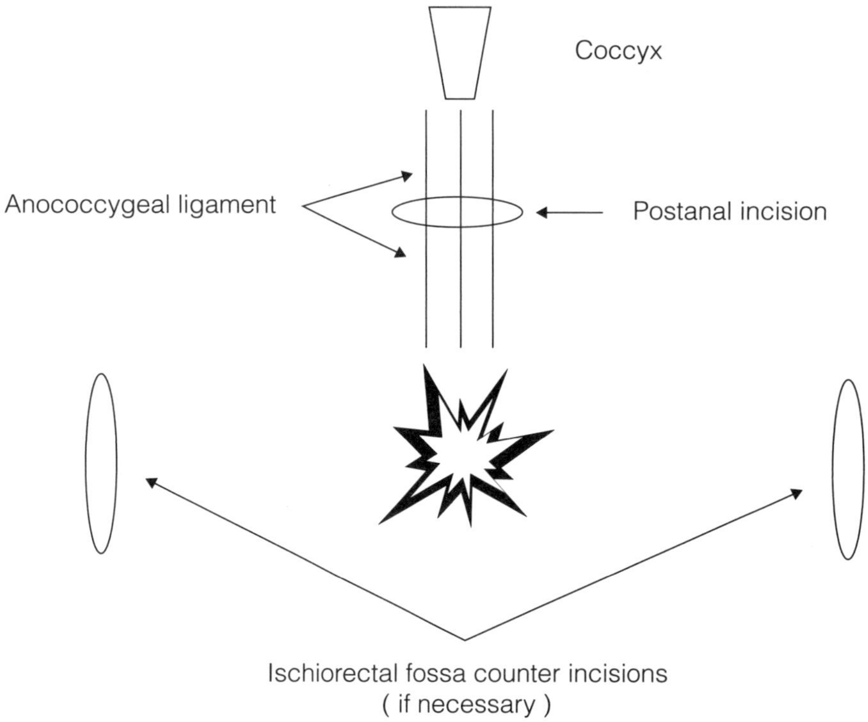

Etiology

Anatomical studies, Doppler blood flow analysis and manometry have classified the etiology of anal fissure. The most widely agreed upon unifying pathologic abnormality in the inciting event of the anal fissure is a tear in the anoderm, usually beginning at the dentate line and extending caudally. Pain results in sphincter spasm, causing a functional anal stenosis that inhibits healing and potentiates the spasm.

An explanation for the occurrence of the fissure in the midline, most commonly posteriorly, has been sought, and several theories have been proposed. The first is of a relative deficiency of muscle fibers in the anterior and posterior midline where the sphincter decussates. This would explain why women, having a thinner perineal body, have a higher incidence of anterior midline fissures compared to men (10% vs. 1%).[19] Second, anatomically, the anterior and posterior midlines are relatively fixed by the perineal body and anococcygeal ligament. With eversion of the anal canal upon defecation, these areas experience increased stretch, and may be more prone to tearing. Third, there may be relative ischemia of the midline, especially posteriorly because of a paucity of blood vessels as demonstrated in cadaveric studies.[20] Patients with fissures have been found by manometry to have increased anal canal pressures, and this may exacerbate the ischemia. Schouten and colleagues[21] performed Doppler flow studies on the anal canal of patients with fissures and found a decrement in blood flow to the posterior commissure of patients with fissures compared to controls, and this was associated with increased anal canal pressures. Following sphincterotomy, the blood flow was increased with a concomitant decrease in sphincter tone. In chronic fissures the hypertonic sphincter and relative ischemia results in failure to heal and signs of chronicity such as fibrosis and induration. All of these factors contribute to the poor healing of chronic anal fissures.

Clinical Presentation

The classic history of patients with an acute anal fissure is an episode of constipation, diarrhea or a difficult bowel movement, followed by pain with subsequent bowel movements. The association of constipation and straining is not consistent and may be present in as few as one-third of patients.[22] The pain is typically described as tearing or burning and associated with defecation, although it may persist for minutes to hours afterwards. More than half of patients will also complain of a small amount of bright red bleeding. Discharge and pruritis may also occur, especially as the history becomes chronic. If a patient is found to have a fissure without this characteristic presentation, complicating factors should be sought. Painless fissures occur with tuberculosis, Crohn's disease and sexually transmitted diseases such as syphilis.

Evaluation

The evaluation of a patient with a classic history is straightforward. A gentle external examination must be performed. Inspection may reveal a posterior or anterior midline "sentinel pile," or skin tag overlying the ulcer. The ulcer may not be visible because of the hypertonic sphincter. The buttocks should be spread and the distal anal canal examined. Specific note should be made of features of chronicity such as visible sphincter fibers, indurated edges, sentinel pile and hypertrophied papilla at the dentate line. It may not be possible to perform a DRE with an acute anal fissure due to pain and this may be deferred initially if the diagnosis is clear. In a patient with a consistent history and examination this is the only evaluation necessary. Further investigation such as endoscopy should be determined based on the individual patient characteristics (ie, age, other symptoms) after resolution of the acute episode as bowel preparation and colonic evaluation may be extremely painful and exacerbate the fissure.

If the presentation is atypical, such as locations other than the midline, painless fissures, significant bleeding or gastrointestinal symptoms, additional investigations may be necessary. These may include examination under anesthesia, ulcer biopsy, cultures or endoscopy.

Treatment

To determine appropriate therapy, an attempt to differentiate chronic from acute anal fissure is important. In general, patients with a long history of symptoms (>3 months) or physical findings of chronicity are less likely to respond to nonsurgical treatment. While medical treatment is not contraindicated in chronic cases, the threshold for operation should be lower.[23]

Between 50% and 90% of patients with an acute *fissure-in-ano* will respond to medical therapy.[22] The mainstays of this therapy have been the use of fiber to prevent constipation and hard stools, and sitz baths to decrease sphincter spasm. The additional use of any type of suppository is not helpful, and may be uncomfortable. Topical anesthetics such as lidocaine jelly should be used judiciously because of the risk of hypersensitivity reactions. Recently, there have been several additions to the pharmacological armamentarium. The goal of each is to decrease the spasm of the sphincter, and topical nitroglycerin is one such agent. The strength prescribed is 0.2% (cardiac preparation is 2.0%), applied as needed. The most common side effect is headache.[24] Diltiazem has been used similarly and may be more effective, with fewer side effects.[25,25a,25b] Botulinum toxin, injected into 2 or 4 quadrants to produce a temporary pharmacologic sphincterotomy, has also been used. The initial reports have been promising although cost considerations currently limit its use.[26]

For failures of medical management, surgical therapy is very effective. Again, the primary goal is relaxation of the hypertonic sphincter, allowing the fissure to heal. The Lord procedure, or anal sphincter stretch (4 finger, 4 minute dilation under anesthesia) results in an uncontrolled disruption of the sphincter. This has been shown to be associated with greater sphincter injury based on ultrasound and manometry, as well as clinical continence disturbances, and for these reasons a sphincterotomy is preferred. A lateral internal sphincterotomy is the most commonly performed procedure. It is performed laterally, without fissurectomy, to prevent a "keyhole" deformity. The internal sphincter is divided, either using a closed or open technique, to a level above the apex of the fissure.

Outcome

The success rate for the Lord procedure is 80%-90% but alterations in continence occur in up to 40% of patients. For a properly performed lateral sphincterotomy, the success rate is >95% and major alterations in continence are infrequent. The recurrence rate may be as high as 25% so patients should be counseled regarding use of dietary fiber and avoidance of constipation.[27]

Pilonidal Disease

Definition

Pilonidal disease occurs in the natal cleft and includes the spectrum of acute abscess to chronic sinuses. It begins as a skin infection related to penetration of the midline region by hair or foreign body. The term pilonidal is of latin origin (pilo=hair, nidal=nest).

Epidemiology

Pilonidal disease is a condition primarily affecting young adults from the age of puberty to 40 years. It is associated with obesity, sedentary occupations and hirsutism, as well as affecting those with glabellar hair. Pilonidal disease is also known as "jeep driver's disease" and is a frequent diagnosis in military personnel. It accounted for more lost days than casualties in the Vietnam War, and affected 79,000 members of the US military, with an average hospital stay of 55 days, in World War II. In a Minnesota study of college students undergoing routine physical exams, the incidence was found to be 11% in men and 0.11% in women. A higher percentage of women undergo treatment for the condition, making the male to female ratio 4:1 in the United States for patients seeking medical care.[28]

Etiology

Although an early explanation for pilonidal disease offered by Hodges in 1880 was that of an acquired condition, in the ensuing years the popular theory was that the disease was of congenital origin. It was thought to result from abnormal fusion of the median raphe with dermal inclusion bodies, remnants of the medullary canal, and even a vestigial sex gland similar to the preen gland in birds. Presently, the theory of acquired etiology is generally accepted. Evidence for an acquired origin includes the findings of distended hair follicles, keratin plugs and hair in most pilonidal sinuses. The mechanism of abscess and sinus formation is still being debated. The 2 popular theories are a foreign body reaction to embedded hairs, or hair follicles within the cleft that become distended and plugged, rupturing into the lateral subcutaneous space.

Pathologically, the midline sinus becomes epithelialized, forming the familiar pits and accounting for recurrences. The lateral extensions are usually lined with granulation tissue unless the condition is longstanding. Hair is found in about two-thirds of cases, and is surrounded by foreign-body giant cells. Microbiologic studies often reveal mixed aerobic and anaerobic bacteria, although the majority contain anaerobes.[28,29]

Clinical Presentation

Most patients will initially present with an abscess or relate a history consistent with an abscess that spontaneously decompressed. In the uncomplicated patient not at risk for sacral osteomyelitis, actinomycosis, or granulomatous diseases, the diagnosis is easily made.

Evaluation

Included in the differential diagnosis are cryptoglandular infections, hidradenitis, actinomycosis, granulomatous diseases (ie, syphilis, tuberculosis) and osteomyelitis of the sacrum. A thorough history and physical examination is usually all that is required. On physical examination, the patient is often hirsute, male, with a deep natal cleft and abundant buttocks hair. If the process is acute, erythema and induration lateral to the midline may be present. In the chronic form, sinus pits in the midline are almost always visible. There may be punctate areas of granulation lateral to the midline. Probing of the sinuses or lateral extensions usually leads towards the midline. No further evaluation is needed.

Treatment

The treatment of the acute episode may be either simple incision and drainage, or drainage with unroofing of the lateral extensions by curetting and packing the wound. Antibiotics are often unnecessary but may be used depending on the presence of cellulitis. Approximately 40%-60% of patients will go on to develop additional symptoms if treated with incision and drainage alone.[30]

Many nonsurgical treatments have been suggested. Some physicians have treated pilonidal sinuses by shaving and depilatories alone with reported excellent success. Phenol has been injected in the tracts in an attempt to obliterate the sinus. There are reports supportive of each of these conservative methods. Surgical therapy ranges from the simple to the very complex. Because of the acknowledged poor healing in the midline, most surgeons recommend that any incision, including those for acute drainage, be lateral to the midline. The simplest procedure is a lateral incision with curettage of all granulation tissue to the midline and removal of all hair. The sinus pits should be curetted or excised as well, and the wound left open. An alternative is en bloc excision to fascia with marsupialization of the wound or primary closure in the elective case. The healing time for marsupialization is generally longer than that of simple curettage (12 vs. 4 weeks) and the wound care is greater, but recurrence rates appear to be similar. For very large and complicated sinus tracts and recurrent disease, the use of flaps including Z plasty, sliding flaps and myocutaneous flaps has been described, but these are rarely necessary.

Regardless of the therapy chosen, the mainstays of treatment are adequate hygiene and prevention of growth of hairs in the natal cleft. Hair removal by shaving should be done weekly. More permanent forms of hair removal such as laser ablation and waxing may be beneficial.

Outcome

The many differing descriptions of operative and nonoperative treatment of pilonidal sinus disease indicate the lack of a perfect solution, and up to 35% of patients will develop a recurrence. Interestingly, after the age of 40 the problem generally resolves.[30] Counseling regarding hygiene and hair removal is an underappreciated method of prevention.

Hemorrhoids

Definition

The presence of hemorrhoidal tissue is a normal anatomic finding, as demonstrated by its presence from birth. Hemorrhoidal tissue consists of anal mucosa overlying sinusoids which are blood vessels without muscular walls. Hemorrhoidal tissue occurs in 3 major positions in the anal canal—the left lateral, right anterior and right posterior lateral. They begin at the top of the anal canal and extend to the anal verge. Most internal hemorrhoids are cephalad and are lined by mucosa, and external hemorrhoids are more caudad and covered by anoderm (skin). Hemorrhoidal disease is a pathologic condition of the hemorrhoidal tissue characterized by bleeding, prolapse, mucous discharge, pruritus ani, thrombosis and pain.

Epidemiology

It is estimated that the prevalence of hemorrhoidal disease in the United States approaches 5%, or 10 million people annually. One-third of these patients seek medical help for the condition, and in 1987 surgical hemorrhoidectomies were performed at a rate of 37 per 100,000. The peak age is between 45 and 65, followed by a decline after age 65, and they are more common in men. The true prevalence is difficult to determine because of the differing definitions of hemorrhoidal disease, and the tendency to attribute most anorectal complaints to hemorrhoids.[31]

Etiology

Despite our recognition of hemorrhoidal disease since biblical times, we do not yet have a full understanding of the pathogenesis. Previously they were thought to be varices of the rectal veins. This has subsequently been discounted based on autopsy studies, demonstration that the bleeding is of arterial nature, and the lack of relationship to patients with portal hypertension. When varices related to the portosystemic connection with the inferior rectal veins occur, they are in the rectum and their appearance is quite different. Thomson in 1975 described the sliding anal lining theory. He proposed that there is displacement caudally of the anal cushions, composed of the sinusoids, Trietz's muscle (smooth muscle) and elastic connective tissue of the submucosa. With straining, tenesmus and irregular bowel habits, the sinusoids may dilate, predisposing to prolapse with resultant stretch of the muscle and elastic connective tissue. Ultimately, this supportive tissue breaks down, creating enlarged and lax hemorrhoidal tissue that is easily traumatized.[32]

Predisposing factors may include constipation, diarrhea and conditions which increase intraabdominal pressure (ie, pregnancy, obesity). Anal manometry has demonstrated increased anal canal resting pressure and abnormal pressure waves within the sphincter. The exact contribution these factors have to hemorrhoidal disease is unknown.

Clinical Presentation

It is important to note that of patients being referred or evaluated for hemorrhoidal disease, a significant number will be found to have other anorectal conditions unrelated to hemorrhoids. A thorough history and examination are important despite the seemingly routine nature of the presenting complaints.

The most common reason for presentation with symptomatic hemorrhoidal disease is painless bleeding. This is most often associated with internal hemorrhoids and is often bright red, dripping into the toilet after a bowel movement. Anemia resulting from bleeding hemorrhoids is unusual and other sources of blood loss should be sought. Pruritus may occur as a result of mucous discharge with significant prolapse and skin tags. Uncomplicated hemorrhoidal disease rarely presents with pain. Since internal hemorrhoids are not covered with anoderm, they are insensate unless strangulated. External hemorrhoids are painful when thrombosed or associated with prolapsed, strangulated internal hemorrhoids. Patients with significant complaints of pain not associated with these clinically obvious complications on visual inspection should be closely evaluated for other causes such as fissure or abscess. Patients who do present with thrombosis and strangulation may have urinary retention and obstipation. Perianal sepsis from gangrenous hemorrhoids is extremely rare.

Evaluation

A careful history, especially regarding potential bleeding dyscrasias, liver disease and bowel symptoms should be obtained. Specific inquiries as to the presence of pain, prolapsing tissue and type of bleeding are important. As stated before, many patients who present with the complaint of hemorrhoids will be found to have other anorectal pathology.

External inspection evaluating for fissure, fistula, or abscess, or skin abnormalities such as ulcerations, neoplasms or evidence of pruritis is performed. Skin tags consistent with external hemorrhoids should be noted. An isolated midline skin tag should raise suspicion of a fissure. A DRE to assess tone and possible anorectal neoplasms should be done. Unless they are very large, it is difficult to palpate internal hemorrhoids. The cornerstone to evaluation for hemorrhoids is anoscopy with all quadrants of the anus visualized. When noting the location, the position should be described by using anterior/posterior and left/right locations rather than by using hands on a clock as patient position may vary. Internal hemorrhoids are often graded based on the degree of prolapse as follows: grade 1—internal hemorrhoids present; grade 2—they prolapse but spontaneously reduce; grade 3—they require manual reduction; and grade 4—they are unable to be reduced.

Finally, patients who present with atypical symptoms or significant anemia should undergo investigation of the colon. Patients with significant symptoms of bleeding should have endoscopy of the distal colon or the whole colon if indicated by age, symptoms or family history of cancer or inflammatory bowel disease.

Treatment

Most symptomatic hemorrhoids can be managed without surgical excision, as evidenced by the drop in the number of hemorrhoidectomies performed in the United States in recent years. Initially, medical management should be undertaken. This involves increased fiber intake (20-30 g/day) to attain a soft and bulky stool and reduce straining, and sitz baths for relief of discomfort. For the majority of patients with grade 1 or 2 hemorrhoids and small thromboses, this is usually sufficient. Topical hydrocortisone and preparations containing anesthetics may alleviate pruritus and discomfort. They should be used sparingly because long-term use may cause atrophy of the skin and hypersensitivity reactions. Suppositories are ineffective because they migrate above the anal canal to the rectum. These medications are of no benefit for bleeding and prolapse.

Up to 80% of patients will respond to medical management. For those who don't, many treatments are available. These include banding, sclerotherapy, cryotherapy, infrared and electrocoagulation, use of a laser or surgical excision. The effect of these various techniques is fixation of hemorrhoidal tissue which, based on the sliding anal lining theory, should address the underlying problem. The area of application of the various techniques should be above the hemorrhoidal cushion, because this is where the sliding mucosa originates. It also decreases the chance of significant bleeding as a complication. Other options for treating hemorrhoids are procedures to decrease the tone of the sphincter (dilatation, internal sphincterotomy).[33]

Common sclerosants include tetradecyl sodium, phenol, quinine and urea. They are injected into the submucosal plane above the dentate line under direct vision. Repeat injections are done 3-4 weeks later if necessary. Coagulation and cryotherapy have a similar effect of scarring the mucosa to the sphincter, and are applied similarly. The equipment involved is more elaborate than for the other methods. Banding results in scarring and sloughing of the strangulated tissue. In general, one area is banded in the initial session. If this is well tolerated, banding of additional hemorrhoids may be repeated in 2-3 weeks. Complications are similar for the different techniques, and include pain, bleeding (immediately and at 7-10 days postprocedure when mucosal sloughing occurs), stenosis and failure.

Increased anal tone has been demonstrated in patients with symptomatic hemorrhoids. This is the rationale behind procedures that disrupt the sphincter. There are studies touting anal dilatation and internal sphincterotomy as sole treatment for hemorrhoids, claiming success rates exceeding 75%. This is not the usual standard treatment regimen when used alone, but some authors advocate performing them concomitantly with surgical hemorrhoidectomy for pain relief.[34]

Thrombosed external hemorrhoids will resolve without surgical intervention. Sitz baths, bowel management and occasionally topical anesthetics are usually sufficient. Excision may reduce the course of pain by a few days and may benefit those patients with increasing or severe symptoms. If the pain is decreasing, excision is of marginal benefit and observation is recommended. In patients opting for surgical management, an elliptical skin excision over the thrombosis after injection of local anesthetic with expression of the thrombus is performed.

Generally, the traditional surgical hemorrhoidectomy is reserved for patients with grade 3 and grade 4 hemorrhoids. The basic technique begins with submucosal infiltration of local anesthetic and epinephrine. Hyaluronidase is sometimes used because it allows spread of the anesthetic by inactivating hyaluronic acid, preventing the diffusion of substances, and it also may help reduce swelling. It does shorten the duration of effect of anesthetics, though, and has not been convincingly shown to have any advantage. Care must be taken not to excise an excessive amount of anoderm. Excision is begun with the largest hemorrhoid and carried above the dentate line. A pedicle suture is used and the hemorrhoidal tissue is excised. The wound may be closed or left open to close by secondary intention. At the conclusion of the procedure, there is unlikely to be anal stenosis if a medium Hill-Ferguson retractor can be inserted into the canal. Potential complications include bleeding, anal stenosis, infection and urinary retention. Use of meticulous surgical technique will reduce the rates of bleeding, anal stenosis and infection. Adequate analgesia and limiting intravenous fluid infusion will minimize urinary retention. Use of any surgical technique in patients with inflammatory bowel disease or the immunocompromised must be conducted with caution.

More recently, stapled hemorrhoidectomy or hemorrhoidopexy are being performed. A stapling device similar to that used in transanal colorectal anastomosis is used to excise a circumferential area of distal anal/rectal mucosa proximal to the dentate line above the internal hemorrhoidal cushions. It is minimally effective for significant external disease, although it may decrease the size of tags to some degree. Concerns regarding the procedure include the potential for stenosis and incontinence because of the finding of internal sphincter fibers in the pathologic specimens. To date, theses complications have not been found to occur to any significant degree in clinical studies. The major advantage is that of significantly less pain resulting in earlier return to activities compared to open hemorrhoidectomy.[34a, 34b, 34c, 34d] There are a limited number of practitioners performing stapled hemorrhoidectomies, but as more experience is gained, it will likely prove to be a significant addition to the treatment of hemorrhoids.

Outcome

Medical management will be successful in the majority of cases. When intervention is required, often the simplest technique is the best. Randomized trials and meta-analyses have demonstrated that banding requires fewer applications and is at least as effective as coagulation, sclerotherapy and laser treatments. It may be associated with more initial discomfort, but has excellent patient satisfaction. An additional advantage of banding is that if a patient has significant discomfort, the band can be removed. Each of these techniques is effective, though, if applied correctly.

Surgical hemorrhoidectomy is very effective, and less than 1% of patients will develop significant recurrent symptoms at least in the short term. Anal stenosis and incontinence are rare if appropriate attention is paid to careful technique.[35]

Anal Incontinence

Definition

Anal incontinence has many definitions, accounting for the difficulty in determining its incidence. Clinically, it is the inability to defer defecation and retain gas, liquid or solid stool because of insufficient sphincter control. The degree of incontinence for each patient is variable, and needs to be quantified based on history.

Epidemiology

Alterations in fecal continence are underreported to physicians and thus the true incidence is unknown. Obstetrical injuries leading to gross fecal incontinence fortunately occur in less than 1% of births in the United States. If dehiscence occurs following repair of a fourth-degree injury (10%), 66% of these patients will develop incontinence. Occult anal sphincter injuries are much more common, and have been noted to occur in 35% of primiparous women when looked for with anal ultrasound. Approximately 25% of elderly hospital patients have symptoms of incontinence, and it is the second most common cause of institutionalization. Incontinence was elicited in 2.2% of the population in one survey, one-third of patients were older than 65, and 63% were women. Of patients reporting some degree of fecal incontinence, one-third had restricted their activities, yet only one-third of these patients had discussed the problem with a physician. As explained by Sangwan and Coller, the impact is underappreciated unless one considers the psychological and social consequences of the problem. The effects on self-esteem, and the associated depression, social isolation, skin problems and genitourinary infections cannot be quantified.[36-38a]

Etiology

A basic understanding of the mechanism of continence is necessary to understand the etiology, clinical presentation and treatment. Although incompletely understood, it is known that continence is controlled by a complex mechanism involving mechanical factors, as well as the reflex and central nervous systems. The major components of continence are sphincter integrity, anorectal sensation, reflexes and innervation, rectal compliance and stool consistency. The innervation of the internal anal sphincter (IAS) is via sympathetic and parasympathetic pelvic nerves (nervi ergenti). Pelvic nerves from the sacral plexus and branches of the pudendal nerve (perineal n.) supply the levators. The external anal sphincter (EAS) is supplied by branches of the pudendal nerve (perineal n., inferior rectal n., pudendal n.), similar to the puborectalis. The course of the pudendal nerve is through Alcock's canal, entering the EAS through the posterolateral ischiorectal fossa. A perturbation in any single factor may be compensated for, but alterations in more than one may result in incontinence.

The resting anal tone is primarily provided by the tonic contraction of the smooth muscle of the internal anal sphincter. The puborectalis angle and the hemorrhoidal cushions contribute to maintenance of resting continence. When a fecal bolus enters the rectum, there is inhibition of the IAS with contraction of the EAS. This mechanism allows the rectal contents to descend into the upper anal canal and the sensory epithelium there to "sample" the contents. If its passage is not socially appropriate, the rectum relaxes and the IAS returns to baseline tone. This is termed the rectoanal inhibitory reflex (RAIR). It requires intact anorectal sensation, rectal compliance, and sphincter integrity and function. A noncompliant rectum or diarrhea may overwhelm the EAS, since it is able to maintain maximum squeeze pressure for only 60 seconds. If the sphincter has been injured or denervated, the fecal bolus will pass without control.[39]

The most common cause of surgically-correctable fecal incontinence is traumatic injury. Obstetrical and iatrogenic disruption from previous surgical procedures accounts for the majority of injuries. Perineal trauma, spinal cord injury, radiation, chronic inflammation, prolapse, congenital anomalies and changes due to chronic disease and aging are responsible for most of the remaining cases.

Pudendal nerve injury as a result of stretching as may occur with childbirth or chronic pelvic floor descent with prolapse or constipation has been postulated to contribute to incontinence. Unilateral disruption does not usually result in incontinence because of significant crossover between the nerves. It is common for pudendal nerve dysfunction to occur concomitantly with other injuries, especially following childbirth.

Clinical Presentation
As mentioned previously, there are many degrees of incontinence. Patients may be incontinent to flatus or stool. For those with stool incontinence, it may be described as leakage or gross fecal incontinence. The timing of the incontinence is important, and it may occur only at night, with loose stools, or because of urgency and inability to defer defecation for prolonged periods. The initial complaint may seem inconsequential, such as pruritus related to chronic leakage, and only with further query and investigation is incontinence identified.

Leakage is associated with decreases in anal resting tone. This may occur with sphincter injury (primarily internal), rectal prolapse or surgical procedures such as low anterior resection or coloanal anastomosis. Urgency can be a sign of decreased rectal compliance (radiation, inflammation), loss of anorectal angle, diarrhea and subclinical sphincter injury. Gross fecal soiling generally involves abnormalities in several components of continence.

Evaluation
Much can be elucidated regarding the etiology and potential therapy of fecal incontinence from a detailed history. Information regarding childbirth, trauma, history of pelvic radiation and previous anorectal procedures should be obtained to help determine the source for sphincter disruption. The event may have occurred in the distant past, but compensatory mechanisms may fail due to aging or chronic disease unmasking the original injury. The pattern of incontinence and stool character is also helpful. Patients with gross incontinence usually have a nonfunctioning internal and external sphincter, often with puborectalis and pudendal nerve dysfunction. Leakage is more characteristic of diminished resting tone due to internal anal sphincter failure. Urgency may be related to diarrhea, proctitis, loss of rectal compliance or diminished sphincter tone. Global pelvic floor dysfunction is often associated with urinary incontinence, stress fecal incontinence and inability to defer defecation. It frequently presents in the elderly or chronically ill. A number of fecal incontinence scales have been developed which are useful in quantifying degree of incontinence.

Physical examination begins with the sensory exam. This can be done carefully with a needle, or sharp tip of a broken cotton swab. The perianal skin is stimulated and should result in a reflex contraction of the anus (anal wink). It is important to perform this test at the beginning of the examination prior to other testing. This indicates grossly intact sensation and pudendal nerve function. The perianal skin is examined for asymmetry, scars, gaping of the anus or evidence of fistula. A DRE is performed with attention paid to anal canal length, resting tone, asymmetry, puborectalis function and masses. The patient is asked to squeeze as if attempting to defer a bowel movement. Watching the buttocks for the use of accessory muscles, and noting the squeeze of the EAS (especially anteriorly) as well as the puborectalis are the goals. At a minimum, proctoscopic examination should be carried out. If the patient has significant alterations in bowel pattern, such as diarrhea, excessive mucus, a recent change or has not previously been screened, consideration should be given to complete colon evaluation. If diarrhea is a significant symptom, this should also be completely evaluated.

In a patient with an appropriate history and a clearly defined sphincter disruption on physical examination, further testing may not be necessary. For the remainder of patients, simple saline infusion tests, pudendal nerve terminal motor latency (PNTML) or EMG measurements, properly performed anal manometry and endoanal ultrasound can be helpful adjuncts. The saline infusion test involves instilling warm saline (1500 cc) in the rectum and noting the time to leak and the volume leaked. It can be used to confirm incontinence in unclear cases. Information regarding the integrity of the nerves can be obtained from PNTML and EMG. Incontinence normally requires bilateral pudendal nerve dysfunction as demonstrated by prolonged PNTML. Some studies suggest this test is the best predictor of function following repair.[40] EMG provides information regarding the innervation of the sphincters as well, although it is more painful and difficult to perform. It is possible to measure anal canal resting pressure (RP), squeeze pressure (SP), length, compliance and sensation using manometry. With multiport catheters, the symmetry of the anal canal can be mapped as well. Filling a balloon and measuring the pressure at which the patient first senses the need to defecate assesses compliance and sensation. Finally, in cases of suspected anatomic sphincter injury in which the physical examination is not definitive, anal endosonography may detail and delineate the disruption.

Treatment

The treatment of fecal incontinence is dependent on both degree of incontinence and the etiology. The majority of patients with mild incontinence will respond to nonsurgical therapy such as diet changes and bowel management. Diet changes usually involve bulking agents such as psyllium to prevent diarrhea. If stools are still loose, antidiarrheals may be added and titrated to firmer stools. Once this has been achieved, patients should attempt to adjust their bowel movements so they occur the same time each day, if necessary through the occasional use of enemas and suppositories. Once diet and bowel management have been maximized, perineal strengthening exercises and biofeedback may help.

Surgery may be indicated if conservative measures are inadequate. There are 3 principal options: repair of a sphincter defect, replacement of the sphincter (with autologous tissue or an artificial sphincter), and diversion. Patients with a sphincter disruption may undergo primary repair of the defect. This allows for repair of the sphincter defect as well as bulking of the perineum. Plication of the levators may be performed at the same time, although this is probably not necessary. This repair can be performed despite abnormal PNMTL with good success. Patients with failed sphincter repair or those with neurogenic incontinence may undergo placement of a neosphincter. Anal encirclement procedures using wire and Silastic bands have been used, but the complication rate has been historically high with few successes. Common autologous choices are gracilis or gluteus maximus muscle. Dynamic muscle grafts used for activation of the neosphincter can be created with the placement of stimulating electrodes implanted in a remote site. Clinical trials assessing an artificial sphincter similar to those used in urology have been reported. The activating balloon is placed in the labia or scrotum and inflated and deflated as needed. For patients who fail using these methods or are medically unfit to undergo surgical intervention, a diverting colostomy or ileostomy may be performed. Sacral nerve stimulation, currently approved in theU.S. only for urinary incontinence, also has shown good efficacy for fecal incontinence.

Outcome

Medical management and dietary manipulation are very effective for the majority of patients. For patients who do not have a demonstrable sphincter injury and idiopathic incontinence, several studies have demonstrated an improvement in continence in up to 90% of patients using biofeedback.[41] Overlapping surgical repair of the separated ends of the sphincter is successful in 70%-80% of appropriately selected cases. In patients with neurogenic incontinence or failed sphincter repair, the artificial and autologous sphincters may be effective. Associated complications include infection, erosion and impaction, with overall success rates averaging 50%-60 %.[42-44a]

Rectal Prolapse

Definition

Procidentia is a full thickness prolapse of the rectum through the anus. It must be differentiated from mucosal prolapse that may occur with hemorrhoidal disease.

Epidemiology

Rectal prolapse occurs most frequently in very young children and middle-aged to older women. Most children who develop it are less than 3 years old and it is associated with cystic fibrosis, parasitic infections and congenital abnormalities, such as bladder exstrophy and meningomyelocele. In adults, the incidence with age varies depending on sex. Procidentia is 4-6 times more common in women and the incidence steadily increases after age 40. A few studies have noted an increase in frequency of prolapse with nulliparous women, though the relationship is unclear. Its incidence is evenly distributed throughout all ages in men. There is a well-recognized association of rectal prolapse with institutionalized patients, especially those with psychiatric disorders.[45]

Etiology

Anatomically, there are 2 prevailing theories for the origin of rectal prolapse. The first is the sliding hernia theory, in which the anterior rectal wall intussuscepts through the anal canal because of a defect in the pelvic fascia. The second and more generally accepted mechanism is that of an internal intussusception. Cinedefecography has supported the concept of a lead point in the rectum 6-8 cm above the anal verge. There are several anatomic abnormalities that have been noted in patients with procidentia. They are a deep pouch of Douglas, a patulous anal sphincter, levator ani diastasis, redundant sigmoid colon, failure of rectal sacral fixation and loss of horizontal position of the rectum. It is not clear whether these predispose to or are a result of prolapse.

Functionally, about 50% of patients have a history of constipation and straining. An equal number of patients have incontinence associated with the prolapse. Manometry demonstrates diminished anal pressures in those with incontinence. Otherwise, there is no unifying physiologic abnormality in these patients.

Clinical Presentation

Symptoms depend on the extent of prolapse and whether or not there is associated incontinence. In the early stages, the only complaints may be of mucus discharge or pruritus ani. Most patients will report the extrusion of tissue with bowel movements or increases in intra abdominal pressure such as with coughing. Patients often complain of rectal pressure, incomplete evacuation and tenesmus. As the condition worsens, the mucosa may become ulcerated and friable with associated bleeding. In extreme cases, strangulation and even small bowel evisceration may occur. Incontinence occurs frequently and may be related to a loss in rectal sensation.

Evaluation

When a patient describes symptoms as above, it is important to have a high index of suspicion or the diagnosis can be missed. If a patient is examined in the supine or prone position, early prolapse may not be evident. If the symptoms suggest procidentia and this is not appreciated on initial exam, the patient should be examined over a toilet or while squatting. The presence of prolapse with concentric rings and a normal anal position with a visible sulcus separate rectal prolapse from mucosal prolapse. A DRE usually reveals a patulous sphincter with diminished squeeze pressures. In all patients, evaluation of the distal large bowel must be performed to identify or exclude lesions as potential lead points or sources of obstruction resulting in straining. Proctoscopic examination may identify mucosal friability and rectal ulcers. The rectal ulcerations are usually anterior and characterized pathologically by obliteration of the lamina propria. In the advanced state this is known as colitis cystica profunda. In older patients who are operative candidates, evaluation of the entire colon should be completed. Manometry may predict which patients will have improvement in their continence, but rarely influences therapy. If the clinical scenario is suspicious and prolapse is not identified on physical exam, cinedefecography may identify a procidentia.

Treatment

Because no therapy has been without recurrence and complication, over 200 repairs have been described. The 2 major approaches are abdominal and perineal. The goal of the various interventions is to correct some of the previously described anatomic abnormalities.

Every abdominal procedure addresses the rectal fixation to the sacrum. This may be accomplished by suture pexy, prosthetic material (Ripstein, Ivalon® sponge) or complete mobilization of the rectum with inflammatory adhesion fixation. The addition of sigmoid resection and/or plication of the levators may also be performed. Regardless of the details, posterior mobilization of the rectum to the coccyx is generally performed. If prosthetics are used, resection is usually not performed.

Because of higher recurrence rates, perineal procedures have commonly been reserved for patients too debilitated to undergo a laparotomy. As described for incontinence, encirclement procedures with a wire (Thiersch) or Silastic bands may be used. More commonly, a perineal rectosigmoidectomy (Altemeir) or mucosectomy with sphincter plication (Delorme) are performed. Their use is being reevaluated because several recent studies have demonstrated recurrence rates similar to those for abdominal procedures, with lower morbidity.

Outcome

Functionally, approximately one-half of patients will have improvement in their continence. The degree of improvement seems to be slightly lower for patients with prosthetics. Constipation may also be worsened in patients with prosthetics and those undergoing division of the lateral ligaments.

Most studies have found the lowest recurrence rates (<10%) for abdominal procedures, but at the expense of greater morbidity. Complication rates vary from 20%-30% for the Ripstein procedure to 15% for resection, and include mesh erosion, infection, constipation, anastomotic leak and sacral bleeding. Historically, the perineal procedures have recurrence rates approaching 40%, but with lower morbidity. Recent reports are more favorable, with recurrence rates in the 5%-20% range.[46-48]

The choice of procedure should be guided by the patient's general medical condition as well as their symptoms. Patents with significant constipation should not undergo division of the lateral stalks or placement of prosthetic material. If they are found to have slow colonic transit, consideration should be given to total colectomy. Very ill and debilitated patients benefit from a more limited perineal operation.

Rectovaginal Fistula

Definition

Traditionally, fistulas between both the anus and rectum and the vagina have been grouped together as rectovaginal fistulas, although the majority are really anovaginal fistulas. Regardless of the source, a rectovaginal fistula is a connection between the lumen of the anus or the rectum and the vagina. There are several classification schemes; the most common is based on the level of the vaginal opening. High fistulas open at the cervix, mid fistulas drain through the mid vagina and low fistulas open at the vaginal fourchette. Fistulas may be acquired or congenital, but this discussion will focus on acquired fistulas, since they are by far the most commonly encountered.

Epidemiology

Of all fistulas involving the anorectum, anovaginal and rectovaginal fistulas account for less than 5% of cases. Because of the varying etiologies including birth injury, Crohn's disease and radiation damage, they occur in all ages. Of these specific etiologies they occur in less than 0.1% of vaginal deliveries, 10% of female patients with Crohn's and 5% of female patients receiving radiation.[49]

Etiology

The 5 major causes of ano- and rectovaginal fistulas are trauma, inflammation, infection, radiation damage and neoplasm. The prevailing etiology varies with the population studied, but obstetrical trauma, operative trauma and Crohn's disease are the most frequently encountered.

The most common cause of a traumatic fistula is childbirth injury. They are associated with prolonged labor and pressure on the anovaginal septum, or third and fourth degree tears with associated sphincter disruption. Perineal operations such as treatment of *fistula in ano*, and vaginal hysterectomy usually result in low and mid ano- and rectovaginal fistulas. Abdominal procedures including hysterectomy, especially for endometriosis and following radiation, and bowel resection with low anastomosis, are more likely to result in high and mid fistulas. This may be associated with an anastomotic leak or the use of circular staplers if a portion of the vaginal wall is incorporated. Foreign bodies, forceful penetration and accidental impalement occur infrequently.

Inflammatory bowel disease accounts for 6%-23% of fistulas depending on the population studied. They are much more common in Crohn's disease and following restorative proctocolectomy, especially if pelvic sepsis occurs. The presence of IBD should be considered with recurring fistulas and in patients without other risk factors.

Cryptoglandular infections may cause low ano- or rectovaginal fistulas, and abdominal processes such as diverticulitis and postoperative infections may cause high fistulas. Less common etiologies include sexually transmitted diseases such as lymphogranuloma venereum.

Injury from pelvic irradiation results in fistula in 1%-22% of treated individuals. It occurs 6 months to 2 years following radiation therapy and must be differentiated by biopsy from recurrent cancer. It begins as proctitis followed by ulceration of the anorectal wall. One-third to one-half of patients with ulceration will develop a fistula. Underlying conditions such as diabetes and previous pelvic surgery, especially hysterectomy, increase the risk of fistula development.

Recurrent and primary gastrointestinal and genitourinary cancers may present with a fistula. Less commonly, leukemia and aplastic anemia result in fistulas.

Clinical Presentation

Most ano- and rectovaginal fistulas are symptomatic. Patients may complain of passing stool or flatus from the vagina. Smaller fistulas may be associated with foul vaginal discharge or vaginitis. Depending on the etiology, varying degrees of incontinence may also be present.

Evaluation

A detailed history focusing on a history of trauma, radiation, pelvic surgery, or gastrointestinal complaints should be obtained. This helps to guide the remainder of the evaluation. A DRE usually reveals a palpable anterior midline pit or defect. Visualization of the anal or rectal mucosa may demonstrate a visible fistula or granulation tissue, and this can often be seen on the vaginal wall as well. It is important to assess sphincter tone and the presence of any defects. At a minimum, a proctoscopic examination should be performed to evaluate the bowel mucosa. Patients without an obvious etiology and those with other gastrointestinal symptoms should undergo sigmoidoscopy or colonoscopy. All suspicious lesions and ulcers must be biopsied to evaluate for neoplasm and IBD.

If a fistula is not demonstrated, additional studies may be warranted. Clinical evaluation includes insertion of a tampon with instillation of methylene blue or activated charcoal in the rectum. The tampon is removed and examined for color change. Vaginograms are occasionally helpful, especially with high fistulas. Increasingly, endoanal ultrasound is being used, and may help delineate sphincter disruption as well.

Therapy

At the completion of the evaluation, an attempt to classify the fistula based on location and complexity is helpful in planning operative strategy. Very low fistulas may be amenable to simple perineal procedures whereas high fistulas and those involving the rectum often require an abdominal approach. One classification scheme of fistulas defines *simple* as low to mid vagina, <2.5 cm in diameter, and usually related to trauma or infection. *Complex* fistulas are high, >2.5 cm, associated with abnormal tissues (ie, radiation, IBD, cancer), or have had prior attempts at repair. As the complexity of the fistula increases, so does the complexity of the repair and the chance for failure.[50]

For repair of simple fistulas, perineal procedures are usually appropriate. These can be performed through the anus, vagina, or the perineum. If the fistula is low and not associated with a sphincter defect, simple mucosal advancement flap repair may be performed. For mid fistulas and those associated with sphincter defects, sphincteroplasty and closure of the fistula is commonly used. In this way, healthy tissue is interposed between the anus and vagina and the perineal body is bulked. Anal and vaginal procedures are similar. Either a mucosal advancement flap to cover the opening or a layered closure with coverage of the fistula is done. It is conceptually appealing to repair the fistula from the anal side because this is the high-pressure zone, but both approaches are performed with similar reported results. As an adjunct, or alone, the use of fibrin glue has been evaluated with success rates varying from 50%-80%, although generally lower for rectovaginal fistulas due to the typically short tract. Its greatest benefit is that it does not preclude subsequent repair if it fails.

The 3 primary options for complex and high fistulas are resection, tissue interposition or fecal diversion. Resection of the involved bowel segment with anastomosis to healthy tissues is the goal. This may require mucosectomy with coloanal anastomosis for very low fistulas. It may be necessary to divert with a proximal stoma to allow for healing of the fistula repair. When it is not possible to exclude abnormal bowel or vagina, mobilization of the rectovaginal septum and tissue interposition is an option. This can be done abdominally (omentum, rectus abdominus muscle) in association with a resection, or as a perineal operation (gracilis, sartorius, gluteus, bulbocavernosus). The aim is to prevent apposition of areas of abnormal tissue and allow for closure. For failures or medically unfit patients, diversion may be performed. Repair can be performed in patients with IBD, but their rectal disease must first be medically controlled.

Outcome
If the procedure is properly selected, resolution of the fistula occurs in 70%-88% of patients regardless of the method. Clearly, patients with complex fistulas, including recurrences, have a higher failure rate, although success rates as high as 85%-100% have been reported.[51]

3. Dermatologic Conditions

Condyloma Acuminatum

Definition
Condyloma acuminatum infection of the perianal skin and anal canal occurs as a result of infection with the human papillomavirus (HPV).

Epidemiology
It is estimated that there are 15 million individuals affected with genital HPV (condyloma) in the United States, and 2 million new cases each year.[52] Since many patients have subclinical disease, patients with visible warts may account for only 10% of all cases infected with the virus. It is more common in homosexual males, comprising 45%-90% of all cases, and in immunocompromised patients. One study found 60% of HIV-infected patients to have anal warts, as opposed to 17% of HIV-negative patients. Clinically evident infection increases with declining CD4+ cell counts.[53]

Etiology
The human papillomavirus is the causative agent, and more than 60 types of HPV have been identified. Of the more common subtypes, HPV-6 and HPV-11 are associated with benign condyloma, while types 16 and 18 have more malignant potential. There are other less frequently seen types that have even greater malignant potential.

Clinical Presentation
The incubation period is 1-3 months after initial contact and many patients are unaware of their sexual exposure. The lesions appear as soft, cauliflower-like growths in and around the anal canal. Patients complain of itching, discharge, bleeding and pain. A sexual history should be elicited, although anal receptive intercourse is not required for the development of perianal condyloma.

Evaluation
The external physical examination should include the genitals as well as the perianal area. More importantly, a careful examination of the anal canal must be performed. Only 6% of patients have condyloma isolated to the perianal skin and 11% have intra-anal warts only.[54] It is impossible to eradicate the external disease without addressing the intra-anal component. If treatment has been carried out, 5% acetic acid applied to the perianal skin may

reveal additional lesions. Because of the association with other sexually transmitted diseases, appropriate testing should be performed. Patients with extensive warts and high-risk sexual or other behaviors should undergo HIV testing.

Squamous cell carcinoma is a potential finding as well, especially in the HIV+ patient population. In these cases, generally a firm or ulcerated area may be palpated associated with the lesions. Giant condyloma, or Buschke-Löwenstein tumor, is a locally aggressive squamous cell cancer which may invade fascia and muscle and is associated with condyloma disease. It should be suspected in any large condyloma. All specimens should be removed and all suspicious lesions should be biopsied and sent for pathologic examination.

Treatment

The primary modes of treatment are destruction, excision, immunotherapy, and local pharmacologic agents. Locally caustic agents include podophyllin and bi- or trichloroacetic acid (BCA, TCA). These are applied to the visible lesions (BCA and TCA may be used in the anal canal) every 1-2 weeks. Multiple visits are necessary and their use is not appropriate for extensive disease. Use is limited to patients with minimal disease and as an adjunct following excision. Imiquimod has also been studied and found to be effective, with the advantage of patient self-application. Destruction with electrocautery, cryotherapy or laser is frequently used. Laser therapy has no proven advantage and may have a higher recurrence rate and be associated with more pain. Added to this is the risk potential from aerosolized virus. Each modality may be used on more extensive lesions and in the anal canal, but generally require the operating room for anesthesia.

Operative excision is advantageous for extensive lesions, for lesions in the anal canal, and for obtaining pathologic specimens. It is definitely indicated if carcinoma is suspected. The use of the Cavitron® ultrasonic aspirator (CUSA) for large lesions has been described with very good success. These large lesions are associated with more bleeding and the CUSA may decrease blood loss.

Preparation of vaccine using the patient's own warts has been studied. 5 grams of the patient's wart tissue are needed for vaccine preparation, and the vaccine is injected intramuscularly for 6 weeks. It may be used following local destruction or excision to reduce recurrence, or as primary therapy. There have been no adverse reactions reported. This treatment is not widely available.

Interferon injected systemically or intralesionally may benefit patients with recurrent disease, extensive lesions or disease that has not responded to conventional therapy. Topical 5-fluorouracil has also been used in patients following ablation of lesions to prevent recurrences.

Outcome

Recurrence rates range from 4% with aggressive multimodality therapy to 30% in HIV+ individuals. Recurrence is affected by individual behaviors, extent of disease, and appropriateness of therapy. Generally, recurrences can be minimized by initial eradication of all visible condyloma, including intraanal lesions, followed by periodic examinations and use of adjuncts such as locally caustic agents, interferon, and potentially immunotherapy for very high-risk individuals. Additionally, all partners should be examined and treated.[55]

Hidradenitis Suppurativa

Definition

Hidradenitis suppurativa is a chronic infection of the apocrine glands and may occur in the perineum, axilla, and inframammary creases. It is characterized by sinuses and tracts originating in the apocrine glands and tunneling into the subcutaneous tissues.

Epidemiology

This chronic infection of the apocrine glands occurs in the perianal and genital area in 15% of patients with hidradenitis.[56] It more commonly affects men and African Americans, usually occurring following puberty. The exact incidence is not known.

Etiology

Hidradenitis is a chronic infection of the apocrine glands initiated by keratin obstruction of the gland orifice. Obstruction may occur because of glandular abnormalities, poor hygiene, obesity, excessive sweating or ill-fitting clothing. Suppuration ensues with rupture into the subcutaneous tissue and the formation of pits and multiple tracts. Infection is most commonly by *Staphylococcus*, *Streptococcus* and coliforms. The chronicity leads to thickening and fibrosis of the skin and subcutaneous tissues.

There may be a hormonal influence as well. Empirical evidence for this includes the onset of hydradenitis with puberty, its exacerbation with the use of oral contraceptives, and clinical improvement with progesterone/estrogen manipulation, menses and pregnancy. Abnormalities in the hypothalamo-pituitary axis and elevations in testosterone levels have been demonstrated in patients with the disease.

Clinical Presentation

Patients generally present in their second and third decade with pain, itching and drainage. They may also complain of symptoms in associated areas such as the axillae, inframammary creases and inguinal folds. There is an association with arthritis and Crohn's disease as well. One selected study found a 35% incidence of Crohn's disease in patients with hydradenitis.[57] While this is probably higher than in most populations, it should be considered during evaluation.

Evaluation

The differential diagnosis includes pilonidal disease, Crohn's disease and ischiorectal abscess. Other potential areas of involvement should be inspected. An anoscopic or proctoscopic exam is performed to evaluate for anorectal conditions, such as cryptoglandular abscess, fistula and Crohn's disease.

Treatment

The initial treatment of acute disease with associated abscess formation is incision and drainage. Antibiotics effective against the suspected organisms may be used as an adjunct but are not effective as primary therapy. Unroofing and limited drainage may be effective for initial control of infection, but not for definitive treatment. The gold standard is full thickness, wide surgical debridement to subcutaneous fat. Most debridements, despite the initial appearance, will eventually close by secondary intention and do not need skin graft or flap coverage. If healing does not occur, these techniques may be used.

Outcome

The course is one of recurrence and progression to fibrosis with the extent depending on the area of involvement. Local surgical treatment has a nearly 100% recurrence rate. Even with surgical debridement, up to 50% of patients may require additional surgery and treatment for recurrent symptoms in the surrounding region.[56]

4. Neoplastic Anorectal Disease

Anal Canal and Perianal Neoplasms

Definition

The literature regarding anal canal and perianal neoplasms has been inconsistent because of differences in anatomic definitions of these disorders. The World Health Organization classification scheme is an attempt to clarify the anatomic issues. The anal canal extends from the pelvic floor to the anal verge, or the extent of the internal sphincter. There are 3 types of epithelium: columnar (upper); transitional, including columnar and squamous (middle); and squamous (lower). The anal margin or perianal skin is comprised of squamous epithelium and extends from the lower edge of the anal canal (anal verge) to the hair-bearing perianal skin, which is usually 5-6 cm from the anal verge.

Epidemiology

Malignant anal neoplasms comprise 6% or less of anorectal cancers, and more than 85% are anal canal tumors. The incidence in the United States has increased recently, perhaps due to the spread of HPV and HIV infection. Most patients are in their sixth or seventh decade, with less than 5% younger than 45 years old. Anal canal carcinomas occur more frequently in women, whereas perianal cancers predominate in men. Associated risk factors are anal receptive intercourse and immunocompromise, especially from HIV and HPV infection. Neoplasms associated with immunocompromise are usually squamous cell, occur in younger patients, and are more aggressive with a higher recurrence rate.[58]

Histology

Perianal. Squamous cell cancers are the most frequent histologic type found in the anal margin. Basal cell cancer, adenocarcinoma, verrucous carcinoma or giant condyloma, and Kaposi's sarcoma also occur. Premalignant lesions are Bowen's disease (*in situ* squamous cell cancer), Paget's disease (*in situ* adenocarcinoma), leukoplakia and condyloma.[59,60]

Anal Canal. Epidermoid cancers, most commonly squamous carcinoma, occur most frequently. Other epidermoid cancers include basaloid, cloacogenic, mucoepidermoid and transitional cell. They all tend to follow the same course and are treated similarly. Other histologic types occurring infrequently are melanoma, adenocarcinoma (of the anal glands) and sarcoma.

Clinical Presentation

Perianal. The presentation of premalignant lesions and cancers is usually with pruritus, drainage and minor bleeding. More than one-half of cases are diagnosed 2 years after symptoms develop, and nearly one-third are initially misdiagnosed.

Anal Canal. One-half of patients with anal canal cancer will have bleeding as a complaint. The other nonspecific symptoms of discharge, pruritus and pain may explain why many patients experience a delay in diagnosis. If pelvic pain, changes in bowel habits or incontinence occur, the sphincter is usually involved and the lesions are advanced.

Evaluation

Physical examination is the most important diagnostic modality for anal neoplasms. Additionally, because lymphatic drainage of anal neoplasms can be through the superior hemorrhoidal, internal iliac or inguinal lymphatics, examination of the groin and biopsy or fine-needle aspiration of any suspicious nodes must be performed. Most patients are elderly, and many of the tumors have an associated increased risk of colonic neoplasms, so colonoscopy should be performed as appropriate.

Perianal. Bowen's and Paget's diseases are potentially malignant lesions of the perianal region. They appear as erythematous, eczematous rashes that may ooze. Squamous and basal cell cancers have appearances similar to those located elsewhere on the skin. Verrucous carcinomas, also known as giant condylomas and Buschke-Löwenstein tumors, are large, slowly growing, cauliflower-like masses that may extend into the anal canal and invade fascia. Any perianal skin abnormality that does not respond to appropriate management should undergo biopsy. Bowen's disease and Paget's disease are reported to have a high association with other neoplasms. In Bowen's disease, other potential sites affected include the pulmonary system, gastrointestinal tract, genitourinary system and reticuloendothelial organs. Visceral carcinomas occur in nearly 50% of patients with Paget's disease.[59-62]

Anal Canal. Anal canal tumors may be visible externally and are always within reach of a DRE. When performing the DRE, attention should be paid to fixation, sphincter involvement and size. The groin should be examined for lymphadenopathy. Direct visualization of the tumor using anoscopy and biopsy are performed. Endoanal ultrasound, CT scan and MRI may provide information regarding depth and stage.

Staging

Both anal canal and perianal neoplasms are staged with the TNM system. The T stage is determined by the size of the lesion, and nodal assessment includes the groin, iliac, and perirectal regions. Lesions with nodal involvement or invasion of adjacent structures (not including the sphincter) are categorized as Stage III or greater (see Table 2).

Treatment

Perianal. Although these entities are usually benign, at least 5% of patients with Bowen's disease and up to 40% of patients with Paget's disease will develop invasive cancer if left untreated. Therefore, traditionally, both Bowen's disease and Paget's disease have been treated with wide local excision. The grossly normal-appearing surrounding areas are often involved microscopically. It has been recommended that mapping of the adjacent skin be performed by taking 4 quadrant biopsies 1 cm from the edge of the lesion, extending into the anal canal, until microscopic findings are normal. A second approach is close observation of patients for the development of lesions suspicious for invasion with expectant treatment.

Patients with large invasive cancers not amenable to local excision may require abdominoperineal resection (APR), potentially with chemoradiation.[59,60]

Malignant perianal lesions, including squamous, basal cell and verrucous carcinoma are treated with wide excision to microscopically clear margins. It may occasionally be necessary to perform an APR for large tumors to obtain clear margins. Chemoradiation is appropriate for squamous cell carcinoma and is being evaluated for verrucous carcinomas.

Anal Canal. Local excision is reserved for early lesions <2 cm in size invading only the submucosa. For all other lesions, more aggressive therapy is needed. Historically, APR was performed for anal canal tumors not amenable to local excision. With the recognition that chemoradiation therapy (Nigro protocol) results in improved local control and long-term survival, APR is now reserved for those with residual or recurrent tumor following this regimen.

Outcome

Perianal. In patients with noninvasive Paget's disease or Bowen's disease who undergo complete excision, cure is likely. Long-term follow-up to detect recurrences is recommended. Invasive Paget's disease has a poor prognosis, largely because one-quarter of patients will have metastases at the time of diagnosis. Of those without metastatic disease, aggressive therapy will result in a 60% 5-year survival rate.

Survival rates for appropriately-treated perianal carcinomas, including verrucous, squamous, and basal cell tumors, are greater than 75%. For squamous cell cancers, size is the most important determinant of survival because patients with T1 tumors have a 100% 5-year survival rate vs. only 40% for those with T3 tumors. In patients with Buschke-Löwenstein tumors, death results from extensive local disease rather than distant metastasis, and up to 50% will develop a local recurrence requiring additional surgery.[59-62]

Anal Canal. Squamous cell cancers of the anal canal have an excellent prognosis when discovered prior to nodal involvement and invasion of adjacent structures. In patients with Stage II or lower tumors, survival is 85% or greater. A factor having a negative impact on survival is T4 tumors and lymph node involvement. In patients with recurrence requiring salvage, APR has potential for cure, but long-term disease-free survival is less than 50%. Malignant melanoma, fortunately rare, has a dismal prognosis, with less than 5% 5-year survival.

Screening has potential for improving survival in patients with identifiable risk factors such as a history of anal intercourse or HPV or HIV infection. Testing using methods similar to the Pap smear

Table 2

Staging of Perianal and Anal Canal Neoplasms

Anal canal		**Perianal skin**	
Primary carcinoma (T)		**(T)**	
Tis	*in situ*	Tis	*in situ*
T1	<2 cm in size	T1	<2 cm
T2	2-5 cm in size	T2	2-5 cm
T3	>5 cm in size	T3	>5 cm
T4 invasion of adjacent organ (vagina, bladder, urethra—does not include sphincter)		T4	invasion of extradermal tissue
Regional Lymph Node (N)		**(N)**	
N0	no nodal involvement	N0	no nodal involvement
N1	perirectal lymph nodes	N1	regional nodes (inguinal)
N2	unilateral iliac/inguinal lymph nodes		
N3	perirectal and inguinal nodes or bilateral inguinal or iliac nodes		
Distant Metastasis (M)		**(M)**	
M0	no metastasis	M0	no metastasis
M1	metastasis	M1	metastasis
Stage		**Stage**	
1	T1, N0, M0	1	T1, N0, M0
2	T2-3, N0, M0	2	T2-3, N0, M0
3	T1-4, N1-3, M0	3	T4, N0, M0
	T4, N0, M0		T any, N1, 0
4	T any, N any, M1	4	T any, N any, M1

identifies early lesions prior to the development of invasive cancer, and may have value.[58,61-63]

Retrorectal and Presacral Tumors

Definition

The retrorectal or presacral space lies beneath the peritoneal reflection of the rectum, superior to Waldeyer's fascia, and just anterior to the presacral fascia overlying the presacral veins. The 2 broad classifications of disease are congenital lesions and neoplastic lesions.

Epidemiology

These are uncommon lesions, occurring in less than 1/40,000 people. They may be neoplastic in 95% of patients in the pediatric population, and less than 50% in adults.[64,65]

Classification

The most common congenital lesions are developmental cysts, including epidermoid, mucus-secreting, teratomas and dermoids, and they may be composed of cells from any of the germ layers. Other congenital lesions include anterior sacral meningocele and rectal duplication.

Neoplastic lesions comprise 60% of presacral tumors, and they may be neurogenic, osseous, fibrous, muscular, fatty or one of many other rare types of tumors.

Clinical Presentation

For all types of lesions, symptoms are related to the size of the lesion and the development of infection or carcinoma. Pain is more common with malignant lesions, but may also occur with infection. Cystic lesions may initially be mistaken for cryptoglandular abscesses, and may only be recognized after multiple recurrences. Patients occasionally complain of constipation and incontinence. The cysts may be discovered incidentally on physical exam, or may present during pregnancy with dystocia.

Evaluation

External examination sometimes reveals a dimple posterior to the anus, associated with a developmental cyst. Sphincter tone is assessed because some neurogenic and malignant lesions affect continence. Much can be discerned from DRE, and more than 97% of these lesions can be palpated. Attention should be paid to attributes such as the size, solid or cystic nature, location and fixation. Anoscopy or proctoscopy is performed and the mucosa examined for any abnormalities.

Additional evaluation includes plain x-rays. A malformed or absent sacrum is associated with some congenital lesions and malignant disease can result in destruction of the sacrum. MRI and CT are very helpful in defining the character and size of lesions, and involvement of adjacent structures. Endoanal ultrasound may also be useful. Biopsy has no role in the evaluation of these lesions.

Treatment

All lesions should be excised because of the risk of infection and potential for malignancy. The approach may be parasacral, abdominal or perineal. Complete excision must be performed with care taken not to disrupt cystic masses. For malignant lesions, radiation may be of additional benefit.

Outcome

Patients with completely excised lesions do quite well. Malignant lesions have a poor prognosis and few survivors beyond 5 years.[64,65]

Rectal Cancer

Definition

The rectum begins at the dentate line and extends proximally 13-15 cm to the rectosigmoid junction. It is arbitrarily divided into low (1-5 cm), middle (5-10 cm) and high rectum (10-15 cm). Rectal cancer is discussed separately from colon cancer because its treatment and ultimate outcome are often different, and because overall and disease-free survival rates are historically lower than for colon cancer. This is largely a result of the confined space of the pelvis leading to frequent involvement of contiguous structures and difficulty in completely resecting the tumor. The vast majority of malignant rectal tumors are adenocarcinomas, with carcinoid and lymphoma occurring infrequently.

Epidemiology

More than 35,000 people in the United States are diagnosed with rectal cancer each year. It is more common in developed countries, and in patients with IBD and familial polyp syndromes.

Clinical Presentation

The early symptoms of rectal cancer are often ascribed to benign anorectal disease such as hemorrhoids. The most common presenting symptoms are, in order of prevalence: bleeding, change in bowel habits, abdominal pain, obstruction and pelvic pain. Obstruction and anemia are unusual, and if they occur, they are usually a sign of advanced cancer. Pain is a more frequent complaint than with colon cancer because of the potential invasion of pelvic nerves, and/or adjacent organs. Presence of a bladder fistula implies bladder invasion.

Evaluation

There are many factors that impact the therapy of rectal cancer including the patient's general health, previous history of pelvic irradiation or pelvic surgery, continence and functional status. A thorough history and physical examination must be performed. Examination of the abdomen, liver, supraclavicular and groin lymph nodes, bimanual pelvic exam and DRE are performed. On DRE, sphincter integrity, level of the lesion if palpable, and fixation are assessed. Proctoscopic exam, and eventually colonoscopy with biopsy are performed. Laboratory evaluation includes complete blood count, and carcinoembryonic antigen (CEA) levels. A chest x-ray is obtained to assess for metastatic lesions. Abdominal and pelvic CT scan can provide information regarding liver metastasis, presence of ureter involvement or hydronephrosis, tumor depth (T stage), involvement of adjacent organs and sometimes lymphadenopathy. Endorectal ultrasound is the most sensitive method of determining tumor depth and is routine in many centers. MRI using endorectal coils has also been used with success. All of these modalities are best at determining local invasion or T stage, ranging from a 70% accuracy with clinical exam to >80% for endorectal ultrasound. They are not as accurate in determining lymph node involvement, ranging from 20%-65% in accuracy. CT scan has the advantage of evaluating for metastatic disease and is reasonably accurate for staging T3 and more advanced local disease. For earlier stage tumors (T1-T2), endorectal ultrasound and MRI are more accurate for defining the T stage.[66-68]

Staging

Accurate preoperative staging is very important in rectal cancer because it often determines the need or appropriateness for neoadjuvant chemotherapy, local excision, or rectal resection. The staging of rectal cancer is primarily by the TNM staging system as shown in Table 3. Tumor depth is assessed through clinical exam and radiographic studies, especially endorectal ultrasound. Since the existing modalities are only fair at identifying perirectal lymph node involvement, historical data regarding risk of lymphatic spread based on depth is used (see Table 3). Potential sites of metastatic disease are regional (pelvic walls), liver, lymph nodes (inguinal, inferior mesenteric artery), lung, lumbosacral spine and brain.

Histology of the tumor affects the prognosis as well and should be considered in treatment decisions. Poor prognostic features include poor differentiation and lymphovascular invasion.

For patients undergoing resection, pathologic staging is performed. There is controversy regarding the staging of patients who have reduced tumor size following neoadjuvant therapy. In general, these patients are treated based on their pretreatment stage.

Treatment

An assessment of the intent of surgery (curative vs. palliative), staging, and medical and functional status of the patient must be taken into account when planning therapy for rectal cancer. Although morbidity and mortality of rectal resection has decreased since the era of Miles in the early 1900s, it is still significant. If the tumor is deemed curable, the next decision is the need for local or rectal resection. Generally, only early lower and middle rectal noncircumferential tumors without negative prognostic features are considered for local excision. Local excision can be performed through a transanal route or posteriorly through a parasacral incision (Kraske). The Kraske approach has a high rate of fistula formation and infectious complications and is rarely performed. Final pathologic staging and margins will determine if further treatment is needed, including rectal resection and/or chemoradiation.

For tumors requiring rectal resection, the next decision regards the use of neoadjuvant therapy. Numerous studies favor the use of preoperative chemoradiation for downstaging and improved local control and survival for stage 2 and greater tumors. Postoperatively, tissues are relatively ischemic and chemoradiation is not as effective. Additionally, avoiding radiation exposure to the anastomosis and reservoir is appealing from a healing and functional perspective when reconstructive operations are used.[67-72]

The options for rectal resection include sphincter preservation or APR. With the advent of circular staplers which allow for very low anastomoses, recognition that a distal margin of 1-2 cm is adequate, and effective adjuvant therapy, an APR should be necessary in less than 10% of rectal cancers. An APR is reserved for very low tumors in which a 1 cm distal margin is not possible, sphincter invasion, and patients with preexisting poor sphincter tone and continence. In the remaining tumors, low anterior resection with colorectal or coloanal anastomosis is possible. There is improved function when a neoreservoir is created, utilizing a colonic J pouch. The decision to use a temporary diverting stoma is influenced by the patient's general medical condition, nutrition, history of pelvic radiation, level of the anastomosis and technical details of the operation.

Technical. Patients undergo bowel preparation prior to surgery. If there is potential for a stoma, preoperative stoma site marking is important. In the operating room, patients undergoing local excision may be placed in the supine or prone position, largely depending on tumor location. For most abdominal cases, the perineal portion is performed in the lithotomy position. A DRE is performed to reassess tumor depth and location.

For rectal resection, the key technical details are the use of sharp mesorectal excision (TME) under direct visualization, obtaining a distal margin of >1 cm, paying attention to radial margins, and en bloc resection of involved pelvic structures. It was initially demonstrated by Heald, and subsequently confirmed by numerous other studies, that TME decreases the risk of local recurrence and increases survival.[73] The use of a 1 cm margin is supported by evidence that there is rarely distal spread of rectal cancer, there is no increase in local recurrence or decreased survival in patients with this margin, and in tumors with distal spread beyond 1 cm survival is poor regardless of the margin obtained.[74] Obtaining free radial margins does influence outcome, and it may require taking pelvic sidewall and contiguous structures. En bloc excision and pelvic exenteration can also improve survival and should be performed in cases of curative surgery. The "no touch" technique of vessel ligation prior to tumor manipulation has not been shown to influence outcome and is unnecessary. High ligation of the inferior mesenteric artery is not necessary from an oncologic standpoint because outcome is not improved, but it is frequently beneficial in terms of colon mobilization and a tension-free anastomosis. At the time of rectal division, instillation of a tumoricidal agent such as Betadine® through a rectal catheter may reduce tumor implantation at the anastomosis and decrease local recurrence.

In cases of local excision, adequate margins must also be obtained. When the specimen is removed, it is oriented and pinned so that accurate margins can be assessed and reported.

Adjuvant Therapy. Chemotherapy is used in tumors with metastatic disease, including to lymph nodes. It may also be of benefit in tumors with adverse histologic features and invasion of perirectal tissues (Stage T3). It may be administered pre- or postoperatively. The common agents are 5-fluorouracil, leucovorin, and recently, oxaliplatin.

Radiation therapy can be used in rectal cancer for local control with excellent results. It may also be administered pre- or postoperatively. Adverse sequelae include radiation proctitis, loss of compliance, fistula and stricture.[67,69-71]

Palliative. Untreated rectal cancer may lead to fistulas, incontinence, ureteral invasion and obstruction, colon obstruction, pelvic nerve and sacral invasion with severe pain, and anemia. For these reasons, treatment including resection for palliation is usually undertaken. Alternative therapies may also be beneficial in patients with a limited life span or who are medically unfit to undergo surgery. Options

Table 3

Rectal Cancer Staging, Lymph Node Involvement and Survival

Primary carcinoma (T)		Lymph node involvement
Tis	*in situ* (intraepithelial/lamina propria invasion)	
T1	submucosal invasion	~10%
T2	muscularis propria invasion	~20%
T3	perirectal fat invasion	~40-60%
T4	invasion of adjacent structure	>80%

Regional Lymph Node (N)	
N0	no nodes
N1	1-3 perirectal lymph nodes
N2	>3 regional lymph nodes
N#	metastasis to node along named vascular trunk

Distant metastasis (M)	
M0	no metastasis
M1	metastasis

Stage		Dukes' classification	5-year survival
1	T1-2, N0, M0	A	75%-85%
2	T3-4, N0, M0	B	55%-77%
3	T1-4, N1-2, M0	C	30%-44%
4	T any, N any, M1	D	<25%

include chemoradiation as primary therapy, fulguration using laser or electrocoagulation, intracavitary radiation, and stenting with metallic expandable protheses.[67,69,75,76]

Outcome
The 2 primary goals of surgery for rectal cancer are control of local disease for symptom control and complete resection of tumor. Stage for stage, rectal cancer has a worse prognosis than colon cancer. As shown in Table 3, survival decreases markedly in patients with lymph node metastases. Oncologic goals of surgery are a distal margin of greater than 1 cm, clear radial margins, TME and en bloc resection of involved organs. Compromise of any of these tenets is associated with a poor outcome. If these goals are accomplished, local recurrence should occur in less than 10% of patients.

Complications of therapy are frequent. Bladder dysfunction (40%), sexual dysfunction (15%-40%), small bowel obstruction, anastomotic leak and stricture commonly occur, but can be minimized by careful surgical technique. Perineal wound problems such as nonhealing, sinuses and fistulas can complicate APR. Overall, nearly 18% of patients undergoing

APR will develop chronic perineal wound problems, and the rate may be higher in patients receiving radiation therapy.[67,69]

5. References

1. Nivatvongs S, Gordon PH. Surgical anatomy. In: Gordon PH, Nivatvongs S, eds. *Principles and Practice of Surgery for the Colon, Rectum and Anus*. 2nd ed. St. Louis, MO: Quality Medical Pub; 1999.

2. Jorge JMN. Anorectal anatomy and physiology. In: Beck DE, Wexner SD, eds. *Fundamentals of Anorectal Surgery*. 2nd ed. London, England: WB Saunders; 1998.

3. Seow-Choen F, Nicholls RJ. Anal fistula. *Br J Surg*. 1992;79:197-205.

4. Vanheuverzwyn R, Delannoy A, Michaux JL, Dive C. Anal lesions in hematologic diseases. *Dis Colon Rectum*. 1980;23:310-312.

5. MacKeigan JM. Anal fistula. *Sem Colon & Rectal Sur*g. 1990;1:211-218.

6. Parks AG. Pathogenesis and treatment of fistula-in-ano. *Br Med J*. 1976;1:463.

7. Vasilevsky CA, Gordon PH. The incidence of recurrent abscess or fistula-in-ano following anorectal suppuration. *Dis Colon Rectum*. 1984;27:126-130.

8. Gordon PH. Anorectal abscesses and fistula-in-ano. In: Gordon PH, Nivatvongs S, eds. *Principles and Practice of Surgery for the Colon, Rectum and Anus*. 2nd ed. St. Louis, MO: Quality Medical Pub; 1999.

9. Winslett MC, Allan A, Ambrose NS. Anorectal sepsis as a presentation of occult rectal and systemic disease. *Dis Colon Rectum*. 1988;31: 597-600.

10. Parks AG, Gordon PH, Hardcastle JE. A classification of fistula-in-ano. *Br J Surg*. 1976;19: 511-513.

11. Ramanujam PS, Prasad ML, Abcarian H, Tan AB. Perianal abscesses and fistulas: a study of 1023 patients. *Dis Colon Rectum*. 1984;27: 593-597.

12. Scoma JA, Salvati EP, Rubin RJ. Incidence of fistulas subsequent to anal abscesses. *Dis Colon Rectum*. 1974;17:357-359.

13. Cirocco WC, Reilly JC. Challenging the predictive accuracy of Goodsall's rule for anal fistulas. *Dis Colon Rectum*. 1992;35:537-542.

14. Lockhart-Mummery HE. Anal lesions in Crohn's disease. *Br J Surg*. 1985;75:S95 S96.

15. Alexander-Williams J, Buchmann P. Perianal Crohn's disease. *World J Surg*. 1980;4:203-208.

16. Hanley PH. Anorectal abscess fistula. *Surg Clin North Am*. 1978;58:487-503.

17. Christensen A, Nilas L, Christiansen J. Treatment of transsphincteric anal fistulas by the seton technique. *Dis Colon Rectum*. 1986;29:454-455.

18. Fleshman JW. Fissure-in-ano and anal stenosis. In: Beck DE, Wexner SD, eds. *Fundamentals of Anorectal Surgery*. 2nd ed. London, England: WB Saunders; 1998.

19. Surrell, JA. Anal fissure. *Sem Colon Rectal Surg*. 1990;4:207-210.

20. Klosterhalfen B, Vogel P, Rixen H, Mittermayer C. Topography of the inferior rectal artery: a possible cause of chronic, primary anal fissure. *Dis Colon Rectum*. 1989;32:43-52.

21. Schouten WR, Briel JW, Auwerda JJA, De Graaf E. Ischemic nature of anal fissure. *Br J Surg*. 1996;83:63-65.

22. Hananel N, Gordon PH. Re-examination of clinical manifestations and response to treatment of fissure-in-ano. Dis Colon Rectum. 1997;40:229-233.

23. Lock MR, Thomson JPS. Fissure-in-ano: the initial management and prognosis. *Br J Surg*. 1977;65:355-358.

24. Richard C, Gregoire R, Plewes A, et al. A randomized, controlled trial comparing topical nitroglycerin and internal sphincterotomy in the treatment of chronic anal fissure. *Dis Colon Rectum*. 1999;42:A13.

25. Antropoli C, Perroti P, Rubino M, et al. Nifedipine for local use in conservative treatment of anal fissures. *Dis Colon Rectum*. 1999;42:1011-1015.

25a. Kocher HM, Steward M, Leather AJ, Cullen PT. Randomized clinical trial assessing the side-effects of glyceryl trinitrate and diltiazem hydrochloride in the treatment of chronic anal fissure. *Br J Surg*. 2002 Apr;89(4):413-417.

25b. Griffin N, Acheson AG, Jonas M, Scholefield JH. The role of topical diltiazem in the treatment of chronic anal fissures that have failed glyceryl trinitrate therapy. *Colorectal Dis*. 2002 Nov;4(6):430-435.

26. Jost WH, Schimrigk K. Botulinum toxin in therapy of anal fissure. *Lancet*. 1995;345:188-189.

27. Jensen SL, Lund F, Nielson OV, Tange G. Lateral subcutaneous sphincterotomy vs. anal dilatation in the treatment of fissure-in-ano in outpatients: A prospective randomized study. *Br Med J*. 1984;289:528-530.

28. Allen-Mersh TG. Pilonidal sinus: finding the right track for treatment. *Br J Surg*. 1990;77:123-132.

29. Nivatvongs, S. Pilonidal disease. In: Gordon PH, Nivatvongs S, eds. Principles and *Practice of Surgery for the Colon, Rectum and Anus*. 2nd ed. St. Louis, MO: Quality Medical Pub; 1999.

30. McLaren CA. Partial closure and other techniques in pilonidal surgery: an assessment of 157 cases. *Br J Surg*. 1984;71:561-562.

31. Johanson JF, Sonnenberg A. Prevalence of hemorrhoids and chronic constipation. An epidemiologic study. *Gastroenterology*. 1990;98:380-386.

32. Thomson WHF. The nature of hemorrhoids. *Br J Surg*. 1975;62:542-552.

33. Moesgaard F, Nielsen ML, Hansen JB, Knudsen JT. High fiber diet reduces bleeding and pain in patients with hemorrhoids. *Dis Colon Rectum*. 1982;25:454-456.

34. Schouten WR, vanVroonhoven TJ. Lateral internal sphincterotomy in the treatment of hemorrhoids: A clinical and manometric study. *Dis Colon Rectum*. 1986;29:869-872.

34a Ho YH, Cheong WK, Tsang C, et al. Stapled hemorrhoidectomy—cost and effectiveness. Randomized, controlled trial including incontinence scoring, anorectal monometry, and endoanal ultrasound assessments at up to three months. *Dis Colon & Rectum*. 2000;43:1666-1775.

34b. Singer MA, Cintron JR, Fleshman JW, et al. Early experience with stapled hemorrhoidectomy in the United States. *Dis Colon & Rectum*. 2002;45:360-367.

34c. Hetzer FH, Demartines N, Handschin AE, Clavien PA. Stapled vs excision hemorrhoidectomy: long-term results of a prospective trial. *Arch of Surg*. 2002;137:337-340.

34d. Dixon M, Stamos M, Grant S, et al: Stapled Hemorrhoidectomy: A Review of Our Early Experience. *Am Surgeon*. (In Press)

35. Johanson JF, Rimm A. Optimal nonsurgical treatment of hemorrhoids: a comparative analysis of infrared coagulation, rubber band ligation and injection sclerotherapy. *Am J Gastroenterol*. 1992;87:1601-1606.

36. Nelson R, Norton N, Cautley E, Furner S. Community-based prevalence of anal incontinence. *JAMA*. 1995;274:559-561.

37. Johanson JF, Lafferty J. Epidemiology of fecal incontinence: the silent affliction. *Am J Gastroenterol*. 1996;91:33-36.

38. Sangwan YP, Coller JA. Fecal incontinence. *Surg Clin North Am*. 1994;74:1377-1398.

38a. Sultan AH, Kamm MA, Hudson CN, Thomas JM, Bartram CI. Anal-sphincter disruption during vaginal delivery. *N Engl J Med*. 1993 Dec 23;329(26):1905-11.

39. Jorge JMN. Anorectal anatomy and physiology. In: Beck DE, Wexner SD, eds. *Fundamentals of Anorectal Surgery*. 2nd ed. Philadelphia, PA: WB Saunders; 1998.

40. Wexner SD, Marchetti F, Jagelman D. The role of sphincteroplasty for fecal incontinence reevaluated: a prospective physiologic and functional review. *Dis Colon Rectum*. 1991;34:22-30.

41. Enck P, Daublin G, Lubke HJ, Strohmeyer G. Long-term efficacy of biofeedback training for fecal incontinence. *Dis Colon Rectum*. 1994;37:997-1001.

42. Sitzler PJ, Thomson JPS. Overlap repair of damaged anal sphincter. *Dis Colon Rectum*. 1996;39:1356-1360.

43. Wexner SD, Gonzalez-Padron A, Rius J, et al. Stimulated gracilis neosphincter operation. Initial experience, pitfalls, and complications. *Dis Colon Rectum*. 1996;39:957-964.

44. Wong WD, Jensen LL, Bartolo DCC, Rothenberger DA. Artificial anal sphincter. *Dis Colon Rectum*. 1996;39:1345-1351.

44a. Wong WD, Congliosi SM, Spencer MP, et al. The safety and efficacy of the artificial bowel sphincter for fecal incontinence: results from a multicenter cohort study. *Dis Colon Rectum*. 2002;45(9):1139-1153.

45. Kupfer CA, Goligher JC. One hundred consecutive cases of complete prolapse of the rectum treated by operation. *Br J Surg*. 1970;57:481-487.

46. Watts JD, Rothenberger DA, Buis JG, Goldberg SM, Nivatvongs S. The management of procidentia: 30 years experience. *Dis Colon Rectum*. 1985;28:96-102.

47. Eisenstat TE, Rubin RJ, Salvati EP. Surgical treatment of complete rectal prolapse. *Dis Colon Rectum*. 1979;22:522-523.

48. Gordon PH. Rectal procidentia. In: Gordon PH, Nivatvongs S, eds. *Principles and Practice of Surgery for the Colon, Rectum and Anus*. 2nd ed. St. Louis, Missouri, MO: Quality Medical Pub; 1999.

49. Senagore A. Treatment of acquired anovaginal and rectovaginal fistulas. *Sem Colon Rectal Surg*. 1990;1:219-223.

50. Lowry AC. Rectovaginal fistulas. In: Beck DE, Wexner SD, eds. *Fundamentals of Anorectal Surgery*. 2nd ed. Philadelphia, Pennsylvania, PA: WB Saunders; 1998.

51. Rothenberger DA, Goldberg SM. The management of rectovaginal fistulae. *Surg Clin North Am*. 1983;13:451.

52. Murphy R. Sexually transmitted diseases. In: Shulman S, Phair J, Sommers H, eds. *The Biological and Clinical Basis for Infectious Diseases,* 4th ed. Philadelphia,PA. WB Saunders; 1992.

53. Breese P, Judson FN, Penley KA, Douglas JM. Anal human papillomavirus infection among homosexual and bisexual men: prevalence of type-specific infection and association with human immunodeficiency virus. *Sex Transm Dis*. 1995;22:7-14.

54. Sohn N, Robilotti JG. The gay bowel syndrome, a review of colonic and rectal conditions in 200 male homosexuals. *Am J Gastroenterol*. 1977;67:478-484.

55. Swerdlow DB, Salvati EP. Condyloma acuminatum. *Dis Colon Rectum*. 1971;14:226-229.

56. Culp CE. Chronic hidradenitis suppurativa of the anal canal: a surgical skin disease. *Dis Colon Rectum*. 1983;26:669-676.

57. Tsianos EV, Dalekos GN, Tzermias C, Merkouropoulos M, Hatzis J. Hidradenitis suppurativa in Crohn's disease. A further support of this association. *J Clin Gastroenterol*. 1995;20:151-153.

58. Myerson RJ, Shapiro SJ, Lacey D, et al. Carcinoma of the anal canal. *Am J Clin Oncol*. 1995;18:32-39.

59. Cleary RK, Schaldenbrand JD, Fowler JJ, Schuler JM, Lampman RM. Perianal Bowen's disease and anal intraepithelial neoplasia. Review of the literature. *Dis Colon Rectum*. 1999;42:945-951.

60. Beck DE. Paget's disease and Bowen's disease of the anus. *Semin Colon Rectal Surg*. 1995;6:143-149.

61. Nivatvongs S. Perianal and anal canal neoplasms. In: Gordon PH, Nivatvongs S, eds. *Principles and Practice of Surgery for the Colon, Rectum and Anus*. 2nd ed. St. Louis, MO: Quality Medical Pub; 1999.

62. Beck DE, Wexner SD. Anal neoplasms. In: Beck DE, Wexner SD, eds. *Fundamentals of Anorectal Surgery*. 2nd ed. London, England: WB Saunders; 1998.

63. Tanum G, Tveit K, Karlsen KO, Hauer-Jensen M. Chemotherapy and radiation therapy for anal carcinoma. *Cancer*. 1991;67:24

64. Jao SW, Beart RW, Spencer RJ, Reiman HM, Ilstrup DM. Retrorectal tumors. Mayo Clinic experience. *Dis Colon Rectum*. 1985;28:644-652.

65. Stewart RJ, Humphreys WG, Parks TG. The presentation and management of presacral tumours. *Br J Surg*. 1986;73:153-155.

66. Wong WD, Orrom WJ, Jensen LL. Preoperative staging of rectal cancer with endorectal ultrasonography. *Perspect Colon Rectal*. 1990;3:315-334.

67. Gordon PH. Malignant neoplasms of the rectum. In: Gordon PH, Nivatvongs S, eds. *Principles and Practice of Surgery for the Colon, Rectum, and Anus*. 2nd ed. St. Louis, MO: Quality Medical Pub; 1999.

68. Kim D, Wong WD, Bleday R. Rectal carcinoma: Etiology and evaluation. In: Beck DE, Wexner SD, eds. *Fundamentals of Anorectal Surgery*. 2nd ed. London, England: WB Saunders; 1998.

69. Chandler PJ, Orkin BA. Rectal carcinoma: Operative treatment. In: Beck DE, Wexner SD, eds. *Fundamentals of Anorectal Surgery*. 2nd ed. London, England: WB Saunders; 1998.

70. Heriot AG, Kumar D. Adjuvant therapy for resectable rectal and colonic cancer. *Br J Surg*. 1998;85:300-309.

71. Freedman GM, Coia LR. Adjuvant and neoadjuvant treatment of rectal cancer. *Sem Onc*. 195;22:611-624.

72. Minsky B, Cohen A, Enker W, et al. Preoperative 5-fluorouracil, low-dose leucovorin, and concurrent radiation therapy for rectal cancer. *Cancer*. 1994;73:272-278.

73. Heald RJ, Husband EM, Ryall RDH. The mesorectum in rectal cancer surgery: The clue to pelvic recurrence? *Br J Surg*. 1982;69:13-16.

74. Pollet WG, Nicholls RJ. The relationship between the extent of distal clearance and survival and local recurrence rates after curative anterior resection for carcinoma of the rectum. *Ann Surg*. 1984;198:159-163.

75. Fritsch A, Seidl W, Walzel C. Palliative and adjunctive measures in rectal cancer. *World J Surg*. 1982;6:569-577.

76. Arnell T, Stamos MJ, Takahashi P, Ojha S, Sze G, Eysselein V. Colonic stents in colorectal obstruction. *Am Surg*. 1998;64(10):986-988.

6. Questions

Note: Questions may have one, more than one or no correct responses.

1. A 28-year-old male presents with pain and perianal swelling. On physical examination he has induration and erythema left and lateral of the anus. There is no fluctuance or induration on DRE. Appropriate management includes:

   A. Oral antibiotics and sitz baths.

   B. Incision and drainage of a perianal abscess without antibiotics.

   C. Incision and drainage of a perianal abscess with primary fistulotomy if a fistula is identified.

   D. Observe and wait for spontaneous drainage of the abscess.

2. A 35-year-old female undergoing chemotherapy for leukemia develops perianal pain. Physical examination of the area does not demonstrate erythema, induration, or other skin changes. DRE is normal except for severe tenderness. Appropriate management includes:

   A. Observation without antibiotics.

   B. Observation and broad-spectrum antibiotics.

   C. Bedside incision and drainage of involved area.

   D. Exam under anesthesia with debridement or drainage as needed.

3. A 56-year-old female is seen with the complaint of bleeding per rectum for several years. She states the bleeding is only with bowel movements, is painless, drips into the toilet bowl and is never mixed with the stool. She is healthy, without family history of cancer and has not had previous evaluation of her colon. Her only abnormality is iron-deficiency anemia. On anoscopy she has grade 2 internal hemorrhoids. Appropriate evaluation includes:

   A. Physical examination including DRE and anoscopy, along with reassurance that no further evaluation or treatment is needed other than stool softeners.

   B. Rigid proctoscopy to 15 cm and if no abnormalities are found, stool softeners and hemorrhoid banding.

   C. Flexible sigmoidoscopy and if normal, hemorrhoid banding.

   D. Colonoscopy and if normal, hemorrhoid banding.

4. An 18-year-old male complains of pain with each bowel movement, which continues for several hours following. There is a small amount of blood on the toilet paper after a bowel movement, otherwise no bleeding. He denies constipation or straining. Aside from the pain, his bowel function is normal. On examination, he is found to have a painful fissure in the anterior midline. A DRE is difficult because of pain and a hypertensive sphincter. This history is most consistent with:

   A. Potential IBD because the fissure is not posterior and he has no history of straining or constipation.

   B. Painful internal hemorrhoids.

   C. *Fissure in ano.*

   D. *Fitula in ano.*

5. Common features of pilonidal disease include:

A. Infecting organisms are limited to gram-positive organisms such as *Staphylococcus* and *Streptococcus*.

B. If adequate surgical excision is performed, recurrence is the exception.

C. Resolution of symptoms is seen during the fifth decade.

D. There is an increased risk of cancer in the involved area.

6. A 45-year-old female is referred with stool incontinence. She has a history of a fourth degree obstetrical injury 10 years ago, but only in the last 2 years has developed urgency, incontinence to gas, and liquid stool. DRE demonstrates an intact anal wink, a left anterolateral sphincter defect with diminished squeeze pressures, and an intact puborectalis squeeze. Initial management may include:

A. Diet management.

B. Biofeedback.

C. Overlapping sphincter repair.

D. placement of an artificial sphincter.

7. A 65-year-old female has a multiyear history of constipation and straining, and has recently developed rectal prolapse with leakage and pruritus, requiring manual reduction. Further evaluation should include:

A. Nothing beyond a physical examination.

B. Colonoscopy.

C. Colonic transit study.

D. Manometry.

8. Further evaluation of the above patient is without abnormality except reduced resting and squeeze sphincter pressures. Potential therapy may include:

A. Medical management with dietary fiber and counseling regarding straining.

B. Perineal rectosigmoidectomy.

C. Ripstein rectopexy (mesh).

D. Sigmoid resection with suture rectopexy.

9. An abdominoperineal resection (APR) is generally indicated in which situations:

A. Anal melanoma with lung metastases.

B. A T3, N1 rectal cancer 8 cm from the anal verge.

C. A patient who has received chemoradiation for squamous cell anal cancer found to have residual tumor on post-therapy biopsy.

D. A T2 rectal cancer 4 cm from the anal verge in an obese, blind elderly female.

10. Adjuvant therapy in rectal cancer:

A. Should always include radiation therapy.

B. Is more effective if given after surgery when the pathology and stage is known.

C. May be used in patients who have had radiation for other pelvic malignancies as long as it wasn't for rectal cancer, and was more than 20 years previously.

D. Is not necessary if a local excision is performed.

Answers

1. B., C.
This patient has an anal abscess based on history and physical examination. Antibiotics may be used as an adjunct if significant cellulitis is present after incision and drainage of the abscess. The use of antibiotics without drainage can make identification of the abscess more difficult, and may create a more complex abscess.
B.: This is appropriate for an otherwise healthy individual who is not immunocompromised or systemically ill. Most anorectal suppuration can be treated in this manner.
C.: The decision as to whether to perform a fistulotomy at the time of incision and drainage is based on the ability to identify the internal opening, the experience of the surgeon and the understanding that nearly one-half of anorectal abscesses will not recur or become fistulas. A primary fistulotomy may be safely performed at the initial surgery if these criteria are met.
D.: This is never appropriate therapy. Some patients will present following spontaneous drainage, and if complete drainage has occurred, no further intervention other than follow-up is necessary.

2. B., D.
Patients with significant immunosuppression may not mount a response, eg, patients with neutropenia, those taking immunosuppressant drugs and those with AIDS may not mount an inflammatory response. Therefore, the typical findings of an infection (ie, swelling, erythema, purulence) may not be present. In the setting of perianal pain without evidence of an external hemorrhoid thrombosis or obvious fissure, it should be assumed that a perianal infection exists and appropriate broad-spectrum antibiotics begun.
B.: There is controversy in the literature as to whether surgical intervention or antibiotics and observation are the optimal treatment. Observation with broad-spectrum antibiotics may be adequate, but close follow-up is required and if improvement is not rapid, surgery should be performed.
C.: Because these patients are unable to mount an adequate immune response and their primary complaint is of pain, an adequate bedside examination without sedation is rarely adequate.
D.: Examination under anesthesia to evaluate for the presence of pus or necrotic tissue is appropriate. Extensive debridement should not be performed unless necrotic tissue is identified. It is safe to make incisions to look for purulence, and failure to do so may result in an inadequate examination.

3. D.
Although the bleeding described is very typical of internal hemorrhoids, the presence of iron-deficiency anemia is very unusual for hemorrhoids. In addition, her age mandates evaluation of her colon. While diet management may be sufficient for treatment of her hemorrhoids, it is important to evaluate for concomitant colonic lesions.
B.: Again, proctoscopy is not sufficient to evaluate for iron-deficiency anemia.
C.: Flexible sigmoidoscopy is adequate in combination with occult blood testing or contrast enema for a screening examination, but not for a patient with symptomatic bleeding and anemia. A full colon evaluation is required.
D.: This is the most appropriate therapy if another source of anemia is not identified (including gynecologic and gastroduodenal sources). Banding is very effective for management of bleeding internal hemorrhoids.

4. C.
Although 90% of fissures occur in the posterior midline, 10% occur anteriorly. In a patient with typical symptoms and a typical appearance on examination, an anterior location does not mandate evaluation for IBD. Many studies demonstrate that less than one-half of patients will have a history of straining or constipation, so this does not mandate evaluation either.
B.: Internal hemorrhoids are not painful unless they are strangulated or gangrenous. It is important to remember that only 30% of patients who present with "hemorrhoids" will be found to have hemorrhoids as the source of their complaints.
C.: This is the most likely diagnosis, and if he responds to medical treatment, no further evaluation is necessary.
D.: *Fistula in ano* is not painful. If there is an abscess associated with the fistula, this may be painful and incision and drainage is necessary.

5. C.
Although traditionally thought to involve only skin organisms, cultures are usually mixed and contain anaerobes. It is unusual to require antibiotics, and most acute infections respond to drainage. The presence of anaerobic organisms is common, and in and of itself does not challenge the diagnosis of pilonidal infection.
B.: Recurrent pilonidal disease is not uncommon, even with adequate surgical excision. Because it may be related to hair growth and hygiene, it is very important to counsel patients regarding hair removal and adequate cleaning of the area. Without patient compliance, recurrence is the rule.
C.: Because there may be a hormonal link, pilonidal disease tends to resolve in the fifth decade, and frequently begins after puberty. It may become quiescent during pregnancy as well.
D.: At one time it was believed that there is an increased risk of cancer, but this has not been conclusively demonstrated.

6. A., C.
Her history and physical examination is consistent with an obstetrical sphincter disruption. The reason for the new onset of symptoms could be a change in the character of her bowel movements (ie, diarrhea), an anorectal lesion that is compromising her rectal compliance or a generalized weakening of her pelvic floor. After evaluation for diarrhea or colorectal lesions, diet management is the first line of treatment and may be very effective, even in the face of a sphincter injury.
B.: Biofeedback may be of most benefit in patients with idiopathic and neurogenic incontinence. The improvement in patients with anatomical sphincter defects is much less predictable.
C.: This is very effective treatment for sphincter defects. Even in patients demonstrated to have pudendal nerve abnormalities, as is often the case in obstetrical injuries, success approaches 80%-90%.
D.: Because of the significant associated risks including infection, erosion, impaction, and the need for patient training, the use of neosphincters is reserved for patients who have failed repairs, and have neurogenic or idiopathic incontinence.

7. B., C.
Given her age, a general physical examination and determination of her medical status as well as evaluation of the remainder of her colon should be performed. This will help to determine appropriate treatment of the prolapse.
B.: Assuming she is a potential medical candidate for abdominal surgery, evaluation of her colon for concomitant neoplasms or a rectosigmoid source of straining should be performed. If she is not a candidate for an abdominal procedure because of prohibitive medical risks, colonoscopy is unnecessary and only the rectosigmoid needs evaluation.
C.: Given the long history of constipation, a colonic transit study should be considered. Patients with very slow colonic transit times may be candidates for colectomy with iliorectal anastomosis.
D.: Whether or not to perform manometry depends on the patient's history and physical examination. There is no study which will conclusively determine which patients will have resolution of constipation or incontinence. Manometry may be used as an adjunct and may aid in predicting which patients will have improvement of their incontinence, but is generally not required.

8. B., D.
A. This patient is symptomatic with pruritus drainage and a need for manual reduction. Although counseling is appropriate, unless she is not an operative candidate, surgical therapy should be performed.
B. Recent studies support the use of the perineal rectosigmoidectomy as primary therapy. There may be a higher recurrence rate, but there is significantly less morbidity and mortality. This is one surgical intervention that could be considered in this patient.
C. The use of prosthetic materials, especially a circumferential wrap such as the Ripstein, has been shown to worsen constipation. In patients with significant symptoms of constipation, prosthetics should be avoided. If prosthetics are used, circumferential wraps should not be performed
D. This would be an excellent choice in this patient. Because of her history of constipation, avoidance of prosthetics and sparing the lateral ligaments is recommended.

9. C.
The survival in a patient with metastatic melanoma is very limited and APR should be avoided. If significant perineal symptoms are present, consideration for a colostomy should be given.
B.: Generally, tumors at this level are amenable to a low anterior resection. This avoids the problems of perineal wounds, permanent stoma and reduces the risk of urinary and sexual dysfunction.
C.: Salvage APR for patients who fail chemoradiation therapy for anal canal squamous cancer is an accepted therapy. There is potential for cure with this procedure.
D.: Although a LAR with a coloanal anastomosis is a significant undertaking, this patient may have better function. Patients with poor vision and dexterity and obesity have difficulty managing stomas. Every consideration should be given to performing an anastomosis. Alternatively, patients with incontinence or dementia may be better served with a stoma rather than a perineal colostomy.

10. All responses are false.
Although radiation therapy is of benefit in reducing local recurrence in rectal cancer, it is not without complications. Potential adverse sequelae include radiation proctitis, stricture, small bowel injury, cystitis, loss of rectal compliance, and ureteral stricture. For these reasons, it should only be used in cases where its benefit exceeds the risks. Tumors with an increased risk of local recurrence include those that are Stage >T2 and have unfavorable pathologic features. Patients who have had previous pelvic surgery, hysterectomy, and previous radiation may or may not be candidates for radiation.
B.: There is evidence that preoperative radiation therapy does not have an adverse effect on the technical performance of the surgery, and may have better oncologic effect than postoperative radiation. This may be a result of the undisturbed blood supply of the tumor preoperatively, which maximizes the radiation effects. Additionally, functional results may be better since the anastomosis and rectal reservoir are spared radiation.
C.: Radiation effects are cumulative and permanent. If the maximum dosage has been given, regardless of the timing or the primary pelvic organ, additional significant external beam radiation may not be given without significant risk
D.: Local excision may be used for early tumors as well as for palliation. In early tumors with unfavorable pathologic features (<T2) consideration should be given to radiation with or without chemotherapy. For tumors >T2, local treatment options, even with adjuvant therapy, are suboptimal treatment. For palliation, radiation may be beneficial alone or in conjunction with local excision.

Chapter 14: Principles of Laparoscopic Surgery

Peter F. Crookes, MD

Contents

1. Introduction

The ability to inspect, dissect and resect abdominal viscera using laparoscopic techniques has transformed the perception and practice of surgery not just for surgeons but for patients and their referring physicians. Laparoscopy has not enabled the performance of operations that were hitherto impossible, but it has allowed many operations to be performed with a dramatic reduction in the cascade of changes seen after conventional major surgery: pain, metabolic stress, the prolonged need for pain medications and the subsequent delay in resumption of GI motility, atelectasis and other pulmonary problems, and the disruption of normal activities of daily living such as driving, eating, socializing and working. It has extended the spectrum of patients to whom surgery can be offered, permitting procedures on pregnant or very elderly patients. The economic effects of laparoscopic surgery are hard to measure, but it generally agreed that the greater direct costs of these procedures compared with their open equivalents is more than compensated for by the reduction in hospital stay and reduction of time lost from work.

The underlying concept of laparoscopy is not new: it has been a well-known tool of gynecologic surgeons for decades, but its use was confined to direct inspection and biopsy of lesions or simple manipulations such as the application of rings to the fallopian tubes for sterilization. The advance responsible for the explosive development of laparoscopy was the ability to view the surgical image on a video screen, allowing the participation of an assistant.[1] Surgical concepts of exposure, retraction, hemostasis, dissection and even newly discovered anatomic relationships were applied to the growing repertoire of surgical procedures amenable to the laparoscopic approach. The techniques were developed for use in the peritoneal cavity, but were rapidly extended to the thorax and later still to potential spaces such as the properitoneal space in the lower abdomen to repair groin hernias, the retroperitoneal space to approach the lumbar spine or kidney, and the anterior neck to locate parathyroids or mobilize the cervical esophagus. Consequently, a whole range of hollow organ and solid organ surgery is primarily approached laparoscopically. Laparoscopic Nissen fundoplication and other lower esophageal operations are now routine, and laparoscopic excision of colon and stomach, division of adhesions and excision of the major solid organs (spleen, adrenal, liver and pancreas) are also common.

This chapter shall give an overview of the surgical principles unique to, or highlighted by, laparoscopy. For specific operative details of most major operations the reader is referred to the chapter relevant to the organ in question.

Indications and Contraindications for Laparoscopic Surgery

The indications for laparoscopy are either diagnostic or therapeutic. Diagnostic laparoscopy is performed to elucidate the cause of abdominal symptoms when the clinical picture is not sufficiently clear or when a nontherapeutic laparotomy would not be justified. A common example is when ovarian or tubal pathology is suspected but appendicitis cannot be ruled out. A related use of laparoscopy is in the staging of abdominal malignancy, where detection of metastatic or locally unresectable disease would spare the patient the risks of a nontherapeutic laparotomy.

Therapeutic laparoscopy is performed with the same intent as any other conventional surgical procedure aimed at curing or palliating the patient's disease. The list of surgical procedures amenable to the laparoscopic approach is expanding all the time, and it is becoming common to think of laparoscopy as being the default method of abdominal surgery and then seek reasons why it should not be done.

There are few absolute contraindications to laparoscopic surgery unless the patient is unfit for surgery of any kind. The most common is inexperience of the surgeon. Uncorrected coagulopathy is also very dangerous. Relative contraindications include the following:

Generalized Peritonitis
In most patients a laparotomy will be required to deal with the problem. However a preliminary laparoscopy may lead the surgeon to the site of the problem and allow a smaller and more directed incision to be made.

Multiple Previous Surgical Procedures

1 or 2 previous operations, especially in a part of the abdomen remote from the focus of the intended surgery, rarely preclude a laparoscopic procedure. However, multiple previous abdominal procedures may render it unsafe to approach the problem laparoscopically, especially if they were followed by infection or if postoperative radiation therapy was given. Adhesions can be lysed laparoscopically, but when they are dense and extensive, the procedure is more time consuming and no safer than an open operation.

Severe Pulmonary Disease

Laparoscopy imposes more stress on the lungs than a laparotomy because of the presence of the CO_2 pneumoperitoneum, the upward pressure on the diaphragm, and the frequent need for the Trendelenburg position.[2] It may nevertheless be less risky to perform the procedure laparoscopically because the alternative may be respiratory failure because of postoperative pain after an open operation. We have performed a laparoscopic Nissen fundoplication in a lung transplant candidate who was characterized by high CO_2 levels even at rest, because it was felt important to remedy the cause—gastroesophageal reflux—prior to transplantation.[3] Provided renal function is adequate, the buildup of CO_2 may be compensated by the kidneys and severe acidosis will not develop.

Prior Incisional Hernia Repair or Abdominoplasty

Patients with a "tummy-tuck" or other abdominoplasty, or with a large mesh repair of an incisional hernia often have an unyielding abdomen in which the pressure rises abruptly before an adequate working space has been established. This may render the performance of a laparoscopic operation unsafe if not impossible.

Certain morbid conditions greatly increase the risk of laparoscopic procedures, depending on the operation. Cirrhosis of the liver makes laparoscopic cholecystectomy hazardous. The liver cannot easily be retracted by pushing the fundus of the gallbladder superiorly, and the coexistence of portal hypertension and coagulopathy also combine to increase the risk. Although some groups have reported low morbidity following laparoscopic cholecystectomy in cirrhotics, it should only be performed by highly experienced surgeons.[4] Similarly, aortic aneurysm increases the danger of both initial entry and the necessary manipulation.

Pregnancy has also been regarded as a relative contraindication to laparoscopy, but recent evidence suggests that provided the intraperitoneal pressures are kept below 12 mm Hg to avoid reduction in venous return and uterine blood flow, laparoscopic surgery can be performed with no greater risk than open surgery. It is important to remember that at 20 weeks gestation, the fundus of the uterus is at the umbilicus and is at risk not just from attempts at insertion, but also during the subsequent manipulation. Consequently, the trocars are often placed 2-3 cm above the umbilicus. The situation most often applies to cholecystectomy or appendectomy, since purely elective surgery is not relevant in pregnant patients. If operation is necessary during pregnancy, if possible it should be performed during the second trimester.[5]

Extreme obesity also increases the difficulty of laparoscopy and the risk of complications, but it should be remembered that the risk of open surgical procedures in these patients is also correspondingly elevated. Indeed, one of the most rapidly growing areas in the field of laparoscopic surgery is the development of laparoscopic banding operations for morbid obesity. Special long trocars and other instruments are available for use in obese patients, and the trocars are often placed closer than normal to the site of the pathology to allow for the greater abdominal dimensions. It is critical to secure the obese patient to the operating table because of the frequent need for steep head-up or head-down positions to allow the operation to be accomplished.[6,7]

Finally, there is growing concern that laparoscopic resections for malignancy are complicated by an unacceptable incidence of port site metastasis. The magnitude of the problem may have been initially overestimated, but it appears to be a problem unique to the laparoscopic approach. Many experimental studies have attempted to define the factors responsible but there is not yet a consensus.[8] At present it appears there is a move away from performing curative laparoscopic cancer resections, and use of laparoscopic procedures is restricted to staging or palliation of malignancy, and more focused on nonmalignant disease.

Patient Understanding and Informed Consent

The lay public often has quite unrealistic ideas about what can be achieved by laparoscopic surgery. A patient being prepared for a laparoscopic operation should be aware that conversion to an open procedure may be necessary. They should be given a realistic assessment of the risks, especially when relatively new procedures are being offered. Ethical problems may arise when a surgeon performs a laparoscopic procedure that is new to the surgical community, or simply new to that surgeon. In such a rapidly changing field, the border between innovation and experimentation may become blurred. If the surgical result is disappointing, the patient may complain not just about the surgeon's ineptitude, but of a more fundamental error—violating the contract between doctor and patient, thus making the patient an unknowing guinea pig. This is not a problem faced by trainee surgeons, but it becomes highly relevant once in practice. Surgeons intending to extend the borders of laparoscopic surgery usually present their ideas to ethics committees of their local hospitals or to committees of national societies. The broad perspective provided by such governing bodies helps prevent the surgeon from overlooking an important legal or ethical issue, sensitizes him or her to aspects of patient care that could be overlooked in the drive to accomplish the technical aspects of the treatment, and provides some grounds for legal defense if the surgeon should be sued by a patient displeased with the result of the operation.

Anesthesia and Laparoscopic Surgery

It is commonly imagined that the reduction of pain and the smoother postoperative recovery of patients after laparoscopic procedures can make a poor-risk patient into a low-risk one if only the operation can be performed laparoscopically. This is a misconception. It is undeniable that the metabolic stress imposed by a laparoscopic operation is less than that of the same operation performed by open surgery.[9,10] However, the laparoscopic environment adds stresses of its own. The insufflation of CO_2 for prolonged periods may exceed the ability of the patient to compensate if there is preexisting lung disease. Similarly, the prolonged use of the Trendelenburg position reduces the ventilatory capacity of the patient and tidal volumes often have to be increased by up to one third. The increased intraabdominal pressure coupled with the Trendelenburg position also puts the patient at higher risk of aspiration. In the postoperative period, the typical reduction in forced expiratory volume seen after open surgery is attenuated, from about 50% to 25%, but the effect is still sizeable.[11]

Preoperative nasogastric and bladder catheterization are standard in most major laparoscopic procedures in the pelvis and lower abdomen, both to guard against aspiration and to reduce the chance of visceral injury. The frequent changes in position of the operating table necessitate special care in positioning and securing the patient. The bony prominences must be carefully padded to protect against skin necrosis and peripheral neuropraxia.

Special considerations apply to intraoperative monitoring in laparoscopic cases. Even minor laparoscopic procedures generally require general anesthesia and may produce major complications if monitoring is inadequate. The increased tendency for CO_2 retention and the increased difficulty of ventilation makes capnography and pulse oximetry essential. For long procedures, the need to obtain serial blood gas estimations makes it worthwhile to insert an arterial line.

The Operating Room Environment

A good image requires a telescope, a camera a bright light source, and an image processor to transform the camera input into an image on the video screen. The operating room (OR) should have trained personnel to set up and adjust the equipment to maximize the image quality because once the procedure has started, the scrubbed surgeon and assistants cannot interrupt the operation to make these adjustments. Most operating suites have a dedicated person to service, connect and act as troubleshooter for laparoscopic equipment. The need to perform emergency laparoscopic procedures outside of regular working hours mandates the presence of trained OR personnel capable of operating the equipment when such a specialist is off duty. Attempting to perform off-hours laparoscopic procedures when the OR staff is unfamiliar with the equipment is an exercise in frustration at best and dangerous at worst. The surgeon must nevertheless be familiar with the basic connections and setup of the equipment to be able to offer guidance to the OR circulating staff when adjustment is required. At the senior level, surgeons are likely to be involved in selecting and budgeting for new or replacement equipment. They are likely to be besieged by manufacturer's representatives urging the purchase of new or modified laparoscopic tools, and should be aware of the operating principles of the various aids to laparoscopy in order to guide the rational selection of equipment for the OR.

Operating Room Setup

Choose the largest OR available. Older operating suites were not designed with the needs of modern surgery in mind. When bulky laparoscopy carts are added to the array of equipment needed for monitoring, anesthesia administration, fluid warming, patient warming, suction/irrigation devices and electrocautery, the environment can become crowded and chaotic. Modern ORs have ceiling-mounted moveable monitors and plenty of space for all of the additional equipment required. The circulating nurse must have immediate access to a tray of conventional surgical instruments and be ready to expedite the conversion to an open procedure if it should be required in a hurry.

Figure 1

Conventional setup for upper GI surgery

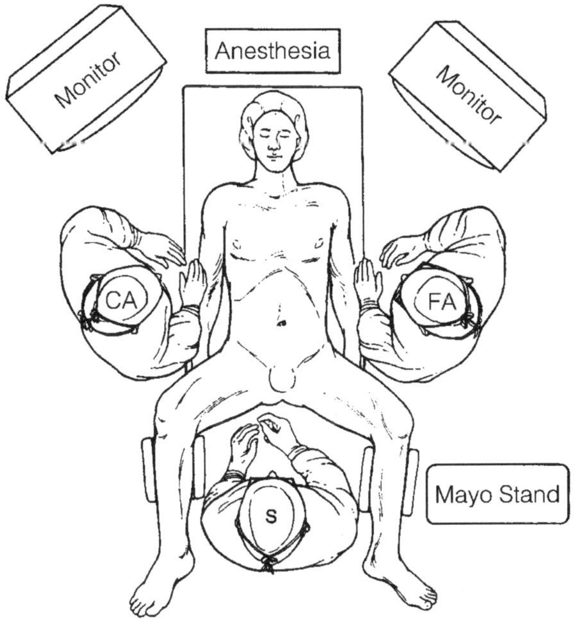

(S, surgeon; FA, first assistant; CA, camera assistant)
Reprinted with permission from Katkhouda N. Advanced Laparoscopic Surgery: Techniques and Tips. *Philadelphia, PA: WB Saunders; 1998.*

Most procedures require 2 monitors because the surgeon and the first assistant are on opposite sides of the table. Hand-eye coordination is best when the direction of each person's instruments coincides with his or her optical axis. Hence, for upper abdominal operations, the monitors are positioned on either side of the patient's shoulders. When approaching the esophageal hiatus, the patient is in the modified lithotomy position with the hips and knees slightly flexed, and the surgeon operates from between the legs as shown in Figure 1. For lower abdominal operations, the monitors are situated on either side of the patient's feet. For certain operations restricted to a small area, such as appendectomy or hernia repair, a single monitor at the foot of the operating table is sufficient, as shown in Figure 2.

2 electrocautery leads are used: one conventional Bovie electrode for the initial skin incision and as a backup in case the operation must be converted to an open procedure, and a separate lead for connection to a laparoscopic dissector, scissors, hook or spatula. A combined suction/irrigation device is essential. Advanced procedures commonly use harmonic shears for dissecting vascular structures such as the gastrosplenic omentum or the lateral peritoneal attachments of colon or spleen. The operating foot pedals for these instruments must be positioned close to the surgeon's dominant foot.

In recent years, concern has been expressed about evacuating the CO_2 from the atmosphere of the operating room. It is hypothesized that liberation of the insufflated gas especially after production of smoke or water droplets could enhance the liberation of viral particles or other infectious agents into the atmosphere of the OR. At present, there is no agreed upon means of evacuating smoke from the OR, and the only masks with sufficiently fine particle filters tend to be uncomfortable.[12,13]

Figure 2

Conventional setup for hernia repair

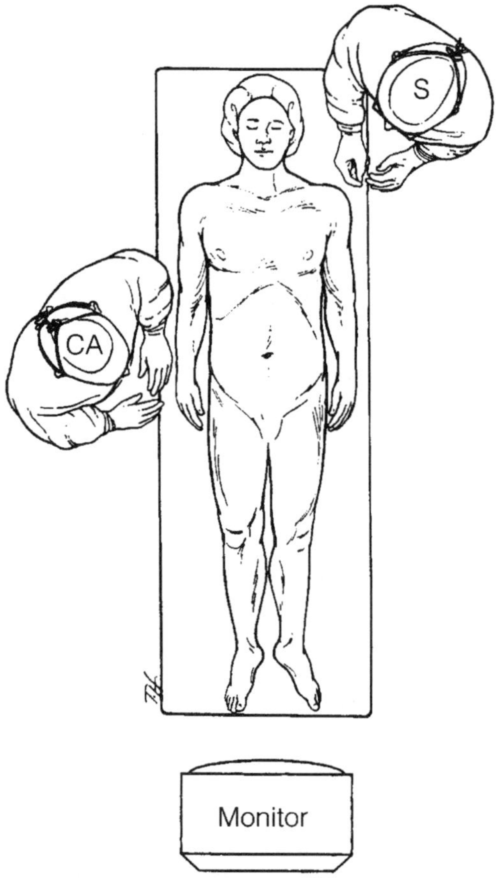

(S, surgeon; CA, camera assistant)
Reprinted with permission from Katkhouda N. Advanced Laparoscopic Surgery: Techniques and Tips. *Philadelphia, PA: WB Saunders; 1998.*

Understanding the Equipment

All laparoscopic procedures depend on the provision of a high-quality image of the relevant structures displayed on a video monitor. To do this requires a camera attached to a long rigid telescope. Initially, the telescope was 10 mm in diameter and had a lens perpendicular to the axis of the scope (the so-called 0° scope). The angle of the scope is determined by the plane of the tissue being inspected. The use of a telescope with a view at 30° to the plane of the tissue allows the scope to see "around the corner" into otherwise inaccessible sites. A 45° telescope is available but offers little additional advantage. These angled scopes have reduced transmission and a more restricted angle of view than the 0° scope. Recently, 5 mm telescopes have begun to take the place of the 10 mm scope, and uses are being found for even smaller (2-3 mm) telescopes, so-called minilaparoscopy. These smaller scopes have poorer optical resolution and a smaller field of vision, and are much more fragile than the conventional 10 mm instrument. They should not be used by the novice until he or she is totally familiar with routine laparoscopic procedures using standard equipment.

Most cameras have a single computer chip for transmission of the image. The color definition often has to be supplemented by software to modify the color and enhance the contrast—so-called digital painting. More elaborate cameras containing 3 chips have better image quality but are heavy and harder for an inexperienced assistant to control.

The most common image problem facing the surgeon is fogging or smearing of the lens. The latter is preventable by taking care during insertion not to bang up against omentum or falciform ligament, but fogging is a frequent nuisance. The best way to prevent it is to keep the telescope warm. Keep a Thermos® flask or a hot water bath nearby in which to dip the telescope, and dry and polish the end rapidly before it has time to cool off. The addition of fog reduction materials is of little value if the scope is allowed to cool.

2. Gaining Access to the Abdomen

The initial step in all laparoscopic procedures is insertion of a trocar which will accommodate the camera and allow insufflation of gas. It is most conveniently positioned in the umbilicus because the absence of subcutaneous fat or muscle in this site makes entry through a small incision easy. The lower border of the umbilical fold is used for lower abdominal procedures and the upper border is used for surgery in the upper abdomen. 2 methods of placing this initial port are popular, usually termed the open and closed methods.

Open Method

A curved incision large enough to admit the trocar is made in the umbilical fold and deepened until fascia is reached. Retracting the umbilical fold upwards with a towel clip may help define the fascia better. Scissors or electrocautery is used to divide the fascia longitudinally and stay sutures of 0 Vicryl™ are inserted into each cut edge. By holding up the properitoneal fat with 2 long narrow tonsil forceps the peritoneum is divided, and the operator's little finger inserted to ensure that nothing is adherent to the abdominal wall. The Hasson trocar is then inserted to its maximum extent and the stay sutures looped round the ears of the flared trocar sheath to establish a seal and prevent its dislodgment. The gas is then connected and the camera inserted when the pneumoperitoneum is established.

Closed (Veress Needle) Method

The skin on either side of the umbilicus is elevated with towel clips and a 2 mm incision made in the umbilical fold. A Veress needle is then carefully advanced through this incision into the peritoneal cavity. 2 distinct clicks are felt as the blunt needle penetrates first the fascia and then the peritoneum. There are several clues to help the surgeon know that the needle is in the peritoneal cavity. A syringe is attached and aspiration attempted. If blood or fluid is encountered, injury to an intraabdominal viscus is suspected. If aspiration is negative, 10 cc of air is then injected. If the air can be recovered, the needle is not in the peritoneal cavity, but in a small loculus formed by either extraperitoneal fat or the omentum. If the air cannot be aspirated, the CO_2 is then connected. The maximum flow through a Veress needle is about 2 L/min, so approximately 2 minutes are necessary to establish a pneumoperitoneum. If the pressure rises abruptly, reaching the threshold of 14 mm Hg after only a few hundred cc of CO_2 has been injected, the needle may be in the properitoneal space. A slow rise in pressure over 2 minutes combined with visible and percussible signs of pneumoperitoneum are signs that it is safe to proceed. A curved 1.5 cm incision in the umbilicus is then made, the skin elevated with towel clips and the trocar inserted directly. The trocar should be held in the palm of the dominant hand with the middle finger extended along the shaft to act as a brake if the fascia should suddenly give way, allowing the trocar to advance rapidly. The trocar may be rotated clockwise and counterclockwise, but should not be rocked back and forth because this will open up the planes of the abdominal wall and allow gas insufflation into these layers. Once inserted, the central obturator is removed and the air vent momentarily opened to ensure that CO_2 can escape. The gas is then connected to the Luer lock attachment on the trocar and the camera inserted.

The choice of method is to some extent a matter of personal preference and training, because with practice both methods are rapid and safe. The open method is generally preferred in the complicated case where there has been previous surgery or where a nonumbilical site for camera insertion is needed. Generally, a site in the quadrant most remote from the site of the previous surgery is chosen. For operations on the esophageal hiatus, the camera needs to be 4-6 cm superior to the umbilicus and often just to the left of the midline in order to avoid smearing of the camera lens by the dependent falciform ligament. Adequate vision and retraction to create these extraumbilical port sites is critical. Narrow (1 cm) S-shaped retractors are available to enable the assistant to retract the skin and fat to expose the fascia without the retractors themselves obscuring field of vision. It is also helpful to have the long extension on the Bovie electrocautery so that the shaft and the surgeon's hand do not get in the way. In obese patients, it may be necessary to use the camera light cord, or even wear a headlight to illuminate the depths of the wounds.

Insertion of Secondary Ports

The sites chosen for additional ports is crucial to the success of the operation. Improper positioning of the operating ports leads to inadequate vision and retraction, and the instruments may end up "fighting" with other retractors or with the camera. For most commonly performed laparoscopic operations, the siting of the ports has now become more or less standardized, but it is nevertheless helpful to understand the logic which has led to the emergence of these broadly agreed upon measures. The most important concept is that of *triangulation*, a technique which ensures that the tips of the instruments in the surgeon's 2 hands focus on the area to be dissected, such that they form the apex of a triangle: the camera is sited between and behind these 2 arms. This is shown diagrammatically in Figure 3. If the operator's 2 ports are too close together, the angle will be too acute and the instruments will hit the camera or each other. If the angle is too obtuse one of the instruments will be pointing toward the camera and the movements will then be reversed, causing awkwardness akin to the problem of writing by looking in a mirror. With practice the counterintuitive movements can be overcome, but it is much simpler to plan the port insertion correctly to start with. The presence of a pneumoperitoneum can alter the proposed site, especially near the costal margin, so the sites should only be marked when the abdomen is distended. It is also important to avoid putting the trocars too close to the structure to be removed. This is a common error in appendectomy. A site too close to the appendix makes it difficult to maneuver the instrument to exert traction on the appendix to allow its dissection.

Figure 3

The concept of triangulation, showing the camera looking toward the apex of the triangle formed by the working instruments

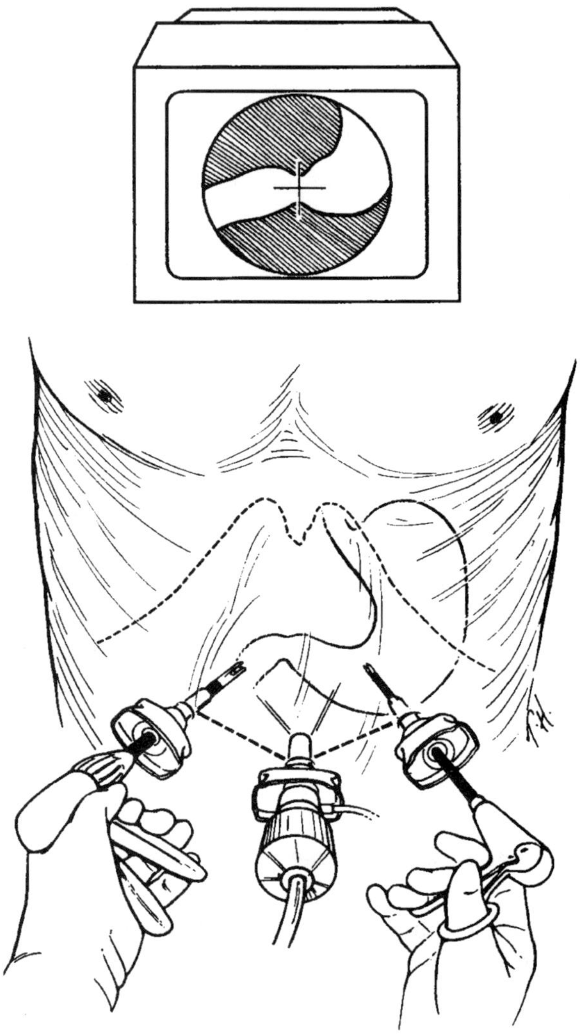

Reprinted with permission from Katkhouda N. Advanced Laparoscopic Surgery: Techniques and Tips. *Philadelphia, PA: WB Saunders; 1998.*

Choice of Trocar Size

Most procedures are performed with 5 mm and 10-11 mm ports. The smaller ports are designed to accommodate grasping forceps, dissecting forceps, scissors and cautery hooks. The larger 10 mm ports are still necessary to accommodate linear stapling instruments and larger Babcock grasping forceps with large jaws. Suturing is also much easier using a 10 mm port because of the ease of introducing a curved needle into the larger opening. In recent years many instruments have been modified to fit into narrower trocars, including Babcock forceps and cameras, so that many operations can be performed entirely with 5 mm instruments with a corresponding reduction in incisional pain. However, this drive for smaller incisions should be tempered by common sense. The difference between a laparoscopic procedure performed using 10 mm ports and one using 5 mm ports is still much smaller than that between using 10 mm ports and the same operation performed by conventional open surgery. Operations involving a lot of retraction and dissection are much harder to perform using the flimsier instruments needed for the smaller incision.

Minilaparoscopy

Advances in computer chip technology have allowed the development of cameras and telescopes which produce acceptable images even with a diameter of only 2-3 mm. Today the technique is most valuable when the key question is whether or not there is any significant pathology in the abdomen at all. In the patient whose abdomen is not evaluable, such as a patient in the ICU, or in the presence of severe burns, head injury or intoxication, formal exploration may be hazardous, and noninvasive methods, such as CT scanning or peritoneal lavage, insensitive. In these patients, the ability to confirm or refute such major processes as perforated viscus, intraperitoneal bleeding or ischemic bowel is valuable. A portable cart with the equipment necessary for lighting and insufflation can be brought to the bedside. Local anesthesia and mild sedation are adequate and the abdomen can be insufflated with nitrous oxide to reduce pain further. Manipulation, dissection and exploration are difficult with these fragile instruments, but it is usually possible to rule in or rule out catastrophic conditions in the abdomen such as those mentioned above.

Technique of Additional Trocar Insertion

The course of the inferior and superior epigastric arteries should be thoroughly known by all laparoscopic surgeons. The proposed site of insertion should be confirmed by observing the site where pressure by the assistant's finger indents the peritoneum. The camera is then advanced towards this point and the abdominal wall transilluminated: the presence of any underlying vessel will become obvious. An incision of sufficient length to accommodate the trocar is made with a number 11 blade. For a 10 mm trocar to fit snugly, the total length of the wound edge must equal the trocar's circumference, ie, 30 mm. The length of the wound is therefore half the circumference of the trocar, or 1.5 times the diameter. Make the incision cleanly without any sawing motion in the fat. Tonsil forceps may be used to spread the subcutaneous tissue down towards the fascia. When the trocar is inserted, the tip may push the peritoneum away from the abdominal muscle layer instead of penetrating it. This often happens near the bladder and near the falciform ligament. It can be prevented by inserting a Babcock forceps and opening the jaws in order to exert pressure on either side of the peritoneum where the trocar is trying to come through. This keeps the peritoneum in contact with the fascia and allows it to be penetrated directly. It also helps prevent the entire abdominal wall from being pushed towards the viscera and reduces the chance of inadvertent visceral injury.

Closure of the Trocar Sites

Closure after open insertion of the Hasson trocar is easily performed by simply tying the previously placed stay sutures. Traction on the suture on one side may reveal suboptimal placement of the stay suture on the other, and at the end of the procedure it is easy to insert an additional suture if required. Closure of the fascia at other trocar sites depends on the size and type of trocar used. Incisional hernia and bowel entrapment are sometimes reported after use of 10-12 mm ports, especially in the lower abdomen, but almost never through 5 mm sites. Among 10 mm trocars, some have a sharp pyramidal cutting blade that may lacerate the muscle and fascia, and entry ports made with these instruments should be formally closed. Many modern disposable trocars have blades that push the fascia aside, and closure of the fascia may be unnecessary if these are used. Similarly, the Storz "corkscrew" trocar sheath merely "worms" its way through the tissues, causing little bleeding, and does not require fascial closure.

Closure of the port sites can be done from the outside by grasping the fascial edge with a Kocher clamp and putting a suture just behind the clamp to emerge in the wound. The suture is then used as a retractor to facilitate placing the clamp on the other fascial edge and repeating the procedure on the other side. There are several devices which can be used to insert a suture from the peritoneal side under direct vision. The simplest has a long offset needle which is flush with the shaft of the introducer but which when rotated comes to lie at a distance so that it can be used to pick up the peritoneum as it is pulled back under laparoscopic vision. It then emerges in the subcutaneous tissue where a length of 0 Vicryl is threaded onto it. The introducer with its needle is then re-inserted into the abdomen, rotated through 180° and the opposite edge of the trocar wound caught with the needle. The threaded needle is then brought out through fascia on the opposite side of the initial suture, detached from the needle, which is then rotated so as to lie flush with its introducer, and it is removed together with the trocar, under vision. The 2 ends of the suture are then tied.

Closure of the skin is an often-neglected part of the operation, but remember that it is the only bit of the surgical procedure the patient sees. Patients often complain about puckered or dimpled skin wounds, and with a little care in mobilizing the subcutaneous tissue it is not hard to make the wounds cosmetically acceptable.

3. Important Concepts in Laparoscopic Surgery

The Pneumoperitoneum and the Working Space

The peritoneal cavity is essentially a potential space. Proper visualization of its contents demands the creation of a pneumoperitoneum. The most common gas in use is CO_2, because its solubility greatly reduces the danger of gas embolism. It has the disadvantage of accumulating in the tissues and causing acidosis when levels exceed the capacity of the lungs to eliminate the excess. In most procedures this process is rarely of significance, but patients with pulmonary disease who are predisposed to retain CO_2 are at risk of serious acidosis. Other gases such as helium and nitrous oxide have been tried with limited success. Regardless of the nature of the gas, it is necessary to be able to create an uncrowded working space in which to visualize, manipulate, and dissect the intraabdominal organs safely (see Figure 4). As a rule of thumb, 2 L of gas must be insufflated without reaching the safe limit of intraperitoneal pressure. This limit is usually set at 14 mm Hg. If the pressure reaches that level before 2 L can be inserted, it is unlikely to be possible to perform the procedure. This is often the situation in small bowel obstruction or in some excessively obese patients. During any operation, when the pressure exceeds the set threshold of 14 mm Hg, an alarm will sound and gas will stop flowing. The most common reason for alarm activation is kinking of the rubber tube at a point just before it connects to the trocar.

Several practical points must be kept in mind. A spare gas cylinder must always be immediately available in case the first cylinder runs low during the procedure. Advanced procedures using extracorporeal suturing cause damage to the plastic diaphragms of the trocars and lead to gas leakage. It is wise to have 2 simultaneous insufflators at this stage in the procedure to prevent frustrating loss of pneumoperitoneum.

Laparoscopic Instruments

Contrary to popular belief, the majority of laparoscopic operations can be performed with a relatively small range of instruments. The basic tray should include grasping forceps, dissecting forceps, scissors, needle holders, knot pushers, hooks, a liver retractor and a suction/irrigation device. Many surgeons now use a system in which a generic handle can be attached to a variety of interchangeable

Figure 4

(A) Inadequate working space with consequent risk of damage to adjacent viscera.
(B) adequate working space

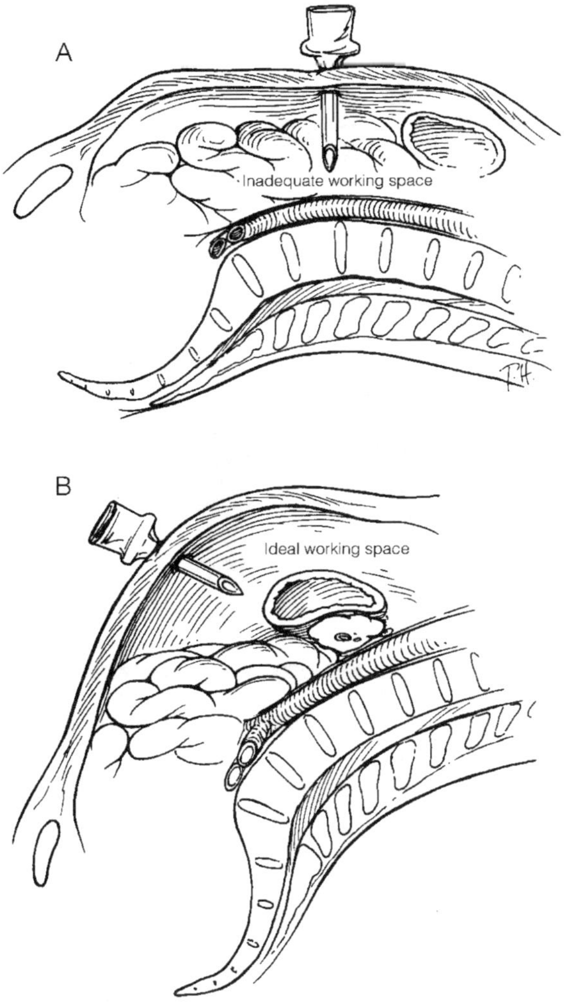

Reprinted with permission from Katkhouda N. Advanced Laparoscopic Surgery: Techniques and Tips. *Philadelphia, PA: WB Saunders; 1998.*

instruments with identical stems that fit into the handle. Scissors and grasping forceps can be used with the same kind of handle. The handle is equipped with rings to allow manipulation by the operator's thumb and fingers, a post for attachment of electrocautery, a knob accessible to the operator's index finger to rotate the shaft and a lever to activate a lock or ratchet. Although the range of instruments may be small, reusable instruments must be kept in good condition and discarded promptly when they no longer function properly. Recent publicity about the inappropriate reuse of hospital equipment designed for one-time use has alerted administrators to the necessity of providing adequate supplies of disposable instruments to reduce the temptation to reuse materials to save money.

Laparoscopic Suturing

The earliest laparoscopic operations did not involve suturing. Cholecystectomy, appendectomy and hernia repair can be accomplished without it. But more complex procedures involving restoration of function often depend on suturing. The major reason for the difficulty of laparoscopic suturing is the lack of 3-dimensional perspective and limitation of the sense of touch. Although these difficulties provided a stimulus for the development of improved methods of clipping and stapling, the ability to suture remains a fundamental surgical tool. Most surgeons now use the same needles and sutures in laparoscopic surgery as they do in open surgery. For suture of the GI tract, the SH needle is preferred. A heavier needle and suture, such as 0 Ethibond®, is useful for suturing bulky structures like the diaphragmatic crura.

Learning to insert sutures accurately requires much practice. The major steps are now standardized. Insert the suture by grasping the suture about 1-2 cm away from the needle, and drag the needle down the trocar into the abdomen. Use the left hand to steady the needle so it looks like a smile with the attached suture towards the surgeon's right hand port. The needle driver then releases the suture and picks up the needle one-third of the way towards the point. A common error is to have the table too high so that the surgeon's arms are at shoulder level during these maneuvers, which can become very tiring. Drop the table or stand on a stool in order to be comfortable. Use a blunt atraumatic grasper in the left hand to present the tissue to be sutured, either by holding it up or by pushing against it to allow the needle to be driven through the chosen spot. Practice is necessary to gain skill in closing and releasing the ratchet of the needle driver without accidentally dislodging the needle.

Much of the difficulty in suturing arises through the awkwardness of tying knots. Early techniques emphasized the use of preformed slip knots, but nowadays standard knotting techniques are routinely practiced. Both extracorporeal and intracorporeal knotting methods are widely used. The extracorporeal technique is certainly easier and is adequate for most procedures. After placing the needle and bringing it through the tissue, the suture is grasped just below the needle and brought out through the same port through which it was inserted. The 2 ends of the suture are now available to the surgeon to form the first throw of a surgeon's knot. This is then pushed down with a knot pusher, which acts much as the surgeon's finger is used to push the knot down when tying in a deep cavity in open surgery. The number of throws depends on the frictional characteristics of the material: for braided material like silk or Ethibond, 3 throws are sufficient, but 5 should be used on slippery monofilament materials like Prolene®.

Intracorporeal suturing is initially harder to learn because the springy suture material often does not lie exactly the way the surgeon desires, and there is no maneuver corresponding to the surgeon's ability in open surgery to hold the crossed threads and supinate the hand so as to bring the free end through the loop. However, intracorporeal suturing inflicts less tissue trauma because the long suture ends are not dragged through the tissues, and surgeons who have mastered it find that when used exclusively, it is actually quicker than extracorporeal knotting. Cut the suture 6 inches from the needle. Place the stitch as described above, and prepare the knot by bringing the needle towards the free end of the suture so that it looks like a smile to the surgeon, as illustrated in Figure 5. Grasp the needle with the needle driver and use the curve of the needle to facilitate the winding motion of forming the loop around the left hand grasper, which then picks up the free end of the suture and pulls it through the loop. The same procedure is then repeated from left to right in reverse to create a square knot.

Preformed loops with slip knots (endoloop) are still useful for ligating stumps such as the cystic duct, appendix and mesoappendix. They are cheaper to use than linear staplers in appendectomy, and are useful in cholecystectomy when the surgeon is faced with a wide cystic duct the endoclip cannot quite accommodate. If the patient is going to require

Figure 5

Intracorporeal knot tying

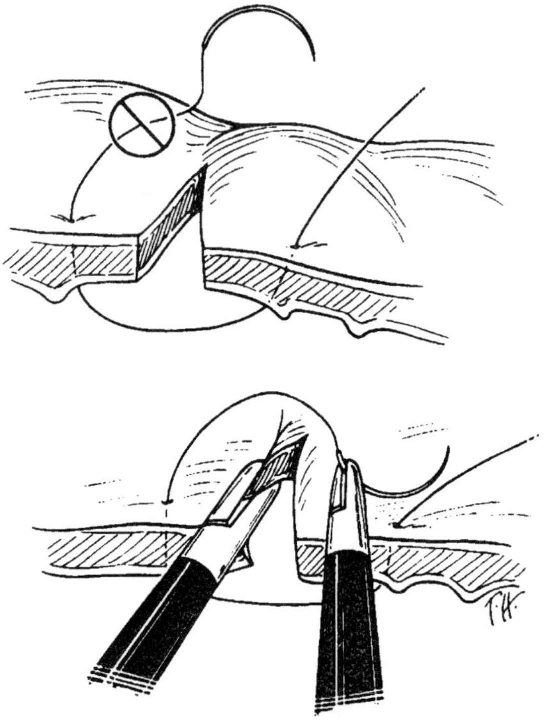

Upper figure shows incorrect approach; lower figure shows correct approach with the tip of the needle on the side of the loose end, allowing the surgeon to form a loop more easily. Reprinted with permission from Katkhouda N. Advanced Laparoscopic Surgery: Techniques and Tips. *Philadelphia, PA: WB Saunders; 1998.*

a postoperative ERCP, an endoloop is a wise precaution because it is more secure than a clip.

Retraction in Laparoscopic Surgery

Gravity is the most helpful retractor in laparoscopic surgery. When operating in the supracolic compartment (biliary tract, foregut, spleen) the table should be in the reverse Trendelenburg position, and it should be in the head down position for operations in the lower abdomen or pelvis. Visualization of the appendix is aided by putting the right side up, and similarly with left-sided organs such as the spleen, putting the left side up allows other attached organs to fall away, as illustrated in Figure 6.

The most frequently retracted organ is the liver. Several different kinds of liver retractors are available. All elevate the left lateral segment against the anterior abdominal wall in order to expose the upper lesser curvature of the stomach and the diaphragmatic hiatus. The trocar can be either in the right subcostal position (retraction from below) or close to the xiphoid (retraction from above). From either approach, the surface of the liver is frequently lacerated by the retractor and the instrument frequently slips during the procedure. 3 major types of liver retractor are available: one device with 5 radiating blades slightly curved at their ends, a second type which is like a hinged rectangle or rhomboid that opens into a diamond shape when extended, and third a triangular flat balloon which gets stiff when inflated. The balloon type is the least traumatic to the liver but is also least effective in providing exposure.

Portions of the gastrointestinal tract requiring retraction are usually held out of the way by Babcock forceps. Care must be taken not to close the ratchet too aggressively or retract too vigorously, or a perforation will result.

Hemostasis

As in open surgery, large or named vessels will ideally be identified, exposed and controlled before being divided. The ability to control such vessels has been transformed by the use of the harmonic scissors. This instrument generates high frequency ultrasound waves of sufficient energy to cause coagulation, but the focus of the device is so precise that it does not cause destruction of adjacent tissue. It is most widely used in division of the short gastric vessels of the greater curvature and fundus during fundoplication, but the vascular peritoneum of the lienorenal ligament and the radially disposed arterial supply of the adrenal gland are also ideal applications for its use. It generates steam rather than smoke and fogs up the environment less than electrocautery.

For larger vessels, the size of the cystic artery or larger, division between clips is preferable. 2 clips are placed on each side of the vessel, except in the case of organ removal, in which case 1 clip is placed on the side of the vessel being excised. The splenic artery and vein present a particular problem because of their size, tortuosity and proximity to structures

Figure 6

Using gravity to facilitate exposure

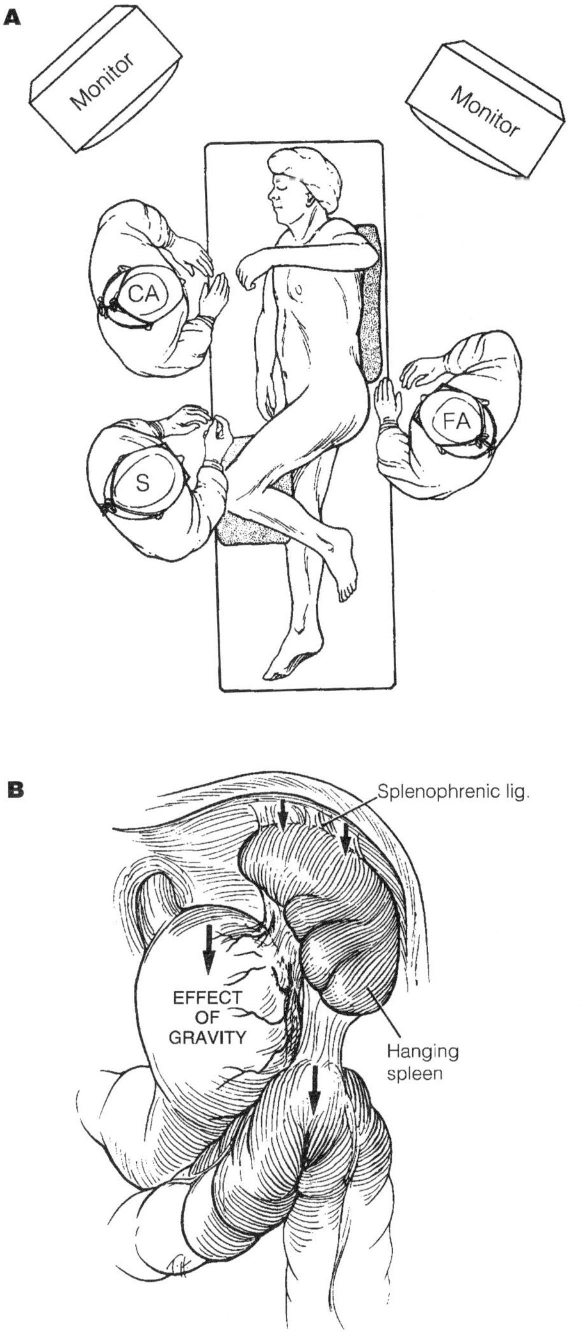

(A) Patient positioning, (B) view of the major advantages of the reverse Trendelenburg and left side positions. Tension is put on the splenic pedicle and the splenic flexure of the colon, and the stomach and small bowel fall out of the way. Reprinted with permission from Katkhouda N. Advanced Laparoscopic Surgery: Techniques and Tips. *Philadelphia, PA: WB Saunders; 1998.*

such as the pancreatic tail. The simplest approach to these vessels is to divide them with the linear stapler/cutter. As in open surgery, it is important to avoid panic and resist the temptation to apply clamps, clips or electrocautery blindly in a pool of blood. Much greater damage can be caused this way.

Diffuse bleeding in laparoscopic surgery is much more annoying than in open surgery. Blood staining the tissues absorbs light and renders the whole operative field much darker, obscuring the details of the structures being dissected. Every effort must be made to prevent unwanted hemorrhage and to deal with it promptly when it occurs. Small gauze sponges can be inserted through a 10 mm trocar and used to mop up surface bleeding as in open surgery. This is particularly helpful in dangerous areas such as the esophageal hiatus.

Finger-Assisted and Hand-Assisted Laparoscopic Surgery

When normal tissue planes are obscured and distorted by inflammation and edema, normal laparoscopic dissecting techniques can fail. In this situation, the surgeon often longs to be able to insert a finger to use its tactile sensitivity to break up adhesions or liberate loops of bowel. This can often be done by removing the trocar from a 10 mm port close to the affected area and inserting the index finger while observing with the camera. The finger fits snugly enough to maintain the pneumoperitoneum, and the camera allows the surgeon to see what he or she is doing. Once the necessary liberation has been performed, the trocar is reinserted and the operation can proceed as planned.[14]

A similar situation on a larger scale occurs with excision of large solid organs, especially the spleen, or in donor nephrectomy. In this case a 4-5 cm transverse incision is made and the surgeon's entire hand and wrist inserted into the abdomen to assist the dissection. A specially-designed sleeve (Pneumosleeve®) can be used to surround the port and keep the CO_2 from escaping.

There are many situations in which a procedure can be performed partly by laparoscopy, but a larger incision must be made in order to complete it. Many colon resections fall into this category: the dissection is done laparoscopically, but then a precisely-directed small incision is made to exteriorize the 2 bowel ends, which are then anastomosed in the conventional way and the completed anastomosis dropped back into the peritoneal cavity. This combination gives the patient the advantages of both approaches while adding little to the trauma of surgery.

Leaving the Abdomen: Specimen Removal and Peritoneal Toilet

Specimens should be placed in a bag before removal to protect against contamination of the wound and to ensure that as much as possible they are removed intact. Several types of specimen bags are available. They come tightly rolled up and are introduced into the abdomen, and when inflated through an attached port the bag straightens out and the mouth opens. The specimen is placed in the bag and the neck closed by pulling the attached suture. The trocar and bag are removed together under direct vision. As the pursestrung neck of the bag presents itself at the skin, it is gently pulled and rocked back and forth, gently forcing the bag through the opening by a process resembling amebic diapedesis. The trocar is subsequently reinserted to complete the clean up and closure process. Large specimens like the spleen have to be morcellated and placed in a bag before removal, and the involved port site must be enlarged slightly to allow safe removal.

The surgeon should keep in mind the motto of many landlords giving instructions to their short-term tenants: "leave this place as you would like to have found it." Evacuation of blood, bile, irrigation fluid and pus should be meticulous. Gallstones spilled during cholecystectomy may cause an intraabdominal abscess if not removed, and it may require a separate bag or a very large sucker to retrieve all the spilled stones.[15]

Major Complications During Laparoscopic Surgery

Many complications specific to individual operations will be described in the relevant chapters of this book. Some general complications that may occur in any laparoscopic procedure are described below.

Major Hemodynamic Instability
This is usually heralded by a lot of activity and whispering at the top end of the table, and it rapidly emerges that for some reason the patient "is not doing well." Hypotension, tachycardia or other arrhythmia, desaturation or difficulty in maintaining ventilation are the most important features. Faced with this alarming situation, the following possibilities should be considered, and one chosen based on the preoperative condition of the patient and the nature of the operation being performed.

Intraoperative myocardial infarct is usually associated with ST segment changes and ectopic activity. A 12-lead ECG will show it most clearly, but it may also be visible on the monitor. ***Pulmonary embolus,*** characterized by tachycardia, desaturation and high right-sided pressures may occur, especially in an old or immobile patient or a younger female on oral contraceptives.

Pneumothorax may occur during surgery on the esophagus in which the pleura is inadvertently opened allowing the CO_2 to enter the pleural cavity. The anesthesiologist will notice that it is harder to ventilate the patient. It may be necessary to insert a chest drain or to reduce the pressure of the gas. If pneumothorax is due to a lung injury, it will get worse with positive pressure ventilation and a chest drain will be necessary.

Gas embolism is the most potentially catastrophic event. It is more likely to occur in situations where the insufflation pressure has been permitted to rise, or when there is extensive soft tissue dissection with the potential for open veins, such as in retroperitoneal procedures. It may also occur at the start of the procedure when the Veress needle is placed in a vein. It can be detected because it will lead to an immediate drop in end-tidal CO_2, the result of an abrupt reduction of pulmonary perfusion, and it may be associated with a "mill wheel" murmur over the precordium, though in practice the amount of noise and chaos produced by the situation in the OR generally precludes hearing anything so subtle.

It generally takes a few minutes before the cause of the abrupt instability becomes apparent. During this interval, the insufflation should be stopped and the pneumoperitoneum released. If the patient is in the head up position, the table should be turned to a horizontal position. Minor episodes of hypotension may respond to these simple measures, but if a major gas embolism has occurred the patient should be placed in a head-down position and turned on the left side. If a CVP line is present it can be used to attempt to aspirate air from the right side of the heart.

Complications from Port Site Insertion
Hemorrhage, either in the form of an expanding hematoma at a port site or constant dripping of blood into the abdomen, is an irritating problem which rarely causes complications from blood loss, but it makes the operation much more difficult and leaves the patient with an enormous bruise. The most common cause is accidental puncture of one of the epigastric arteries. Once it is recognized, it should be treated promptly to limit the size of the hematoma and to allow the operation to proceed unimpeded. A stout Prolene suture on a Keith needle can be passed alongside the trocar into the abdomen and brought out the other side, and the ends tied over a gauze roll. This should allow the bleeding to be tamponaded. The suture can be cut a day or two later before the patient goes home.

Conclusion: Maintaining and Developing Laparoscopic Skills

The established surgeon, whether in academic or in private practice, is a lifelong learner, and nowhere is this concept as vital as in the rapidly developing field of laparoscopic surgery. Surgeons who commonly use laparoscopic techniques, or who would like to do so, benefit immensely from being affiliated with one of the major organizations dedicated to this field. In the USA, the major organizations are the Society of American Gastrointestinal Endoscopic Surgeons (SAGES) and the Society of Laparoendoscopic Surgeons. Similar large societies exist in Europe and Latin America. In an environment where there is little formal opportunity to develop new skills after residency or fellowship, contact with fellow surgeons struggling with the same problems is a rewarding experience.

By its very nature, laparoscopic surgery is highly dependent on advanced technology, and for this reason is changing more rapidly than perhaps any other field of surgery. As one might expect in this environment, dissemination of information commonly takes place over the Internet rather than in traditional surgical journals. Several Web sites, including those of the surgical societies mentioned above, and others in the public domain such as ***Laparoscopy.com***, are useful sources of information about novel techniques and also give the surgeon information about the expectations and misconceptions of the lay public.

4. References

1. Litynski GS. *Highlights in the History of Laparoscopy*. Frankfurt, Germany: B Bernert Verlag; 1996.

2. Shantha TR, Harden J. Laparoscopic cholecystectomy: anesthesia related complications and guidelines. *Surg Laparosc Endosc*. 1991;1:173-178.

3. Tsai P, Peters J, Johnson W, Cohen R, Starnes V. Laparoscopic fundoplication 1 month prior to lung transplantation. *Surg Endosc*. 1996;10:668-670.

4. Sleeman D, Namias N, Levi D, et al. Laparoscopic cholecystectomy in cirrhotic patients. *J Am Coll Surg*. 1998;187:400-403.

5. Lachman E, Schienfeld A, Voss E, et al. Pregnancy and laparoscopic surgery. *J Am Assoc Gyn Laparosc*. 1999;6:347-351.

6. Robinson SP, Hirtle M, Imbrie JZ, Moore MM. The mechanics underlying laparoscopic intraabdominal surgery for obese patients. *J Laparoendosc Adv Surg Tech A*. 1998;8(1):1-8.

7. Schirmer BD, Dix J, Edge SB, Hyser MJ, Hanks JB, Aguilar M. Laparoscopic cholecystectomy in the obese patient. *Ann Surg*. 1992;216:146-152.

8. Pearlstone DB, Feig BW, Mansfield PF. Port site recurrences after laparoscopy for malignant disease. *Sem Surgical Onc*. 1999;16:307-312.

9. Frazee RC, Roberts JW, Okeson GC, et al. Open cholecystectomy versus laparoscopic cholecystectomy: a comparison of postoperative pulmonary function. *Ann Surg*. 1991;213:651-654.

10. Glaser F, Sannwald GA, Buhr HJ, et al. General stress response to conventional and laparoscopic cholecystectomy. *Ann Surg*. 1995;221:372-380.

11. Ortega AE, Richman MF, Hernandez M, et al. Inferior vena caval blood flow and cardiac hemodynamics during carbon dioxide pneumoperitoneum. *Surg Endosc*. 1996;10:920-924.

12. Baggish MS, Poiesz BJ, Joret D, Williamson P, Refai A. Presence of human immunodeficiency virus DNA in laser smoke. *Lasers Surg Med*. 1991;11:197-203.

13. Divilio LT. Improving laparoscopic visibility and safety through smoke evacuation. *Surg Laparosc Endosc*. 1996;6:380-384.

14. Katkhouda N, Mason RJ, Mavor E, et al. Laparoscopic finger-assisted technique (fingeroscopy) for treatment of complicated appendicitis. *J Am Coll Surg*. 1999;189:131-133.

15. Birkett DH. Spilled cells, spilled clips, spilled stones. New problems or old challenges. *Surg Endosc*. 1995;9:269-271.

5. Questions

1. The more rapid return of GI function after laparoscopic surgery compared with open surgery is linked to:

A. Reduced manipulation of tissue with the laparoscopic approach

B. More frequent use of preoperative bowel preparation

C. Reduced need for pain medication

D. Earlier removal of the nasogastric tube

2. Absolute contraindications to a laparoscopic operation include:

A. Coagulopathy responding to fresh frozen plasma and vitamin K administration

B. Inexperience on the part of the surgeon

C. Lung disease causing dyspnea at rest

D. Morbid obesity

3. Compared with open surgery, patients undergoing laparoscopic surgery have:

A. Decreased risk of aspiration

B. Decreased catecholamine response

C. Increased venous return to the heart

D. Decreased risk of peripheral nerve injuries

4. The major source of bleeding during laparoscopic Nissen fundoplication is from:

A. Accidental aortic damage caused while dissecting the esophageal hiatus

B. The short gastric arteries

C. The left lobe of the liver

D. Accidental injury to the spleen

5. During laparoscopic cholecystectomy the cystic duct is too wide to be safely occluded with a single clip. The correct solution is to:

A. Place an additional clip from the other side of the cystic duct

B. Tie the cystic duct with an Endoloop

C. Convert to open cholecystectomy to make the closure secure

D. Insert a T-tube in the common bile duct

6. The harmonic scalpel differs from the Bovie electrocautery in which respect?

A. It generates more heat over a smaller area

B. It can be used for sealing large vessels such as the splenic artery

C. It requires a separate grounding pad

D. It cannot be used for dissecting like the Bovie electrocautery can

7. Sudden cardiovascular collapse immediately upon insufflation with the Veress needle suggests:

A. Myocardial infarct

B. Tension pneumothorax

C. CO_2 embolism

D. Bowel perforation

8. CO_2 insufflation for pneumoperitoneum is limited by:

A. The solubility of CO_2 leading to systemic hypercarbia

B. The reduction in venous return produced by intraabdominal pressures greater than 14 mm Hg

C. Shoulder pain produced by stimulation of the diaphragm by dissolved CO_2 in the postoperative period

D. The risk of elevating the CO_2 concentration in the operating room

9. In performing laparoscopic exploration in a patient with previous abdominal surgery the safest approach is to:

A. Open part of the original scar carefully and insert the Hasson trocar under direct vision

B. Put the trocar just below the costal margin where adhesions are unlikely

C. Insert the trocar in the quadrant of the abdomen furthest from the previous operative site

D. Use the umbilicus regardless of the location of the scar from the previous surgery, and divide the adhesions under direct vision

10. The treatment for gas embolism includes:

A. Steep head-down tilt of table

B. Aspiration of air via a central line, if present

C. Turn right side of patient up

D. All of the above

Answers

1. C.
The major advantage of the laparoscopic approach appears to be the reduced need for opiates. The administration of postoperative opiate medications is known to delay the return of GI function. The manipulation of the tissues is effectively the same as in open surgery, and early removal of the nasogastric tube is a consequence rather than a cause of accelerated return of GI function.

2. B.
Coagulopathy certainly makes laparoscopy more dangerous, but when it responds to correction in the short term it is more properly described as a risk factor than an absolute contraindication. Lung disease may contraindicate prolonged operations where CO_2 buildup would be hazardous, but it is also a risk factor, not a contraindication. An inexperienced surgeon is an absolute contraindication. It is much wiser to do the operation open than compromise the patient's safety.

3. B.
Many studies have shown that the catecholamine response to laparoscopic surgery is less than that for comparable open surgery. Most of these studies have looked at cholecystectomy. The risk of aspiration may actually increase, and venous return to the heart is decreased by the pneumoperitoneum. Peripheral nerve injuries may actually be more common in laparoscopic surgery because of the frequent changes in position often required.

4. C.
Aortic damage has been reported to occur during insertion of the crural sutures, and the short gastric arteries occasionally give problems, but this has been reduced by the increasing use of the harmonic scalpel for this part of the operation. Splenic damage is similarly reduced by use of this method of dividing the gastrosplenic ligament. But liver lacerations from retractor-induced injury are common, because it is necessary to hold up the left lateral segment of the liver firmly during the procedure, and the body habitus of patients needing laparoscopic Nissen fundoplication is associated with a bulky, fatty liver.

5. B.
Additional clips are not helpful for a wide cystic duct. An Endoloop is the best solution because it affords security in case a postoperative ERCP is required, which is frequently the case when the cystic duct is wide. It is acceptable to use a "stick tie" suture through and around the cystic duct, but it is more awkward to perform. It is quite unnecessary to convert to an open operation or insert a drainage tube.

6. A.
The major advantage of the harmonic scalpel is that it generates enough heat to coagulate the enclosed blood vessels, but the heat is precisely focused so it is not disseminated to nearby tissues. It should not be used on large named blood vessels. It generates high frequency ultrasound waves and requires no grounding pad, and has a reversible blade which can be used to dissect as well as coagulate.

7. C.
The occurrence of sudden collapse before the operation has actually begun suggests gas embolism. Tension pneumothorax and myocardial infarct may cause similar catastrophic changes but are unlikely in otherwise healthy patients before surgery begins. A bowel perforation is unlikely to produce changes of this rapidity.

8. A.
CO_2 accumulates in the body during laparoscopic operations but can be compensated by several storage and buffering mechanisms. In patients with limited compensating mechanisms, particularly patients with advanced lung disease, hypercarbia and consequent respiratory acidosis limit the duration of CO_2 insufflation. Atmospheric CO_2 is unaffected.

9. C.
All the other solutions are dangerous because they increase the risk of causing injury to a structure which is likely to be adherent, but which cannot be seen or dealt with through the small incision. Consequently, the safest method is to insert the trocar at the site least likely to contain adhesions.

10. D.
All of these maneuvers help localize the gas in the apex of the right ventricle and limit the functional right ventricular outflow obstruction.

Chapter 15: Bariatric Surgery

Brian R. Smith, MD
Ninh T. Nguyen, MD

Contents

1. Introduction

Obesity is a chronic disease that has become a major nutritional health problem in most industrialized countries. Obesity among Unites States adults is increasing at an alarming rate. Data from the National Health and Nutrition Examination Survey (NHANES) demonstrated that the prevalence of obesity in adults increased from 22.9% in 1988-1994 to 30.5% in 1999-2000; morbid obesity (body mass index [BMI] ≥ 40) also increased from 2.9% to 4.7%, respectively.[1] Overweight children and adolescents in the United States are also increasing in number. According to the NHANES report, the prevalence of overweight individuals among 12-19 year-olds increased from 10.5% in 1988-1994 to 15.5% in 1999-2000.[2,3]

The health implications of obesity include increased risk for coronary artery disease, hypertension, hyperlipidemia, insulin-resistant type II diabetes mellitus, sleep apnea, stroke, arthritis of the weight-bearing joints and increased prevalence for selected types of cancer. The risk for developing these comorbidities is proportional to the degree of obesity. The relative risk of death is increased substantially with increasing BMI, particularly in patients with BMI >35 kg/m^2.[2,4] Obesity contributes to approximately 300,000 premature deaths each year as a result of health-related complications.[5] Treatment of obesity-related comorbidities is also costly. In the United States, it has been estimated 9.1% of the national health expenditure.[6] The mean annual total health care costs for patients with a BMI of 35 or higher is 44% greater than the annual costs for patients with BMI of 20 to 24.9. Bariatric surgery has been shown to substantially improve or resolve many common obesity-related comorbid conditions, including type II diabetes, hypertension, sleep apnea, and hyperlipidemia. A recent report of 10-year outcomes from the observational Swedish Obese Subjects demonstrated marked benefits favoring surgery compared to matched control subjects treated medically, including recovery from diabetes, lipid abnormalities, sleep apnea and quality of life.[8]

Since the 1991 National Institutes of Health consensus conference, bariatric surgery has become an acceptable option for the treatment of morbid obesity.[9] Nonsurgical treatment for severe obesity includes a combination of low-calorie diet, behavioral therapy, exercise program, and/or pharmacotherapy. However, limited success has been reported. In long-term follow-up, most patients failed to maintain their reduced body weight. Even with pharmacotherapy, patients who respond to therapy usually regained weight when their treatment was stopped. A randomized controlled trial that compared bariatric surgery with a nonsurgically treated control group demonstrated that at 24 months of follow-up, the mean difference in weight loss greatly favored surgical therapy.[10]

Several bariatric operations have been introduced in the past four decades. These operations encompass a spectrum from restrictive to malabsorptive procedures. Roux-en-Y gastric bypass (GBP) is the most commonly performed operation for obesity. With the advent of a laparoscopic approach, the public now views bariatric surgery as a less invasive operation with less postoperative pain and a faster recovery. In addition, laparoscopic adjustable gastric banding was approved for clinical use by the Food and Drug Administration in June 2001 and has become an increasingly popular alternative to gastric bypass. This chapter provides an overview of the indications for bariatric surgery, facility requirements, patient selection, commonly performed bariatric surgical procedures and their results, and the role of laparoscopy in bariatric surgery.

2. Definitions of Obesity

Severe obesity is defined as being twice the ideal body weight as calculated from the Metropolitan Life Insurance height/weight tables. A more precise method for classification of obesity is BMI, which is calculated by dividing the weight in kilograms by the height in meters squared. The classification of obesity as reported by the American Society for Metabolic and Bariatric Surgery is as follows:

• Overweight:	BMI 25 ≤27
• Mild obesity:	BMI 27 ≤30
• Moderate obesity:	BMI 30 ≤35
• Severe obesity:	BMI 35 ≤40
• Morbid obesity:	BMI 40 ≤50
• Super obesity:	BMI 50 ≤60
• Super-super obesity:	BMI >60

3. Indications and Contraindications for Surgery

The indications for surgery follow the guidelines set forth by the 1991 National Institutes of Health Consensus Development Conference Panel for the treatment of severe obesity.[9] The panel recommended that patients seeking treatment for severe obesity should consider a comprehensive nonsurgical program as the first treatment option, and subsequent bariatric surgery could then be considered for well-informed and motivated patients with acceptable operative risks. The criteria for bariatric surgery are as follows:

1. Patients who have failed multiple attempts at nonsurgical means of weight loss.
2. Well-informed and motivated patient who understand the risks and benefits of the procedure.
3. Have a long history of severe obesity (more than 5 years) without an endocrine cause for obesity.
4. Have acceptable operative risks and no significant psychiatric illnesses.
5. Have a BMI exceeding 40 kg/m^2, or a BMI between 35 and 40 kg/m^2 with associated obesity-related health conditions such as severe sleep apnea, Pickwickian syndrome, obesity-related cardiomyopathy, disabling joint disease, diabetes mellitus, hypertension or hyperlipidemia.
6. Able to participate in long-term follow-up.

In 2004, a bariatric Consensus Conference Panel convened regarding the state of bariatric surgery, with findings and recommendations which included:[11]

1. A multidisciplinary team including a surgeon, anesthesiologist, dietician, nurse and experienced office personnel should be used in the care of the bariatric surgery patient.
2. Candidates should have attempted to lose weight by nonoperative means but should not be required to complete formal nonoperative obesity therapy as a precondition for the operation.

3. Candidates should have a comprehensive medical evaluation before the operation; evaluation by subspecialists is not routinely needed but should be available if indicated.

4. The surgical team should be receptive to change in selecting operative procedures and concepts and the introduction of new operative approaches.

5. Standard of care for bariatric surgery includes use of laparoscopic and open techniques.

6. Additional experience should be obtained with extending the benefits of bariatric surgery to adolescents.

7. Considerations should be given to extending the benefits of bariatric surgery to patients with BMI 30-34.9, who have a condition that can be cured or markedly improved by substantial and sustained weight loss.

8. Because bariatric surgery can be cost-effective in less than 4 years, in comparison with nonoperative management, critical examination of the cost-to-benefit ratio is indicated.

9. Increased clinical investigation, basic research and education in the obesity field are strongly recommended. Advanced age, previous abdominal operations, or previous bariatric procedures that are functionally ineffective or have failed for anatomic or technical reasons are not necessarily contraindications. In contrast, active substance abuse and certain psychiatric disorders (schizophrenia, borderline personality disorder, uncontrolled depression) should be considered absolute contraindications for bariatric surgery.

4. Preoperative Evaluation

Morbid obesity is often associated with numerous medical comorbidities. These comorbidities are often exacerbated by obesity and often improve or resolve after weight loss. Common comorbidities associated with morbid obesity include:

1. Hypertension
2. Hyperlipidemia
3. Type II diabetes mellitus
4. Gastroesophageal reflux
5. Arthritis of the weight-bearing joints
6. Infertility
7. Urinary stress incontinence
8. Cardiovascular disease
    - Coronary artery disease
    - Left-ventricular hypertrophy
    - Pulmonary hypertension
9. Lower extremity venous stasis
10. Respiratory insufficiency
    - Obesity hypoventilation syndrome
    - Obstructive sleep apnea
11. Certain cancers

The preoperative evaluation should include a complete medical history and physical examination, assessment of the patient's operative risk, assessment of obesity-related comorbidities, and education about the surgical options and risks/benefits of the operation. All comorbid conditions that are listed should be recognized and treated or optimized before surgery is undertaken, and monitored for improvement and/or resolution after surgery.

5. Facility Requirements

In order to perform bariatric surgery, the health care facility must be able to accommodate the morbidly obese patient in all aspects, starting with a system for evaluation to follow-up. The institution performing bariatric surgery should have a bariatric surgical team, skilled staff, appropriate operating room equipment and sufficient institutional resources. A bariatric surgical team consists of experienced surgeons and physicians, anesthesiologists, nurses and nutritionists. Specialists in the field of cardiology, pulmonology, endocrinology and psychiatry should be available. The operating room must have operating tables and ancillary equipment to accommodate morbidly obese patients. The operating room staff should also be familiar with the equipment, instruments and procedures for management of morbidly obese patients. The hospital facility should have beds, commodes, chairs and wheelchairs to accommodate the morbidly obese. In addition, radiology should be capable of handling the radiologic needs of morbidly obese patients.

6. Bariatric Operations

Several different bariatric operations are commonly performed for the treatment of morbid obesity. The five most commonly performed procedures are listed below in order of frequency:

1. Roux-en-Y gastric bypass
2. Adjustable gastric banding
3. Vertical sleeve gastrectomy
4. Vertical banded gastroplasty
5. Biliopancreatic diversion and/or duodenal switch

Vertical banded gastroplasty, vertical sleeve gastrectomy and the adjustable gastric band are purely restrictive operations. Roux-en-Y gastric bypass is also a restrictive operation but with a malabsorptive component. Biliopancreatic diversion and the duodenal switch operations are malabsorptive procedures. There have been five randomized trials comparing weight loss among surgical procedures. In two studies, gastric bypass was compared to vertical banded gastroplasty and weight loss outcomes favored gastric bypass at 12 and 36 months.[12] There have been no randomized trials comparing outcomes of gastric bypass vs. adjustable gastric band or gastric bypass vs. duodenal switch.

7. The Laparoscopic Approach to Bariatric Surgery

The laparoscopic approach to bariatric surgery was introduced in the early 1990s. Laparoscopic bariatric surgery is performed through 5-6 abdominal ports with the creation of carbon dioxide pneumoperitoneum. Specialized instruments including mechanical staplers, grasping instruments, ultrasonic shears and suturing devices are used to perform the operation without the need for the traditional abdominal incision. Laparoscopic gastric banding was first reported in 1993.[13] Subsequently, laparoscopic vertical banded gastroplasty (VBG) and Roux-en-Y gastric bypass (GBP) were described in 1994.1[14,15] By 2000, laparoscopic biliopancreatic diversion had been reported.[16]

Wound infection and late incisional hernia following open bariatric surgery can be as high as 11.5% and 20%, respectively.[17] The laparoscopic approach to bariatric surgery was first developed in an effort to reduce the morbidity of the surgical wound. However, many other benefits of the laparoscopic approach have been identified. In a randomized trial comparing laparoscopic vs. open GBP, Nguyen and colleagues reported that laparoscopic GBP was associated with less postoperative pain, a shorter length of hospitalization, decreased need for intensive care unit stay and faster recovery (Table 1).[18] In addition, the laparoscopic approach to gastric bypass has been shown to reduce the host's systemic stress responses, improve postoperative pulmonary function, decrease the incidence of venous thromboembolism and decrease the host's operative trauma compared to the open approach.[19-22]

The role of laparoscopic bariatric surgery in patients with compromised cardiac, renal, hepatic and respiratory function is unknown and further studies are needed. The adverse consequences of pneumoperitoneum include carbon dioxide absorption and the effects of increased intraabdominal pressure on the various body systems. Carbon dioxide absorption can result in hypercarbia, hypercapnia and systemic acidosis. The increased intra abdominal pressure has been shown to depress cardiac function, reduce respiratory compliance and increase airway pressure, reduce intraoperative urinary output and alter postoperative hepatic transaminases.[23] Patients with potential impediment to laparoscopic bariatric surgery include those with large ventral hernia, patients with android body habitus and patients with BMI greater than 60.

Table 1

Laparoscopic versus Open Gastric Bypass

Clinical Parameters	Laparoscopic	Open
Operative time	+ + +	+ +
Blood loss	+	++
Length of hospitalization	+ +	+ + +
Requirement for intensive care stay	+	+ +
Postoperative pain	+	+ +
Days to return to work	+ +	+ + +
Days to return to normal activities	+	+ +

8. Patient Selection for Laparoscopic Bariatric Surgery

Patient selection for laparoscopic bariatric surgery depends on the surgeon's experience with the laparoscopic technique. Surgeons inexperienced in laparoscopic bariatric surgery should select patients with low BMI (less than 45), patients with gynecoid body habitus, female patients and patients without prior abdominal surgery or only previous lower abdominal surgery. Male patients tend to have more central obesity and intra abdominal fat deposition, which makes laparoscopic exposure of the operative field more difficult. As surgeons gain experience in laparoscopic bariatric surgery, the selection criteria for the laparoscopic approach can be broadened to patients with higher BMI, male patients and patients with android body habitus.

9. Laparoscopic Gastric Bypass

Trocar Position

The patient is placed in a supine position. The surgeon stands on the patient's right side and the assistant on the patient's left side (Figure 1). The initial access is through an abdominal incision at the left midclavicular line above the umbilicus. Pneumoperitoneum is introduced through a Veress needle, and a 12 mm trocar is placed at this site and used as the camera port. Four additional trocars are placed, including a 5 mm trocar at the left anterior axillary line below the subcostal margin for the assistant surgeon. A 5 mm trocar is placed at the right midclavicular line below the right subcostal margin and a 12 mm trocar is placed close to the midline above the umbilicus (Figure 2). Occasionally, the falciform ligament is divided to provide a free space for placement of the 12 mm trocar. A fifth trocar is placed at the patient's right anterior axillary line below the costal margin for retraction of the left lobe of the liver.

Figure 1

Room set-up for laparoscopic bariatric surgery

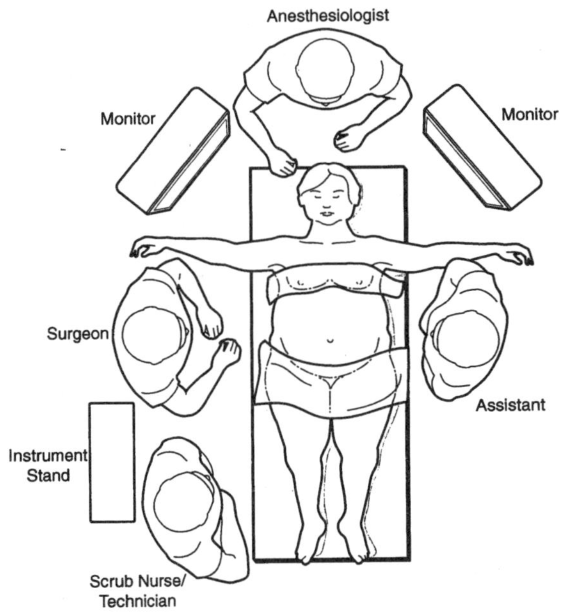

Figure 2

Abdominal port position for laparoscopic gastric bypass

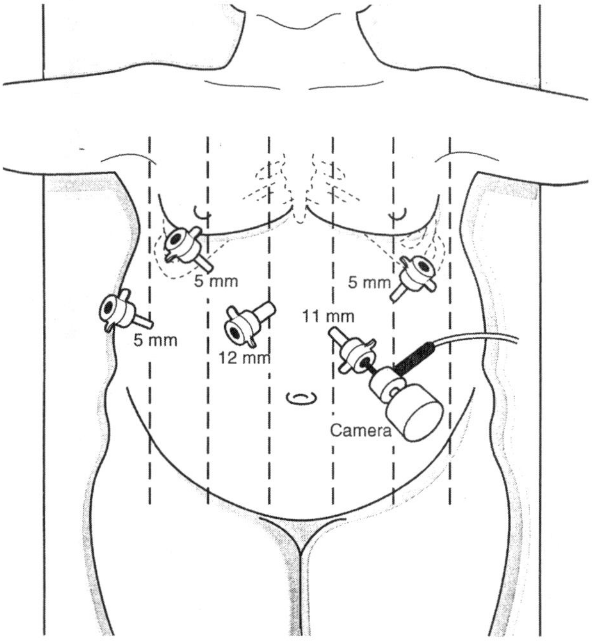

Figure 3

Division of the jejunum and its mesentery

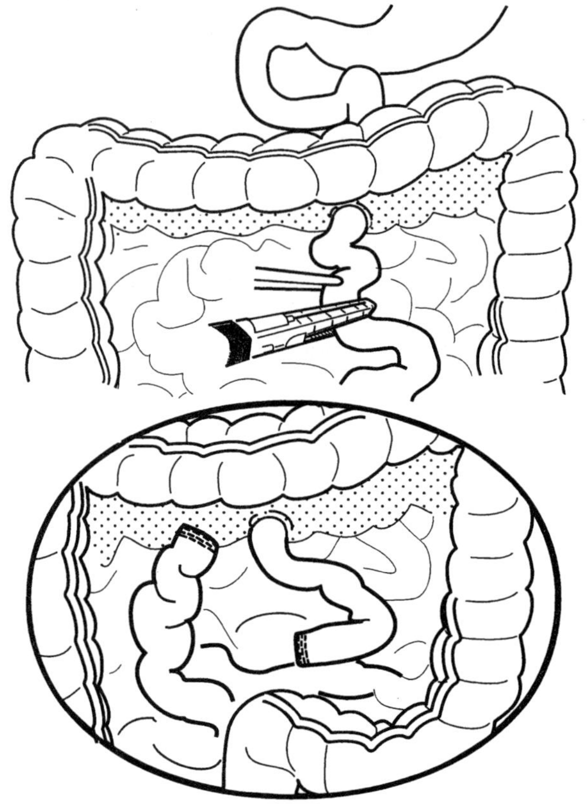

Jejunojejunostomy

The jejunum and its mesentery are divided 40 cm distal to the ligament of Treitz (Figure 3). The Roux limb is measured to the desired length (75-150 cm based on BMI). We routinely perform a 75 cm Roux limb for patients with BMI <50 and 150 cm Roux limb for patients with BMI ≥50. A single stay suture approximates the two loops of small bowel for creation of the side-to-side jejunojejunostomy. An enterotomy is created in both limbs of the small bowel. The anastomosis is created with a single application of a 60 mm 3.5 mm (blue) linear stapler (Figure 4). The remaining enterotomy defect is sutured closed (Figure 5). An anti-obstruction suture is placed to prevent postoperative angulation of the Roux limb. The jejunojejunostomy mesenteric defect is closed with interrupted sutures to prevent postoperative internal herniation.

Route of the Roux Limb

The Roux limb can be brought to the gastric pouch in a retrocolic retrogastric (Figure 6) or antecolic antegastric route. One advantage of retrocolic retrogastric route is the short distance to the gastric pouch and therefore less tension is present on the gastrojejunostomy. One disadvantage of the retrocolic technique is the possible injury to the middle colic vessel during creation of the transverse mesocolon defect. The advantages of the antecolic technique are the elimination for the need to create a transverse mesocolon defect or the need for closure of both the transverse mesocolon and the Petersen hernia defects.

Gastrojejunostomy

The key features for creation of the gastrojejunal anastomosis are creation of a small gastric pouch (15-20 mL) based on the lesser curvature of the stomach, preservation of the blood supply to the gastric pouch from the left gastric vessels and creation of a tension-free anastomosis. There are many

Figure 4

Laparoscopic jejunojejunostomy with the linear stapler

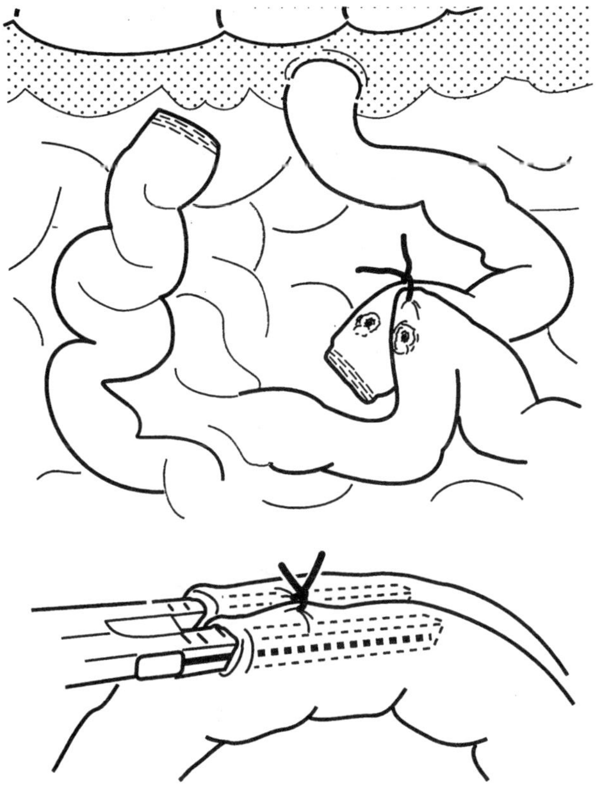

Figure 5

Closure of the enterotomy defect with interrupted sutures

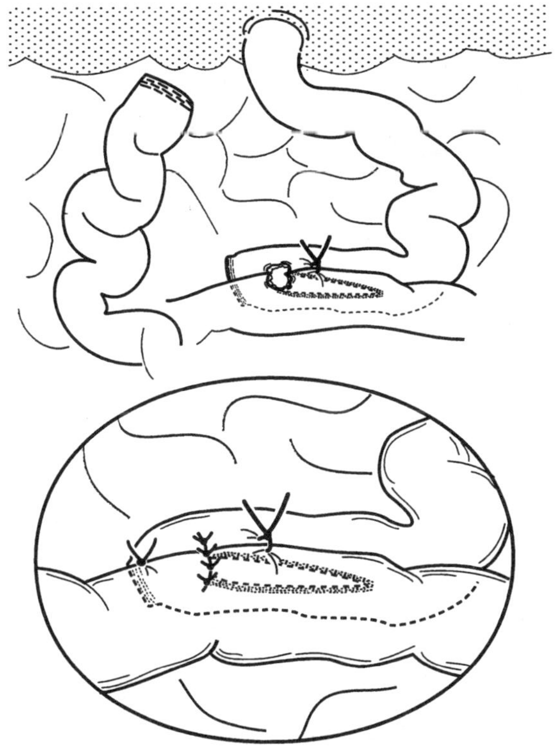

methods for creation of the gastrojejunostomy, including the hand-sewn technique and the linear and circular stapled technique. In addition, the circular technique has variation in the method for introduction of the anvil; the anvil can be placed transorally or transabdominally. The individual technique for creation of the gastrojejunostomy is often based on the surgeon's preference and experience with a particular technique. Our preferred method for creation of the gastrojejunostomy is the circular stapled technique with the anvil placed transabdominally. The anvil is inserted transabdominally through an enlarged trocar site. An anterior gastrotomy is created on the lesser curve of the stomach. The anvil, attached to a ski needle, is positioned through the gastrotomy and penetrates the anterior gastric wall approximately 1 cm below the gastroesophageal junction (Figure 7). Multiple applications of the linear stapler are then applied adjacent to the anvil transversely, and then superiorly towards the angle of His to create the gastric pouch (Figure 8). The circular stapler is inserted transabdominally, placed through the jejunal Roux limb, and attached to the anvil for creation of the gastrojejunostomy (Figure 9). Reinforcement sutures are placed circumferentially around the anastomosis to minimize tension (Figure 10).

Postoperative Care

Patients are extubated in the operating room, transferred to the recovery room and then taken to the surgical ward. A nasogastric tube is not routinely used for postoperative drainage. Postoperative pain is controlled with intravenous morphine sulfate using a patient-controlled analgesia method. Patients are encouraged to ambulate on the operative night as well as to perform incentive spirometry

Figure 6

Retrocolic retrogastric placement of the Roux limb

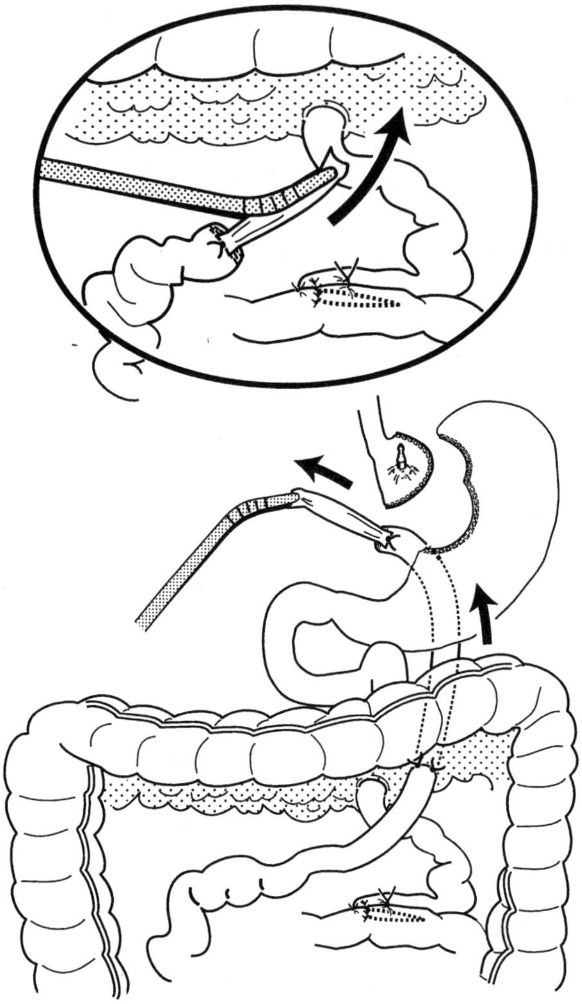

Figure 7

Transabdominal placement of the anvil in preparation for a circular stapled gastrojejunostomy

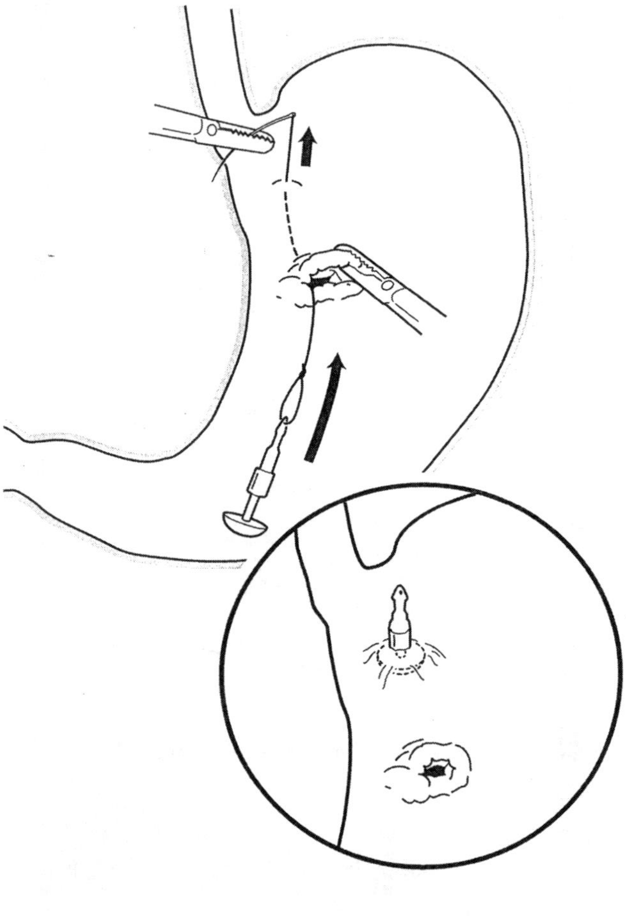

and deep-breathing exercises. A gastrograffin contrast study is performed on the first or second postoperative day. Clear liquids are started after confirmation of an intact anastomosis without evidence of contrast leak or obstruction. Patients are discharged home, often on POD 2, when they can tolerate oral fluid.

Results

Results of laparoscopic GBP are listed in Table 2.[18,24-33] The mean BMI in these series ranged from 43 to 52 kg/m^2. Mean operative times ranged from 90 to 260 minutes. Operative blood loss during laparoscopic GBP was consistently low, ranging from 115 to 137 mL. Conversion rates ranged from 1.1% to 6.9%. Mortality rates were low, ranging from 0%-1.1%. Early perioperative complications included anastomotic stricture, anastomotic leak, wound infection, early bowel obstruction, deep venous thrombosis and gastrointestinal hemorrhage. Late complications included bowel obstruction from internal hernia and anastomotic stricture.

Weight loss after laparoscopic GBP is thought to be equivalent to that after open GBP, as the only difference between the two techniques is the method of access. Long-term weight loss after laparoscopic

Figure 8

Creation of the gastric pouch with multiple applications of the linear staplers

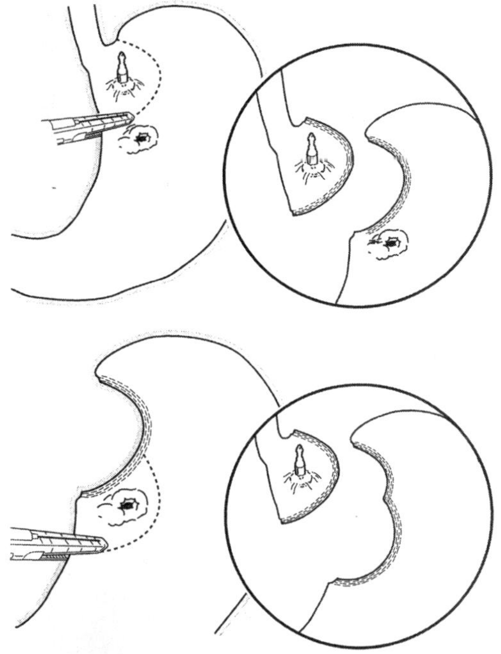

Figure 9

Creation of a circular stapled gastrojejunostomy

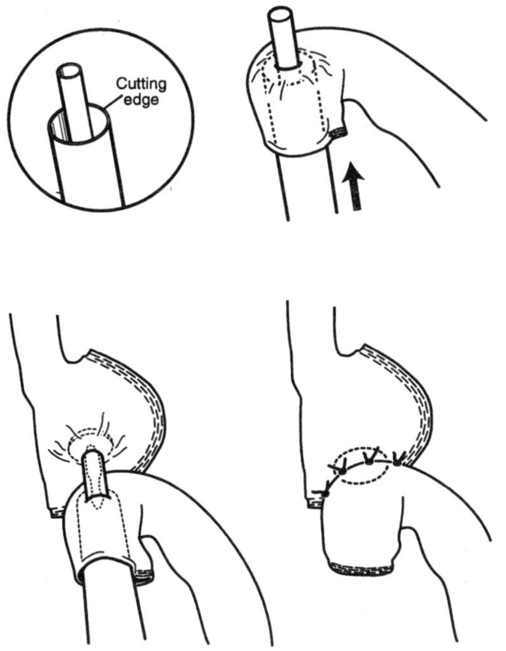

Figure 10

Completed laparoscopic Roux-en-Y gastric bypass

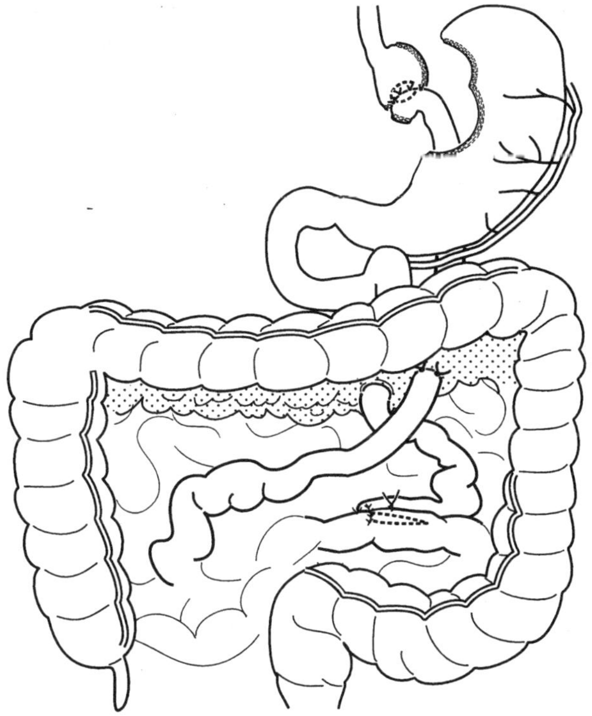

Table 2

Selected Series of Laparoscopic versus Roux-en-Y Gastric Bypass

Published Series	Year	N	Mean BMI	OR Time (min)	Conversion	Leaks	Mortality	Excess Body Weight Loss
Lugan et al[32]	2004	53	49	186	8%	3.7%	3.7%	—
Westling et al[31]	2001	30	41	235	23%	0	0	—
Biertho et al[30]	2003	456	49	—	1.9%	0.6%	0.4%	75% (1.5 y)
Ballesta-Lopez et al[29]	2005	600	44	119	0.5%	3.8%	1.1%	68% (2 y)
Oliak et al[27]	2002	300	51	141	1%	1.3%	1%	—
Higa et al[28]	2001	1500	—	—	1.3%	0.9%	0.2%	62% (3 y)
Nguyen et al[18]	2001	79	48	225	2.5%	1.3%	0%	68% (1 y)
Schauer et al[24]	2000	275	48	260	1.1%	4.4%	0.4%	83% (2 y)
Wittgrove et al[25]	2000	500	—	90	—	2.2%	0%	>80% (5 y)
Marema et al[26]	2005	1077	8	95	—	0.6%	0.1%	—
Sundbom et al[33]	2004	25	44	150	0%	4%	0%	—

OR: operative time; BMI: body mass index

GBP has been reported by Wittgrove et al[25] at more than 80% of excess body weight loss at five years. In addition, gastroesophageal reflux, diabetes and sleep apnea were eliminated in more than 98% of patients.[25] There have been 4 randomized trials comparing the outcomes of laparoscopic vs. open gastric bypass.[18,31-33] Results from these trials are reported in Table 2.

10. Laparoscopic Adjustable Gastric Banding

Technique

The laparoscopic adjustable gastric banding (LAGB) is performed using five abdominal trocars similar to the trocar position for laparoscopic GBP. With the patient in a reverse Trendelenburg position, the left lobe of the liver is retracted anteriorly using a self-retaining retractor. A balloon suction catheter is placed transorally, advanced into the stomach, and inflated to 15 mL by the anesthesiologist. The balloon is pulled back and lodged at the gastroesophageal junction. The equator of the balloon serves as a landmark for placement of the gastric band.

There is now only one accepted method for placement of the gastric band. The esophagogastric technique, otherwise known as the *pars flaccida technique*, begins with the dissection on the right crus of the diaphragm posterior to the esophagus. A retroesophageal tunnel is created toward the angle of His. Dissection then takes place at the angle of His just proximal to the first short gastric vessel, where a window for the band is created between the stomach and diaphragm. The gastric band and its tubing are inserted into the peritoneum through a 15 mm trocar. An atraumatic, articulating instrument is passed through the dissected retroesophageal plane and exits at the angle of His. The band tubing is inserted into the opening of the articulating instrument. The instrument is withdrawn from the tunnel, and the band is pulled into position around the gastric cardia. The band is securely closed using the buckle on the band. To prevent band slippage, three anterior gastrogastric sutures are placed on the anterior aspect of the band. The gastric band tubing is removed through the left midclavicular trocar and connected to an implantable port. The access port is placed above the anterior rectus fascia.

There are currently two adjustable gastric bands on the market, the Lap-Band® (Allergan, Irvine, CA), and the Realize® Band (Ethicon, Cincinatti, OH). Both bands have buckles on the band and are applied in a similar fashion.

Postoperative Management

Patients are extubated in the operating room, transferred to the recovery room and then to the surgical ward. A gastrograffin contrast study is performed on the first postoperative day. Clear liquids are initiated and the patient is discharged. Adjustments to the band can be performed postoperatively by percutaneous access of the subcutaneous port in an office setting, typically without the need for fluoroscopy.

Results

Results of laparoscopic LAGB are listed in Table 3.[34-43] The operative time ranged from 60 to 105 minutes. Conversion to open laparotomy occurred in 08.3%. Mortality was low, ranging from 0%-0.6%. Perioperative complications included gastric perforation and bleeding. Late complications included food intolerance, band slippage, pouch dilatation and band erosion. Esophageal dilatation has also been reported.[44] Weight loss after laparoscopic ASGB has been reported to be 54% at 5 years and 58% at 8 years.[34,36,37]

Table 3

Selected Series of Laparoscopic Adjustable Silicone Gastric Banding

Selected Series	Year	N	Mean BMI	OR Time (min)	Conversion	Mortality	Band Removal	Excess Body Weight Loss
Weiner et al[37]	2003	984	47	--	0%	0%	59%	(8 y)
Angrisani et al[41]	2002	1853	44	--	3.1%	0.5%	--	--
Favretti et al[42]	2002	830	46	--	2.7%	0.6%	--	--
O'Brien et al[36]	2002	709	--	56	1%	0%	1.7%	54% (5 y)
Szold et al[43]	2002	715	43	78	0.8%	0%	4.4%	--
Zinzindohoue et al[39]	2002	500	44	105	2.4%	0%	--	55% (3 y)
Cardiere et al[40]	2000	652	45	80	3.8%	0.1%	2.0%	62% (2 y)
Dargent[35]	1999	500	43	--	1.9%	0%	6.0%	64% (3 y)
Ceeten et al[38]	2003	625	40	80	0.3%	0%	--	47% (3 y)
Biertho et al[34]	2005	824	43	--	8.3%	0.3%	6%	55% (5 y)

OR: operative time; BMI: body mass index

OR: operative time; BMI: body mass index

11. Laparoscopic Vertical Sleeve Gastrectomy

Laparoscopic vertical sleeve gastrectomy (VSG) has become an increasingly common and popular operation over the last five years. The procedure originated as part of a duodenal switch operation and later evolved into a staging procedure for super-obese and/or high-risk operative patients. These individuals would undergo an initial operation consisting entirely of a vertical resection of the lateral aspect of the gastric body and fundus. It was eventually realized that many of these patients ultimately did not need to go on to a second stage, as weight loss from the initial sleeve was sufficient.

The operation begins with mobilization of the greater curvature of the stomach and division of the short gastric vessels. Using a linear laparoscopic stapler, the greater curve of the stomach is transected approximately 6 cm proximal to the pylorus, with successive staples fired cephalad and parallel to the lesser curve and against a 42 French bougie. The resected stomach is removed through one of the large port sites. Operative time for this procedure is generally 1-2 hours. Postoperative care is similar to that of laparoscopic gastric bypass with an upper gastrointestinal study on the first postoperative day and initiation of a clear liquid diet with a negative study for leak or obstruction. Patients typically are discharged on the first or second postoperative day after ambulating and tolerating oral analgesics.

The largest published VSG study to date included 216 patients and found a 59% excess weight loss at 1 year.[45] Complications include staple line leak, nausea and vomiting, pulmonary embolism and hemorrhage. Studies documenting long-term results for VSG are due out in the near future.

12. Laparoscopic Vertical Banded Gastroplasty

The VBG operation consists of constructing a small gastric pouch based on the lesser curvature of the stomach and a restricted outlet due to a prosthetic band. The VBG is a purely restrictive bariatric procedure with no malabsorptive component. The mechanism of weight loss is primarily related to caloric restriction. The VBG originally became popular because it is a relatively simple operation and has low operative risk. Short-term results have been reported to be excellent; long-term results, however, are less favorable.[46-51] Current experience of laparoscopic VBG is limited to certain centers in Europe and the United States. The mean BMI in these series ranged from 41 to 55 kg/m^2, and operative time for this procedure was generally short. Conversion rates to laparotomy ranged from 0%-25%. Operative mortality was zero in most series. Early complications included outlet stenosis and staple-line leak; late complications included staple-line fistula, band erosion, stoma stenosis, food intolerance and pouch dilation. Weight loss after VBG varied between reports. Morino et al[50] reported a 61% excess weight loss at 4 years. In contrast, Kalfarentzos et al[51] reported only a 37% excess weight loss at five years. The advantages of laparoscopic VBG are its reversibility, preservation of the gastrointestinal tract and maintained absorption of micronutrients. Disadvantages of VBG included lower weight loss compared to Roux-en-Y GBP, long-term weight gain, high revision rate and development of maladaptive eating behavior.

13. Laparoscopic Biliopancreatic Diversion

Biliopancreatic diversion (BPD) was developed by Scopinaro in the late 1970s.[44] The small bowel is divided 250 cm proximal to the ileocecal valve and a subtotal gastrectomy leaving a 400 mL gastric remnant is performed. The distal (alimentary) limb is connected to the proximal gastric pouch. The proximal limb (biliopancreatic limb) is connected end-to-side to the ileum 50 cm proximal to the ileocecal valve. This operation is considerably more complex and technically more difficult than the previously described operations. The role of malabsorption procedures in the treatment of morbid obesity is limited to certain centers; they comprise less than 15% of bariatric operations. These procedures may have a role in treating patients who are extremely obese (BMI >60) or who have failed other bariatric operations. Rabkin et al[52] reported the largest study on laparoscopic duodenal switch with 345 patients. The mean BMI was 50. The mean operative time was 201 minutes. Conversion occurred in 2% of patients and there was no operative mortality. The mean percent of excess weight loss at 2 years was 91%.

14. Lap Band vs. Lap Gastric Bypass

There have been three case-controlled studies comparing the outcomes of LAGB with laparoscopic GBP. Jan et al[53] reported the outcomes of 219 patients who underwent laparoscopic GBP with 154 patients who underwent banding. One death occurred in each group. The incidence of major and minor complications is similar. However reoperation rate was higher in the Lap-Band group and early weight loss was greater with gastric bypass. Weber et al[54] reported that laparoscopic GBP was superior to Lap-Band in a matched control study of 103 Lap-Band patients and 103 laparoscopic gastric bypass patients. Body mass index at 2 years decreased from 48.0 to 36.8 kg/m^2 in the Lap-Band group and from 47.7 to 31.9 kg/m^2 in the gastric bypass group. In addition, the gastric bypass procedure achieved a significantly better reduction in obesity-related comorbidities. Lastly, Biertho et al[30] reported a comparative study of 1200 cases (456 gastric bypasses vs. 805 Lap-Band). Excess body weight loss at 18 months was superior in the gastric bypass group.

15. References

1. Odgen CL, Carroll MD, Curtin LR, et al. Prevalence of overweight and obesity in the United States, 1999-2004. *JAMA.* 2006;295:1549-1555.

2. Ogden CL, Flegal KM, Carroll MD, Johnson CL. Prevalence and trends in overweight among US children and adolescents, 1999-2000. *JAMA.* 2002;288(14):1728-1732.

3. National Center for Health Statistics. Chartbook on Trends in the Health of Americans. Hyattsville, MD: Public Health Service;2006.

4. Calle EE, Thun MJ, Petrelli JM, Rodriguez C, Health CW Jr. Body-mass index and mortality in a prospective cohort of US adults. *N Engl J Med.* 1999;341(15):1097-1105.

5. Allison DB, Fontaine KR, Manson JE, Stevens J, VanItallie TB. Annual deaths attributable to obesity in the Uniteds States. *JAMA.* 1999; 282(16):1530-1538.

6. Finkelstein EA, Fiebelkorn IC, Wang G. National medical spending attributable to overweight and obesity: How much, and who's paying? Health Affairs Web Exclusive. 2003;W3:219-226.

7. Quesenberry CP, Caan B, Jacobson A. Obesity, health service use, and health care costs among members of a health maintenance organization. *Arch Intern Med.*1998;158(5):466-472.

8. Karason K, Lindroos AK, Stenlof K, Sjostrom L. Relief of cardiorespiratory symptoms and increased physical activity after surgically induced weight loss: results from the Swedish Obese Subjects study. *Arch Intern Med.* 2000; 160:1797-1802.

9. NIH Conference:Gastrointestinal surgery for severe obesity: consensus development conference panel. *Ann Intern Med.*1991;115(12):956-961.

10. Andersen T, Stokholm KH, Backer OG, Quaade F. Long-term (5-year) results after either horizontal gastroplasty or very-low-calorie diet for morbid obesity. *Int J Obes.*1988;12:277-284.

11. Buchwald H. Bariatric surgery for morbid obesity: health implications for patients, health professionals, and third-party payers. *J Am Coll Surg.* 2005;200:593-604.

12. Maggard MA, Shugarman LR, Suttorp M, et al. Meta-analysis: surgical treatment of obesity. *Ann Intern Med.* 2005;142:547-559.

13. Catona A, Gossenberg M, La Manna A, Mussini G. Laparoscopic gastric banding: preliminary series. *Obes Surg.* 1993;3(2):207-209.

14. Wittgrove AC, Clark GW, Tremblay LJ. Laparoscopic gastric bypass, Roux-en-Y: preliminary report of five cases. *Obes Surg.* 1994; 4(4):353-357.

15. Hess DW, Hess DS. Laparoscopic vertical banded gastroplasty with complete transection of the staple-line. *Obes Surg.* 1994 4(1):44-46.

16. Ren CJ, Patterson E, Gagner M. Early results of laparoscopic biliopancreatic diversion with duodenal switch: a case series of 40 consecutive patients. *Obes Surg.* 2000;10(6):514-523.

17. Kellum JM, DeMaria EJ, Sugerman HJ. The surgical treatment of morbid obesity. *Curr Probl Surg.* 1998;35(9):791-858.

18. Nguyen NT, Goldman C, Rosenquist CJ, et al. Laparoscopic versus open gastric bypass: a randomized study of outcomes, quality of life, and costs. *Ann Surg.* 2001;234(3):289-291.

19. Nguyen NT, Lee SL, Goldman C, et al. Comparison of pulmonary function and postoperative pain after laparoscopic versus open gastric bypass: a randomized trial. *J Am Coll Surg.* 2001;192(4):469-476.

20. Nguyen NT, Lee SL, Anderson JT, Palmer LS, Canet F, Wolfe BM. Evaluation of intraabdominal pressure after open and laparoscopic gastric bypass. *Obes Surg*. 2001;11(1):40-45.

21. Nguyen NT, Goldman CD, Ho HS, Gosselin RC, Singh A, Wolfe BM. Systemic stress response after laparoscopic and open gastric bypass. *J Am Coll Surg*. 2002;194(5):557-567.

22. Nguyen NT, Hinojosa MW, Fayad C, et al. Laparoscopic surgery is associated with a lower incidence of venous thromboembolism compared with open surgery. *Ann Surg*. 2007;246:1021-1027.

23. Nguyen NT, Wolfe BM. Physiologic effects of pneumoperitoneum in the morbidly obese. *Ann Surg*. 2005;241(2):219-226.

24. Schauer PR, Ikramuddin S, Gourash W, Ramanathan R, Luketich J. Outcomes after laparoscopic Roux-en-Y gastric bypass for morbid obesity. *Ann Surg*. 2000;232(4):515-529.

25. Wittgrove AC, Clark GW. Laparoscopic gastric bypass, Roux-en-Y 500 patients: technique and results, with 3-60 month follow-up. *Obes Surg*. 2000;10(4):233-239.

26. Marema RT, Perez M, Buffington CK. Comparison of the benefits and complications between laparoscopic and open Roux-en-Y gastric bypass surgeries. *Surg Endosc*. 2005;19:525-530.

27. Oliak D, Ballantyne GH, Davies RJ, et al. Short-term results of laparoscopic gastric bypass in patients with BMI ≥60. *Obes Surg*. 2002;12:643-647.

28. Higa KD, Ho T, Boone KB. Laparoscopic Roux-en-Y gastric bypass: technique and 3-year follow-up. *J Laparoendosc Adv Surg Tech*. 2001;11(6):377-382.

29. Ballesta-Lopez C, Poves I, Cabrera M, Almeida A, Macias G. Learning curve for laparoscopic Roux-en-Y gastric bypass with totally hand-sewn anastomosis: analysis of first 600 consecutive patients. *Surg Endosc*. 2005;19:519-524.

30. Biertho L, Steffen R, Ricklin T, et al. Laparoscopic gastric bypass versus laparoscopic adjustable gastric banding: a comparative study of 1,200 cases. *J Am Coll Surg*. 2003;197:536-547.

31. Westling A, Gustavsson S. Laparoscopic vs. open Roux-en-Y gastric bypass: a prospective, randomized trial. *Obes Surg*. 2001;11:284-292.

32. Lugan JA, Frutos D, Hernandez Q, et al. Laparoscopic versus open gastric bypass in the treatment of morbid obesity: a randomized prospective study. *Ann Surg*. 2004;239:433-437.

33. Sundbom M, Gustavsson S. Randomized clinical trial of hand-assisted laparoscopic versus open Roux-en-Y gastric bypass for the treatment of morbid obesity. *Br J Surg*. 2004; 91:418-423.

34. Biertho L, Steffen R, Branson R, et al. Management of failed adjustable gastric banding. *Surgery*. 2005;137:33-41.

35. Dargent J. Laparoscopic adjustable gastric banding: lessons from the first 500 patients in a single institution. *Obes Surg*. 1999;9(5):446-452.

36. O'Brien PE, Dixon JB. Lap-Band® outcomes and results. *J Laparoendosc Adv Surg Tech*. 2003;13:265-270.

37. Weiner R, Blanco-Engert R, Weiner S, Matkowitz R, Schaefer L, Pomhoff I. Outcome after laparoscopic adjustable gastric banding – 8 years experience. *Obes Surg*. 2003; 13(3):427-434.

38. Ceelen W, Walder J, Cardon A, et al. Surgical treatment of severe obesity with a low-pressure adjustable gastric band: experimental data and clinical results in 625 patients. *Ann Surg*. 2003; 237:10-16.

39. Zinzindohoue F, Chevallier JM, Douard R, et al. Laparoscopic gastric banding: a minimally invasive surgical treatment for morbid obesity: prospective study of 500 consecutive patients. *Ann Surg*. 2003; 237(1):1-9.

40. Cadiere GB, Himpens J, Vertruyen M, Germay O, Favretti F, Segato G. Laparoscopic gastroplasty (adjustable silicone gastric banding). *Semin Laparosc Surg*. 2000;7(1):55-65.

41. Angrisani L, Furbetta F, Doldi SB, et al. Lap Band: adjustable gastric banding system: the Italian experience with 1863 patients operated on 6 years. *Surg Endosc*. 2003;17(3):409-412.

42. Favretti F, Cardiere GB, Segato G, et al. Laparoscopic banding: selection and technique in 830 patients. *Obes Surg*. 2002;12(3):385-390.

43. Szold A, Abu-Abeid S. Laparoscopic adjustable silicone gastric banding for morbid obesity: results and complications in 715 patients. *Surg Endosc*. 2002;16(2):230-233.

44. DeMaria EJ, Sugerman HJ, Meador JG, et al. High failure rate after laparoscopic adjustable silicone gastric banding for treatment of morbid obesity. *Ann Surg*. 2001; 233(6):809-818.

45. Lee CM, Cirangle PT, Jossart GH. Vertical gastrectomy for morbid obesity in 216 patients: report of 2-year results. *Surg Endosc*. 2007;21:1810-1816.

46. Naslund E, Freedman J, Lagergren J, Stockeld D, Granstrom L. Three-year results of laparoscopic vertical banded gastroplasty. *Obes Surg*. 1999;9(4):369-373.

47. Azagra JS, Goergen M, Ansay J, et al. Laparoscopic gastric reduction surgery: preliminary results of a randomized, prospective trial of laparoscopic vs. open vertical banded gastroplasty. *Surg Endosc*. 1999;13(6):555-558.

48. Suter M, Giusti V, Heraief E, Zysset F, Calmes JM. Early results of laparoscopic gastric banding compared with open vertical banded gastroplasty. *Obes Surg*. 1999;9(4):374-380.

49. Gerhart CD. Hand-assisted laparoscopic vertical banded gastroplasty: report of a series. *Arch Surg*. 2000;135(7):795-798.

50. Morino M, Toppino M, Bonnet G, Rosa R, Garrone C. Laparoscopic vertical banded gastroplasty for morbid obesity: assessment of efficacy. *Surg Endosc*. 2002;16(11):1566-1572.

51. Kalfarentzos F, Kechagias L, Soulikia K, Loukidi A, Mead N. Weight loss following vertical banded gastroplasty: intermediate results of a prospective study. *Obes Surg*. 2001; 11(3):265-270.

52. Rabkin RA, Rabkin JM, Metcalf B, Lazo M, Rossi M, Lehman-Becker LB. Laparoscopic technique for performing duodenal switch with gastric reduction. *Obes Surg*. 2003;13(2):263-268.

53. Jan JC, Hong D, Pereira N, Patterson EJ. Laparoscopic adjustable gastric banding versus laparoscopic gastric bypass for morbid obesity: a single-institution comparison study of early results. *J Gastrointest Surg*. 2005;9:30-41.

54. Weber M, Muller MK, Bucher T, et al. Laparoscopic gastric bypass is superior to laparoscopic gastric banding for treatment of morbid obesity. *Ann Surg*. 2004;240(6):975-983.

16. Questions

1. The most common bariatric operation performed in the US is:

A. Gastric banding

B. Roux-en-Y gastric bypass

C. Vertical banding gastroplasty

D. Biliopancreatic diversion

2. The cost of obesity in the US is estimated to be:

A. 9% of national health expenditure

B. 20% of national health expenditure

C. 6% of national health expenditure

D. 1% of national health expenditure

3. Among subjects who successfully lose a substantial quantity of weight by medical treatment, what percent maintain the weight loss for more than a few years?

A. 20%

B. 15%

C. 50%

D. 5%

4. A useful indicator of obesity is the body mass index (BMI), which is calculated by:

A. Kg/m^2

B. m^2/kg

C. Lbs/ft

D. m/kg

5. All of the following are indications for bariatric surgery except:

A. Patient who has failed medical attempts and has a BMI of 40 with no comorbid conditions

B. Patient with a BMI of 36 with severe diabetes mellitus

C. Patients with a BMI of 55 with no comorbid conditions

D. Patient with a BMI of 45 and active substance abuse

6. All of the following are usually involved in the care of a patient undergoing bariatric surgery except:

A. Cardiologist

B. Endocrinologist

C. Psychiatrist

D. Pulmonologist

E. All of the above

7. The advantages of laparoscopic bariatric surgery to open surgery include:

A. Reduction in perioperative morbidity

B. Reduction in wound infection

C. Shorter length of hospital stay

D. Earlier return to activities of daily living and work

E. All of the above

8. The length of the Roux limb of gastric bypass depends on:

A. BMI of the patient

B. Height of the patient

C. Gender

D. Intraabdominal fat content

9. Which one of the following is the most common late complication after laparoscopic Roux-en-Y gastric bypass?

A. Anastomotic leak

B. Internal hernia

C. Anastomotic stricture

D. Gastrointestinal bleeding

10. Which one of the following bariatric operations is considered a purely restrictive procedure?

A. Roux-en-Y gastric bypass

B. Laparoscopic adjustable gastric banding

C. Duodenal switch

D. Biliopancreatic diversion

Answers

1. B.
Of all the bariatric procedures, Roux-en-Y gastric bypass is the most commonly performed operation. In a survey of the membership of the American Society for Bariatric Surgery, it was found that 70% of all bariatric operations were Roux-en-Y GBP.

2. A.
The cost of obesity in the US is estimated to be at 9.1% of the national health expenditure. The major source of the cost arises from treatment of obesity-related comorbidity (CAD, type II diabetes, hypertension).

3. D.
All current modes of medical treatment for morbid obesity are ineffective at maintaining the weight loss.

4. A.
BMI is calculated by dividing the weight in kilograms by the square of height in meters.

5. D.
Active substance abuse and certain psychiatric disorders (schizophrenia, borderline personality disorder and uncontrolled depression) should be considered contraindications for bariatric surgery.

6. E.
All candidates should have a comprehensive medical evaluation before the operation. Evaluation by a specialist should be available if indicated.

7. E.
All of the above are the advantages of laparoscopic bariatric surgery compared to open surgery.

8. A.
Most surgeons base the length of the Roux limb on the patient's BMI.

9. C.
Anastomotic stricture occurs in the range of 4%-20% after laparoscopic GBP. Treatment consists of endoscopic balloon dilation.

10. B.
Adjustable gastric banding and vertical banded gastroplasty are considered purely restrictive operations.

Chapter 16: Abdominal Aortic Aneurysms

Samuel E. Wilson, MD

Contents

1. Atherosclerotic Aneurysms

Definition

An aneurysm is a localized dilation of a blood vessel, usually an artery, to greater than 150% of its normal diameter. Arterial aneurysms are found throughout the vascular tree. Aortic aneurysms are typically acquired, true aneurysms, affecting all 3 layers of the arterial wall (intima, media and adventitia). Traumatic aneurysms are most often false. Abdominal aortic aneurysms (AAA) are typically fusiform, but about 10% or less are saccular.

History

The French surgeon Dubost accomplished the first successful repair of an abdominal aortic aneurysm in 1951, replacing the aneurysm with a homograft. Surgical pioneers, particularly DeBakey, not only made AAA repair a safer operation, but developed the modern technical methods for open repair. Replacement of the aorta with a homograft was formed to be associated with late complications, which led to the development of prosthetic graft material. Voorhees is credited with the first use of synthetic graft material. Since 1957, Dacron® (Dupont Company, Inc.) has been the primary material used for synthetic aortic grafts. Beginning in the early 1990s, endovascular aneurysm repair (EVAR) dramatically reduced the morbidity and mortality, so that today the majority of patients with abdominal aneurysms have an endovascular procedure. Improvements in technique, devices, graft material and intensive care management have made aneurysm repair available to nearly all reasonably fit patients.

Epidemiology

Abdominal aortic aneurysms most frequently affect the elderly, and rupture of AAAs is the 10 leading cause of death in older men. The incidence of abdominal aortic aneurysms of all sizes has increased over the past 5 decades. In men, the incidence increases rapidly after age 55; in women, after age 70.[45] The incidence of AAA in a large screening study is shown in Table 1.

Table 1

Prevalence of Abdominal Aortic Aneurysms 4 cm or Larger Detected by Screening Men

Age (yrs)	Never Smoked (No.)	Prevalence of AAA (%)	Smokers (No.)	Prevalence of AAA (%)
50-54	1152	0	4359	0.3
55-59	1481	0	5819	0.9
60-64	2985	0.2	11,119	1.5
65-69	4198	0.2	14,129	1.9
70-74	4679	0.5	13,008	2.5
75-79	254	0.8	5669	2.7

From Lederle FA, Johnson GR, Wilson SE, et al. Ann Int Med. *1997;126:441-449.*

Pathogenesis and Risk Factors

Various studies have identified risk factors independently associated with abdominal aortic aneurysms, although their findings are sometimes contradictory. Generally, mean aortic diameter has been found to increase with age, male gender and height.[27] The effect of each of these variables, however, is quite small. For example, aortic diameter increases an average of 0.3 cm every 10 years. Nearly all height and weight groups are within 1 cm of gender means. Gender variance is also quite minimal, ie, 0.23-0.35 cm.[27,36,39]

Atherosclerotic disease was previously thought to be the foremost etiologic factor contributing to the development of aortic aneurysms, but recent research has challenged this belief.[47] The exact mechanism of aneurysm formation remains unknown, but the pathogenesis is likely related to factors that either increase intraluminal expansile forces (eg, hypertension), decrease arterial wall resistance to these forces (eg, histolytic enzymes) or are an inherited defect in arterial wall structural proteins.

The Aneurysm Detection and Management (ADAM) study of over 70,000 veterans showed that a history of tobacco smoking was the single factor most closely related to the development of AAA (Table 2). The mechanism by which smoking might lead to the development of aneurysms through accelerated deterioration of collagen and elastin remains speculative.[26] Atherosclerosis, coronary artery disease, elevated serum cholesterol level and a family history of AAA were all independently associated with AAA development in the ADAM study. A negative association existed between diabetes and AAAs.

About 10%-15% of aneurysm patients have a genetic predisposition, which is both an X-linked and autosomal dominant inheritance. This genetic defect results in decreased type III collagen content in arterial walls.

Chronic obstructive pulmonary disease (COPD) is associated with increased levels of elastase in the blood. Patients who have COPD show an increased risk of developing AAAs; however, tobacco may be the common etiologic agent in both diseases.[1]

Patients who develop aneurysms have different characteristics than those who develop aortoiliac occlusive

Table 2

Characteristics of 73,451 US Veterans 50-79 Years of Age Screened for Abdominal Aortic Aneurysms

Characteristic	Value
Mean age, years	66.2
Male, %	97.2
Race	
White, %	87.0
Black, %	8.2
Other, %	4.9
Height, cm	176.4
Weight, kg	84.8
Family history of AAA, %	5.1
Smoking history, %	75.5
Currently smoking, %	18.7
Years smoking	30.1
Hypertension, %	55.1
Hypercholesterolemia, %	52.3
Coronary artery disease, %	39.0
Claudication, %	6.7
Cerebrovascular accident, %	11.5
Atherosclerosis, %	46.0
Deep venous thrombosis, %	7.4
Diabetes, %	18.1
Chronic obstructive pulmonary disease, %	14.4
Cancer, other than skin, %	12.4

From: Lederle FA, Johnson GR, Wilson SE et al. Prevalence and associations of abdominal aortic aneurysms detected through screening. Ann Int Med. *1997;126:441-449.*

disease (Leriche's syndrome). Those with aneurysms are more likely to be older, male, tall and have a family history of aneurysms. Collagenase is increased in the aortic wall of patients with aneurysms, but not in those with occlusive disease. Patients with aneurysms also have elevated levels of serum elastase compared to the general population and those with occlusive disease.[7]

Infrequent causes of AAA include infection, syphilis, arteritis, connective tissue disorders and trauma.

Men are more frequently affected by AAA than women at a ratio of 4:1. The recognition that AAAs are primarily a disease of the elderly, ie, it affects approximately 2% of the male population over 60 years old, has led to proposals for screening programs using ultrasound in the population over 60 years of age.

Natural History

Over 50 years ago, Estes reported 102 patients with AAA, 63% of whom died due to aneurysm rupture.

Only 19% were alive after 4 years. Patients with symptomatic aneurysms had an even poorer prognosis, with 80% dead within 1 year. In addition to death from aneurysm rupture, these patients were also at increased risk due to cardiac, cerebral and renal comorbidities.[16] These data, derived from unoperated patients with large aortic aneurysms before vascular surgery became routine, have little value in management of today's smaller aneurysms, but do emphasize the danger of the untreated aneurysm.

Aneurysm enlargement and rupture is the ultimate outcome of a progressively expanding aneurysm should the patient live long enough (Table 3). The average growth rate is 0.2-0.4 cm/year, but this may vary from patient to patient and from year to year. Overall, the rate of growth is related to size, ie, larger aneurysms grow faster. 80% of aneurysms grow and 15%-30% expand by at least 0.5 cm/year.[3] It is critical to identify those aneurysms that are enlarging rapidly because these have the greatest chance of rupturing.

The risk of AAA rupture is related to size as measured by maximum diameter (Table 4). Aneurysms less than 4 cm rarely rupture. The Aneurysm Detection and Management study found that the annual rate of rupture in aneurysms measuring 4-5.4 cm was 0.6%.[29] In contrast, 20% of AAAs larger than 7 cm rupture within a year. Risk factors for rupture include large

Table 3

Expansion Rate of AAAs Related to Size (cm/year)

Investigator	<3 cm	3-4 cm	4-5 cm	5-6 cm	>6 cm	Overall
Nevit	.21	.26	.46			.32
Berstein	.22	.39	.36	.43	.64	.42
Gilmaker	.22	.15	.43	.44	.91	.38
Delin		.54		.47	.70	.53
Serepetti			.48			.48
Totals	.21	.27	.42	.43	.75	.41

From Hollier LH, Taylor LM, Ochsner J. Recommended indications for operative treatment of abdominal aortic aneurysms. J Vasc Surg. *1992;15:1046-1053.*

initial diameter, elevated blood pressure, and history of chronic obstructive pulmonary disease. Nonetheless, it is important to remember that an aneurysm may rupture at any size (Table 5).

In addition to rupture, other complications may arise in the untreated AAA. These include:

- Distal embolization of the peripheral vascular system
- Infection by *Staphylococcus* spp, Gram-negative organisms and yeast
- Aortoenteric fistula
- Aortocaval fistula
- Thrombosis
- Chronic coagulopathy

A marked improvement in operative survival rates over the last four decades and particularly with advent of EVAR should lead the primary care physician to refer most patients with AAA for evaluation for open or endovascular repair. 20 years ago, only half of primary care physicians would refer elderly patients for AAA repair, and only 25% would send an elderly patient for consultation if the aneurysm were greater than 8 cm.[37] Today, we believe the great majority of patients seek assessment by a vascular surgeon.

Diagnosis

AAAs are usually asymptomatic when diagnosed. Physical examination may reveal a pulsatile upper abdominal mass. When symptoms are present, eg, a leak or rupture, evaluation and treatment are urgent. The classic symptoms of rupture include back or abdominal pain, a pulsatile abdominal mass and hemodynamic instability.

Many modalities have evolved to assist clinical diagnosis in identifying and characterizing AAAs. Historically, cross table lateral abdominal radiographs were used to find the eggshell-like calcification of the aortic wall and estimate size. Today, ultrasound and CT scanning have emerged as the primary screening and diagnostic tools, respectively.[44] The ideal test for AAA

Table 4

Relation of Size to Rupture Among 473 Unoperated AAAs at Autopsy

Size	No. AAA	No. Ruptured	% Ruptured
<4 cm	201	19	9.5
4-5 cm	64	15	23.4
5-7 cm	83	21	25.3
7-10 cm	68	31	45.6
>10 cm	43	26	60.5
Unknown size	14	6	
Total	473	118	24.9

From Darling RC III, Brewster DC, Darling RC. Circulation. *1977;56:164.*

Table 5

Rate of Rupture for AAAs

Investigator		1 year	% Ruptured 3 years	% Ruptured 5 years
Kremer	<5 cm	0	0	NA
Cronenwett[12]	<6 cm	3	9	15
Nevitt	<5 cm	0	0	0
	>5 cm	5	NA	25
Johansson	<5 cm	0	0	7.1
	>5 cm	NA	NA	43.8
Gilmaker	<5 cm	2.5	2.5	2.5
	>5 cm	8.7	28	NA

From Darling RC III, Brewster DC, Darling RC. Circulation. *1977;56:164.*

would be sensitive, specific, have minimal interobserver and intraobserver variability, and have few side effects. CT angiography comes closest to meeting these criteria in patients who have normal renal function.

Accurate measurement of diameter is essential; a difference of only a few millimeters can alter treatment course. Ultrasound, although sensitive and specific, is operator dependent. Interobserver operator variance of 0.5 cm or more may be seen in one-third of patients. Ultrasound also tends to underestimate aneurysm size and is less accurate in measuring the aneurysm's relationship to surrounding structures, most importantly the renal arteries.[12]

CT scans are accurate in measurement of size and have virtually no false negative results. A high degree of precision can be obtained, but to do so requires standardization of the definition of AAA diameter and the expertise of an experienced radiologist. Intraobserver variance is minimal (90% <0.2 cm) and although it is less than that of ultrasound, it may be significant (>0.5 cm in 17%).[28A] CT scan can generally provide sufficient information regarding the proximal extent of the aneurysms. (Computed tomographic angiogram CTA) and three-dimensional CT technologies are widely used in preoperative assessment.

MRI scans have poorer resolution than CT scans. MRI, however, does not require the use of intravenous and oral contrast agents, and should be considered in patients with allergies or impaired renal function.

Angiography's role in AAA diagnosis has progressively decreased over the years. Angiography underestimates aneurysmal diameter and instead measures intraluminal size. Angiography is used selectively, eg, when other vascular anomalies are suspected (renovascular hypertension or mesenteric ischemia), the extent of the aneurysm is not well demarcated on other studies or if peripheral vascular procedures are being considered in addition to aortic repair (Table 6). Claudication, pain at rest and absence of lower extremity pulses may prompt one

Table 6

Indications for Arteriography

Renovascular disease
Chronic mesenteric ischemia
Iliac artery and femoropopliteal occlusive disease
Juxta suprarenal AAA, if not seen clearly on CT
Horseshoe kidney
Prior colectomy
Thoracoabdominal extension
Endovascular graft placement

From Sternberg WC, Gonze MD, Garrard CL. Abdominal and thoracoabdominal aortic aneurysms. Surg Clin North Am. *1998;78:827-843.*

to obtain preoperative angiography. Angiography is invasive and is associated with morbidity and mortality. A calibrated aortogram and/or 3-dimensional CTA are obtained prior to endovascular repair.

Over 95% of AAAs occur below the level of the renal arteries. The inferior mesenteric artery (IMA) is usually the only mesenteric vessel of significance arising from the aneurysm. Prominent collateral circulation and stenosis (or occlusion of the IMA at its origin from the aneurysm wall) often renders it nonessential. When the superior mesenteric artery is occluded, the IMA forms important collaterals to the small bowel; therefore, it must be preserved by reimplantation to the aortic replacement graft.

Evaluation

Abdominal aortic aneurysms, often found in patients who have chronic obstructive pulmonary disease and coronary atherosclerosis, are associated with significant comorbidities; therefore, preoperative assessment of patients is essential in order to reduce perioperative morbidity and mortality.

Atherosclerosis is a systemic disease. Evaluation of the entire vascular system, beginning with a detailed history and physical examination, is crucial before proceeding with AAA repair. Prior history of cerebrovascular accidents, transient ischemic attacks and amaurosis fugax or a carotid bruit suggests that the carotid and vertebral arteries should be evaluated. A report of angina pectoris, palpitations or family history of coronary artery disease may indicate that a detailed cardiac assessment is appropriate. Lower extremity claudication, pain at rest, ischemic changes or an abnormal ankle brachial index may prompt investigation into treatable peripheral vascular disease.

Over 50% of postoperative deaths after AAA repair are due to events related to myocardial ischemia. Identification of patients in need of preoperative medical, surgical intervention or perioperative invasive monitoring may lessen this risk. One-third of patients have known cardiac disease; 1 in 20 will need surgical revascularization or angioplasty. Goldman and others describe 5 high-risk criteria for adverse cardiac events at the time of major surgery:

- Age greater than 70 years
- Diabetes mellitus
- History of ventricular arrhythmia
- Q waves on ECG or myocardial infarct within 6 months
- History of angina pectoris

Patients with these adverse clinical variables have higher risk of experiencing a postoperative cardiac ischemic event, compared to those who have none of the criteria.

Preoperative evaluation with treadmill or dipyridamole-thallium nuclear imaging stress tests may be beneficial in determining cardiac risk. They have been shown to have a greater predictive value of adverse outcome than clinical markers alone.[15] The tests may be of most benefit in those patients deemed to be at moderate risk, ie, those having one or two of Goldman's criteria. In these patients, if the stress test is normal the cardiac risk is similar to patients with no criteria. If the stress test is positive, however, such patients have a 30% risk of an adverse cardiac outcome. Patients meeting 3 or more criteria generally do not benefit from a stress test, if only because the majority will fail. These patients should be considered for coronary angiography if AAA repair is planned.

Indications for Surgery

Any patient who has AAA rupture is considered for emergent repair unless the clinical situation is hopeless. Likewise, patients with a symptomatic or rapidly expanding aneurysm should undergo early repair. Guidelines for repair of aortic aneurysm are shown in Table 7. The actual indications for surgery in a contemporary vascular practice are shown in Table 8.

Complex aneurysms causing embolization, thrombosis, and fistula to IVC or duodenum, or those associated with intra abdominal occlusive disease, should be repaired. The urgency of this repair depends on the acuity and severity of symptoms. Dissecting, mycotic, false or saccular aneurysms should also be evaluated for repair.

For typical infrarenal, fusiform AAA, the results of the UK Small Aneurysm Trial and US Aneurysm Detection and Management study allow surgeons to

Table 7

Guidelines for AAA Repair

Symptomatic aneurysms
Saccular aneurysms
Size 5.5 cm or greater in patients with manageable risk factors
Size >5 cm in low-risk patients
Size 4-5 cm in young, low-risk patients

From Brewster DC, Cronennett JL, Mallett JW, et al. Guidelines for the Treatment of Abdominal Aortic Aneurysms. J Vasc Surg. *2003; 37:1106-1117.*

Table 8

Indications for Surgery Found in the Kingston Study

AAA greater than 5 cm	87%
Diameter increased >0.5 cm/6 months	16%
Pain	5%
Coexistent occlusive disease	2%
Iliac or femoral aneurysm requiring treatment	3%
Peripheral embolism	1%

From Brown ZP, Pattenden R, Guelius JR. Selective management of small abdominal aortic aneurysms: the Kingston study. J Vasc Surg. *1992;15:21-27.*

make more rational decisions for the patient who has a small aneurysm. Lowering the threshold for repair by 1 cm would result in a doubling of the number of patients to be considered for repair. It is important to remember that two-thirds of patients in the small aneurysm trials required operation during the follow-up period. If an operation on an aneurysm is postponed because of its small size, close regular monitoring of the AAA size is required.[6] Repeat ultrasound examination should be done every 6 months to 1 year; patient compliance with this monitoring is crucial. During the observation period, any correctable risk factors should be addressed so that if the aneurysm is enlarging and needs repair, the patient is prepared.

Relative contraindications for repair include severe irreversible CAD, malignancy limiting life expectancy to less than 2 years, and severe dementia. Recent myocardial infarction (<6 months previously), intractable congestive heart failure and severe angina pectoris are reasons to delay the operation in order to improve the patient's preoperative status. Patients who are poor candidates for open repair may be considered for endovascular repair.

Combined Procedures

The choice to perform an additional nonvascular intra abdominal operation at the time of AAA repair remains controversial. Several disorders may be considered for repair at the time of AAA repair, including cholelithiasis, hernias and neoplasms.

Ouriel found that patients with cholelithiasis have an increased risk of developing acute cholecystitis after AAA repair if a cholecystectomy is not performed. 9 of 11 patients had 1 episode within 3 years, and 2 had acute cholecystitis in the immediate postoperative period. One of these patients died after the development of biliary sepsis.[33] If cholecystectomy is planned, the aneurysm should be resected and the retroperitoneum closed prior to removing the gallbladder. This decreases the risk of contamination and graft infection.

Inguinal hernias can be repaired via the preperitoneal space using the midline incision by direct suture or by patching the defect with mesh (similar to the technique used in laparoscopic repair). These procedures involve limited risk of contamination.

If an unsuspected intra abdominal tumor is discovered at the time of scheduled repair, first address the most critical condition. All symptomatic, dissecting, expanding and ruptured aneurysms, for instance, should be treated first. If a near-obstructing gastrointestinal tumor is found during elective AAA repair it should be resected and the AAA repair delayed, especially if the aneurysm is small. Small gastrointestinal tumors should be resected at a later date if the AAA is large and the risk of rupture exceeds the risk of delaying resection of the tumor. A few surgeons advocate combined AAA repair and gastrointestinal procedures, but the risk of graft infection deters most surgeons from taking this action. With preoperative CTA, undiagnosed tumors are now unusual.

Asymptomatic renal artery stenosis is often found in patients with AAAs. When these lesions are left unrepaired, some patients show increased systolic blood pressure and demonstrate the need for additional antihypertensive medications at late follow-up. Despite these findings, since there is no difference in survival rate, need for dialysis, or serum creatinine level, repair of asymptomatic, noncritical renal artery stenosis[53] is not recommended.

Aneurysms of the renal artery that are believed to be caused by arteritis or medial necrosis are multiple in one-quarter of patients; these are most often saccular and therefore at risk of rupture. These patients may have hypertension, abdominal or flank pain, a bruit or hematuria. Some controversy exists about repair of calcified renal artery aneurysms, but most vascular surgeons recommend repair if the aneurysm is greater than 1.5-2.0 cm in diameter or symptomatic. Reconstruction of the vascular system is preferable to nephrectomy. Simultaneous repair of aortic and renal artery aneurysms carries a greater risk of mortality than performing only the repair of the aortic aneurysm.[3]

Anesthesia

Patients with COPD may benefit from use of an epidural catheter, which significantly improves postoperative pain control and pulmonary status. Invasive monitoring, including arterial line and pulmonary artery wedge monitoring may be indicated for the patient who has a known or suspected cardiac disorder. Preoperative antibiotics are generally given, and many surgeons order a mechanical bowel preparation.

A cell saver may be employed to reinfuse shed blood and reduce the risk from transfusion of bank blood, although some surgeons do not encounter sufficient blood loss to justify the expense and possible complications of blood salvage. Autologous and donor-directed blood can reduce the need for the use of bank blood.

Operative Approach

In open repair, the transperitoneal approach is most commonly used for access to the infrarenal aortic aneurysm. The benefits of this approach include the ability to conduct a full abdominal exploration, evaluation of colonic viability prior to closure, simple incision and closure, shorter operative time and better exposure of the iliac arteries distally.

Most surgeons reserve the posterolateral retroperitoneal approach for patients with high-risk comorbidities or special anatomical considerations. This approach may also be considered in patients with extensive adhesions, ostomies, intra abdominal infection and possibly previous surgical procedures. Some surgeons prefer this approach in inflammatory or juxta-renal aneurysms. Proponents claim certain physiologic advantages, including minimal gastrointestinal tract manipulation, improved pulmonary function, reduced intensive care and shortened hospital stay.

Technique for Open Repair

Prior to proceeding with the operation, it is important to evaluate the lower extremities for pulses, ischemic changes or any abnormalities. The patient is placed in the supine position and prepped from the xiphoid to the knees.

Through a midline incision the peritoneum is entered and the abdomen inspected for any unsuspected pathology. The transverse colon is then retracted superiorly and the small bowel is packed to the right. Most surgeons use self-retaining retractors to maintain this exposure.

The abdominal aorta is exposed to the proximal neck of the aneurysm by division of the retroperitoneum and ligament of Treitz to the left renal vein. This vein may need to be mobilized and divided (rarely) if the infrarenal neck is too short to cross-clamp the aorta. An anomalous retroaortic left renal vein is found in less than 2% of patients. Infrequently, the inferior vena cava may be found to the left of the aorta or there may be a duplication of the vena cava. In this case, the vena cava may pass over the aorta at the level of the renal vessels. These anomalies may be identified on CT scan and extra care is required to avoid injury. Some surgeons obtain circumferential control of the artery at the neck, but most only dissect the lateral walls due to the venous bleeding that may be encountered from a posterior dissection.

Once adequate proximal dissection has been completed, the distal extent of the aneurysm is evaluated. If there are no aneurysms, the common iliac arteries are exposed. The parasympathetic nerves are anterior to the left common iliac artery and should be preserved. If an aortoiliac graft is needed, the external and internal iliac arteries are exposed. The iliac veins lie behind the arteries, are hazardous and their tributaries are fragile. Utmost care should be taken to avoid injury.

An intravenous heparin bolus (75-100 U/kg) is given prior to cross-clamping the exposed vessels. The distal clamps may be placed first to reduce the risk of embolization of atheromatous plaque, although blood loss may be minimized by clamping proximally first, thus decompressing the aneurysm. The aneurysm is opened and plaque and debris are removed. Back-bleeding from the lumbar arteries is controlled with transfixion ligatures, typically 2-0 silk sutures. The aneurysmal sac is left in place to be closed around the graft.

A preclotted or gelatin-impregnated knitted or a woven Dacron straight graft is used if the iliac arteries are not involved, and a bifurcation graft is used to repair disease that extends to the iliac arteries. The proximal anastomosis is performed in an end-to-end fashion with nonabsorbable suture (3-0 Prolene®) in a running manner. The cross-clamp should then be placed distal to this anastomosis so that the integrity can be assessed and repair sutures placed, if needed. The distal anastomosis is then completed in a similar manner.

A bifurcated graft may be required if the iliac arteries are aneurysmal or have significant atherosclerotic disease. Within the abdomen, a bypass can be made to the external iliac arteries. If needed, bilateral femoral dissections will provide access for complete iliac bypass. Perfusion of at least one internal iliac artery is recommended.

Prior to opening all clamps, the graft should be flushed free of debris. Back-bleeding from both iliac arteries should be demonstrated. After removal of the clamps, acidosis and hypotension may be seen. These complications can be avoided by slowly opening the clamp over a few minutes and by coordinating closely with the anesthesiologist to accomplish unclamping. After the aneurysm is repaired, the femoral pulses are palpated to assure distal perfusion.

Perfusion of the left colon needs to be evaluated. The inferior mesenteric artery can generally be oversewn; however, in less than 2% of patients, this may cause serious ischemia of the sigmoid colon. Indications that collateral circulation is adequate include back-bleeding from the IMA, pulsatile flow to the colonic arcade after ligation and the presence of one patent hypogastric artery. If there is doubt regarding the viability of the colon, the IMA should be reimplanted using a Carrel patch. The incidence of left colon ischemia and subsequent infarction is higher in patients with ruptured aneurysm, likely due to prolonged hypotension or operative interruption of mesenteric collaterals during dissection in the retroperitoneal hematoma.

By closing the aneurysm sac and retroperitoneum, the aortic graft is isolated from the bowel. Generally, drains are not used. Next, the linea alba and skin should be reapproximated in the standard fashion, making sure to take generous bites of fascia.

Postoperative Management and Complications

AAA repair is a major operation that is associated with significant postoperative complications. Many patients spend at least the first 24 hours in an intensive care setting before being transferred to the ward.

Most patients can be extubated soon after completion of an uncomplicated operation. Aggressive pulmonary management is required to avoid respiratory complications. Adequate pain control is essential in order to facilitate patient participation, and continuous epidural blocks are very useful in this effort. Pneumonia frequently complicates the postoperative course and preventive efforts are well worthwhile.

Patients with preexisting cardiac disease need to be followed closely to avoid volume overload. This is especially true on postoperative day 3, when third space fluid mobilization is anticipated. Central venous monitoring may help guide the judicious use of intravenous diuretics. Early cardiac complications include ischemia, arrhythmia and congestive heart failure.

A nasogastric tube is usually placed intraoperatively and can be removed within 24 hours. Diet may be resumed as soon as bowel sounds are present. An aggressive work-up is indicated if the suspicion of colonic ischemia arises. This may be manifested by bloody stool or sepsis. Early evaluation with endoscopy is indicated; in most cases, the ischemia involves the mucosa. These patients can be treated with supportive measures, including antibiotics. Transmural ischemia may be indicated by signs of peritonitis, acidosis or deteriorating clinical status. Full thickness necrosis of the colonic wall causes contamination of the peritoneal cavity, thereby placing the graft at risk of infection. Resection of gangrenous bowel, colostomy and creation of a Hartman's pouch is required. Other gastrointestinal complications include bleeding, cholecystitis, ascites, obstruction and *Clostridium difficile* colitis.[48] Some of these complications are related to intraoperative visceral hypoperfusion.

Bleeding from the graft may occur at a suture line or through interstices of the graft. Close monitoring of hemoglobin level and coagulation factors are mandatory if bleeding is suspected. Re-exploration should be performed if bleeding persists after any coagulopathy has been corrected. The arterial system to the lower extremities should be evaluated to ensure that postoperative emboli or thrombi have not developed. Acute lower limb ischemia manifested by digital cyanosis is likely due to microembolization.[23] However, it is associated with an increased mortality and amputation rate. Graft thrombosis is a rare, late complication that affects 1%-2% of patients. Treatment depends on whether the thrombosis is acute or chronic. Collateral circulation may have developed to obviate the need for reoperation. Deep venous thrombosis occurs in 10% of patients after vascular reconstruction. Low-dose anticoagulants or prophylaxis with a sequential compression stocking and early ambulation are helpful.[18]

Graft infection is a serious but rare complication that, in most series, occurs in less than 1% of patients soon after surgery. Conservative treatment consists of removal of the graft and extra-anatomical restoration of blood flow, usually with an axillobifemoral graft. Antibiotics cannot usually treat a graft infection, although new work indicates that a graft infection secondary to the low virulence *Staphylococcus epidermidis* may be treated by excision, debridement and *in situ* replacement in addition to antibiotics. Untreated infected grafts are at a high risk of hemorrhage at the anastomotic site. Graft infection is associated with a 25%-50% mortality. The presence of bacteria in an intraluminal thrombus does not appear to be a factor in the development of graft infection, therefore, routine intraoperative cultures are unnecessary unless clinical aortitis exists. Pseudoaneurysms may develop at the suture lines in approximately 1% of patients, presenting as a painful or pulsatile mass. These aneurysms are usually associated with graft infection and may rupture. Diagnosis can be confirmed with angiography or CT scan, and repair is required.

A communication from the aortic anastomosis to the duodenum may cause an aortoenteric fistula, usually a late complication (Table 9). The breakdown is most often at the proximal anastomosis and the overlying duodenum. Sudden and massive bleeding requires emergent intervention. If the patient is stabilized, esophagogastroduodenoscopy can be performed. Induction of anesthesia may induce vascular collapse, so this may be done in the operating room with the patient prepared for immediate exploration. Confirmation of the diagnosis should lead to laparotomy, removal of the graft, repair of the intestine and extra-anatomical bypass. Several case reports have shown successful management by endoluminal graft placement, but there is limited follow-up.

Table 9

Late Graft-Related Complications After AAA Repair in 1087 Patients Over 12 Years

Complication	Number	Incidence, %
Aortoenteric fistula	10	0.9
Pseudoaneurysm	14	1.3
Bowel ischemia	4	0.4
Graft infection	3	0.3
Total	31	2.8

From Plate G, Hollier LA, O'Brien P, Pairolero PC, Cherry KJ, Kazmier FJ. Recurrent aneurysms and late vascular complications following repair of abdominal aortic aneurysms. Arch Surg. *1985;120:590-594.*

Injury to the sympathetic nerve plexus results in sexual dysfunction. Sexual dysfunction preoperatively is common in aneurysm patients and should be noted in medical record to obviate medico-legal issues. Retrograde ejaculation has been reported in up to two-thirds of patients, and impotence in up to one-third of patients.[50] Spinal cord ischemia is infrequent in elective AAA repair. The anterior spinal syndrome is manifest by paraplegia, incontinence, and loss of pain and temperature sensation.

Morbidity and Mortality

The mortality rate associated with open AAA repair has progressively decreased. Improvements and refinement of operative techniques were initially responsible for lowering death rates. Subsequently, decreased mortality is attributed to advances in anesthesia and other postoperative care. Most centers report a mortality rate of less than 5%, and two-thirds of deaths in the perioperative course are associated with comorbidities related to diffuse atherosclerosis and chronic respiratory disease, specifically myocardial infarction, congestive heart failure cerebrovascular accidents, renal failure, and pneumonia. In patients over 80 years of age, postoperative mortality may be 10% for open surgery.

Long-term survival is age dependent. Patients under 70 years of age can expect a 70%-80% survival rate at 5 years, 50% at 10 years, and 20%-25% at 15 years. Studies have demonstrated that in high-volume institutions, or where surgery is performed by experienced vascular surgeons, improved short-term survival and fewer complications are achieved.

Although open abdominal aortic aneurysm repair remains a useful operation, it is giving way to endovascular repair, unless there is a contraindication to EVAR (usually anatomic). Today, few dispute that all aneurysms of sufficient size should be repaired unless strong contraindications are present. The available data indicate that identification and early aortic reconstruction of abdominal aortic aneurysms 5 cm or more will save lives and improve the quality of life. Patients with aneurysms of less than 5 cm need to be treated on a case-by-case basis, taking into account the growth rate of the aneurysm, the patient's general medical condition and age.

2. Ruptured Abdominal Aortic Aneurysms

Epidemiology

Rupture is the most common lethal complication of abdominal aortic aneurysm. Patients with ruptured abdominal aortic aneurysms are, on average, older than those who present with nonruptured aneurysms, 75 vs. 68 years of age. The male-to-female ratio of patients with rupture is 7.8:1, which is higher than the ratio observed for patients without rupture.[11,19-21]

AAAs are diagnosed in only one-third of patients who have ruptured abdominal aortic aneurysms, and emergent repair carries a high mortality and morbidity. Of approximately 50% of AAA patients who arrive at the hospital with rupture, roughly 50% will survive emergency repair. The overall survival rate is only 20%-25%. Patients who present in shock have a very poor prognosis.

Presentation

Although it is obvious in many patients, the diagnosis of a ruptured abdominal aortic aneurysm requires a high index of suspicion because its presentation is not always typical. The classic triad of sudden onset of abdominal or flank pain, hypotension and a pulsatile abdominal mass is found in only half of patients who have ruptured aneurysms. Older patients with hemodynamic instability and abdominal pain should have ruptured aneurysm considered in the differential diagnosis.

Diagnosis

Early diagnosis of ruptured aneurysm, and repair before onset of shock, is favorable to a successful outcome. Management of ruptured AAA is labor intensive, requiring involvement of all hospital resources including critical care during the recovery period. Emergent operation depends on coordination of prehospital, emergency room, radiology, anesthesia, and surgery staff. An operation should not be delayed for confirmatory tests if the patient is unstable and presents with signs and symptoms consistent with rupture.

The resuscitation, evaluation and testing should be done simultaneously. A brief history and physical can be obtained concurrently with the securing of large-bore IV access and the drawing of blood for typing and cross-matching. Radiographs and an electrocardiogram should only be done if time permits. If ultrasound is available in the emergency room, it may quickly confirm the diagnosis. Patients should not go to the radiology department for additional studies unless they are stable and the diagnosis is uncertain after initial screening. The patient should be taken to the operating room without delay once the diagnosis is confirmed. Although open operation has been the standard treatment, there are now case series of ruptured AAAs having been treated by endovascular graft placement. The availability of an endovascular team, EVAR equipment and a patient with relatively stable vital signs would afford the best circumstances for endovascular repair of a ruptured aortic aneurysm.

Operative Procedure

Uncontrollable hypotension can result on initiation of anesthesia; induction of general anesthesia should not be started until the patient is prepped and draped and the operative team is gowned. After conventional laparotomy, proximal control should be obtained quickly, often at the diaphragmatic hiatus. Compression of the proximal aorta may be done if cross-clamping cannot be performed safely and quickly. Once vascular control has been obtained, aggressive resuscitation can proceed. Prosthetic tube or bifurcation grafts are used in the standard manner with a nonporous, woven Dacron® graft. Anticoagulation is often unnecessary.

Complications

Postoperative complications are common after repair of ruptured aneurysm. Respiratory failure is seen in 50% and renal failure in 30% of patients. Both complications are associated with mortality rates greater than 50%. Myocardial failure is responsible for 12% of deaths. There is a higher incidence of transmural left colonic ischemia after ruptured aneurysm repair. This incidence was as high as 18% in the Harborview experience.[21] Increased left colon infarction rates are likely to be worsened by prolonged hypotension. Resection may be required in the postoperative period for full thickness necrosis.

Mortality

Mortality after repair of AAA rupture remains high, even in the most advanced centers. Outcome has been associated with 2 sets of variables:

Patient-dependent
- Age >76 years
- Medical condition and comorbidities
- Delay in presentation
- Hypotension
- Operative findings—location and size of aneurysm, free vs. contained rupture

Physician-dependent
- Time to diagnosis, transfer to the operating room and technical performance of the operation
- Resuscitation
- Hemodynamic status, temperature, coagulopathy, urine output and acid-base balance at completion of surgery
- Technical complications at operation
- Experience of the surgeon and medical center

Mayo Clinic surgeons identified preoperative factors associated with a higher mortality, including hypotension, low hematocrit, high APACHE II score and a history of chronic obstructive pulmonary disease.[19] Preoperative cardiac arrest is associated with a very poor outcome, and some centers consider cardiac arrest a contraindication to attempting surgical repair.

3. Inflammatory Aortic Aneurysms

Epidemiology

About 5% of aortic aneurysms are considered to be inflammatory. They typically present at a younger age (62.2 years vs. 68.2 years) and are more frequently seen in males.[46] In the past, many cases of inflammatory aneurysms were not suspected preoperatively, but were noted at the time of repair; however, with preoperative CT they are usually detected.

Etiology

The precise cause of inflammatory aneurysms remains unclear. A distinct inflammatory process unrelated to atherosclerosis affecting the aortic wall may lead to aneurysm formation. On the other hand, inflammatory aneurysms may be at the extreme end of the clinical spectrum of inflammation and fibrosis seen in atherosclerotic aneurysms. Aneurysms which do not demonstrate gross evidence of inflammation often feature varying degrees of chronic inflammatory changes and fibrosis. Inflammation resolves after aneurysm repair, which supports the belief that the inflammation does not cause the aneurysm; it is a reaction to it.

Patients with atherosclerotic aneurysms and inflammatory aneurysms share a similar history of smoking, chronic obstructive pulmonary disease, and cardiovascular disease. Inflammatory aneurysms may have a slightly lower risk of rupture due to thick encasing of the aneurysm by the reactive process, but often this process is not completely circumferential.

Presentation

The most common complaint is back or abdominal pain. A triad of chronic pain, weight loss, and an elevated erythrocyte sedimentation rate may be found in a minority of patients with inflammatory aneurysms. Ureteral obstruction is rare in standard AAAs, but is seen in 20% of patients with inflammatory AAAs.[38] Pain and ureteral obstruction are highly suggestive of an inflammatory aneurysm.

Diagnosis

On imaging, the aortic wall is thickened at the aneurysm site but the posterior wall is typically spared from the inflammatory process, ie, the changes are seen in the anterior and lateral periaortic space. CT scan demonstrates soft tissue inflammation surrounding the aorta and is the best mechanism of detecting inflammatory aneurysms preoperatively. Angiography does not differentiate atherosclerotic aneurysms from inflammatory aneurysms. Excretory pyelography or CT should be performed if ureteral obstruction is considered EVAR is the preferred repair..

Operative Procedure

At operation, inflammatory aneurysms appear encased in a thick, dense, pearly-white, fibrotic process. The inflammation spreads in all directions and may involve the entire retroperitoneum to include, in some patients, the duodenum, inferior vena cava and ureters. The posterior wall of the aorta is typically spared, and up to 20% of patents have evidence of chronic rupture.[38]

Certain modifications of a standard abdominal aortic aneurysm repair will help to avoid complications. Preoperative steroids have been used but are associated with a theoretical risk of rupture through the posterior wall. Some surgeons advocate the retroperitoneal approach. Ureteral stents can be inserted if the patient has obstruction. Dissection should be kept to a minimum to prevent injury to associated inflamed and friable structures. Infrarenal proximal control can be obtained in most cases, but suprarenal or supraceliac control may be required to avoid significant dissection. I have found the most difficult step to be dissecting the duodenum off the inflammatory aneurysm. The inflammation may extend to the common iliac arteries; however, the external iliac arteries are usually spared. If involved, the common iliac arteries should be oversewn and anastomosis made to the external iliac. Prosthetic graft placement is performed in the standard manner. In patients in whom the aneurysmal sac cannot be closed over the graft, the retroperitoneum or omentum can be interposed to isolate the graft. Endovascular repair, where appropriate, would avoid many of the difficulties of open surgery.

Table 10

Inflammatory vs. Atherosclerotic Aneurysms

	Inflammatory	Atherosclerotic	Statistical Significance
Age (mean), years	62.2	68.2	$P < 0.01$
Sex (m/f)	26/4	330/126	$P < 0.01$
History of smoking, %	77	74	NS
COPD, %	47	50	NS
Diabetes	3	7	NS
Previous abdominal surgery	43	40	NS
Occlusive arterial disease	53	52	NS
Myocardial infarction	13	9	NS

From Sterpetti AV, Hunter WJ, Feldhaus RJ. Inflammatory aneurysms of the abdomincal aorta: incidence, pathologic and etiologic considerations. J Vasc Surg. *1989;9:643-650.*

Complications

The operative time and blood loss are similar to those of ordinary aneurysm repair if dissection is kept to a minimum. Morbidity and mortality rates are similar to those that occur after repair of noninflamed aneurysms. Most cases of ureteral obstruction resolve after repair of the aneurysm. Steroids can be tried if obstruction persists.

4. Traumatic Aortic Aneurysms

Epidemiology

High-speed, deacceleration traffic accidents resulting in traumatic aortic aneurysm and rupture are responsible for 15%-20% of blunt trauma deaths. 90% of aortic transections are fatal at the accident scene. Survival depends on the formation of a false aneurysm contained by the adventitia and retroperitoneal structures. The adventitia is responsible for 60% of aortic tensile strength. Trauma is the most common cause of aortic aneurysms in younger age groups. Patients are typically in their 20s or 30s and atherosclerosis does not play a role. An unsuspected aneurysm may rupture suddenly or may be discovered years after the traumatic event. A history of sudden deceleration injury should arouse the suspicion of acute aortic transection. There is a 2-fold increase in aortic transection when a patient is ejected from the vehicle.

Presentation

Injury to the aorta requires significant deceleration injury. Mechanisms include automobile and other vehicular accidents or falls from significant heights. Direct blows to the chest are not associated with deceleration and are rarely associated with aortic injury.

Internal organs continue to move in rapid deceleration; the result is that the suspended heart and great vessels tear at their fixed points. The most frequent site of disruption is the segment distal to the left subclavian artery. Thoracic aortic injuries are 20 times more common than abdominal injuries. More proximal injuries tend to be associated with direct trauma.

The diagnosis must be considered in patients who have experienced major decoration injury regardless of evidence of external injury. Patients often present with significant associated injuries, eg, head injury, extremity and pelvic fractures, and abdominal injuries that may be life-threatening and require immediate intervention. Once stabilized, radiologic evaluation of the mediastinum and aorta may be obtained.

Physical findings can include hypertension in the upper extremities, shock, a harsh systolic murmur, anuria, paraplegia or absent femoral pulses.

Diagnosis

History is the most important initial clue to diagnosis of this injury. Screening AP chest x-ray provides the following radiographic signs:

- Widening of the mediastinum
- Apical pleural cap
- Deviation of the trachea to the right
- Deviation of the esophagus to the right (seen when nasogastric tube is inserted)
- Indistinct tracheal stripe
- Obliteration of the aortic knob
- Depression of the left bronchus
- Pleural effusion
- Clavicle or first rib fracture

Many diagnostic tests to screen for aortic injury have emerged, including high-resolution spiral CT scanning, ultrasound and transesophageal echocardiogram. In the presence of clinical or radiographic findings consistent with transection, CTA or aortography should be obtained. The high mortality rate associated with failure to diagnose the injury justifies liberal use of invasive testing.

Treatment

Most patients with traumatic transection of the aorta do not reach the hospital alive. Rupture of a contained transaction is unpredictable, so operation should begin as soon as it is safe to proceed. A small number, roughly 2%, survive and develop chronic pseudoaneurysm. They are also at risk of rupture and should undergo repair when diagnosed.

Other critical injuries may require prior or simultaneous treatment. If repair is delayed, judicious use of beta-blockers and hypotensive agents may be indicated.

Intubation with a double lumen endotracheal tube is helpful for exposure. Patients are evaluated for EVAR versus open repair. In open repair, the descending thoracic aorta is exposed using a left lateral thoracotomy. Proximal and distal control should be obtained without disrupting the hematoma. If the operation is performed expeditiously, bypass may not be necessary; however, occurrence of visceral vessel and spinal ischemia may be reduced with bypass.

Once control is obtained the hematoma should be opened. The aorta is repaired either primarily or with Dacron graft. Typically, primary repair is not feasible due to undue tension on the suture line.

Complications

Complications include bleeding, phrenic nerve injury, recurrent laryngeal nerve injury and false aneurysms at suture lines. Other complications associated with nontraumatic aneurysm repair, such as respiratory or renal failure, can be seen. If the patient was hemodynamically unstable, higher rates of visceral and spinal cord injury can be anticipated.

Results

Long-term results have been excellent following repair of transection. Operative mortality is less than 10% in acute cases and less than 5% in chronic transections. Nonetheless, many patients succumb to other injuries.

5. Thoracoabdominal Aortic Aneurysms

The pathogenesis, natural history and epidemiological considerations of thoracoabdominal aortic aneurysms are similar to those of abdominal aortic aneurysms.

Natural History

Without treatment, thoracoabdominal aortic aneurysms (TAAAs) tend to increase in size and rupture. Unless comorbid conditions make the patient an unacceptable operative risk, aneurysms larger than 6 cm should be repaired. Risk factors for rupture include larger aneurysm size, increased patient age, history of COPD and symptoms.

Classification

Crawford and associates developed a widely accepted classification system for TAAAs. This classification system has allowed for uniformity in reporting and helps plan the appropriate operative repair. The categories are:

- Type I—Aneurysms involving the descending thoracic aorta from the left subclavian artery to the upper abdominal visceral vessels, not involving the renal arteries
- Type II—Aneurysms originating at the left subclavian artery and descending below the renal arteries into the abdomen
- Type III—Aneurysms starting in the distal thoracic aorta and involving the abdominal aorta
- Type IV—Aneurysms involving the abdominal aorta from the diaphragm to the aortic bifurcation

Presentation

Patients with TAAA are often asymptomatic. The aneurysm is usually noted when the patient has radiological procedures performed for other conditions. If the aneurysm has ruptured, the patient will often present in shock or complain of back or upper abdominal pain.

Diagnosis

TAAAs are initially evaluated with thoracic and abdominal CT angiograms. An aortogram branches and provides valuable information regarding visceral artery stenosis and a "road map" to reconstruction.

Operative Considerations

As with AAA, optimization of cardiac and pulmonary function is essential prior to proceeding with TAAA repair. This may require additional diagnostic and therapeutic procedures. Preoperative angiographic localization of the artery of Adamkiewicz has been advocated by some to aid in selective reimplantation, but this is not always possible due to difficulty in identification.

Mesenteric and spinal ischemia are the major complications of TAAA repair. Preoperative planning and intraoperative technical considerations, such as monitoring of spinal fluid pressure, may significantly lower the complication rate. By maintaining blood pressure, replacing blood products in a timely fashion, and preventing hypothermia and acidosis, the anesthesiologist plays a vital role in this operation. Experience is growing with endovascular repair of thoracoabdominal aneurysms at specialized centers.

Operative Technique

For the open repair, the left chest, abdomen and groin can be accessed with the patient in the right lateral decubitus position. A thoracoabdominal incision is made. For type I and II aneurysms, the incision is extended to the 5th or 6th intercostal space. For type III and IV aneurysms, the incision is carried to the 8th intercostal space. The aneurysm is exposed in the retroperitoneal plane, the diaphragm is divided, and proximal and distal control is obtained. Temporary extracorporeal femoral or axillofemoral bypass may be instituted to perfuse the abdominal viscera while the thoracic portion of the aneurysm is repaired. Rapid repair with selective visceral cold perfusion is an alternative method.

In an attempt to decrease resistance to spinal cord flow, cerebrospinal fluid drainage by a lumbar drain may be maintained throughout the operation and for at least 48 hours postoperatively. Some reports indicate that paraplegia and paraparesis can be decreased when lumbar drainage is used. Epidural cooling may extend permissible spinal cord ischemic time, thereby allowing for intercostal artery reimplantation. Patent intercostal arteries from T7 to L4 should be implanted when feasible. Emphasis should be placed on arteries at the level of T11-L1, which serves to revascularize the artery of Adamkiewicz in the majority of patients.[41] Selected early results with endovascular repair show a lower incidence of paraplegia.

Complications

Intraoperative coagulopathy is a common complication. Excessive bleeding causes loss of clotting factors, reperfusion acidosis, and hypothermia. Concurrent replacement of blood products and maintaining core body temperature are essential to suppress this complication. Segmental reperfusion and the use of bicarbonate may decrease acidosis. Close communication with the anesthesiologist is essential. Coagulopathy can persist into the postoperative period. Hemostatic parameters should be monitored frequently. Reoperation for bleeding is associated with a higher mortality rate.

Neurologic complications are much more frequently seen in TAAA than in AAA repair. Paraplegia or paresis is a complication of TAAA repair in approximately 15% of patients, and 25% of these arise more than 24 hours after the operation. Type II and dissecting aneurysms have a higher incidence of this complication. Reimplantation of intercostal arteries, CSF drainage, sequential clamping, bypass and more recently, endovascular repair, may reduce the incidence of this complication. No pharmacological agent has been shown to be of benefit at this time.

6. Popliteal Aneurysms

The occurrence of popliteal aneurysms is strongly associated with the abdominal aortic aneurysms.[24] About one-third of the time, AAAs are found in patients with popliteal aneurysms, and almost 10% of patients with AAAs have popliteal aneurysms. For this reason, when aortic aneurysms are found the possibility of coexistent popliteal artery aneurysms should be considered, and vice versa.

Epidemiology

The true incidence of popliteal aneurysms is unknown. Lawrence et al estimates that in hospitalized patients, femoral or popliteal aneurysms are found in 4.85 per 100,000 patients.[24] They often go undetected in life and are not routinely sought in postmortem examination. They are thought to be second only to AAAs in frequency and account for 70% of peripheral aneurysms.[14] Over 90% occur in male patients and they are bilateral in up to half of the cases.

History

Popliteal aneurysms, once typically found in postillions, were the first aneurysms to be diagnosed and treated. The early attempts at surgical repair of popliteal aneurysms were directed at large, painful and expanding aneurysms. Initially, the direct approach to the artery via the popliteal fossa was used to repair the aneurysm. Hunter is credited with treating this aneurysm by ligating the superficial femoral artery in the mid-thigh. Proximal ligation relies on sufficient collateral flow to maintain limb viability and is not in use today. Interposition or bypass with a vein segment or prosthetic graft is the preferred treatment today.

Anatomical Variants

Of the 2 types of popliteal aneurysms, the most common type occurs in the elderly patient with atherosclerotic disease. The aneurysm lies in the proximal popliteal fossa, large and sometimes multilobular. They are often bilateral. The second variety is often seen in younger active men who do not have atherosclerotic disease. These aneurysms are smaller, unilateral and more rounded. They are much more difficult to find on physical exam, since they are more concealed behind the knee. These aneurysms may be due to local mechanical distortions or injury.

Natural History

One-third of patients are asymptomatic at diagnosis (Table 11). Popliteal aneurysms are complicated by thrombosis and distal embolization, which cause symptoms of occlusive vascular disease. Compression of adjacent neurovascular structures may cause edema or neuropathy in the case of a large aneurysm.

There is a significant incidence of thromboembolic complications and subsequent frequent amputations. In patients selected for conservative management, 24% experience complications at 1 year and 68% at 5 years.[13] For this reason, conservative management is not recommended, except in selected patients.

Surgical Indications and Methods

All patients with acute complications (acute thrombosis or embolism) of popliteal aneurysms require emergent treatment to salvage the limb. Increasing evidence supports elective repair of asymptomatic aneurysms greater than 2 cm to avoid critical ischemia.[43] In patients with multiple aneurysms, AAA should be treated first, followed by repair of the popliteal aneurysm.

The popliteal aneurysm can be ligated and bypassed with saphenous vein or prosthetic graft. A medial approach allows for harvesting of the saphenous vein through the same excision and provides suitable proximal exposure, but does require division of medial muscles and tendons. The posterior approach is ideal for popliteal aneurysms, but exposure is limited if there is proximal or distal extension, and a separate excision may be needed if a saphenous graft is used.

Patients who present with acute ischemia require intraoperative infusion of thrombolytic agents prior to bypass excision of the aneurysm.

Elective endoluminal graft stenting of popliteal aneurysms is a less invasive technique than operation. This approach remains investigational and long-term results are unknown. Stents across joints may fracture over time because of continued stress.

Table 11

Presenting Symptoms Associated with Popliteal Artery Aneurysms

	Incidence, %
No symptoms	37.2
Rupture	1.4
Limb ischemia	55.0
Local compression	6.5

From Dawson I, Sie RB, van Bockel JH. Atherosclerotic popliteal aneurysm. Br J Surg. *1997;84(3):293-299.*

Outcome

Compared to outcomes with repair in the emergency setting, elective reconstruction offers higher long-term patency and higher limb survival rates. 5 year patency rates range from 75%-80%. Limb survival rates should exceed 90% at 5 and 10 years. A higher patency rate and limb survival is obtained by using saphenous vein, rather than prosthetic graft, as the interposition or bypass material. The probability of developing aneurysms in other locations is increased in patients with popliteal aneurysms, and long-term surveillance is required.

7. Endovascular Aortic Aneurysm Repair

History

In 1991, Parodi described the first transfemoral aortic aneurysm exclusion using balloon-expandable stents to fix a fabric graft inside the aneurysm.[35]

Types of Devices

Two groups of grafts are available:

1. ***Covered stents***–stents covered by prosthetic graft material.

2. ***Stent graft devices***–grafts are fixed at both ends or supported throughout their length by wire forms.

Bifurcation grafts of modular designs allow for more customization according to anatomical variances.

Components of Graft Devices

1. ***Delivery system***–introduces sheath and delivery catheters small and flexible enough to navigate the femoral and iliac artery while not kinking when deployed.

2. ***Prosthetic graft***–must be strong and durable, yet compact in order to fit within the delivery system. Polyester (Dacron) and PTFE are the preferred materials at this time. Material should not be porous to serum.

3. ***Attachment systems***–must provide a tight seal so as to prevent leakage and to anchor the graft to the aortic wall to prevent migration. Methods to accomplish this have either utilized a series of hooks or barbs or have relied on the intrinsic expansile forces of the stents (Nitinol®). Late detachment has been reported and the ideal attachment technique remains to be determined.

Technical advances over the first decade have led to simpler devices with extended application. Each system has advantages and disadvantages. Currently, due to anatomical limitations, endovascular devices are a feasible alternative in great majority of patients. Development and clinical trials to perfect available devices and create alternatives are ongoing. In addition, improvised grafts, which allow for customization, are occasionally used. Suprarenal wire attachment has simplified the problem of the short AAA neck.

Patient Selection

Initially, only high-risk patients who were deemed nonoperative candidates for open repair were considered for the endovascular technique. As experience with the procedure has broadened, more patients with AAA are being considered for endovascular repair. Periodic follow-up imaging requirements must be taken into account when making decisions regarding endovascular repair.

Certain anatomic variations of the patient's aneurysm limits universal application. Specific limitations vary depending upon the device used and will change with new developments such as suprarenal attachment.

Preoperative Evaluation

The combination of angiography and dynamic CT (CTA) provides accurate measurement of arterial morphology to evaluate for inclusion criteria and allow for proper sizing of the graft. Precise fitting of the graft is essential to reduce the incidence of migration and leak. Routine preoperative cardiopulmonary and vascular evaluation should be performed on all patients, although the possibility of conversion to open technique is not over 5%. Procedures are often performed in a specialized operating room with cineradiography and appropriate technical support.

Technique

Access is obtained via unilateral or bilateral exposure and control of the common femoral or distal external iliac artery. The patient should be heparinized systemically. An on-the-table aortogram identifies the precise location of the renal and iliac arteries. The graft is inserted and proximal fixation is obtained by stent expansion. The distal end or limbs of the graft are deployed and fixed by various techniques depending upon the type of graft utilized. A completion angiogram is performed to confirm location of the graft, exclusion of the aneurysm (no leak) and lack of technical complications (ie, kinking, spiraling). Endoleak or imprecise fit may be alleviated with additional stent placement.

Results/Benefits

A successful deployment will result in exclusion of the aneurysm and unobstructed distal arterial flow. Aneurysm size often decreases with a successful procedure. Reported success rates vary but exceed 90% in most series, and mortality rates range from 0%-5%. The most common failure modes are endoleak, migration, distal embolization and thrombosis of the graft. Endoleak rates are approximately 20% at 30 days, but decrease significantly by 6 months.

A CT and duplex ultrasound within 1 to 2 weeks of the procedure should be performed to evaluate for endoleak or migration. Additional evaluation should be done at 3-6 months, and then annually. At this writing, follow-up should be planned indefinitely, although some surgeons have lessened the frequency of imaging.

In large part, early enthusiasm regarding the potential benefits of endovascular grafting has been realized. Boyle noted improved respiratory function and pain control.[4] White has reported decreased blood loss and shorter intensive care stays.[19] The EVAR (UK) trial and DREAM (Dutch) trial both confirmed significantly lower 30-day mortality rates with EVAR than with open repair (by one-third that of open repair).[55,56]

A review by Moore reported a 6 year (1992-98) single site prospective comparison of open vs. endovascular aneurysm repairs. His group reported significantly lower surgical time, blood loss, blood replacement, ICU and hospital stay. Statistically non-significant but lower rates of myocardial infarction, respiratory failure and colon ischemia were seen as well. 5 year survival were equal. Overall hospital costs were lower in the endovascular group. The cost of additional preoperative testing and long-term follow-up imaging were not considered in this study.[31]

Complications

Endoleak is the most common cause of "failure" after an endovascular repair; it has been reported in up to 20% in some studies, and all devices to date have been shown to have this complication to some extent. The treatment depends upon the origin of the leak and the impact on AAA shrinkage. Conservative management may be considered in type II endoleaks that seal spontaneously by 6 months in 50% of patients. Other leaks can be treated with endovascular supplementary stenting. Conversion to an open procedure is associated with a higher morbidity and mortality, and can result in an operation in a high-risk patient who would not ordinarily be considered for elective open repair.

Endoleak Classification[52]

Postoperative endoleak is defined as the persistent flow of blood in the aneurysm sac outside the graft. A review of approximately 700 endovascular procedures at the Cleveland Clinic documented a 23% incidence of endoleak at any time in the postoperative period.[42] Type I endoleaks are attachment site leaks, type II endoleaks are caused by back perfusion of the AAA sac from patent aneurysm sac side branches (typically the IMA and lumbar arteries), type III endoleaks result from graft defects (suture holes, fabric tears, separation of modular components) and type IV endoleaks are caused by graft porosity.[49] Endoleak (particularly Type I) can lead to endotension, subsequent aneurysm expansion and rupture. Therefore, endoleak after endovascular abdominal aortic aneurysm repair should be monitored closely, and if persistent or associated with aneurysm enlargement, should be corrected.

Endoleak Treatment

Type I and Type III endoleaks should be treated soon after they are discovered; they should not be observed for a prolonged interval. When feasible, endovascular placement of overlapping extension grafts or cuffs yields an overall 97% success rate. If endovascular treatment of type I and III endoleaks is not possible, open repair (consisting of stent graft extraction and traditional AAA repair) may be indicated.[17]

The presence of an early Type II endoleak alone does not warrant treatment. These endoleaks should be observed, as they may not lead to aneurysm enlargement, or they may spontaneously thrombose within the first post operative year.[34] Type II endoleaks are treated when the aneurysm continues to enlarge or has failed to contract 12 months after the initial endovascular repair. Type II leaks in patients with a shrinking aneurysm sac are not treated.[42]

Treatment of type II endoleak involves selective embolization of the arteries feeding the endoleak, embolization of the aneurysm sac or both.[40]

Embolization may be carried out by the transarterial (via the IMA or lumbar arteries) or translumbar approach.[22] Coil-induced thrombosis of the aneurysm sac via a translumbar puncture was shown to have a 92% success rate.[2] Selective embolization of feeding vessels is also employed to correct type II endoleaks.

Other Complications

Other device-related complications include arterial dissection or rupture, renal and bowel infarction, stenosis, embolization, graft infection, incision infection, graft migration and rupture. As with open repairs, systemic complications include pneumonia, myocardial infarction, other cardiac morbidities and renal failure. The procedure is associated with radiation exposure and considerable intravenous contrast load. Some studies have shown that complication rates decrease with experience and technical improvements in endografts.[10,31]

Information is accumulating on long-term results of endovascular aortic aneurysm repair for example, 5-year outcomes.Because of concomitant cardiovascular disease and malignancy supervening, it is unlikely there will be a significant survival advantage with either technique. Nevertheless, the initial survival advantage at 1 month provides an opportunity for an expanded lifespan. EVAR has been the most significant advance in vascular surgery over the last 50 years.

Table 12

Clinical Results of Endograft Repair of Abdominal Aortic Aneurysm

Authors Year	Device	No. of pts.	Peri operative Mortality	Successful Deployment	Endoleak First 30 days	Endoleak at 12 mo	Endoleak at 24 mo
Moore et al, 2003[31]	Ancure®	573	10 (1.7%)	531 (92.7%)	130 (42.2%)	79 (30.3%)	55 (24.4%)
Carpenter et al, 2003[8]	Lifepath®	182	0 (0%)	178 (98%)	21 (12%)	N/A	N/A
Matsumura et al, 2003[30]	Excluder®	235	2 (1%)	235 (100%)	39 (22%)	40 (17%)	47 (20%)
Zarins et al, 2003[54]	AneuRx®	1193	22 (1.8%)	1182 (99.1%)	147/1056 (13.9%)	132/951 (13.9%)	129/772 (16.7%)

8. Pharmacotherapy of Abdominal Aneurysms

Recognition that aortic inflammation and proteolytic degradation of the extracellular matrix are key mechanisms in formation of aortic aneurysms has spurred interest in pharmacotherapy.[57] Since many aneurysms are below the threshold for intervention when discovered, a pharmacological method of preventing growth would have major application. Several strategies for prevention of aneurysm growth have shown promise in animal models, and generally fall into the categories of hemodynamic management, suppression of inflammation and inhibition of protease activity.[58] With regard to hemodynamic control, propanolol does not appear to inhibit aneurysm expansion, although animal data shows that angiotensin-converting enzyme inhibitors have a slowing effect on growth. A small, randomized clinical trial showed doxycycline, an antimicrobial, to slow growth leading the authors to call for a larger trial.[59] Also, coenzyme A reductase inhibitors (statins) may promote tissue stabilization by diminishing pro-inflammatory signaling and prevent extracellular matrix degradation.[60]

9. References

1. Anderson DW, Edwards TK, Ricketts MH. Multiple defects in type III collagen synthesis are associated with the pathogenesis of abdominal aortic aneurysms. *Ann NY Acad Sci*. 1996;800:216-228.

2. Baum RA, Carpenter JP, Golden MA, et al. Treatment of type 2 endoleaks after endovascular repair of abdominal aortic aneurysms: comparison of transarterial and translumbar techniques. *J Vasc Surg*. 2002;35:23-9.

3. Benjamin ME, Hansen KJ, Craven TE. Combined aortic and renal artery surgery. A contemporary experience. *Ann Surg*. 1996;223(5):555-565.

4. Boyle JR, Thompson JP, Thompson MM: Improved respiratory function and analgesia control after endovascular AAA repair. *J Endovasc Surg*. 1997;4:62-65.

5. Brewster DC, Cronenwett JL, Hallett JW, et al. Guidelines for the treatment of abdominal aortic aneurysms: Report of a Subcommittee of the Joint Council of the American Association for Vascular Surgery and Society for Vascular Surgery. *J Vasc Surg*. 2003;37:1106-1117.

6. Brown ZP, Pattenden R, Guelius JR. Selective management of small abdominal aortic aneurysms: the Kingston study. *J Vasc Surg*. 1992;15:21-27.

7. Cannon DJ, Read RC. Blood elastolytic activity in patient with aortic aneurysms. *Ann Thorac Surg*. 1982;34:11-15.

8. Carpenter JP, Brewster DC, Kwolek C, et al. Multicenter trial results of the lifepath system for endovascular aortic aneurysm repair (EVAR). [Abstract]. Chicago, Illinois. *Society for Vascular Surgery*. June 8, 2003.

9. Cerveira JJ, Cohen JR. Laparoscopic assisted abdominal aortic aneurysm repair. *Surg Clin North Amer*. 1999;79:541-550.

10. Chuter TAM, Risberg G, Hopkinson BR. Clinical experience with a bifurcated endovascular graft for aortic aneurysm repair. *J Vasc Surg*. 1996; 24:655-665.

11. Crawford, ES, Saley SA, Babb JW III. Infrarenal abdominal aortic aneurysm; factors influencing survival after operations performed over a 25-year period. *Ann Surg*. 1981;193:699-709.

12. Cronenwett JL, Sargent SK, Wall MH. Variables that affect the expansion rate and outcome of small abdominal aortic aneurysms. *J Vasc Surg*. 1990;11:260-269.

13. Dawson I, Sie RB, van Bockel JH. Atherosclerotic popliteal aneurysm. *Br J Surg*. 1997;84(3):293-299.

14. Dent TL, Lindenauer SM, Ernst CB. Multiple atherosclerotic arterial aneurysms. *Arch Surg*. 1972;105:338-344.

15. Eagle KA, Coley CM, Newell BA. Combining clinical and thallium data optimizes preoperative assessment of cardiac risk before major vascular surgery. *Ann Int Med*. 1989;110:859-866.

16. Estes JE. Abdominal aortic aneurysm: a study of one hundred two cases. *Circulation*. 1950;2:258.

17. Faries PL, Cadot H, Gautam A, et al. Management of endoleak after endovascular aneurysm repair: Cuffs, coils, and conversion. *J Vasc Surg*. 2003;37:1155-1161.

18. Fletcher JP, Batiste P. Incidence of deep vein thrombosis following vascular surgery. *Intl Angiology*. 1997;16(1):65-68.

19. Gloviczki P, Pairolero PC, Mucha P Jr. Ruptured abdominal aortic aneurysms: care should not be denied. *J Vasc Surg*. 1989;15:851.

20. Hoffman M, Avellone JC, Pleecha GR. Operation for ruptured abdominal aortic aneurysms: a community-wide experience. *Surgery*. 1982;91:597.

21. Johansen K, Kohler TR, Nicholls SC. Ruptured abdominal aortic aneurysm: the Harborview experience. *J Vasc Surg*. 1991;13:240-247.

22. Kasirajan K, Marek JM, Lansfeld M. Technique and results of transfemoral superselective coil embolization of type II lumbar endoleak. *J Vasc Surg*. 2003;38:61-66.

23. Kuhan G, Raptis S. "Trash foot" following operations involving the abdominal aorta. *Aust NZ J Surg*. 1997;67:21-24.

24. Laurence PF, Lorenzo-Rivero S, Lyon JL. The incidence of iliac, femoral, and popliteal artery aneurysms in hospitalized patients. *J Vasc Surg*. 1995;22:409-415.

25. Lawrence DD, Charnsangavec C, Wright KC. Percutaneous endovascular graft: Experimental evaluation. *Radiology*. 1987;163:357-360.

26. Lederle FA, Johnson GR, Wilson SE. Prevalence and associations of abdominal aortic aneurysms detected through screening. *Ann Int Med*. 1997;126:441-449.

27. Lederle FA, Johnson GR, Wilson SE. Relationship of age, gender, race, and body size to infrarenal aortic diameter. *J Vasc Surg*. 1997;26:595-601.

28. Lederle FA, Wilson SE, Johnson GR. Variability in measurement of abdominal aortic aneurysms. *J Vasc Surg*. 1995;21:945-952.

29. Lederle FA, Wilson SE, Johnson GR, et al. Immediate repair compared with surveillance of small abdominal aortic aneurysms. *N Engl J Med*. 2002;346:1437-1444.

30. Matsumura JS, Brewster DC, Makaroun, MS, et al. A multicenter controlled clinical trail of open versus endovascular treatment of abdominal aortic aneurysm. *J Vasc Surg*. 2003;37:262-271.

31. Moore WS, Keshyap VS, Vescera CL: Abdominal Aortic Aneurysm: A 6-year comparison of endovascular versus transabdominal repair. *Ann of Surg*. 1999;231:289-306.

32. Moore WS, Matsumura JS, Makaround MS, et al. Five-year interim comparison of the Guidant bifurcated endograft with open repair of abdominal aortic aneurysm. *J Vasc Surg*. 2003;38:46-55.

33. Ouriel K, Ricotta JJ, Adams JT. Management of cholelithiasis in patients with abdominal aortic aneurysms. *Ann Surg*. 1983;198:717.

34. Parent FN, Meier GH, Godziachvili V. et al. The incidence and natural history of type I and II endoleak: a 5-year follow-up assessment with color duplex ultrasound scan. *J Vasc Surg*. 2002;35:474-481.

35. Parodi JC, Palmaz JC, Barone HD. Transfemoral intraluminal graft implantation of abdominal aortic aneurysm. *Ann Vasc Surg*. 1991;5:499-499.

36. Pedersen OM, Aslaksen A, Vik-Mo H. Ultrasound measurement of the luminal diameter of the abdominal aorta and iliac arteries in patients without vascular disease. *J Vasc Surg*. 1993;17: 596-601.

37. Pertacek MR, Lawson JD, Rhea WG Jr. Resection of abdominal aortic aneurysms in the over-80 group. *South Med J*. 1980;73:579.

38. Pennell RC, Hollier LH, Lie JT. Inflammatory abdominal aortic aneurysm: a thirty-year review. *J Vasc Surg*. 1985;2:859-869.

39. Pleumeekers HJCM, Hoes AW, van der Does E. Aneurysms of the abdominal aorta in older adults: the Rotterdam study. *Am J Epidemiol*. 1995; 142:1291-1299.

40. Rhee SJ, Ohki T, Veith FJ, et al. Current status of management of type II endoleaks after endovascular repair of abdominal aortic aneurysms. *Ann Vasc Surg*. 2003;17:335-344.

41. Safi HJ, Miller CC III, Carr C. Importance of intercostal artery reattachment during thoracoabdominal aortic aneurysm repair. *J Vasc Surg*. 1998;27:58-68.

42. Sampram ESK, Karafa MT, Mascha EJ. et al. Nature, frequency, and predictors of secondary procedures after endovascular repair of abdominal aortic aneurysm. *J Vasc Surg*. 2003;37: 930-936.

43. Sarcina A, Bellosta R, Luzzani L. Surgical treatment of popliteal artery aneurysms. A 20-year experience. *J Cardiovasc Surg*. 1997;38(4): 347-354.

44. Scott RA, Ashton HA, Day DN. Abdominal aortic aneurysms in 4237 screened patients: prevalence, development and management over 6 years. *Br J Surg*. 1993;80:1122-1125.

45. Spouge AR, Stephame RW, Wooley B. Abdominal sonography in asymptomatic executives: prevalence of pathologic findings, potential benefits, and problems. *J Ultrasound Med*. 1996;15:763-767.

46. Sterpetti AV, Hunter WJ, Feldhaus RJ. Inflammatory aneurysms of the abdominal aorta: incidence, pathologic and etiologic considerations. *J Vasc Surg*. 1989;9:643-650.

47. Tilson MD. Aortic aneurysms and atherosclerosis. *Circulation*. 1992;85:378-379.

48. Valentine RJ, Hagino RT, Jackson MR. Gastrointestinal complications after aortic surgery. *J Vasc Surg*. 1998;28:404-411.

49. Wain RA, Marin MS, Ohki T, et al. Endoleaks after endovascular graft treatment of aortic aneurysms: classification, risk factors, and outcome. *J Vasc Surg*. 1998;27:69-78.

50. Weinstein MH, Machleder HI. Sexual function after aortoiliac surgery. *Ann Surg*. 1975;181:787.

51. White GH, May J, McGahan T. Historic control comparison of outcome for matched groups of patients undergoing endoluminal versus open repair of abdominal aortic aneurysms. *J Vasc Surg*. 1996;23:201-212.

52. White GH, Yu W, May J. Endoleak as a complication of endoluminal grafting of aortic aneurysms: Classification, incidence, diagnosis, and management. *J Endovasc Surg*. 1997;4:152-168.

53. Williamson WK, Abou-Zamzam AM Jr., Moneta GL. Prophylactic repair of renal artery stenosis is not justified in patients who require infrarenal aortic reconstruction. *J Vasc Surg*. 1998;28:14-20.

54. Zarins CK et al. The US AneuRx Clinical Trial: 6-year clinical update 2002. *J Vasc Surg*. 2003;37:904-908.

55. EVAR Trial Participants. Comparison of endovascular repair with open repair in patients with abdominal aortic aneurysms (EVARI trial). *Lancet*. 2004;364:843-848.

56. Prinssen M, Verhoeven ELG, Buth J, et al. A randomized trial comparing conventral and endovascular repair of abdominal aortic aneurysms. *N Engl J Med*. 2004;351:1607-1618.

57. Dawson J, Choke E, Sayed S, Cockerill G, Roftus I, Thompson MM. Pharmacotherapy of abdominal aortic aneurysms. *Curr Vasc Pharmacol*. 2006; 4(2):129-149.

58. Baxter BT, Terrin MC, Dalman RL. Medical management of small abdominal aortic aneurysms. *Circulation*. 2008; 117(14):1883-1889.

59. Mosorin M, Juvonew J, Biancari F, et al. Use of doxycycline to decrease the growth rate of abdominal aortic aneurysms: a randomized double-blind, placebo-controlled pilot study. *J Vasc Surg*. 2001; 34(4):606-610.

60. Aoki H, Yoshimura K, Matsuzaki M. Turning back the clock: regression of abdominal aortic aneurysms via pharmacotherapy. *J Mol Med*. 2007; 85(10):1077-1088.

10. Questions

1. In men over age 60, the incidence of aortic dilatation greater than 4 cm detected by ultrasound screening is:

A. 0.05%

B. 5%

C. Approximately 0.5%

D. Between 1% and 2%

2. Aortic aneurysm is most closely associated with which of the following:

A. History of smoking

B. Diabetes mellitus

C. Hypertension

D. Female gender

3. CT angiogram is indicated in preoperative evaluation of aortic aneurysm when endovascular repair is planned:

A. To measure the exact diameter of the aneurysm neck

B. To determine extent of iliac aneurysms

C. In patients whose systolic blood pressure would exceed 160 mm Hg without antihypertensives

D. To measure length of the aneurysm neck

E. All of the above

4. The most accurate and cost-effective screening method for aortic aneurysm is:

A. Careful physical examination

B. Computed tomography

C. Abdominal ultrasound

D. Technetium flow study

5. One advantage of the retroperitoneal approach for aortic aneurysm repair is said to be:

A. Easier access to iliac arteries

B. Shorter operation time

C. Decreased blood transfusions

D. Improved postoperative pulmonary function

6. Which of the following aortic replacement grafts requires preclotting?

A. Woven Dacron

B. Protein-impregnated Dacron

C. Knitted Dacron

D. PTFE

7. An anatomical characteristic precluding endovascular aneurysm repair by infrarenal graft attachment is:

A. Proximal neck larger than 1.5 cm

B. Distal neck less than 1.5 cm

C. Heavily calcified, tortuous iliac arteries

D. Maximum aneurysm diameter greater than 6 cm

8. Control of an aortocaval fistula is most safely accomplished by:

A. Caval ligation

B. Direct suture of the defect after aortic clamping and opening of aneurysm

C. External localization of fistula site and careful dissection of IVC from aorta, followed by suture closure

D. Transfemoral application of a fibrin glue-coated, detachable balloon

9. Complications of untreated atherosclerotic (non-inflammatory) aortic aneurysms may include all of the following except:

A. Distal embolization

B. Rupture

C. Aortoduodenal fistula

D. Obstruction of ureters

10. A type I endoleak after endograft repair:

A. Does not occur with new generation grafts

B. Has no morbid consequences

C. Is caused by a patent IMA

D. May result in further aortic enlargement or graft migration

Answers

1. D.
Researchers of the ADAM study found that male veterans over the age of 60 had aortic dilatation of at least 4.0 cm in 1.4% of subjects.

2. A.
The ADAM study noted that patients who had a history of smoking were 5.57 times more likely to have an aortic aneurysm of 4 cm or more than nonsmokers, and that those with a family history of aneurysm were twice as likely to have the disease as those without a family history of aneurysm. Furthermore, hypertension has been known to have a weaker association with aortic aneurysm. Diabetes mellitus was found to have a negative correlation with aortic aneurysm.

3. E.
Endovascular repair requires accurate knowledge of the AAA neck diameter and length in order to select a prosthesis. Renal artery stenosis may be responsible for unmanageable hypertension. Iliac aneurysms may prevent good distal attachment site.

4. C.
Abdominal ultrasound is a cheap and effective method of screening large populations for aortic aneurysm. Male patients should be screened if they are smokers, or have a family history of aneurysm or high blood pressure.

5. D.
Access to the right iliac artery may be more difficult with the retroperitoneal approach, and the operation time and blood loss is not significantly decreased in using this method. Nonetheless, improved postoperative pulmonary function in the absence of a long midline incision is the expected result.

6. C.
The only graft needing preclotting is knitted Dacron.

7. C.
For infrarenal attachment, clinically available endovascular grafts require a proximal neck 1.5 cm in length distal to the renal arteries. Bifurcation grafts do not require a distal aortic neck. Heavily calcified tortuous iliac arteries would prevent introduction of an endoluminal graft and aortic diameter is a relative restriction. Endografts with suprarenal attachment are now in clinical trial.

8. B.
Control of an aortic caval fistula is most safely obtained by direct suture from inside the aneurysm sac.

9. D.
Atherosclerolic aneurysms rarely cause ureteral obstruction. This complication may be seen with an inflammatory aneurysm.

10. D.
Untreated type I endoleaks may result in further aortic enlargement and require correction. Type II endoleaks may be safely observed for a year expecting spontaneous closure.

Chapter 17: Extracranial Vascular Disease

Jeffrey L. Ballard, MD, FACS

Contents

1. Carotid Bifurcation Lesions

The natural sequela of an untreated critical atherosclerotic lesion of the carotid artery is associated with significant morbidity and mortality. A stroke can have a devastating impact on the life of its victim and family, as well as the economic resources of our already taxed health care system. Appropriately selected, carotid artery reconstruction has a positive effect on the occurrence of stroke, and now it is widely recognized that successful surgical or endovascular therapy has greater impact on morbidity and mortality compared to medical management alone. However, implicit in this approach is knowledge of the natural history of both symptomatic and asymptomatic carotid artery lesions. Risks and benefits of extracranial carotid artery reconstruction must be carefully analyzed so that vascular specialists can adopt precise operative techniques and appropriate methods of perioperative management.

Natural History

Understanding the incidence and natural history of extracranial vascular disease in a given population forms the basis for therapy. Management schemes that encompass diagnosis, treatment and prevention stem from this knowledge base.

Cerebral Infarction

Several population studies have emphasized different aspects of stroke incidence.[1,2] The Rochester, Minnesota study demonstrated an alarming progression of stroke risk with advancing age.[3] In the age group from 55 to 64 years, the cerebral infarction rate was 277 per 100,000 population per year. However, this figure escalated to 1786 per 100,000 per year in the over age 75 group. In addition, men had a 1.5 time greater risk of stroke than women in all age groups. An Australian study demonstrated an overall stroke incidence of 330 per 100,000 per year for all ages, and this included recurrent events.[4] In the United States, there are approximately 160 new strokes per 100,000 population per year.[1,2]

Stroke remains the #3 US killer after heart disease and cancer. In 2003, for instance, cerebrovascular disease (ie, stroke) was responsible for over 150,000 US deaths. The death rate following an initial stroke has been reported to be as high as 38%.[1,2] For survivors, there is a significant rate of ongoing neurologic dysfunction and an alarmingly high rate of recurrent cerebral infarction in the same anatomic region. Pooled data from several studies demonstrate the recurrent stroke rate per year to be approximately 9%, and this rate is highest in the first 12 months following the initial event.[1,2] Clearly, these data underscore the significant morbidity and mortality associated with cerebral infarction.

Stroke-in-evolution deserves special mention, as its natural history is quite dismal.[1,2] This syndrome is heralded by a mild-to-moderate cerebral infarct that progresses within hours or days to a major infarct. There can also be a waxing and waning pattern of signs and symptoms with incomplete recovery, eventually leading to a significant fixed deficit. In these cases, watchful waiting is associated with significant morbidity and mortality.

Mentzer and colleagues showed that conservative management resulted in complete recovery or mild residual deficit in only 23% of 263 pooled cases of stroke-in-evolution.[5] 62% of patients had moderate-to-severe neurologic dysfunction and overall mortality was approximately 15%. On the other hand, emergent endarterectomy in their small series of 17 patients resulted in complete recovery in 12 (70%). The others remained unchanged after surgery, and no patient had worsening of their preoperative deficit.

Transient Ischemic Attacks

Although generally considered benign, episodes of transient cerebral ischemia may herald subsequent stroke or other neurologic disability. In this regard, it is extremely important to distinguish focal neurologic events from "global" symptoms, such as dizziness or vertigo. This is because the ultimate stroke risk is greater following a true transient ischemic attack (TIA) than for the latter.

Transient focal neurologic deficits can occur in either the anterior or posterior cerebral circulation. Signs are usually quite definite, and a skilled examiner can readily wade through the murk of described symptoms to make an accurate diagnosis. TIAs completely resolve by 24 hours regardless of their severity or duration. In the past, events that lasted longer than 24 hours but resolved like a TIA were termed reversible neurologic deficits or RINDs.[6]

However, this term has fallen out of favor because events that last this long invariably produce some cell death, even though it may be subclinical.[6]

Carotid-based TIAs clearly indicate instability of the plaque lesion. Similar to recurrent cerebral infarction, stroke risk is highest in the first year after diagnosis.[1,2] Pooled data demonstrate this risk to be 11%-16%.[1,2] In subsequent years, the risk tapers to 5%-9%, so that at the end of 5 years 30%-35% of untreated patients with TIA will have had a stroke. In the Rochester, Minnesota study, stroke rates following a TIA were 23%, 37% and 45%, respectively, at 1, 3 and 5 years.[3]

A pattern of repeated TIAs with complete recovery is termed *crescendo TIAs*. This pattern usually occurs over the course of days, although some patients will report increasing frequency of the same transient ischemic episode over the course of weeks. Left untreated, stroke risk of crescendo TIAs is at least that of any other TIA and probably much higher, though data on this particular subset is sparse. In our vascular practice, patients with crescendo TIAs referable to a carotid bifurcation lesion are immediately admitted to the hospital and heparinized after confirming that a head CT scan is negative for intracerebral bleeding. Urgent carotid endarterectomy is performed shortly thereafter. In our experience, patients with true carotid-based crescendo TIAs have all had an uneventful recovery using this algorithm.

Asymptomatic Carotid Lesions

Prospective natural history data demonstrate an annual stroke incidence of approximately 4% ipsilateral to an asymptomatic carotid artery stenosis >50%.[1,2] However, when the stenosis progresses to greater than 70%, the stroke risk increases significantly. Roederer and colleagues reported the risk of ischemic symptoms to be 35% within 6 months and 46% at 1 year for lesions that progressed to severe stenosis.[7] Another study of critical asymptomatic lesions demonstrated a combined TIA and stroke rate of 22% within 1 year of diagnosis.[1,2]

Asymptomatic ulcerated plaque lesions also carry a similar stroke risk.[8-10] Moore and colleagues were the first to demonstrate that deep or complex ulcerative lesions were associated with a 5%-8% stroke risk per year.[9,10] Therefore, these ulcerative lesions should be treated like any other severe stenosis even if the carotid artery happens to be minimally diseased otherwise. In our experience, it is distinctly unusual to have deep and/or complex ulceration at the carotid bifurcation without an associated moderate-to-severe stenosis.

2. Pathology

The overwhelming majority (~90%) of lesions that affect the extracranial cerebrovascular system are the result of progressive atherosclerosis. This disease process characteristically occurs at the carotid bifurcation and more specifically at the proximal portion of the internal carotid artery. Symptoms are usually the result of debris embolization from plaque rupture or platelet/thrombus aggregate embolization from an ulcer. Secondary pathologic entities responsible for carotid lesions that may require treatment include fibromuscular dysplasia, coils and kinks, aneurysms, dissection, arteritis, radiation injury and recurrent carotid artery stenosis.

Fibromuscular Dysplasia

This nonatherosclerotic process has been recognized as an entity that can cause cerebrovascular symptoms since its first description in 1964.[1,2] It is wise to remember that fibromuscular dysplasia (FMD) of the carotid artery is associated with intracranial aneurysms (~30% incidence) and FMD of other arteries such as renal (most common) and external iliac (third most common after carotid artery). Of the 4 described histologic variations (intimal fibroplasia, medial hyperplasia, medial fibroplasia and perimedial dysplasia), the most common pattern affecting the carotid arteries is medial fibroplasia.[1,2] In this variant, arterial media smooth muscle is replaced with fibrous connective tissue. This process may result in 1 severe focal stenosis or a series of tight stenoses that appear angiographically as a "string of beads." Aneurysmal dilation of the arterial wall can occur as well. Although the exact cause of symptoms is debatable, there can be embolism, dissection or cerebral hypoperfusion due to hemodynamically significant stenoses in series or one severe focal lesion.

Coils and Kinks

Coils are generally discovered incidental to a more proximal severe internal carotid artery stenosis. Normally, the extracranial carotid system is somewhat kinked in early stages of development.[1,2] If the carotid artery does not straighten during descent of the heart and great vessels into the mediastinum, then loops or coils may persist above the level of the carotid bifurcation.[1,2] The fact that this occurs at an embryologic level explains the relative high incidence of bilaterality (~50% of cases). An asymptomatic loop or coil does not warrant treatment. However, those that are associated with cerebrovascular symptoms do require reconstruction.

Kinks, which also may be congenital, are more likely than coils to cause cerebrovascular symptoms, because they are usually associated with atherosclerotic plaque. An angle less than 90 degrees may significantly reduce prograde cerebral blood flow or be associated with distal embolization.[1,2] Therefore, these lesions should be reconstructed. Kinks with less severe angulation do not require treatment unless neck rotation, flexion or extension cause symptoms.

Aneurysm

Carotid aneurysms may cause a myriad of symptoms. Mechanisms responsible for neurologic dysfunction include thrombosis (rare), rupture (rare), embolization (frequent) or compression of adjacent structures such as cranial nerves.[1,2] Most are fusiform; however, saccular aneurysms do occur and these are frequently associated with a history of neck trauma. Mycotic aneurysms may occur as a result of bacterial seeding of an atherosclerotic lesion. *Staphylococcus aureus* is the usual pathogen, but fortunately, these aneurysms are exceedingly rare now that there are effective treatments for syphilis and peritonsillar abscess.[1,2] Pseudoaneurysms may form if there is suture line disruption, infection or other technical defect not adequately addressed during a previous carotid procedure.

Dissection

Dissection of the carotid artery is an acute event that may occur spontaneously or secondary to blunt neck trauma. In the former situation, the pathologic entity may be atherosclerosis, FMD or cystic medial necrosis. Dissections afflict all age groups but particularly young adults (25-45 years old) and may account for 5% or more of ischemic strokes in this age group.[11] Unilateral dissection of the internal carotid artery (ICA) occurs with a reported incidence of 2%-3% in closed neck injuries.[11]

Dissection occurs when an intimal tear is followed by intramedial hemorrhage. Direct inspection at surgical exploration shows a moderate cylindrical dilation and sharply demarcated dark blue discoloration of the dissected segment. On microscopic examination of excised segments, the dissection is in the outer layer of the media with a characteristic double lumen. A pseudoaneurysm may form between the media and adventitia, or hemorrhage and thrombosis around the intima may slowly occlude the vessel. Embolization may also occur distally, leading to a variety of presenting symptoms. Fortunately, spontaneous resolution of the process on anticoagulant medication is the rule and it is rare that the patient requires operative reconstruction of the dissected vessel.[11]

Angiographic findings are classified as follows: type A involves a short segment of the cervical internal carotid artery not extending to the skull base, type B extends to the petrous canal and type C demonstrates occlusion.[11] Intracranial angiography can supply additional important information regarding collateral cerebral blood flow and evidence of embolic phenomenon.

Spontaneous dissection may occur without symptoms. However, the usual presentation includes sudden severe neck pain or unilateral temporal headache. Cranial nerve dysfunction or Horner's syndrome may accompany these symptoms.[1,2,11] Direct compression is the mechanism for dysfunction of cranial nerves IX, X, XI or XII and it is presumed that disruption of periadvential sympathetic fibers is the etiology of Horner's syndrome.[1,2,11]

In the blunt trauma setting, one must maintain a high index of suspicion in order to make the diagnosis. Clinical findings suggestive of dissection include significant hematoma of the neck, Horner's syndrome, cranial nerve dysfunction, TIA or limb paresis in an alert patient.[11] In essence, the primary indication for further imaging of the cervical carotid artery in blunt trauma cases is any neurological deficit that cannot be explained by head CT scan findings.

Arteritis

Giant cell arteritis may cause cerebral dysfunction due to extra- or intracranial arterial involvement. Generalized malaise symptoms and an elevated sedimentation rate may be accompanied by tenderness over the affected carotid artery.[1,2] This arterial inflammation, which typically affects an older age group, is characterized histologically by giant cell and lymphocyte infiltration of the media.[1,2] Clinical improvement with steroid therapy alone is the rule, although normalization of the sedimentation rate may lag behind clinical recovery.

Aortic arch branch vessel disease from Takayasu's arteritis can also cause cerebral dysfunction. Similar to giant cell arteritis, symptoms improve with corticosteroid therapy. However, a younger patient is usually seen with this entity. Operative treatment, if needed, is best effected by arterial bypass as severe arterial inflammation generally precludes endarterectomy.[1,2]

Radiation Injury

Cervical radiation is known to cause accelerated atherosclerosis of the cervical carotid artery.[1,2] Interestingly, this process usually lags years behind radiation therapy and affected areas are not in the usual proximal internal carotid artery location. Extensive common carotid artery lesions are not uncommon. In these cases, there is injury throughout the vessel wall. Layers affected include the endothelium, ground substance, elastic lamina and smooth muscle.[1,2] Grossly, the vessel is fibrotic and cordlike. Standard endarterectomy techniques may be difficult to perform in this setting and in many instances, carotid reconstruction with a vein graft is the best option.

Recurrent Carotid Stenosis

Reported range for recurrent carotid stenosis varies from 1%-21%, at least one-third of which may progress to severe lesions.[1,2] Within the first 18 months to 2 years following endarterectomy, the pathologic lesion accounting for recurrent disease is usually exuberant smooth muscle proliferation (AKA myointimal hyperplasia). After this time, recurrent lesions through the previous endarterectomy site are usually atherosclerotic in nature. Clamp injury proximal or distal to the operative site may also contribute to the incidence of late restenosis. However, these lesions are not really "recurrent" and in all likelihood were missed at the time of the original procedure.

Early carotid restenosis from myointimal hyperplasia appears as a concentric smooth surface on gross inspection. This surface morphology appears to have a lower risk for debris embolization.[1,2] Therefore, most investigators do not intervene unless the recurrent lesion is severe. Furthermore, re-do endarterectomy is precluded in these cases by the dense accumulation of myointimal fibroplasia. An endarterectomy plane is unable to be affected, thus patch angioplasty or carotid artery graft replacement are frequently employed for these remedial procedures.

Late carotid re-stenosis should be treated like any other atherosclerotic carotid lesion. In our practice, re-do endarterectomy is recommended when symptomatic patients have moderate or severe lesions and asymptomatic patients have severe lesions. Unlike recurrent myointimal hyperplastic lesions, an endarterectomy plane can usually be established so that the procedure can be completed in the usual fashion.

3. Clinical Evaluation

A thorough medical history and physical examination are paramount for appropriate diagnosis and selection of treatment options. This should include an assessment of associated risk factors, detailed review of cerebrovascular symptoms or pattern of disease progression, and personal review of the diagnostic imaging study or studies. It is extremely helpful to have the patient or a family member recreate any acute event. For instance, there may only be a subtle difference in the patient's perception of dysarthria vs. aphasia. However, the former points toward a right carotid lesion and the latter toward a left carotid lesion. From the examiner's perspective, one must be able to clinically locate the lesion and deduce the likely etiology of the presenting symptom(s).

Physical examination is problem focused, with emphasis on the cardiac, peripheral vascular and neurological systems. Obviously, if the patient has already recovered from a TIA or stroke, the physical examination is less likely to guide therapy. On the other hand, accurate and repeated examination is critical in helping to decide when an improving stroke patient has reached their plateau of recovery. This is important because endarterectomy before this time may worsen the situation, or waiting too long may increase the risk for recurrent stroke.

Common Clinical Syndromes

3 distinct clinical syndromes are the usual impetus for patient referral to a vascular specialist. They can be categorized as patients with stroke, patients with TIA, and patients with asymptomatic but high-grade stenoses or deep ulceration.[1,2] Often an auscultated bruit in an otherwise asymptomatic patient leads to carotid duplex ultrasound with the serendipitous finding of a severe stenosis. Other asymptomatic patients may have disease progression as demonstrated by serial duplex ultrasound examination.

A TIA or stroke is usually the result of cerebral emboli and less commonly from acute arterial thrombosis. Ipsilateral transient monocular blindness (or amaurosis fugax) is usually described as a shade coming down over the eye. Alternatively, this event may be described as a cloudy veil that the patient can barely see through. Some patients experience transient monocular total visual loss. Cortical events usually occur in the middle cerebral artery (MCA) distribution. These produce contralateral motor and sensory dysfunction. The patient will frequently describe the motor dysfunction as limb weakness, paralysis or clumsiness.[1,2] Loss of sensation or paresthesias may affect the contralateral side of the face or one or both of the contralateral extremities. Broca's aphasia is a result of ischemia in the distribution of the superior MCA branch in the dominant (usually left) hemisphere.[6] This is characterized by reasonable speech comprehension but difficult speech output. Ischemia of the inferior MCA branch in the dominant hemisphere produces a different type of aphasia, called fluent or Wernicke's, that is characterized by poor comprehension as well as nonsensical speech.[6] Dysarthria, which is a motor disturbance of articulation, is a nondominant hemisphere symptom that is often confused with aphasia.[1,2,6]

Other stroke patterns are less common. Unilateral infarction in the anterior cerebral artery distribution typically results in lower extremity motor dysfunction with sparing of the face and upper extremity.[6] Bilateral infarction causes disabling behavioral and cognitive impairment. Infarction in the posterior cerebral artery distribution results in contralateral homonymous hemianopsia.[6] Fortunately, sparing of central vision allows for functional vision despite loss of half the visual field. Cortical blindness can occur with bilateral PCA infarction. Arterial ischemia in the basilar artery distribution causes pontine infarction, which may be fatal if the vessel occludes acutely.[6] These patients look like the "lights are on, but nobody's home" and will appear to be alert despite loss of significant midbrain function. Cerebral ischemia in the distribution of the lenticulostriate or thalamoperforate arteries is termed lacunar infarction. Occlusion or rupture of these end arteries results in pure motor (usually) or pure sensory (less common) strokes.[6] Most patients who demonstrate a lacunar stroke pattern (AKA lacunae) on CT scan have severe chronic, and often uncontrolled, hypertension.[1,2,6]

4. Diagnostic Modalities

The paradigm for the diagnostic evaluation of the cervical carotid system continues to evolve with time, and has also been driven by technological advances in treatment. Just a few years ago, arteriography had essentially been eliminated from the preoperative work-up of patients with cerebrovascular symptoms. However, increasing utilization of carotid angioplasty and stent deployment has lead to resurgence in the number of carotid arteriograms performed in the U.S. and arteriography is still considered by many surgeons to be the gold standard carotid imaging study. Even so, there are a few compelling reasons for not necessarily obtaining an arteriogram prior to every endarterectomy. Selection of patients for carotid endarterectomy (CEA) based on arteriography exposes the patient to arteriographic-related complications, a small diagnostic procedure stroke/death risk, and adds to the overall cost of the procedure.[12-18]

Duplex ultrasonography (DU) has been shown by many authors to accurately and noninvasively detect lesions at the carotid bifurcation.[14-25] This diagnostic test exposes the patient to a negligible risk of stroke and death. Further, it is repeatable, reproducible and is generally well-tolerated by all patients. Its diagnostic data, like that of arteriography, can be obtained in an outpatient setting, but the procedure cost is significantly less. CEA based solely upon DU is appropriate if the technical aspects of the ultrasound evaluation are satisfactory, if the study of the carotid bifurcation is as accurate as a comparable arteriogram and if the study provides all the necessary information for safe surgery.[14-25]

The vascular groups at Cedars-Sinai Medical Center, UCLA and the University of Illinois at Chicago predicted a diminishing role for carotid arteriography as early as 1986.[14,15,21] In a more recent study, Dawson et al,[19] demonstrated that clinical assessment and duplex scanning alone were sufficient for the preoperative evaluation of at least 93% of candidates for CEA. Others have also confirmed that DU of the carotid bifurcation is as accurate as a comparable arteriogram, and typically is a better imaging modality than either CT or magnetic resonance (MR) angiography.[14-25]

In a retrospective case series analysis of all patients who had CEA over a 2-year period at a university teaching hospital, there was excellent agreement between DU and arteriography in the detection of internal carotid artery (ICA) occlusion or stenosis >45% in the 165 patients who had both imaging studies performed before CEA.[25] The accuracy of DU compared to arteriography was 99.4%, while the sensitivity and specificity were 99.4% and 100%, respectively. Concordance between DU and arteriography decreased somewhat when stenotic ICA lesions were further stratified into 2 groups (moderate, 45%-70% and severe, 70%-99%). However, in surgical practice, whether a symptomatic ICA stenosis is moderate or severe does not change the clinical indication for CEA.[26] On the other hand, accuracy in separating an ICA occlusion from a 98%-99% stenosis, or in defining a 60%-70% asymptomatic ICA stenosis from one that is less severe, is essential.

In the experience cited above, 1 symptomatic severe ICA stenosis and 1 asymptomatic severe ICA stenosis were misread by DU as occluded and moderate, respectively.[25] A correct surgical plan for CEA was made only after arteriography. 16 other symptomatic ICA stenoses, read as moderate by DU, were demonstrated to be severe by arteriography, although CEA was already clinically indicated in each case. 6 type "C" ulcers not well-visualized by DU were associated with high grade carotid stenosis, which was already accurately diagnosed by DU. This finding is not entirely unexpected as DU is primarily designed to detect flow-limiting lesions.[27]

Arteriography remains the study of choice for delineating ulcerative plaque lesions as well as imaging of aortic arch branch and intracerebral vessels.[28] Nonetheless, refinements in high-resolution B-mode ultrasound imaging and in CT angiography have facilitated the diagnosis of ulcerative carotid bifurcation lesions. In addition, clinically evident disease of the proximal great vessels can usually be deduced by careful patient history and physical examination as well as indirect clues from DU.[28] Finally, there is an extremely low incidence (1.5%-2.0%) of associated intracranial aneurysms in patients with typical cerebrovascular symptoms.[29] Most of these are saccular microaneurysms with little clinical relevance. Lack of significant synchronous aortic arch branch or intracranial lesions demonstrated by arteriography has allowed us to comfortably eliminate this and other diagnostic studies, such as CT or MR angiography from the usual preoperative work-up of elective CEA patients.

Compelling as the above data appear, there are still some circumstances in which carotid arteriography is particularly useful.[15,18,20,23] This is true if there is inadequate ultrasound imaging of the carotid bifurcation, and of particular importance when symptoms are referable to an unsatisfactorily imaged carotid bifurcation. A suggestion of more proximal or distal disease that is beyond the imaging capabilities of DU also warrants further interrogation by arteriography, as does planning for carotid artery stent deployment (Section 9). In our current vascular practice, we do not routinely obtain arteriograms to confirm duplex diagnosed ICA occlusion or to image recurrent stenotic carotid lesions that are undergoing open repair.

Complications of Diagnostic Modalities

Stroke, transient cerebral ischemia, contrast induced nephrotoxicity, local arterial complications and death are occasionally associated with carotid arteriography.[12-18] In fact, carotid arteriography accounted for one-half of the perioperative neurologic morbidity (1.2%) associated with the Asymptomatic Carotid Atherosclerosis Study (ACAS).[1,2,30] Although mortality associated with carotid arteriography is extremely low (0%-0.6%), nonfatal complications can be quite disabling. Transient neurologic events were the most common nonfatal complication noted in a review of 8 prospective studies that included a combined total of 2227 cerebral arteriograms.[31,32] In that review, there was a 4.1% neurologic complication rate and permanent disabling stroke rate of 1.0%.[31] Therefore, despite anecdotal evidence to the contrary, the above data suggest that an accurate stroke risk of carotid arteriography is ~1.0%. This is not an insignificant percentage, particularly when one considers the detail with which surgical results are scrutinized and the small margin of error acceptable for CEA.

Use of nonionic contrast agents has greatly decreased the incidence of acute renal failure and generalized nephrotoxicity associated with arteriography. However, the incidence of post-arteriography, contrast-induced nephrotoxicity is not insignificant for patients with diabetes, particularly if there is preexisting renal insufficiency.[32] Elderly patients (>70 years) and those with congestive heart failure are at risk for acute pulmonary edema, in addition to contrast-induced nephrotoxicity. Clinically significant local complications of arteriography such as pseudoaneurysm, hemorrhage, hematoma, arterial thrombosis, arteriovenous fistulae and nerve injury are troublesome. The total incidence of these complications ranges from 0.1%-5%.[31,33-36]

5. Surgical Considerations and Technique

General Considerations

The purpose of carotid artery surgery is to eliminate recurrent neurologic symptoms or to prevent stroke. Despite Eastcott's initial report detailing the operative repair of a carotid artery lesion in 1954, the proper role of carotid artery surgery has undergone a long-tested journey.[30,37-40] Since the natural history of both symptomatic and asymptomatic carotid lesions has become less controversial, risks and benefits of carotid artery reconstruction must be carefully analyzed so that surgeons continue to adopt appropriate criteria for patient selection and safe operative techniques, as well as methods of perioperative management.

No area of carotid artery surgery has been as controversial as the use of proper techniques for cerebral protection during the critical phase of carotid artery clamping necessary to perform carotid endarterectomy. Historic and current methods employed for cerebral protection include type of anesthesia (ie, regional vs. general), induced hypertension, hypercarbia or hypocarbia, and the use of a temporary inlying or outlying intraluminal carotid shunt. Although some surgeons continue to advocate cervical block anesthesia and have reported excellent results with this technique, the majority of surgeons prefer general endotracheal anesthesia.[41-47] Besides providing a motionless operative field, general anesthesia decreases the metabolic demand (oxygen consumption) of brain tissue. The concept that systemic hypertension increases blood flow has been questioned by many investigators.[48-50] Most now believe that the detrimental effects of induced hypertension on myocardial oxygen consumption outweigh the minimal improvement in regional cerebral blood flow in patients with poor collateral circulation. Similarly, the general cerebrovascular effect of hypercapnia was, at one time, an appealing method of intraoperative management. However, current consensus suggests that while hypercapnia may increase blood flow in the normal brain, it decreases flow to ischemic brain because of vasomotor paralysis in areas of cerebral ischemia (the so-called reversed Robin Hood phenomenon).[51,52] In fact, recent data suggest that because of this cerebral "steal" effect, higher cerebral perfusion pressures are required to maintain normal cerebral metabolism with increasing hypercapnia.[53,54]

Hypocapnia, on the other hand, causes cerebral vasoconstriction, which depresses overall cerebral blood flow, reduces potential collateral flow and probably increases the risk of cerebral ischemia.[50,53]

Despite a greater understanding of cerebral physiology and refinements in the technique of carotid artery surgery, the various maneuvers to protect the brain from ischemia during carotid artery clamping have been used either routinely without reliance upon a monitoring technique, or selectively with precision monitoring. Generally, normocapnia and normotension (intraoperative blood pressure is maintained at average "normal" preoperative levels) are maintained to maximize cerebral protection. Consensus has not yet emerged in regards to local vs. general endotracheal anesthesia, but this issue stirs less emotion than the debate over the use of intraluminal carotid artery shunts. At times, the arguments for and against carotid artery shunting has left the realm of logic and science and bordered on religious philosophy.

The controversy concerning the use of an indwelling shunt during carotid endarterectomy has 3 main schools of thought: routine shunting, no shunting and selective shunting. Those surgeons who routinely use shunts,[54-60] a school of thought most arduously advocated early on by Javid et al[54] and recently by Flanigan et al,[55] believe that routine shunting improves surgical results because cerebral protection allows extended operative time and therefore achievement of the best possible technical result. In addition, routine shunting may decrease the frequency of technical problems associated with the occasional use of a shunt and remove the operative indecision inherent in the application of the various criteria for selective shunting. Surgeons who do not use shunts, a school of thought which has been ardently supported by Baker et al,[61] and a concept also supported by others,[62-66] have emphasized the dangers of shunt-induced thrombosis, embolization and intimal dissection. These investigators have proposed that the physical presence of a shunt impairs satisfactory technical performance of carotid artery surgery. A third group of surgeons, represented by Woodworth et al,[67] Wylie et al[68] and Sundt et al,[69,70] selectively use an indwelling temporary shunt. This selective use of a shunt is based on criteria which try to determine abnormalities in intraoperative cerebral perfusion or hypoperfusion.[56,67-76] The selective criteria for shunt use include abnormal intraoperative electroencephalography,[69-71,73,74] decreased cerebral blood flow,[69] preoperative neurologic deficit,[67] intraoperative neurologic deficit with test carotid occlusion in awake patients,[41-43,75,76] poor back bleeding, low internal carotid artery back pressure (stump pressure)[67,68,72,75] and contralateral carotid occlusion.[56,61,62]

Detailed discussion of each of these methods is beyond the scope of this review and the interested reader is referred to Chapter 41 in Moore's *Surgery for Cerebrovascular Disease* (2nd edition).[77]

Standard Endarterectomy

Indications for carotid endarterectomy were recently agreed upon by a consensus conference of the American Heart Association Stroke Council.[26] These were divided into recommendations for symptomatic and asymptomatic patients. Table 1 demonstrates surgical indications for a good risk-symptomatic patient if the surgeon's morbidity and mortality rate is less than 6%. Table 2 demonstrates indications for asymptomatic patients if the surgeon's morbidity and mortality rate is <3%.

Technique

The common carotid artery bifurcates approximately 2.5 cm below the angle of the mandible.[78] Normally, the sternocleidomastoid muscle, the posterior belly of the digastric muscle and the omohyoid muscle bind the carotid bifurcation. Thus, a skin incision placed along the anterior border of the sternocleidomastoid muscle will facilitate exposure of the carotid sheath. The common facial vein will come into view as the incision is deepened. This vessel courses superficial to the carotid bifurcation to join the internal jugular vein. It serves as an important landmark during the dissection. Several small vessels coursing toward the sternocleidomastoid muscle are nutrient branches from the superior thyroid artery and vein. These vessels should be ligated and divided to avoid troublesome postoperative bleeding.

In the typical carotid dissection, the common carotid artery should be exposed above the level of the omohyoid muscle. Once this vessel is isolated, further distal dissection along its medial aspect

Table 1

Indications for CEA in Low-Risk Symptomatic Patients[a]

A. Proven indications
   1. One or more TIAs in previous 6 months with an ipsilateral carotid stenosis ≥70%
   2. Mild stroke with carotid stenosis ≥70%

B. Acceptable but not proven indications
   1. TIAs in previous 6 months and a moderate stenosis (50%-69%)
   2. Stroke-in-evolution and a stenosis ≤70%
   3. Mild or moderate stroke in previous 6 months and a stenosis 50%-69%
   4. Symptomatic carotid stenosis ≤70% combined with required coronary bypass grafting

C. Uncertain indications
   1. TIAs with carotid stenosis ≤50%
   2. Mild stroke with carotid stenosis ≤50%
   3. Acute carotid thrombosis with symptoms

D. Proven inappropriate indications
   1. Moderate stroke with mild (≤50%) stenosis, patient not receiving aspirin
   2. Single TIA, mild stenosis, and patient not receiving aspirin
   3. High-risk patient with multiple TIAs and mild stenosis, not receiving aspirin
   4. High-risk patient, mild or moderate stroke, mild stenosis, not receiving aspirin
   5. Global ischemic symptoms with mild stenosis
   6. Asymptomatic patient with acute internal carotid dissection, receiving heparin

[a] *These criteria for surgeons with a morbidity and mortality rate <6%.*

Table 2

Indications for CEA in Asymptomatic Patients

A. Proven indications
   1. Stenosis ≥70% (some surgeons have lowered this threshold to ≥60% following ACAS publication, however this author continues to use a cut-off of 70% stenosis for this group)

B. Uncertain indications
   1. High-risk patient and/or surgeon with a morbidity and mortality rate of greater than 3%, combined carotid/coronary operations, or nonstenotic ulcerative lesions

C. Proven inappropriate
   1. Facility and/or surgeon combined stroke morbidity and mortality ≥5%

facilitates exposure of the superior thyroid and external carotid arteries. Dissection in the "V" of the carotid bifurcation should be avoided because this area is extremely vascular. It is wise to expose and dissect out the internal carotid artery well above the level of gross atherosclerotic disease. This dissection is usually 1 to 2 cm above the bifurcation, and thereby avoids the highly vascular carotid sinus tissue.

The descending branch of the hypoglossal nerve (AKA ansa cervicalis) is located anterior and parallel to the sternocleidomastoid muscle. If this branch is followed upward, the main hypoglossal nerve trunk can be located. Division of the descending branch of the hypoglossal nerve near its origin allows the main nerve trunk to be displaced upward and forward, thus providing higher exposure of the internal carotid artery. A nutrient vein and artery associated with the sternocleidomastoid muscle course in immediate relation to this nerve at this level. Care should be taken to avoid injury to the underlying hypoglossal nerve when these vessels are ligated and divided. This maneuver allows the nerve to retract superomedially and out of harm's way. Division of this artery/vein "sling" about the hypoglossal nerve facilitates exposure of the internal carotid artery under the posterior belly of the digastric muscle.

Arteriotomy should be created just proximal to carotid bulb and anterolateral to the carotid flow divider. This incision is then lengthened distally under direct vision through the diseased ICA to a point at which there is normal appearing intima. It is critical not to make this arteriotomy on the anteromedial aspect of the ICA near the carotid sinus, as this is a relatively fixed area that is hard to reapproximate without creating a focal narrowing that is at risk for restenosis. It is wise to find the correct endarterectomy plane at the level of the carotid bulb. Thereafter, endarterectomy first proceeds proximally and the specimen is excised sharply at the level of the common carotid artery using angled Potts scissors. Everting the external carotid artery into the carotid bulb facilitates endarterectomy at this level. Then, at the mid-to-distal ICA, one must carefully find the plaque transition point between the diseased segment to be removed and the remaining nondiseased intimal surface. This is the critical step in the performance of a technically sound CEA, and, if done correctly, tacking sutures are rarely required. Meticulous care is then taken to ensure that there are no remaining loose areas of media through the endarterectomized surface. In our practice, bovine pericardial patch angioplasty reapproximates the arteriotomy, and intraoperative duplex ultrasound scanning completes the procedure.

Exposure of the High Internal Carotid Artery

One of the most difficult vascular exposures is the high internal carotid artery.[78] The surgeon must contend with a limited visual field and vital nerve structures within a confined space. This is frequently made more difficult by a space-occupying vascular lesion or the presence of vascular injury with hemorrhagic staining and displacement of the tissues. Structures that overlie the high ICA in the neck include the facial nerve, parotid gland, ramus of the mandible, and mastoid and styloid processes. The hypoglossal nerve, glossopharyngeal nerve, digastric and stylohyoid muscles, and occipital and posterior auricular arteries cross the ICA in the distal neck, and at this level the vessel courses progressively deeper to enter the petrous canal of the temporal bone.

Exposure routinely begins at the level of the common carotid artery proximal to the carotid bifurcation. The omohyoid muscle serves as a landmark for the proximal extent of this exposure. The dissection continues distally, protecting the vagus nerve, which lies immediately behind the internal carotid artery. The hypoglossal nerve is exposed and the descending branch is divided in order to displace the hypoglossal nerve forward. It becomes evident that one is now working in a progressively narrowing triangle with inadequate space to perform any major vascular reconstructive procedure. The digastric and stylohyoid muscles are divided to facilitate this exposure. The styloid process and the stylohyoid ligament are excised. The glossopharyngeal and the superior laryngeal nerves must be identified and preserved.

Anatomic dissection in human cadaver specimens demonstrates that division of the posterior belly of the digastric muscle will facilitate exposure of the internal carotid artery to the middle of the first cervical vertebra. Anterior subluxation of the mandible improves exposure to the superior border of the first cervical vertebra. The addition of styloidectomy to the above maneuvers extends the exposure cephalad approximately 0.5 cm.[79] Fisher and associates[80] described a unique technique of wire fixation of the mandible to hold its subluxed position during the operative procedure. The 12-15 mm of space obtained converts the triangle described above into a narrow rectangle. In the discussion of Fisher's paper, Stanley suggested that a towel clip placed on the angle of the mandible through two small stab incisions would allow the subluxation to be fixed by minimal retraction. Dossa et al[81] also suggested that temporary mandibular subluxation can be accomplished in a safe and expeditious manner using diagonal interdental/Steinman pin wiring. With any of these techniques, it is important to avoid dislocation of the mandible, since serious injury can occur to the temporomandibular joint, and even to the contralateral internal carotid artery.

In situations requiring more room for reconstruction, transection of the mandibular ramus with either translocation or temporary removal of the condyle and ramus fragment will afford wider exposure. In these cases, arch bars and wires are used to immobilize the mandible following induction of anesthesia. The usual carotid endarterectomy incision is extended posteriorly to a point behind the ear. The carotid bifurcation and internal carotid artery are exposed, as described previously. The mandibular ramus of the facial nerve is protected. The angle of the mandible is exposed and the periosteum elevated toward the mandibular notch anteriorly and posteriorly. The mandibular ramus is divided vertically using a power saw posterior to the foramen of the inferior alveolar artery and nerve. The posterior bone fragment is gently rotated out and upward as the pterygoid muscles are divided, thus allowing its removal. The bone fragment is preserved in chilled lactated Ringer's solution until it is replaced following arterial reconstruction.

Once the mandibular ramus is removed, the digastric and stylohyoid muscles are divided and the dissection is continued to the base of the skull. Care should be taken to protect the hypoglossal, glossopharyngeal and vagus nerves, which are in immediate relation to the high internal carotid artery. The mandibular fragment is returned to its anatomic location following completion of internal carotid artery reconstruction and interrupted nonabsorbable sutures close the temporomandibular joint capsule. A thin titanium plate is used to stabilize the reapproximated mandibular fragment. The cervical fascia and platysma muscle are reapproximated, followed by routine skin closure.

Open Balloon Angioplasty

This technique was often used in the past for FMD lesions of the carotid artery, before the widespread use of percutaneous balloon angioplasty. Indications for open balloon angioplasty of FMD lesions included those that caused stroke or were associated with severely decreased cerebral blood flow due to a series of stenoses or 1 focal critical stenosis. Other treatment options include carotid artery resection with end-to-end reconstruction or autologous vein interposition graft, ICA dilation with rigid dilators and operative closed balloon angioplasty. Open balloon angioplasty is the safest operative dilation approach, as significant complications have been described with the other mechanical or balloon techniques.[82]

Correction of Coils and Kinks

Symptoms usually prompt diagnosis of this problem. Therefore, indications follow those of any other symptomatic carotid lesions. A severely stenotic coil or kink also warrants treatment, although the true stroke risk is really unknown.

Technique

A number of techniques are useful to correct nonstenotic coils and kinks, none of which are applicable to every situation. For a redundant ICA without significant stenosis, the following procedures can be used: segmental ICA resection with primary reanastomosis; transection of the proximal ICA with translocation of the distal ICA to a more proximal location on the carotid bulb; and segmental common carotid artery resection with primary anastomosis.[1,2] All of these procedures are designed to shorten the redundant ICA. In this author's experience, it is much easier to resect and re-anastomose a segment of common carotid artery, as the anastomosis is larger and exposure is generally better. This maneuver requires a little extra mobilization of the external carotid artery and division of at least the superior thyroid artery.

If there is a severe stenosis at a kink, for instance, then a longitudinal arteriotomy should be made anterolateral to the carotid flow divider and opened distally beyond the disease level to fully assess the underlying atherosclerotic plaque lesion. In these circumstances, endarterectomy may or may not be required. However, patch closure will eliminate the stenosis and mechanically straighten out the kinked vessel.

External Carotid Endarterectomy

Indications

Some symptomatic patients may have severe external carotid artery (ECA) stenosis in conjunction with ipsilateral ICA occlusion. There is stagnant blood flow in the carotid bulb and turbulent blood flow in the proximal ECA due to the stenosis. In these cases, debris from the stump of the occluded ICA may be prone to embolization. Amaurosis fugax is commonly associated with this syndrome. Cortical events are also possible because there are numerous collateral pathways that connect ECA branches with the intracranial ICA. ECA endarterectomy with obliteration of the blind ICA stump is the procedure indicated for these symptomatic cases. Asymptomatic cases do not warrant treatment.

Technique

The carotid bifurcation is exposed in the fashion previously described. However, before proceeding any further, a continuous wave Doppler probe should be positioned over the mid-ICA to confirm its occlusion. This author usually creates an arteriotomy over the anteromedial aspect of the carotid bulb (almost exactly opposite of the arteriotomy used for standard CEA), and then extends this into the ECA. This incision specifically avoids the very vascular carotid sinus tissue at the crotch of the bifurcation. Endarterectomy requires neat feathering of the specimen away from the ECA similar to the technique described earlier for the ICA. Obliteration of the blind ICA stump after endarterectomy precedes Dacron® patch closure. This is accomplished by placing horizontal mattress sutures of polypropylene across the ICA stump under direct vision until it is closed. A smooth flow surface that tapers into the ECA is affected by this maneuver.

Alternatively, the occluded ICA can be divided flush with the carotid bulb and ligated distally. At the base of the transected ICA, an arteriotomy is extended distally through the ECA stenosis and proximally into the bulb as needed. Patch closure creates a widely patent ECA and a smooth taper between the distal common carotid artery and ECA. This author does not use this technique because troublesome bleeding is often encountered during surgical manipulation at or near the carotid sinus. A third surgical option, which has been used with success by this author, involves the creation of an arteriotomy in the usual location for a standard CEA and carrying it into the occluded ICA. The ICA is then transected 2-3 cm distal to the bulb. Endarterectomy proceeds through the transected ICA and eversion endarterectomy is accomplished at the level of the ECA. The remaining endarterectomized ICA adventitia is then folded down and trimmed to reapproximate the carotid bulb. This requires a bit of ingenuity to fashion a new carotid bulb, but the advantage is that this is an autologous reconstruction.

Obviously, the most feared complications of CEA are stroke and/or death. However, there are other important complications that also warrant discussion. These are perioperative oscillations in blood pressure, intracerebral hemorrhage, technical defects, cranial nerve injury, hematoma and wound infection.

Blood Pressure Oscillations

Manipulation of the carotid sinus during endarterectomy can cause perioperative hypotension and/or hypertension. It has been suggested that after endarterectomy, the newly compliant carotid bulb affects the baroreceptor mechanism leading to these shifts in blood pressure.[1,2] Some authors have also implicated type of anesthesia as a causative factor. However, the hypothesis that general anesthesia is associated with more blood pressure oscillations than local anesthesia has not been prospectively studied. Whatever the mechanism, there is no question that poorly controlled hypertensive patients have a significant incidence of blood pressure fluctuations with CEA.[1,2]

In a study of 100 consecutive CEAs, Bove et al.[83] noted significant intraoperative hypotension in 28% and hypertension in 19%. There was a higher stroke rate in this group compared to those who were normotensive throughout the procedure. In addition, bradycardia may develop during surgical manipulation of the carotid bulb. This can be associated with significant decrease in blood pressure. Local injection of 1% lidocaine into the soft tissue at the "V" in the carotid bifurcation will promptly resolve this problem.

Blood pressure oscillations may persist into the immediate postoperative period. Atropine, nitroprusside (Nipride®) and phenylephrine (Neosynephrine®) or norepinephrine (Levophed®) are all useful to treat persistent bradycardia, hypertension and hypotension, respectively. Small boluses of these medications are usually all that is needed and resolution is usually affected before the patient is ready to leave the recovery room. On rare occasion, continuous drip of one of these drugs may require ICU monitoring until the pressure oscillations stabilize.

In this early postoperative period, one would typically opt for a fluid bolus or dopamine to treat hypotension and nitroglycerine to treat hypertension, as opposed to the agents mentioned above. However, in this circumstance hypotension is not usually the result of hypovolemia. Therefore, a fluid bolus is not likely to correct the problem and may in fact tip a marginal patient into congestive heart failure. Similarly, dopamine is not usually effective at low doses. It is most effective in this situation at levels that stimulate alpha-adrenergic receptors like the more direct acting agents, phenylephrine or norepinephrine. Furthermore, nitroglycerine is not the drug of choice for quick and effective control of severe hypertension after CEA. Nitroglycerine affects venous capacitance vessels more than arterial vessels, and the agent is not as easy to titrate as is nitroprusside.

Intracerebral Hemorrhage

This rare but well described complication appears to be caused by post-CEA loss of autoregulation within the brain that leads to dramatic cerebral hyperperfusion.[84-87] In a series of 2362 consecutive CEAs performed at the Mayo Clinic, this complication occurred in 14 (0.6%) patients.[87] The most distressing aspect of this problem is that it typically occurs days (even 5 to 7 days later in a few reports) after an uneventful CEA. A consistent preoperative finding that has been described in nearly all reported cases is a patient history of severe longstanding cerebral ischemia due to a very high-grade carotid stenosis. This has also been reported to occur in the interim between staged CEAs in patients with severe bilateral lesions.

The syndrome of cerebral hyperperfusion is heralded by severe ipsilateral headache followed by seizures and temporary or permanent focal neurologic deficits.[84-87] Unfortunately, death from massive cerebral hemorrhage is the usual outcome. It has been suggested that strict perioperative blood pressure control in at-risk patients may minimize the incidence of this complication.[84-87] However, this practice should be routine for all patients having CEA anyway. At the very least, a high index of suspicion should be maintained in all at-risk patients, and possibly, a longer period of postoperative in-hospital monitoring would be required to ensure that blood pressure is well-controlled prior to discharge.

Technical Complications

These problems can be avoided altogether by meticulous surgical technique and by imaging the reconstructed carotid artery following endarterectomy. The only way to ensure clean proximal and distal endpoints is to directly inspect them at the time of CEA. This means that the arteriotomy must be carried beyond the disease in the ICA and at least through the carotid bulb proximally. Careful attention to the transition between the atherosclerotic plaque being removed and the remaining nondiseased ICA virtually eliminates the need for tacking sutures. Finally, the endarterectomized surface should be thoroughly inspected for evidence of loose fragments or any other debris that may be at risk for embolization.

Postreconstruction imaging with duplex ultrasound will ensure a technically perfect result. The detailed gray-scale images and blood flow velocity data supplied by this sensitive and specific modality are truly invaluable.[22] This author always images the proximal and distal clamp points in addition to the CEA site because a flap can occur in these areas that is otherwise inconspicuous by gross inspection. Intraoperative arteriography is a less desirable imaging modality for a variety of reasons. These include the fact that forceful intra-arterial injection of contrast may cause distal embolization or dissection, the angiocatheter may cause a dissection plane in the proximal remaining atherosclerotic plaque, the image is in a single plane and often, overlying instruments or operating table interfere with a complete image. However, this is still better than simply using a continuous wave Doppler probe. This frequently used modality is not specific enough to be relied upon and the inexperienced operator may not appreciate subtle changes in signal intensity that may indicate residual disease or clamp injury.

Cranial Nerve Injury

Important cranial and somatic nerves are at risk for injury during carotid endarterectomy.[78] The mandibular ramus of the facial nerve is vulnerable to injury due to head position. Turning the head away from the carotid artery to be operated upon draws the mandibular ramus well below the mandible and increases the possibility of facial nerve injury. Nerve damage by retraction (usually) or surgical dissection (rarely) can cause temporary or permanent dysfunction. The great auricular nerve (C2, C3 dermatomes) should be protected in its location on the sternocleidomastoid muscle just anterior to and below the ear. Damage to this nerve can cause numbness of the posterior aspect of the auricle and a distressing postoperative occipital headache on the operated side. The spinal accessory nerve is at risk if the superior aspect of the dissection is inadvertently directed lateral to the internal jugular vein. Here, the nerve is vulnerable as it courses through the sternocleidomastoid muscle. Vigorous retraction on the superior aspect of this muscle may also result in nerve paresis.

The surgeon must also be constantly aware of the location of the vagus nerve and its branches. It lies within the carotid sheath between the common carotid artery and the internal jugular vein. Normally, it is directly behind the internal carotid artery at its origin. Care must be taken to prevent injury to the nerve at this vulnerable location. Additional care is required to prevent vagus nerve injury during re-do carotid exposure, as the nerve, encased in scar tissue, frequently courses anterior to the carotid bifurcation. The superior laryngeal nerve arises from the vagus nerve above the carotid bifurcation, passes behind the internal carotid artery, and descends medial to the superior thyroid artery. Mobilization of this vessel should be done at its origin so as not to injure the more medially located superior laryngeal nerve or its external branch. The external branch of the superior laryngeal nerve may sometimes pass between branches of the superior thyroid artery or be adherent to it.

The hypoglossal nerve is usually visualized during routine endarterectomy and is at particular risk for injury during high ICA exposure. The glossopharyngeal nerve is also vulnerable to injury if the dissection is carried near the skull base, and especially if styloidectomy is performed to help this exposure. Table 3 lists the location and tests for function of the important nerves encountered during carotid endarterectomy, with special remarks.

Table 3

Regional Nerves Encountered During Carotid Endarterectomy

Nerve Branch	Location Encountered	Test for Function	Remarks
Mandibular ramus of facial nerve (cranial nerve VII)	Deep to platysma muscle; can be 5–10 mm below inferior margin of mandible	Ask patient to show teeth; check for paralysis of lower lip	Gentle use of metal retractors on mandible; nerve is pulled down when head is rotated to opposite side for operative exposure
Great auricular nerve (C2-C3 dermatomes)	Anteromedial surface of sternocleidomastoid (SCM) muscle anterior and below ear	Anesthesia of ear and adjacent scalp	Causes disturbing occipital headache when damaged
Cutaneous cervical nerve (C2-C3 dermatomes)	Subcutaneous on deep fascia	Anesthesia of skin below mandible	Warn patient preoperatively regarding possible sensory loss
Glossopharyngeal nerve branch (cranial nerve IX)	Between external and internal carotid arteries (carotid sinus nerve)	None	Manipulation of nerve may cause bradycardia and/or hypotension; atropine IV or local infiltration of nerve with lidocaine will relieve circulatory changes
Vagus nerve (cranial nerve X)	Within carotid sheath; between internal jugular vein and common carotid artery; directly behind internal carotid artery	Indirect laryngoscopy for vocal cord function	Dissect "right on" distal common and internal carotid arteries and avoid "past pointing" with vascular occluding clamps
External branch of superior laryngeal nerve (branch of cranial nerve X)	Adjacent and medial to superior thyroid artery	Loss of function of cricothyroid muscle	Inability to produce high tones
Hypoglossal nerve (cranial nerve XII)	Main nerve trunk crosses the internal and external carotid arteries 1-2 cm above carotid bifurcation; sternocleidomastoid artery and vein branches sling around nerve	Extended tongue deviates to side of injured nerve	Visualize descending branch first and follow up to main nerve trunk; careful individual ligation of SCM muscular arterial and venous branches to preserve dry operative field

The value of cranial nerve protection during carotid surgery is emphasized by the classic reports of Evans and associates[88] and Hertzer and colleagues.[89] Evans and associates prospectively studied the incidence of cranial nerve injury during carotid surgery. Prior to and following carotid endarterectomy, surgeons as well as a speech pathologist made observations regarding cranial nerve function. There was a 4% incidence of preoperative vagus nerve dysfunction when a surgeon made the evaluation. However, a 30% incidence of preoperative vagus nerve dysfunction was noted when the evaluation was made by a speech pathologist. Two days postendarterectomy, surgeon evaluation demonstrated a 14.6% incidence of vagus nerve deficit, whereas the speech pathologist reported a 35% incidence of superior laryngeal or recurrent nerve dysfunction. These data emphasize the wisdom of a thorough vocal cord evaluation prior to reoperation, or when operating on the second side soon after the first, at which time paresis of cord function may still persist.

In 1999, Ballotta and colleagues[90] reviewed 200 consecutive carotid endarterectomies in Italy. There were 25 (12.5%) cranial nerve injuries in 24 patients. Cranial nerves injured included: hypoglossal (11), recurrent laryngeal (8), superior laryngeal (2), marginal mandibular (2) and the greater auricular (2). Fortunately the deficits were transient, with all but 4 injuries recovering by 6 months. The mean recovery time was 5.8 months with a range of 1 week to 37 months. Forssell and associates91 reviewed 656 consecutive carotid endarterectomy patients in Malmö, Sweden that were pre- and postoperatively examined at the Department of Phoniatrics concerning cranial nerve function. 75 (11.4%) carotid operations resulted in 1 or more cranial nerve injuries. These included 70 hypoglossal, 8 recurrent laryngeal, 2 glossopharyngeal and 2 superior laryngeal injuries. Only 2 (0.30%) nerve injuries were permanent. Frequency of injury increased with a junior surgeon (0.05%), shunt use (0.05%) and patch closure (0.01%).

In summary, cranial nerve injuries are usually caused by direct trauma such as stretch, retraction, clamping or transection. Nerve transection should be rare in experienced hands. Primarily re-approximating the epineurium with fine suture at the time of injury best repairs a transected cranial nerve. Most cranial nerve injuries are transient, with full recovery to be expected within 6 months on average.

Hematoma and Wound Infection

These two complications are not common, but either one can be life-threatening if not recognized and promptly treated. Large cervical hematomas require immediate drainage. In the early postoperative period, any patient complaining of difficulty swallowing or breathing mandates prompt clinical examination. The wound should be opened at the bedside and hematoma evacuated if the patient's breathing is already labored. Formal re-exploration can then proceed urgently. Any obvious bleeding point, which is not usually found, should be repaired or ligated. The wound is then copiously irrigated and reapproximated over a closed suction drain. Waiting to open the neck incision until the patient arrives in the operating room could prove to be disastrous, as obliteration of normal anatomic planes makes emergent intubation extremely difficult at best. In our practice, we do the following to minimize the incidence of postoperative cervical hematomas: anticoagulation effect of heparin is reversed with protamine sulfate and meticulous wound hemostasis is obtained by utilizing thrombin soaked Gelfoam® and silk ligatures. Finally, a small round closed suction drain is liberally used for 24 hours to evacuate the potential space.

Deep wound infections following CEA are extremely rare. However, should one occur, this requires immediate open drainage and wound debridement. Culture-specific intravenous antibiotics will be required for at least 4 to 6 weeks. If a prosthetic patch is in place, the patient is at high risk for patch blow-out, and one may need to consider vein graft replacement of the carotid artery. Superficial infections, which are usually localized stitch abscesses, can be treated expectantly with warm compresses and oral antibiotics. Prophylactic antibiotics are not technically mandatory before CEA. However, this author uses them routinely because prosthetic patch closure is always anticipated.

Stroke and Death

These complications are clearly the most feared. However, in experienced hands, the perioperative incidence of either event usually ranges from 1%-

3%.[1,2,92] In a recent review of our vascular registry, the combined stroke and death rate was 0.68% for 442 consecutive CEAs regardless of the indication.[55] In fact, there were no deaths in this published series. These morbidity and mortality data are well below those recommended by the Stroke Council guidelines and are similar to those reported by other specialized centers of excellence.[1,2,26,92] Unfortunately, pooled data from community surveys indicates that this is not the norm. Combined stroke and death rate in these reviews ranges from 7%-21%.[1,2,92] Data such as these should cause one to question the wisdom of having CEA in nonspecialized centers. This is particularly true for asymptomatic disease, as the operation is for stroke prophylaxis. Thus, it is critical for the patient (and family) to consider surgeon morbidity and mortality rates when deciding to have this procedure.

The usual etiology of post-CEA cerebrovascular events is embolization. Thus, it is unlikely that the clinical course can be ameliorated in most circumstances. However, events that occur due to technical defects such as a flap or dissection, or acute carotid artery thrombosis can be corrected with hope of recovery. Technical defects can only be detected if immediate post-reconstruction imaging is routinely performed after CEA. This adds little time to the procedure and ensures technical perfection. Duplex ultrasound is ideal for this because detailed gray-scale images can be combined with Doppler velocity criteria to fully evaluate the reconstructed carotid bifurcation and clamp sites. Arteriography may be used as well, although images are only obtained in a single plane and the procedure is not noninvasive. Continuous wave Doppler ultrasound is a nonspecific imaging modality that is not recommended for immediate post-reconstruction imaging. It does not facilitate visual detection of technical or other flow-limiting lesions.

Any significant technical defect should be corrected at the time of CEA. Distal defects will require re-clamping of the ICA. However, prograde ICA flow can be maintained during repair of a proximal defect by placing an atraumatic vascular clamp across the carotid bulb proximal to the ECA. Severe kinking or other high-grade stenotic lesion associated with primary closure is best treated by patch angioplasty. We have been impressed that the incidence of duplex ultrasound detected postreconstruction abnormalities is greatly reduced by routine Dacron patch closure of the carotid arteriotomy. However, the modality is quite sensitive. Thus, experience is required to appreciate which lesions need remedial care and which do not. This author re-operates on lesions with peak systolic flow velocities ≥145 cm/sec. In addition, flow-limiting flaps or clamp-induced dissections, particularly those that are not in the direction of prograde cerebral blood-flow, are repaired as these can rapidly lead to arterial thrombosis.

If a patient awakens with a neurologic deficit, it is imperative to rule out arterial thrombosis, as this is a problem that can be remedied. At this point it is wise to remember that it is distinctly unlikely that the carotid artery will have thrombosed in the short interim that just passed prior to extubation if immediate postreconstruction imaging was normal. Therefore, rather than re-open the neck, this author immediately scans the neck to be sure the ICA is open or there is at least end-diastolic flow in the common carotid artery, which indirectly indicates patency of the ICA. Immediate re-operation is planned if the ICA appears to be thrombosed. If a widely patent carotid reconstruction is re-confirmed then emergent head CT scanning is recommended to rule-out intracerebral hemorrhage. Thereafter, anticoagulation and/or antiplatelet therapy is recommended if the head CT does not demonstrate a bleed. This algorithm is pursued with the knowledge that almost all postoperative events are embolic in nature, and therefore not retrievable.

On the other hand, if immediate postreconstruction imaging was not performed, then the neck should be re-opened and the carotid bifurcation grossly inspected for signs of thrombosis. An obviously thrombosed artery requires thrombectomy. However, if the carotid appears to be patent, then on-table duplex ultrasound or arteriographic imaging should be performed to be sure that a technical defect or clamp induced dissection has not been overlooked. This maneuver is helpful because simply re-opening the carotid reconstruction is not an entirely benign procedure. The algorithm proceeds as described above if no defect can be demonstrated.

Hours later or the following day, if there is occurrence of a neurologic event, this author immediately scans the neck as described above. Immediate re-operation is planned if the ICA is occluded or if the patient has repetitive transient events or neurologic deterioration. However, if the ICA is found to be patent, then arteriography is indicated to visualize the aortic arch branches and intracranial cerebrovascular circulation in addition to the operative site. Significant defects or thrombus requires immediate re-operation. Anticoagulation and/or antiplatelet therapy is recommended for minimal defects or negative studies.

7. Surgical Results

As indicated previously, in experienced centers, results of CEA are superb. Combined stroke and death rate ranges from <1%-3%. Hospital stay is usually 1 day or less, and the procedure is well tolerated by all age groups.[25,55,93]

Pooled data demonstrate that CEA for asymptomatic lesions reduces the annual stroke risk from 6.4% to 1.0%.[92] However, since the annual death risk changes very little, the combined stroke and death risk is only reduced from 11.6% to 7.5%. CEA for patients with TIA reduces the annual stroke risk from 8.5% to 2.3%.[92] This is in contrast to the annual stroke risk of ~5.9% with best medical therapy alone. The combined annual stroke/death risk following CEA is reduced from 14.3% to 10.2% in the same group of patients.[92] This reduction in annual stroke and death risk is most dramatic for patients having uncomplicated CEA for completed stroke. In this group of patients, annual stroke risk is reduced from 14.4% to 4.5% after CEA and annual death risk is decreased from 14.6% to 8.3%.[92] Similarly, combined annual stroke/death risk is reduced from 29% to 12.8%.[92]

Results of Randomized Clinical Trials

3 important clinical trials have been completed and thoroughly scrutinized in the medical literature. 2 of these randomized symptomatic patients to surgery vs. best medical therapy, and the other randomized asymptomatic patients to similar treatment strategies. The following is a brief summary of each trial:

The North American Symptomatic Carotid Endarterectomy Trial (NASCET) randomized symptomatic patients with 70%-99% carotid stenosis to either CEA or medical therapy (aspirin).[39] The surgical arm consisted of 300 patients, and there were 295 in the medical treatment arm. The perioperative morbidity and stroke mortality rate was ~5.0%. However, at 18 months the study was halted because the incidence of fatal and nonfatal strokes was 7% in the CEA group compared to 24% in the medical group. This highly statistically significant ($P<0.001$) difference represented an absolute stroke risk reduction of 17% and a relative stroke risk reduction of 71% in favor of CEA. Similarly, mortality risk reduction statistically significantly favored the surgical group. At 18 months, the mortality rate was 12% for patients treated with best medical management compared to 5% for the CEA group. This significant ($P<0.01$) relative risk reduction in mortality was approximately 58% in favor of surgery.

The European Carotid Surgery Trial (ECST) was carried out over 10 years and generally echoes the NASCET findings.[40] In this clinical trial,[2,5,18] symptomatic patients with severe carotid stenosis (70%-99%) were randomized to either CEA or medical management. At a mean follow-up of 3 years, CEA reduced the risk of ipsilateral stroke by >80% compared to best medical management only. This 6-fold risk reduction in subsequent stroke was highly statistically significant ($P<0.0001$) despite what this author considers to be an unacceptably high perioperative combined stroke/death rate of 7.5%.

One important difference between the NASCET and the ECST was the method used to calculate arteriographic degree of carotid stenosis.[2,39,40] The NASCET method compares the diseased ICA diameter to the more normal distal ICA diameter where the walls are in parallel. However, in the ECST, the stenosis through the diseased ICA is compared to the projected diameter of the carotid bulb. Measuring the diameter of an imaginary outline of the nondiseased carotid bulb makes this estimate. Therefore, the European method overestimates the degree of residual stenosis compared to the NASCET. This means that a number of symptomatic patients in the ECST had significant benefit from CEA with moderate stenosis as measured by NASCET criteria.

The Asymptomatic Carotid Atherosclerosis Study (ACAS) randomized 1662 patients with a 60% asymptomatic stenosis to CEA (n=828) or to best medical management (n=834).[30,38,94] This study was conducted in 34 North American medical centers and the degree of stenosis was measured angiographically using NASCET criteria. When the results were published in the Journal of the American Medical Association, the perioperative stroke and death rate was quoted as 2.3%. However, close review of the manuscript demonstrates this rate to include the 1.2% incidence of stroke morbidity and mortality that occurred as a result of the preoperative angiography. The true surgical 30-day combined stroke/death rate was 1.52%. These excellent results after CEA conferred a stroke/death risk reduction of 69% for men and 16% for women. While these results do not seem to be so impressive for women, it is worth noting that the male-to-female ratio in this study was 2:1. Like the NASCET, this study was halted before completion because the results so overwhelmingly favored CEA.

8. Vertebral Artery Lesions

Although natural history data are lacking, it is clear that significant vertebral artery (VA) lesions are associated with embolization and/or hypoperfusion in the posterior cerebral circulation. Hypotension of the basilar artery territory due to flow-limiting stenosis is responsible for ~45% of vertebrobasilar ischemia, and emboli account for another 21%.[95] The remaining causes for arterial ischemia are mixed (21%), or unable to be classified (13%). Symptoms of vertebrobasilar insufficiency are multiple and varied. Pooled data demonstrate these to include dizziness (66% incidence), posterior headache (50%), blurred vision (47%), vertigo (38%), ataxia (31%), tinnitus (31%), dysarthria (31%), diplopia (28%), nausea (25%), syncope (22%), perioral numbness/tingling (16%) and hemispheric TIAs (9%).[95]

The VA is divided into 4 anatomic segments.[95] The first segment (V_1) extends from artery origin to its entry into the bony process of C-6 (can also enter at C-7, C-5 and even C-4). The intraosseous segment to the top of C-2 is known as segment V_2. Segment 3 (V_3) extends from the top of C-2 to the point at which the VA courses through the dura and the last segment (V_4) ends at the contralateral VA with formation of the basilar artery. Arteriography is the most useful diagnostic modality for imaging the vertebrobasilar system. Standard aortic arch views may demonstrate anatomic variants, such as an arch origin of the left vertebral artery proximal to the left subclavian artery, or right vertebral artery origin from the innominate or right common carotid artery.[96,97] However, additional oblique views are needed to completely demonstrate the vertebral artery origins, as these may be overshadowed by the proximal subclavian artery. Arteriographic abnormalities may range from severe origin stenosis or compression in segment V_2 by osteophytes to proximal occlusion with reconstitution of the more distal VA and basilar arteries via occipital artery collaterals.[96,97]

Surgical Indications

These are not nearly as straightforward as those are for carotid occlusive disease. In fact, when a severe VA lesion is ipsilateral to a significant carotid stenosis, the carotid lesion should be repaired first, as this will usually relieve vertebrobasilar symptoms. Clinical symptoms combined with anatomic findings will dictate the appropriate surgical procedure to be performed. Generally agreed to anatomic VA findings that warrant repair include >75% stenosis of the dominant VA, bilateral ICA occlusion with >50% VA stenosis, and any lesion suspected of causing clear-cut symptoms regardless of degree of stenosis.[95] Most VA reconstructions are performed to relieve symptoms associated with a severe stenosis in segment V_1 or for arterial impingement/occlusion in segment V_2.

Proximal reconstructive techniques range from proximal VA transposition to the common carotid artery, other subclavian artery site or stump of the thyrocervical trunk, to bypass from the subclavian artery or thyrocervical trunk to the VA.[96,97] The classic distal reconstruction is a bypass from the common carotid artery to the VA between the C1 and C2 transverse processes using autologous vein graft. Additionally, Dr. Ramon Berguer has championed alternative methods for distal VA reconstruction.[96,97] These include external carotid or occipital artery transposition to distal VA or distal VA transposition to the distal ICA. The interested reader is referred to these chapters in *Rutherford's Textbook of Vascular Surgery* (5th edition), or *Moore's Comprehensive Review of Vascular Surgery* (5th edition), for more details.[96,97]

Surgical Results

Long-term data demonstrate excellent stroke prevention and/or resolution of symptoms after VA reconstruction. Durability of the various reconstructive VA techniques is similar to other arterial reconstructions and these demonstrate superb long-term patency. Pooled data that combines both proximal and distal VA reconstructions demonstrate symptom cure in 85% of patients and symptom improvement in another 7% of patients.[95] Perioperative stroke incidence is remarkably low (<1%) as is the follow-up stroke rate (1.5%) at a mean of 1 year.[95] 10 year survival data indicate that a significant majority (71%) of patients are alive and well after VA reconstruction.[95]

Transient Horner's syndrome, which occurs with an incidence of 33%, is the most common perioperative morbidity associated with proximal VA reconstruction.[95-97] Other reported complications include lymph fistula (3.2%), transient dysphagia (1.9%), subclavian artery thrombosis (1.7%), phrenic nerve injury (1.1%), and, rarely, chylothorax (0.4%).[95] Operative mortality is low (0.5%), 10-year survival is excellent (83%) and the overwhelming majority (93%) of proximal VA reconstructions are still patent 10 years after surgery.[95-97] Sixty-two percent of patients are symptom free at 10 years and another 15% are at least improved. Some patients' (13%) symptoms remain unchanged, with the remaining few (10%) worse at 10 year follow-up.[95-97]

Overall operative mortality for distal VA reconstruction is 3.3%.[95] Graft thrombosis is the most common perioperative complication and rarely, there is injury of the spinal accessory nerve.[95-97] 10-year patient survival (83%) is similar to proximal VA reconstructions and secondary graft patency is approximately 85%.[95-97] Most patients (85%) can expect to be symptom free after distal VA reconstruction.[95-97]

9. Carotid Stenting for Atherosclerotic Lesions

The purpose of carotid artery treatment is to eliminate recurrent neurologic symptoms or to prevent stroke. Carotid endarterectomy has been the mainstay of treatment for the past 50 years. However, recent clinical trials have also confirmed the safety and efficacy of carotid artery stenting.[98-106] Currently, all stents are being used as an off-label device or as part of a clinical trial such as the Carotid Revascularization Endarterectomy vs. Stent Trial (CREST).[107] In general, high surgical risk symptomatic patients with >50% stenosis and asymptomatic high risk patients with >80% stenosis should be considered as candidates for this percutaneous intervention. Appropriate selection of treatment modality is then based on further review of patient risk factors, arterial anatomy and plaque morphology. In experienced hands, results of either carotid endarterectomy or stenting are superb, with a very low incidence of procedural related complications.[98-106]

While endovascular treatment of carotid lesions is still widely debated, the following indications are gaining widespread acceptance:

- Recurrent carotid stenosis
- Postradiation carotid stenosis
- Very distal internal or proximal common carotid artery lesions
- Carotid stenosis associated with technically challenging surgical anatomy such as a high bifurcation or an adjacent tracheostomy
- Prohibitive surgical risk, eg, severe cardiac or pulmonary disease

Catheter-based management of extracranial cerebrovascular disease has evolved since Palmaz® or Wall stents were first deployed across the carotid bifurcation in the early 1990s. This early experience was truly viewed as experimental, and these early devices were problematic with regard to stent deformity, recurrent in-stent stenosis and carotid dissection.[106] In addition, investigators have always been concerned about the potential catastrophic result of embolic debris during catheter manipulation and stent deployment. Fortunately, advances in stent technology (eg, Nitinol® stents and newer model Wall stents), as well as the use of cerebral protection devices, have improved outcomes.[98-106] Occlusive balloon or filter catheters are commonly used today for cerebral protection.[108] Others have championed protection systems that essentially prevent cerebral embolization by intermittent flow reversal within the internal carotid artery or continuous flow reversal by creation of a temporary arteriovenous shunt.[108] The bottom line with these advances is a safer procedure in the hands of experienced endovascular surgeons.

Needless to say, appropriate patient selection is paramount as some risk factors actually are associated with a higher risk of embolic complications.[106] These factors include:

- Age > 80 years
- Heavily diseased aortic arch or hostile arch anatomy
- Significant thrombus at the carotid bifurcation
- Subtotal carotid occlusion, ie, string sign
- Crescendo TIAs or very recent TIA
- Coexistent common carotid stenosis either proximally or at bifurcation
- Severely calcific carotid lesions
- Severe distal internal carotid artery tortuosity
- Previous major stroke or dementia

Diagnostic duplex ultrasound is usually followed by arteriography to assess the anatomy and degree of stenosis at the carotid bifurcation.[106] Arterial diameter is also measured and intracranial lesions or other vascular anomalies are noted, as these will influence the course of the procedure.[106] Carotid stenting is performed in an angiographic suite with the patient awake and mildly sedated. Ready access to intravenous drugs such as heparin, atropine and other pressor agents is mandatory, as it is not unusual for either significant bradycardia or hypotension to occur during the procedure.[106] Cannulation of the external carotid artery via a femoral artery puncture facilitates passage of a working catheter into the common carotid artery. A guide wire is then carefully passed across the lesion in the internal carotid artery. In the typical scenario, the stenosis is predilated with a low profile angioplasty balloon before a cerebral protection device is passed into the distal internal carotid artery.[98-106] This is followed by passage of a second catheter that contains the tightly compressed stent. Finally, the stent is deployed across the lesion and usually "touched up" with an appropriate diameter balloon. The stent and protection device can then be removed together and followed by completion arteriography. Post-procedure anticoagulation is not routine and most patients can be discharged the next day. Antiplatelet therapy, however, is recommended for at least 4 weeks post-procedure and is usually maintained lifelong.

Procedure related complications are usually a result of guidewire and catheter manipulation of the arterial system.[98-106] These complications include:

- Arterial bleeding, hematoma or pseudoaneurysm at the catheter puncture site
- Renal insufficiency or failure secondary to contrast dye
- Carotid dissection or pseudoaneurysm
- Intra-stent thrombus formation
- Recurrent post-stent stenosis of the carotid artery
- Neurologic events either during the procedure or in the early post-treatment period

Clearly, a major neurologic event is the most demoralizing of the aforementioned possible complications. Fortunately, this is usually an uncommon occurrence and clinical results of carotid stenting are at least comparable to contemporary surgical results.[98-106] However, given the track record and proven efficacy of carotid endarterectomy, this procedure remains the current standard of care in nearly all US medical centers.

10. References

1. Moore WS. Fundamental considerations in cerebrovascular disease. In: Rutherford RB, ed. *Vascular Surgery*. 5th ed. Philadelphia, PA: WB Saunders; 1999:1713.

2. Moore WS. Extracranial cerebrovascular disease: the carotid artery. In: Moore WS, ed. *Comprehensive Review of Vascular Surgery*. 5th ed. Philadelphia, PA: WB Saunders; 1998.555.

3. Matsumoto N, Whisnant JP, Kurland LT, et al. Natural history of stroke in Rochester, Minnesota, 1955 through 1969: an extension of a previous study, 1945 through 1954. *Stroke*. 1973;4:20.

4. Wallace DC. A study of the natural history of cerebral vascular disease. *Med J Aust*. 1967;1:90.

5. Mentzer RM, et al. Emergency carotid endarterectomy for fluctuating neurologic deficits. *Surgery*. 1981;89:60.

6. Hughes RL, Anderson CA, Sung GY. Diagnosis, evaluation, and medical management of patients with ischemic cerebrovascular disease. In: Rutherford RB, ed. *Vascular Surgery*. 5th ed. Philadelphia, PA: WB Saunders; 1999:1730.

7. Roederer GO, Langlois YE, Jager KA, et al. The natural history of carotid arterial disease in asymptomatic patients with carotid bruits. *Stroke*. 1984;15:605.

8. Madison FE, Moore WS. Ulcerated atheroma of the carotid artery: arteriographic appearance. *Am J Roentgenol*. 1969;107:530.

9. Moore WS, Hall AD. Ulcerated atheroma of the carotid artery: a cause of transient cerebral ischemia. *Am J Surg*. 1968;116:237.

10. Moore WS, Hall AD. Importance of emboli from carotid bifurcation in pathogenesis of cerebral ischemic attacks. *Arch Surg*. 1970;101:708.

11. Ballard JL, Bunt TJ, Fitzpatrick BC, Malone JM. Bilateral traumatic internal carotid artery dissections: case report. *J Vasc Surg*. 1992;15:431.

12. Toole JF, Baker WH, Castaldo JE. Endarterectomy for asymptomatic carotid artery stenosis. *JAMA*. 1995;273:1421.

13. Collier PE. Carotid endarterectomy: a safe cost-efficient approach. *J Vasc Surg*. 1992;16:926.

14. Wagner WH, Treiman RL, Cossman DV, Foran RF, Levin PM, Cohen JL. The diminishing role of diagnostic arteriography in carotid artery disease: duplex scanning as definitive preoperative study. *Ann Vasc Surg*. 1991;5:105.

15. Goodson SF, Flanigan DP, Bishara RA, Schuler JJ, Kikta MJ, Meyer JP. Can carotid duplex scanning supplant arteriography in patients with focal carotid territory symptoms? *J Vasc Surg*. 1987;5:551.

16. Kraiss LW, Kilberg L, Critch S, Johansen KH. Short-stay carotid endarterectomy is safe and cost-effective. *Am J Surg*. 1995;169:512.

17. Ranaboldo C, Davies J, Chant A. Duplex scanning alone before carotid endarterectomy: a 5-year experience. *Eur J Vasc Surg*. 1991;5:415.

18. Marshall WG, Kouchoukos NT, Murphy SF, Pelate C. Carotid endarterectomy based on duplex scanning without preoperative arteriography. *Circulation*. 1988 Sep;78 (3 Pt 2):I1-15.

19. Dawson DL, Zierler RE, Strandness DE, Clowes AW, Kohler TR. The role of duplex scanning and arteriography before carotid endarterectomy: a prospective study. *J Vasc Surg*. 1993;18:673.

20. Ranger WR, Glover JL, Bendick PJ. Carotid endarterectomy based on preoperative duplex ultrasound. *Am Surg*. 1995;61:548.

21. Moore WS, Ziomek S, Quinones-Baldrich WJ, Machleder HI, Busuttil RW, Baker JD. Can clinical evaluation and noninvasive testing substitute for arteriography in the evaluation of carotid artery disease? *Ann Surg*. 1988;208:91.

22. Ballard JL, Fleig K, De Lange M, Killeen JD. The diagnostic accuracy of duplex ultrasonography for evaluating the carotid bifurcation. *Am J Surg*. 1994;168:123.

23. Dawson DL, Zierler RE, Kohler TR. Role of arteriography in the preoperative evaluation of carotid artery disease. *Am J Surg*. 1991;161:619.

24. Farmilo RW, Scott DJA, Cole SEA, Jeans WD, Horrocks M. Role of duplex scanning in the selection of patients for carotid endarterectomy. *Br J Surg*. 1990;77:388.

25. Ballard JL, Deiparine MK, Bergan JJ, Bunt TJ, Killeen JD, Smith LL. Cost-effective evaluation and treatment for carotid disease. *Arch Surg*. 1997;132:268.

26. Moore WS, Barnett HJ, Beebe HG, et al. Guidelines for carotid endarterectomy. A multidisciplinary consensus statement from the ad hoc committee, American Heart Association. *Stroke*. 1995;26:188.

27. Moore WS. Role of vascular laboratory in the diagnosis and management of patients with cerebrovascular disease. In: Moore WS, ed. *Surgery for Cerebrovascular Disease*. 2nd ed. Philadelphia, PA: WB Saunders; 1996:177.

28. Akers DL, Markowitz IA, Kerstein MD. The value of aortic arch study in the evaluation of cerebrovascular insufficiency. *Am J Surg*. 1987;154:230.

29. Lord RSA. Relevance of siphon stenosis and intracranial aneurysm to results of carotid endarterectomy. In: Ernst CB, Stanley JC, eds. *Current Therapy of Vascular Surgery*. 2nd ed. Philadelphia, PA: BC Decker; 1991:94.

30. National Institute of Neurological Disorders and Stroke. Clinical advisory: carotid endarterectomy for patients with asymptomatic internal carotid stenosis. *Stroke*. 1994;25:2523.

31. Hankey GJ, Warlow CP, Molyneux AJ. Complications of cerebral angiography for patients with mild carotid territory ischaemia being considered for carotid endarterectomy. *J Neurol Neurosurg Psychiatry*. 1990;53:542.

32. Dawson DL. Carotid surgery without arteriography. In: Zierler RE, ed. *Surgical Management of Cerebrovascular Disease*. New York, NY: McGraw-Hill; 1995:313.

33. Mani RL, Eisenberg RL. Complications of catheter cerebral arteriography: analysis of 5000 procedures. II. Relation of complication rates to clinical and arteriographic diagnosis. *Am J Roentgenol*. 1978;131:867.

34. Hessel S, Adams D, Abrams H. Complications of angiography. *Radiology*. 1981;138:273.

35. Earnest F, Forbes G, Sandok B, et al. Complications of cerebral angiography: prospective assessment of risk. *AJR*. 1984;142:247.

36. Dion J, Gates P, Fox A, Barnett H, Blom R. Clinical events following neuroangiography: a prospective study. *Stroke*. 1987;18:997.

37. Eastcott HHG, Pickering GW, Robb C. Reconstruction of internal carotid artery in a patient with intermittent attacks of hemiplegia. *Lancet*. II 1954;267(6846):994-996.

38. Towne JB, Weiss DG, Hobson RW. First phase report of cooperative Veterans Administration asymptomatic carotid stenosis study–operative morbidity and mortality. *J Vasc Surg*. 1990;11(2):252.

39. NASCET Collaborators. Beneficial effect of carotid endarterectomy in symptomatic patients with high-grade carotid stenosis. *N Engl J Med*. 1991;325(7):445.

40. ECST Collaborative Group. MRC European Carotid Surgery Trial: interim results for symptomatic patients with severe (70-99%) or with mild (0-29%) carotid stenosis. *Lancet*. 1991;337:1235.

41. Imparato AM, Ramirez A, Riles T, Mintzer R. Cerebral protection in carotid surgery. *Arch Surg*. 1982;117:1073.

42. Hobson RW, Wright CB, Sublett JW, et al. Carotid artery back pressure and endarterectomy under regional anesthesia. *Arch Surg*. 1974;109:682.

43. Connolly JE, Kwann JHM, Stemmer EA. Improved results with carotid endarterectomy. *Ann Surg*.1977;186(3):334-342.

44. Connolly JE. Carotid endarterectomy in the awake patient. *Am J Surg*. 1985;150:159-165.

45. Whittemore AD. Carotid endarterectomy. An alternative approach. *Arch Surg*. 1980;115:940.

46. Riles TS, Kopelman I, Imparato AM. Myocardial infarction following carotid endarterectomy. a review of 683 operations. *Surgery*. 1979;85:249.

47. Imparato AM. Cerebral protection during anesthesia for carotid and vertebral surgery. In: Bernstein EF, Callow AD, Nicolaides AN, Shifrin EG, eds. *Cerebral Revascularization*. London, England: Med-Orion Publishing; 1993:283.

48. Waltz AG. Effect of blood pressure on blood flow in ischemic and non-ischemic cerebral cortex: The phenomena of autoregulation and luxury perfusion. *Neurology*. 1968;18:613.

49. Bloodwell RD, Hallman GL, Keats AS, Cooley DA. Carotid endarterectomy without a shunt: results using hypercarbic general anesthesia to prevent cerebral ischemia. *Arch Surg*. 1968;96:644.

50. Boysen G. Cerebral hemodynamics in carotid surgery. *Acta Neurol Scand* (Suppl). 1973;52:3-86.

51. Youmans JR, Kindt GW. Efficacy of carbon dioxide in the treatment of cerebral ischemia. *Surg Forum*. 1968;19:425.

52. Brawley BQ, Strandness ED, Kelly WA. The physiologic response to therapy in experimental cerebral ischemia. *Arch Neurol*. 1967;17:180.

53. Ferguson GG, Gamache FW. Cerebral protection during carotid endarterectomy: intraoperative monitoring, anesthetic techniques, and temporary shunts. In: Smith RR, ed. *Stroke and the Extracranial Vessels*. New York, NY: Raven Press; 1984:187.

54. Javid H, Ormand CH, Williams SD, et al. Seventeen-year experience with routine shunting in carotid artery surgery. *World J Surg*. 1979; 3:167.

55. Thompson JE, Talkington CM. Carotid endarterectomy. *Ann Surg*. 1976;184:1.

56. Hertzer NR, Beven EG, Greenstreet RL, Humphries AW. Internal carotid back pressure, intraoperative shunting, ulcerated atheroma, and the incidence of stroke during carotid endarterectomy. *Surgery*. 1978;83:306.

57. Browse NL, Ross-Russell R. Carotid endarterectomy and the Javid shunt: the early results of 215 consecutive operations for transient ischemic attacks. *Br J Surg*. 1984;71:53.

58. Hamann H: Carotid endarterectomy. prevention of stroke in asymptomatic (Stage 1) and symptomatic (Stage II) patients? *Thorac Cardiovasc Surgeon*. 1988;36:272.

59. Strawn DJ, Hunter GC, Guernsey JM, Kishore C. The relationship of intraluminal shunting to technical results after carotid endarterectomy. *J Cardiovasc Surg*. 1990;31:424.

60. Schiro J, Mertz GH, Cannon JA, Cintora I. Routine use of a shunt for carotid endarterectomy. *Am J Surg*. 1981;2006;20(4):482-487.

61. Baker WH, Littooy FN, Hayes AC, et al. Carotid endarterectomy without a shunt: the control series. *J Vasc Surg*. 1984;1:50.

62. Baker WH, Dorner DB, Barnes RW. Carotid endarterectomy: Is an indwelling shunt necessary? *Surgery*. 1977;82:321.

63. Ott DA, Cooley DA, Chapa L. Coelho A. Carotid endarterectomy without temporary intraluminal shunt: study of 309 consecutive operations. *Ann Surg*. 1980;191:708.

64. Whitney DG, Kahn EM, Estes JQ, Jones CE. Carotid artery surgery without a temporary indwelling shunt: 1917 consecutive procedures. *Arch Surg*. 1980;115:1393.

65. Reddy K, West M, Anderson B. Carotid endarterectomy without indwelling shunts and intraoperative electrophysiologic monitoring. *Can J Neurol Sci*. 1987;14:131.

66. Morowetz RB, Zeiger EH, McDowell HA Jr. Correlation of cerebral blood flow and EEG during carotid occlusion for endarterectomy (without shunting) and neurologic outcome. *Surgery*. 1984;96:184.

67. Moore WS, Yee JM, Hall AD. Collateral cerebral blood pressure: An index of tolerance to temporary carotid occlusion. *Arch Surg*. 1973;106:520.

68. Hays RJ, Levinson SA, Wylie EJ. Intraoperative measurement of carotid back pressure as a guide to operative management for carotid endarterectomy. *Surgery*. 1972;728:953.

69. Sundt TM Jr, Sharbrough FW, Piepgras DG, et al. Correlation of cerebral blood flow and electroencephalographic changes during carotid endarterectomy with results of surgery and hemodynamics of cerebral ischemia. *Mayo Clin Proc*. 1981;56:533.

70. Sundt TM Jr, Houser OW, Sharbrough FW. Carotid endarterectomy: Results, complications and monitoring techniques. *Adv Neurol*. 1977;16:97.

71. Phillips MR, Johnson WC, Scott M, Et al. Carotid endarterectomy in the presence of contralateral carotid occlusion: the role of EEG and intraluminal shunting. *Arch Surg*. 1979;114:1232.

72. Archie JP Jr. Technique and clinical results of carotid stump back-pressure to determine selective shunting during carotid endarterectomy. *J Vasc Surg*. 1991;13:319.

73. Baker JD, Gluecklich B, Watson CW, et al. An evaluation of electro-encephalographic monitoring during carotid surgery. *Surgery*. 1975;78:787.

74. String ST, Callahan A. The critical manipulable variables of hemispheric low flow during carotid surgery. *Surgery*. 1983;93:46.

75. Kwaan JH, Peterson GJ, Connolly JE. Stump pressure: an unreliable guide for shunting during carotid endarterectomy. *Arch Surg*. 1980;115:1083.

76. Steed DL, Peitzman AB, Grundy BL, Webster MW. Causes of stroke in carotid endarterectomy. *Surgery*. 1982;92:634.

77. Malone JM, Ballard JL. The placement of a carotid artery shunt: argument for its routine use. In: Moore WS, ed. *Surgery for Cerebrovascular Disease*. 2nd ed. Philadelphia, PA: WB Saunders; 1996:347.

78. Ballard JL. Anatomy and surgical exposure of the vascular system. In: Moore WS, ed. *Vascular Surgery: A Comprehensive Review*. 6th ed. Philadelphia, PA: WB Saunders; 2002:45.

79. Mock CN, Lilly MP, McRae RG, Carney WI Jr. Selection of the approach to the distal internal carotid artery from the second cervical vertebra to the base of the skull. *J Vasc Surg*. 1991;13:846.

80. Fisher D, Clagett G, Parker J, et al. Mandibular subluxation for high carotid exposure. *J Vasc Surg*. 1984;1:727.

81. Dossa C, Shepard AD, Wolford DG, Reddy DJ, Ernst CB. Distal internal carotid exposure: a simplified technique for temporary mandibular subluxation. *J Vasc Surg*. 1990;12:319.

82. Ballard JL, Guinn JE, Killeen JD, Smith DC. Operative balloon angioplasty of the carotid artery: a technique in evolution. *Ann Vasc Surg*. 1995;9:390.

83. Bove EL, Fry WJ, Gross WS, Stanley JC. Hypotension and hypertension as consequences of baroreceptor dysfunction following carotid endarterectomy. *Surgery*. 1979;88:633.

84. Piepgras DG, Morgan MK, Sundt TM Jr, Yanagihara T, Mussman LM. Intracerebral hemorrhage after carotid endarterectomy. *J Neurosurg*. 1988;68:532.

85. George SM Jr, Klamer TW, Lambert GE Jr. Cerebral hyperperfusion syndrome: an etiology of seizures following carotid endarterectomy. *J Ky Med Assoc*. 1993;91:451.

86. McCabe DJ, Brown MM, Clifton A. Fatal cerebral reperfusion hemorrhage after carotid stenting. *Stroke*. 1999;30:2483.

87. Reigel MM, Hollier LH, Sundt TM Jr, Piegras DG, Sharbrough FW, Cherry KJ. Cerebral hyperperfusion syndrome: a cause of neurologic dysfunction after carotid endarterectomy. *J Vasc Surg*. 1987;5:628.

88. Evans W, Mendelowitz D, Liapis C, et al. Motor speech deficit following carotid endarterectomy. *Ann Surg*. 1982;196:461.

89. Hertzer N, Feldman B, Beven E, et al. A prospective study of the incidence of injury to the cranial nerves during carotid endarterectomy. *Surg Gynecol Obstet*. 1980;151:781.

90. Ballotta E, Da Giau G, Renon L, et al. Cranial and cervical nerve injuries after carotid endarterectomy: a prospective study. *Surgery*. 1999;125:85-91.

91. Forssell C, Kitzing P, Bergqvist D. Cranial nerve injuries after carotid artery surgery: a prospective study of 663 operations. *Eur J Vasc Endovasc Surg*. 1995;10:445-449.

92. Taylor LM, Porter JM Jr. Carotid endarterectomy. In: *Basic Data Underlying Clinical Decision Making in Vascular Surgery*. St. Louis, MO: Quality Medical Publishing; 1994;182.

93. Wong DT, Ballard JL, Killeen JD. Carotid endarterectomy and abdominal aortic aneurysm repair: are these reasonable treatments for patients over age 80? *Am Surg*. 1998;64:998.

94. The asymptomatic carotid artery stenosis group: study design for randomized prospective trial of carotid endarterectomy for asymptomatic atherosclerosis. *Stroke*. 1989;25:523.

95. Kline RA, Berguer R. Vertebral artery Reconstruction. In: *Basic Data Underlying Clinical Decision Making in Vascular Surgery*. St. Louis, MO: Quality Medical Publishing; 1994:186.

96. Berguer R. Vertebrobasilar ischemia. Indications, techniques, and results of surgical repair. In: Rutherford RB, ed. *Vascular Surgery*. 5th ed. Philadelphia, PA: WB Saunders; 1999:1823.

97. Berguer R. Reconstruction of the supra-aortic trunks and vertebrobasilar system. In: Moore WS, ed. *Vascular Surgery: A Comprehensive Review*. 5th edition. Philadelphia, PA: WB Saunders Co; 1998:598.

98. Yadav JS, Wholey MH, Kuntz RE, et al. Stenting and angioplasty with protection in patients at high risk for endarterectomy investigators. Protected carotid-artery stenting versus endarterectomy in high-risk patients. *N Engl J Med*. 2004;351(15):1493-1501.

99. Roubin GS, New G, Iyer S, et al. Immediate and late clinical outcomes of carotid artery stenting in patients with symptomatic and asymptomatic carotid artery stenosis: a 5-year prospective analysis. *Circulation*. 2001;103:532-537.

100. Veith FJ, Amor M, Ohki T, et al. Current status of carotid bifurcation angioplasty and stenting based on a consensus of opinion leaders. *J Vasc Surg*. 2001;33:S111-S116.

101. Ahmadi R, Wilifort A, Lang W, et al. Carotid artery stenting: Effect of learning curve and intermediate-term morphological outcome. *J Endovasc Ther.* 2001;8:539-546.

102. Brooks WH, McClure RR, Jones MR, et al. Carotid angioplasty and stenting versus carotid endarterectomy: randomized trial in a community hospital. *J Am Coll Cardiol*. 2001;38: 1589-1595.

103. Endovascular versus surgical treatment in patients with carotid stenosis in the Carotid and Vertebral Artery Transluminal Angioplasty Study (CAVATAS): a randomised trial. *Lancet*. 2001;357:1729-1737.

104. Brown M. Meta-analysis of randomized controlled trials of carotid artery stenting vs. carotid endarterectomy [abstract]. 3rd International Course on Carotid Angioplasty and Other Cerebrovascular Interventions. Frankfurt, Germany; October 24-26, 2003.

105. Brooks WH, McClure RR, Jones MR, et al. Carotid angioplasty and stenting vs. endarterectomy for treatment of asymptomatic carotid stenosis: a randomized trial in a community hospital. *Neurosurgery*. 2004;54: 318-324.

106. Scissons RP, Kupinski AM. Carotid Stenting. *Vascular US Today*. 2005;10:19.

107. Hobson RW Jr, Brott T, Ferguson R, et al. CREST: carotid revascularization endarterectomy versus stent trial. *Cardiovasc Surg*. 1997;5:457.

108. Reimers B, Sievert H, Schuler GC, et al. Proximal endovascular flow blockage for cerebral protection during carotid artery stenting: results from a prospective multicenter registry. *J Endovasc Surg*. 2005;12:156.

11. Questions

1. Of the following nerves, which ***one*** is most likely to be injured during carotidendarterectomy?

   A. Recurrent laryngeal nerve

   B. Vagus nerve (X)

   C. Hypoglossal nerve (XII)

   D. Superior laryngeal nerve

   E. Glossopharyngeal nerve (IX)

2. All of the following are true regarding carotid artery exposure ***except*** which one of the following?

   A. The hypoglossal nerve (XII) crosses anterior to the distal internal carotid artery.

   B. The vagus nerve (X) passes posterolateral to the carotid bifurcation.

   C. Distal carotid exposure is safely facilitated by anterior dislocation of the mandible.

   D. Distal exposure may be facilitated by division of the posterior belly of the digastric muscle and the stylohyoid muscle.

   E. Anteriorly, the distal internal carotid artery is covered by the parotid gland, ramus of the mandible, and the styloid process.

3. Middle cerebral artery infarction in the ***dominant*** cerebral hemisphere may result in which of the following deficits?

   A. Broca's aphasia

   B. Wernicke's aphasia

   C. Dysarthria

   D. Right-sided upper and/or lower extremity weakness

   E. Contralateral homonymous hemianopsia

4. Which of the following are ***acceptable*** indications for carotid endarterectomy?

   A. Severe (>70%) right ICA stenosis with ipsilateral 50% siphon stenosis in a 60-year-old male with an episode of right amaurosis fugax 2 weeks previously

   B. Moderate (>50%) ICA stenosis in a 70-year-old female with a mild residual deficit after ipsilateral cerebrovascular accident (CVA)

   C. Mild (15%-49%) internal carotid artery stenosis in a 65-year-old male with CVA referable to the side with mild stenosis, who is not on antiplatelet therapy

   D. A patient with repeated TIAs in the same anatomic distribution over the past 10 days with an ipsilateral carotid stenosis greater than 70%

   E. Stroke-in-evolution in a nonambulatory 88-year-old male with severe ipsilateral carotid stenosis and brain metastases from prostate carcinoma

5. Which of the following statements are ***true*** regarding duplex ultrasound examination of the extracranial cerebrovascular system?

   A. Carotid arteriography is the gold standard for evaluation of the extracranial cerebrovascular system.

   B. Every duplex ultrasound-diagnosed internal carotid artery occlusion must be confirmed with carotid arteriography.

   C. Duplex ultrasound is an invasive modality that is associated with significant patient morbidity.

   D. Numerous investigators have demonstrated duplex ultrasound to be a highly accurate imaging modality for the cervical carotid system.

   E. Duplex ultrasound can detect a carotid bifurcation stenosis of more than 60% as well as it can detect a severe carotid siphon stenosis.

6. Which one of the following indications for vertebral artery (VA) reconstruction is ***incorrect?***

A. Greater than 75% stenosis of the dominant VA with appropriate symptoms

B. Bilateral ICA occlusion with greater than 50% VA stenosis

C. A mild to moderately stenotic VA lesion suspected of causing clear-cut vertebrobasilar symptoms

D. A symptomatic patient with severe distal vertebral artery stenosis and ipsilateral severe proximal internal carotid artery stenosis

E. Severe (>70%) VA stenosis in a 60-year-old male with dense cerebellar infarct

7. The following statements are true regarding the arteriographic evaluation of the vertebral arteries ***except:***

A. Origin stenosis is the most common atherosclerotic lesion seen within segment V_1.

B. Extrinsic compression is the most likely mechanism for arterial stenosis or occlusion in segment V_2.

C. The arteriographic diagnosis of a widely-patent VA contralateral to one that is the etiology of emboli obviates the need to repair the diseased side.

D. The origin of the left VA may arise from the aorta proximal to the left subclavian artery.

E. Complete carotid artery arteriographic images are necessary to help plan the appropriate VA reconstruction.

8. Which of the following statements regarding appropriate treatment of pathologic entities affecting the extracranial carotid system is ***true***?

A. Fibromuscular dysplasia (FMD) lesions of the carotid are best treated by endarterectomy.

B. Carotid artery aneurysms are benign and therefore can be followed expectantly.

C. Urgent endarterectomy is indicated for acute carotid dissection to arrest thrombus propagation and to tack down the dissected portions of the intima and media.

D. Severe symptomatic carotid restenosis 14 months after CEA is best treated by repeat endarterectomy.

E. Prednisone is the best initial treatment for severe common carotid artery stenosis associated with Takayasu's arteritis.

9. Regarding the natural history of carotid bifurcation lesions, which one of the following statements is ***false***?

A. The highest rate of recurrent stroke is within 12 months of the initial event.

B. TIAs are benign and the ultimate stroke risk is negligible.

C. At the end of 5 years, the rate of stroke in untreated patients with carotid-based TIA is 30%-35%.

D. Almost one-quarter of untreated patients with severe asymptomatic carotid stenosis will demonstrate symptoms within 1 year of diagnosis.

E. Stroke-in-evolution has such a dismal prognosis that surgical intervention should be withheld.

10. Which one of the following statements regarding perioperative stroke is ***false***?

A. Most perioperative events after CEA are embolic in nature.

B. If intraoperative postreconstruction imaging was performed in a patient who awakens with stroke, the patient should be ***rescanned*** immediately to rule out carotid artery thrombosis.

C. If intraoperative postreconstruction imaging was not performed in a patient who awakens with stroke, the patient should be ***reexplored*** to rule out carotid artery thrombosis.

D. If a patient has a stroke hours after surgery, then nothing can be done.

E. A patient with bilateral severe ICA stenosis is at risk for postoperative cerebral hyperperfusion syndrome.

Answers

1. C.

The vagus and hypoglossal nerves have the highest reported incidence of injury during carotid endarterectomy. However, recent reports, including 2 from Italy and Sweden, demonstrate that the incidence of hypoglossal nerve injury exceeds that of vagus nerve injury.[90,91] Any cranial nerve injury is debilitating and care must be taken to avoid injury, particularly during re-do carotid exposure, or when operating on the contralateral carotid artery shortly after the first side has been operated on.

2. C.

Structures that overlie the high internal carotid artery in the neck include the facial nerve, parotid gland, ramus of the mandible, and mastoid and styloid processes. The hypoglossal nerve, glossopharyngeal nerve, digastric and stylohyoid muscles, and occipital and posterior auricular arteries cross it. Anterior subluxation of the mandible or transection of the mandibular ramus improves high internal carotid artery exposure to the superior border of the first cervical vertebra. It is important to avoid dislocation of the mandible since serious injury can occur to the temporomandibular joint and even to the contralateral internal carotid artery.

3. A., B., D.

The left cerebral hemisphere is usually dominant. Therefore, cortical events that occur in the middle cerebral artery (MCA) distribution will produce contralateral (right-sided) extremity motor and sensory dysfunction. Broca's aphasia is a result of ischemia in the distribution of the superior MCA branch in the dominant hemisphere.[6] Ischemia of the inferior MCA branch in the dominant hemisphere produces a different type of aphasia, called fluent or Wernicke's, that is characterized by poor comprehension as well as nonsensical speech.[6] Dysarthria, which is a motor disturbance of articulation, is a nondominant hemisphere symptom that is often confused with aphasia.[6] Infarction in the posterior cerebral artery distribution results in contralateral homonymous hemianopsia.[6]

4. A., B., D.

Proven indications for CEA include one or more TIAs in last 6 months with an ipsilateral carotid stenosis >70% or mild stroke with carotid stenosis >70%.[26] Acceptable indications include TIAs in past 6 months and a moderate stenosis (50%-69%), stroke-in-evolution and a stenosis >70% in good risk patient and mild or moderate stroke in past 6 months with an ipsilateral moderate (50%-69%) stenosis.[26] Tandem intracranial lesions should not deter the surgeon from recommending bifurcation endarterectomy for otherwise appropriate indications.[2] It is unlikely that a patient with a symptomatic mild stenosis will receive benefit from CEA and in this setting antiplatelet therapy is best treatment. This is true even if the contralateral carotid artery is occluded. Finally, in a poor surgical risk patient, the benefit of CEA is extremely low, particularly for the clinical syndrome of stroke-in-evolution.

5. D.

The paradigm has changed for the diagnostic evaluation of the cervical carotid system. It is now recognized that arteriography can be virtually eliminated from the preoperative work-up of patients with cerebrovascular symptoms.[25] Many investigators consider duplex ultrasound (DU), and not arteriography, to be the gold standard carotid imaging study and there are compelling reasons for not necessarily obtaining an arteriogram prior to every endarterectomy. DU accurately and noninvasively detects lesions at the carotid bifurcation. This diagnostic test exposes the patient to negligible risk. Numerous investigators have demonstrated that duplex derived information about the carotid bifurcation is as accurate as a comparable arteriogram.[25] However, there are some circumstances in which carotid arteriography is useful. This is true if there is inadequate DU imaging of the carotid bifurcation and of particular importance when symptoms are referable to an unsatisfactorily imaged carotid bifurcation. A suggestion of more proximal or distal disease that is beyond the imaging capabilities of DU also warrants the use of arteriography. With experience, even routine arteriography to confirm duplex diagnosed ICA occlusion or to image recurrent stenotic carotid lesions is unnecessary.

6. D. and E.

Clinical symptoms combined with anatomic findings will dictate appropriate surgical management of vertebral artery lesions. Generally agreed to anatomic VA findings that warrant repair include >75% stenosis of the dominant VA, bilateral ICA occlusion with >50% VA stenosis, and any lesion suspected of causing clear-cut symptoms regardless of degree of stenosis.[95-97] When a severe VA lesion is ipsilateral to a significant carotid stenosis, the carotid lesion should be repaired first, as this will usually relieve vertebrobasilar symptoms. Recovery from a dense stroke is unlikely. Therefore, VA reconstruction in this setting is not indicated, as it will not significantly change the outcome.

7. C.

All answers except C. are correct. Standard aortic arch views may demonstrate congenital anatomic variants such as an arch origin of the left vertebral artery proximal to the left subclavian artery, or right vertebral artery origin from the innominate, or right common carotid artery.[95-97] Severe stenosis within segment V1 is usually due to atherosclerosis of its origin and stenosis and/or occlusion within segment V2 is often due to osteophytic compression.[95-97] A VA lesion suspected of causing clear-cut symptoms should be repaired even if the contralateral VA is widely patent. VA reconstructions may involve the carotid system with bypass and/or transposition.[95-97] Therefore, carotid arteriography is a key component of the preoperative work-up.

8. E.

Answer E. is correct, the rest are false. FMD lesions are best treated by open balloon angioplasty although other mechanical and balloon techniques have been used and are well described.[82] Carotid aneurysms are not benign and they may cause a myriad of symptoms. Mechanisms responsible for neurologic dysfunction include thrombosis (rare), rupture (rare), embolization (frequent) or compression of adjacent structures such as cranial nerves.[1,2] Carotid dissections rarely require operative reconstruction, as spontaneous resolution of the process on anticoagulant medication is the rule.[11] Early intervention can worsen the situation and inability to establish prograde cerebral blood flow may require acute carotid artery ligation. Neointimal hyperplasia is responsible for early carotid restenosis.[1,2] This lesion is generally not amenable to standard endarterectomy techniques. Reconstruction is best effected by patch angioplasty. Arterial lesions associated with arteritis are best treated initially with steroids. Persistent symptoms that are associated with significant lesions are usually reconstructed/bypassed as endarterectomy is generally precluded.

9. B.

Answer B. is incorrect. Pooled data from several studies demonstrate the recurrent stroke rate per year to be approximately 9% and this rate is highest in the first 12 months following the initial event.[1,2] Although generally considered benign, episodes of transient cerebral ischemia may herald subsequent stroke or other neurologic disability. Carotid-based TIAs clearly indicate instability of the plaque lesion. Similar to recurrent cerebral infarction, stroke risk is highest in the first year after diagnosis. Pooled data demonstrate this risk to be 11% to 16%.[1,2] In subsequent years, the risk tapers to 5% to 9% so that at the end of 5 years 30%-35% of untreated patients with TIA will have had a stroke.[1,2] A study of critical asymptomatic lesions demonstrated a combined TIA and stroke rate of 22% within 1 year of diagnosis.[1,2] Mentzer and colleagues showed that conservative management resulted in complete recovery or mild residual deficit in only 23% of 263 pooled cases of stroke-in-evolution.[5] On the other hand, emergent endarterectomy in their small series of 17 patients resulted in complete recovery in 12 (70%).[5]

10. D.

Answer D. is incorrect. Almost all postoperative events following CEA are embolic in nature and therefore, not retrievable. However, if a patient awakens with a neurologic deficit it is imperative to rule-out arterial thrombosis, as this is a problem that can be remedied. At this point, it is wise to remember that it is distinctly unlikely that the carotid artery will have thrombosed in the short interim that just passed prior to extubation if immediate postreconstruction imaging was normal. Therefore, rather than re-open the neck, this author immediately scans the neck to be sure the ICA is open or there is at least end-diastolic flow in the common carotid artery, which indirectly indicates patency of the ICA. Immediate re-operation is planned if the ICA appears to be thrombosed or if intraoperative imaging was not performed. Hours later or the following day, if there is occurrence of a neurologic event, this demands urgent care. This author immediately scans the neck as described above. Immediate re-operation is planned if the ICA is occluded or if the patient has repetitive transient events or neurologic deterioration. However, if the ICA is found to be patent, then arteriography is indicated to visualize the aortic arch branches and intracranial cerebrovascular circulation in addition to the operative site. Cerebral hyperperfusion syndrome is a well-described complication that appears to be caused by post-CEA loss of autoregulation within the brain[84-87] The most distressing aspect of this problem is that it typically occurs days (even 5 to 7 days later in a few reports) after an uneventful CEA. A consistent preoperative finding that has been described in nearly all reported cases is a patient history of severe long-standing cerebral ischemia due to a very high-grade carotid stenosis. This has also been reported to occur in the interim between staged CEAs in patients with severe bilateral lesions.

Chapter 18: Peripheral Vascular Occlusive Disease

Paul M. Anain, MD
David J. Caparrelli, MD
Julie Ann Freischlag, MD

Contents

1. Introduction

Atherosclerotic vascular disease, which involves the infrarenal abdominal aorta, iliac arteries, and lower extremity vessels, is the most common cause of the symptoms of arterial insufficiency or peripheral vascular disease. The management of patients with peripheral vascular occlusive disease should be evaluated and judged on the natural history and epidemiology of the disease.[1] Careful study of the risk factors present in patients with peripheral vascular disease has practical importance in the management of individual patients, allowing for global interventions, including lifestyle modification and medical or surgical interventions. Over the last two decades endovascular treatment, ie, percutaneous transluminal angioplasty and stenting, has replaced open bypass operation as the major intervention for occlusive arterial disease.[31] Bypass operations are now used for patients who have complex obstruction, eg, long segment or below knee femoropopliteal artery disease, or extensive bilateral iliac and common femoral occlusion.

2. Pathogenesis

Arteriosclerosis is regarded as a major factor in the development of peripheral vascular disease. A basic definition of atherosclerosis is "a disease of the arteries in which fatty plaques develop on their inner walls, with eventual obstruction of blood flow."[2] This basic definition does not encompass the entire spectrum of atherosclerotic lesions. Advanced plaques may invade the media, and atheromas at certain stages may produce enlargement of arteries.

The risk factors for atherogenesis and peripheral vascular disease are varied and include both behaviors and genetic predisposition. The main behaviors that can lead to the development of atheromas are the consumption of large amounts of animal fat and cigarette smoking. The effects of factors such as sedentary lifestyle, alcohol consumption and high stress are less clear. Genetic predispositions include male sex, age over 65, diabetes, hypertension, hyperlipidemia and homocystinemia.

3. Fatty Streaks

Fatty streaks are minimally raised, yellow lesions frequently found in the aortas of infants and children. These early lesions have lipid deposition intracellularly in macrophages and in smooth muscle cells.[3] Reports have described the progression of the initial fatty streaks and intermediate lesions thus: Type I lesions in children are the earliest microscopic lesions, consisting of an increase in intimal macrophages with the appearance of foam cells. Type II lesions are grossly visible, and by staining with Sudan III. Foam cells and heterogeneous droplets of extracellular lipids can be seen. Type III lesions are considered intermediate lesions, a bridge between the fatty streaks and the typical atheromatous fibrous plaque, the type IV plaque. The type III plaques are found in areas of the arterial tree prone to atherosclerotic lesions. These susceptible sites are typically exposed to low shear stress, causing increased influx of low-density lipoprotein (LDL).[3,4,5] LDL accumulation may occur, due to:

- alterations in the permeability of the intima;
- increases in the interstitial space in the intima;
- poor metabolism of LDL by vascular cells;
- impeded transport of LDL from intima to media, and;
- increased plasma /LDL concentrations or specific binding of LDL to connective tissue components.[6]

Another event that occurs in the process of atherogenesis is the binding of monocytes to the endothelial lining, with subsequent migration to the subintimal layer to become macrophages.

The complete sequence of events that lead to atherogenesis in peripheral vascular occlusive disease continues to be explored, and it is hoped will lead to the discovery of means to stop the process.[7]

4. Diagnosis

History and Physical Examination

The diagnosis of peripheral vascular occlusive disease and its anatomical location can usually be determined by the history and physical examination. The history should be broad in scope, yet should maintain a focus on the disease process in question and be guided by questions that help make the diagnosis. A brief overall history should start with details of the present illness and include patient age and symptoms, including onset, duration, location, character, and aggravating and alleviating factors. The clinician should determine if pain occurs when walking, how far the patient can walk prior to pain, where pain is most severe (buttock or calves), any pain at rest and history of impotence. Table 1 lists the presenting symptoms of patients with peripheral vascular occlusive disease and categorizes them as either "functional" or "critical" ischemia. Risk factors should also be pursued, including tobacco use (and type: cigarettes, cigars, pipe, chewing or snuff), how many packs per day for how many years, and if and when the patient quit smoking. A past medical history should include risk factors for peripheral vascular disease, including diabetes (is patient on insulin to control it, and if so, how much and for how long), hypertension, hypercholesterolemia (and any medication patient is taking to control it), and personal and family history of peripheral vascular disease. Risk factors that put a patient at high surgical risk should also be elucidated, including the presence of coronary artery disease and pulmonary disease.[8]

The physical examination should confirm that the patient's complaints are due to blockages in the vascular system. A full vascular examination should be performed at the time of initial examination; however, a detailed examination of the extremities should be performed according to the patient's symptoms. Inspection of the lower extremities will often reveal severe muscle atrophy. The skin may be pale, thin, and shiny with hair loss on the toes. Pallor with elevation and rubor with dependency indicates severe ischemia, and persistent rubor is a sign of critical ischemia. Inspection of the toes and feet should be performed to seek tissue necrosis such as open ulcers. Inspection of spaces between the toes should also be performed to reveal hidden ulcers. Frank gangrene is evident when present, and can be dry or wet, meaning that the area of tissue necrosis is infected. Ischemic ulcers are extremely painful and occur distally on the toes, on pressure points such as the lateral or medial malleolus, or in areas of minor trauma. The skin surrounding these ulcers is shiny and atrophic. The ulcer usually has irregular edges and a pale base with little bleeding. Pulses are always absent and there will be associated elevation pallor and dependency rubor. Dangling the foot over the side of the bed may relieve the pain. This should be distinguished from the trophic ulcer in diabetic patients, which is a painless ulcer occurring at pressure points, often the sole of the foot at the metatarsal heads, and there is an obvious associated neuropathy with decreased sensation. The trophic ulcer appears as a punched-out lesion which bleeds easily.

Examination of the pulses must also be performed on each patient. Palpation of the common femoral, popliteal, posterior tibial, and dorsalis pedis arteries should be performed on each leg and compared. This can give insight to the level of disease. Pulses can be graded as either present or absent or on a 4-point scale, with zero representing no pulse, 1+ as barely palpable, 2+ as slightly diminished, 3+ as normal, and 4+ meaning an accentuated pulse. An accentuated popliteal pulse is often the sign of an aneurysm.

Doppler Examination

An integral part of the initial examination should include the use of Doppler ultrasound (US). The simplest test is to use the Doppler to detect flow or locate a vessel when it cannot be palpated and measure the first blood pressure detected when a cuff, usually on the thigh or calf, is deflated. A more detailed noninvasive exam can also be performed with the Doppler. Using graduated blood pressure cuffs, pressure measurements can be obtained at the high thigh, low thigh, calf, ankle and mid foot. The cuff is inflated at each level to the point of vessel occlusion and the Doppler sounds disappear. The cuff is then deflated until the Doppler sounds are first heard to determine the pressure in that segment. More elaborate probes used for this examination are able to configure waveform analysis from the pulse volume recording. The normal peripheral arterial flow pulse is characterized by a rapid acceleration in

Table 1

Symptoms of Peripheral Vascular Occlusive Disease

Functional Ischemia	**Critical Ischemia**
Claudication	Rest pain
Occurs in functional muscle unit	Pain in foot and toes
Thigh, hip or buttock- aortoiliac disease	Persistent; worse at night
Calf-aortoiliac and/or infrainguinal disease	Multilevel, including infrapopliteal disease
Reproducible with exercise	Paresthesias
Relieved with cessation of exercise	Muscle paresis
Impotence (Leriche syndrome)	Ulceration and/or gangrene

early systole that culminates in a sharp peak velocity, followed by a rapid deceleration phase during which velocities fall to zero, a short period of flow reversal in early diastole, and a low-level forward flow phase extending throughout the remainder of diastole. These fluctuations in velocity produce a characteristic triphasic audible Doppler sound. Beyond the obstruction, the flow pulse becomes more rounded, the acceleration phase less rapid, the peak is less well defined, and the reversed flow component disappears, while velocities remain well above baseline levels. The relationship between the ankle (highest of DP or PT) to the arm pressure is the basis of the ankle arm index (AAI).

In the normal vascular system the ankle pressure exceeds the arm pressure by 10-20 mm Hg. A normal AAI ratio is 1.1 or greater. Claudicators will typically have AAIs of 0.8 or less, and the AAI will drop further with exercise. Having the patient do toe raises or walk on the treadmill until symptoms start and then rechecking the AAI can demonstrate this. Ischemic rest pain typically does not occur until the AAI is 0.4 or less, and tissue loss does not occur until the AAI is 0.3 or below. When absolute pressure is less than 35 mm Hg, the prognosis for limb salvage is poor. In patients with diabetes, the vessels of the lower extremity are often calcified, and the vessels will not be compressed by the blood pressure cuff, and therefore will show falsely elevated AAIs.[8]

Diagnostic Angiography

Contrast angiography is performed in order to visualize the arterial anatomy of the lower extremities. The standard femoral angiogram consists of filling the distal aorta and vessels of the legs down to the ankles with contrast media. A routine study also typically includes visualization of the infrarenal aorta and aortic bifurcation. Digital subtraction angiography (DSA) techniques are particularly helpful for visualization of the arteries in the lower calf and foot, and afford improved visualization of delayed, poorly-filled vessels distal to sites of obstruction. It is important that the bifurcation of the superficial and profunda femoral arteries be well visualized. Oblique views may be required to find a significant stenosis in this area. A reduction of a vessel's cross sectional diameter of 75% or more is indicative of a hemodynamically significant lesion.[9] If the significance of a lesion is in doubt, a pressure gradient should be performed across the lesion before and after the administration of papavarine. Gradients that are not hemodynamically significant at rest may become significant after the administration of the vasodilator. A gradient equal to or greater than 15 mm Hg at rest following administration of the vasodilator is regarded as indicative of a significant lesion.[10,11]

Computed tomographic angiography is obtained with an intravenous injection of constrast and may be done preoperatively to localize the extent of the lesion, reserving direct arteriogram for the intervention.

Atherosclerotic disease produces plaques with varying degrees of aortic narrowing, occlusion and aneurysms to the aorta. Arteriograms will show localized or diffuse changes and eccentric or concentric narrowing. With severe stenosis, a rich collateral bed will be present. When a complete occlusion is present, the arteriogram will reveal the level of occlusion and what vessel reconstitutes. In patients with severe disease, delayed films should be obtained in order to locate a suitable patent vessel for a surgical bypass.

Contrast angiography should only be performed on the patient with significant enough disease to warrant intervention. Angiography alone carries a complication rate of less than 5%. Arterial puncture site complications include hematoma, dissections, pseudoaneurysm, arteriovenous fistulas and thrombosis. The frequency of these complications depends on the amount of calcification in the vessel, anticoagulation, the size of the catheter used and attention paid to postprocedure hemostasis. Catheterization complications include arterial dissection, perforation and embolism. The risk of these complications depends on the experience of the angiographer, anatomic variation of the vessels, the vessel catheterized and the intrinsic nature of the vessel. The complications related to contrast media include renal failure, fluid overload, congestive heart failure, transverse myelitis and anaphylactoid reactions. These complications can be minimized by adequate hydration of the patient, careful catheter placement, and appropriate use of a steroid preparation or nonionic contrast for those with known allergy.[12]

5. Aortoiliac Occlusive Disease

While not as common as femoropopliteal disease, aortoiliac disease is common in the middle-aged and elderly. Aortoiliac disease may be severely disabling because of the large number of muscle groups that are affected. The symptoms of aortoiliac disease may involve muscles of the thigh, hip, and buttocks as well as the calf. Some patients with aortoiliac disease only have symptoms of calf claudication, making it difficult to differentiate from femoropopliteal disease. In addition to claudication, males with aortoiliac disease may have difficulty achieving or maintaining an erection because of decreased perfusion of the hypogastric arteries, which causes decreased perfusion to the internal pudendal arteries. The complex of aortoiliac disease is called Leriche syndrome, and consists of thigh or buttock claudication, atrophy of the leg muscles, impotence and decrease in the femoral pulses.[13] Aortoiliac disease is rarely the cause of rest pain or tissue loss. The collateral circulation carried around the obstruction by the gluteal muscles is usually sufficient to adequately perfuse the lower extremities at rest. Disease in these segments may, however, cause ischemia and tissue loss through distal embolization of cardiac or iliac atherosclerotic plaques.[14,15]

The symptoms, progression, and optimal management depend on the extent and distribution of disease. Type I aortoiliac disease is confined to the distal aorta and iliac arteries. Type II manifests more widespread aortic and external iliac artery disease. Patients with type III disease exhibit multilevel symptoms including infrainguinal disease.

Patients with type I disease, approximately 10% of patients with aortoiliac disease, usually have upper leg claudication with absence of more severe ischemic disease. These patients are usually younger, with a low incidence of hypertension or diabetes. Over half these patients are female and have small aortas and iliac vessels. Commonly there is thrombosis of one or both iliac vessels with the potential of thrombosis of the infrarenal aorta. Most patients requiring surgery for aortoiliac disease have diffuse disease. 20%-25% have a type II pattern, with occlusive disease mostly in the abdominal aorta, but also extending into the external iliacs and even into the femorals. About two-thirds of these patients have multilevel disease, including infrainguinal and infrapopliteal disease.

These patients have the more typical disease patterns of diabetes and hypertension associated with coronary artery disease. They also have a more significant pattern of distal ischemia with the possibility of tissue necrosis.[17]

Indications for Intervention

Patients with severe thigh, buttock, and calf claudication should be evaluated for intervention to treat diseased aortoiliac segments. Patients who are having rest pain or have evidence of ischemic ulcerations or tissue loss should be evaluated angiographically for potential intervention.

Procedures

The majority of iliac occlusions are treated successfully by percutaneous transluminal angioplasty usually with stent placement. Open bypass operations are performed for bilateral, diffuse occlusive lesions. The aortobifemoral bypass, although performed much less frequently today, is still an important vascular operation.

For the low-risk patient, a direct aortofemoral bypass is the most durable repair, using synthetic grafts most commonly made of Dacron®. The overall 5-year patency for these grafts approaches 80%, and the 10-year rate is close to 75%. The early mortality for this procedure is less than 3%. The proximal anastomosis can be constructed in either an end-to-end or end-to-side fashion (Figure 1). Both have the same excellent patency rate. The main advantage of the end-to-end anastomosis is that it does not allow reestablishment of blood flow through the diseased distal aorta, thus eliminating the potential for thrombus or atheromas to embolize. The end-to-side anastomosis has the theoretical advantage of keeping the hypogastric vessels perfused through antegrade flow in cases of external iliac disease.

Figure 1

Proximal anastomosis

1A depicts an end-to-end anastomosis of the aorta with an end-to-side anastomosis to the femoral. 1B shows an end-to-side anastomosis of the aortic and the femoral.

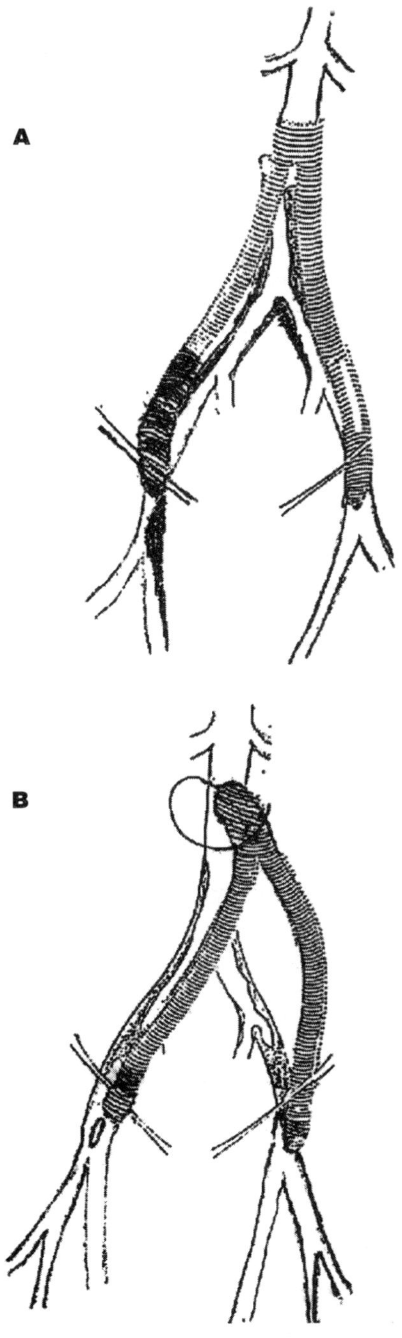

The complications of direct aortoiliac reconstruction may be significant. Both early and late complications occur at a different rate in each patient with this procedure, depending on the comorbid condition of the patient and the surgical technique involved. Early complications include risks from surgery, including myocardial infarction and pulmonary complications. Other operative complications include distal embolization, colonic ischemia and ureteric injury. Late complications include graft limb thrombosis, graft infection and pseudoaneurysm.

The most common cause of perioperative death in these patients is myocardial infarction. There is a well-known association between aortic disease and coronary artery disease. Prior to surgery on the abdominal aorta (both for occlusive and aneurysmal disease), patients should undergo a detailed cardiac examination. Early postoperatively there is a major risk of developing pneumonia, which can be limited by preoperative cessation of smoking and incentive spirometer teaching, along with the use of epidural anesthesia for postoperative pain control. Patients should also have pulmonary function evaluation prior to consideration for aortic surgery. Given the intimate relationship of the ureters to the retroperitoneum and the common iliac arteries, the surgeon must pay particular attention to the location of the ureters. In reoperative surgery, placement of ureteric stents may help the surgeon identify them. Colonic ischemia is also a known complication of aortic reconstruction, occurring in 2% of the cases. This most commonly involves the rectosigmoid colon due to interruption of vascular supply, from ligation of the inferior mesenteric artery, or from embolization. The status of the hypogastric vessels should also be evaluated, with at least one hypogastric being preserved, especially if the inferior mesenteric vessel is sacrificed.

Graft limb occlusion is the most common late complication following aortofemoral bypass. Occlusion rates range from 5%-10% within 5 years.[22] Usually only one limb is affected with severe ischemic symptoms. Reoperation can be either thrombectomy or femoral-femoral bypass. Often thrombosis has occurred because of narrowing of the profunda femoris artery orifice, which may require endarterectomy to maintain patency particularly when the superficial femoral artery is occluded. Anastomotic pseudoaneurysm is also a well-described complication of aortofemoral bypass. The femoral anastomosis is the most common site of pseudoaneurysm, occurring in 1%-5% of patients. Many factors contribute to pseudoaneurysm formation, including tension of the suture line, thin or diseased arterial walls, and poor surgical technique. Diagnosis of an enlarging pseudoaneurysm is an indication for repair. Graft infection is the most serious of all late complications, occurs in less than 1% of aortic grafts, and is usually staphylococcal. The mainstay of treatment is graft removal with extra-anatomic bypass, though some surgeons recommend inline replacement with femoral vein or prosthetic material in selected situations. Recently, some surgeons have been successful in retaining the graft limb, using local revision and debridement, if the infecting organism is *Staphylococcus epidermitis*.

In higher-risk patients or in patients with limited disease, more limited extraanatomic bypasses can be performed. Depending on the location and extent of the disease and the patient's comorbidities, less invasive repairs such as iliofemoral, femorofemoral or axillofemoral bypasses can be performed (see Figures 2 and 3). For high-risk patients with isolated distal iliac or external iliac disease, the iliofemoral bypass is a good alternative that does not subject the patient to the complications of an open aortic procedure. The early mortality of these procedures approaches zero. Recent reports by Whittemore and colleagues[28] show 4-year patency rates for iliac grafts of 96%, and those for the iliac-femoral bypasses of 76%, with better patency when the distal vessels are patent. When patients have disease isolated to one iliac or in patients with bilateral disease and an iliofemoral was performed, a femoral-femoral bypass can be used to revascularize the contralateral limb. For the high-risk patient, this procedure gives quite good results, with patency rates of 60%-80% at 5 years. This procedure is especially beneficial in the high-risk patient because it can be done under local or regional anesthetic.[17]

Figure 2

Femoral-femoral bypass

If one iliac vessel has adequate flow, a femoral-femoral bypass can be performed to supply blood to the side with the occluded iliac.

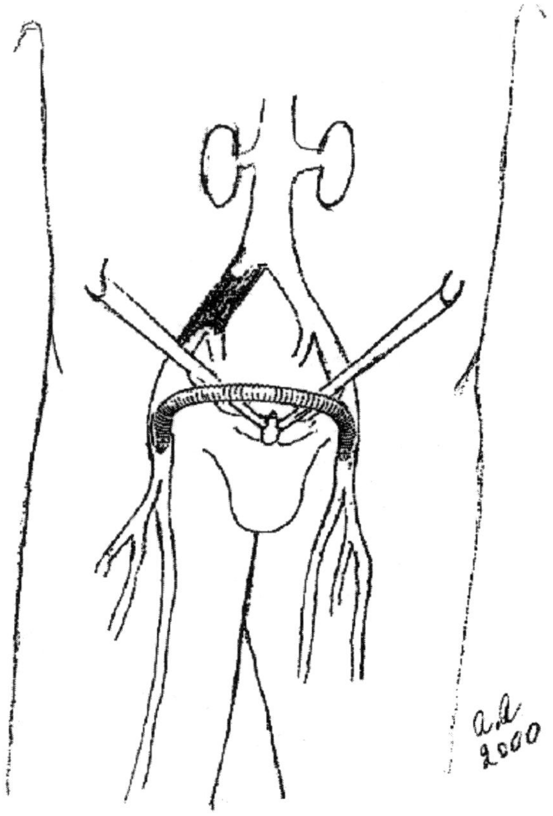

Figure 3

Axillofemoral bypass

The axillofemoral bypass can be performed to one or both femoral arteries. The arm with the highest blood pressure should be used as the donor side.

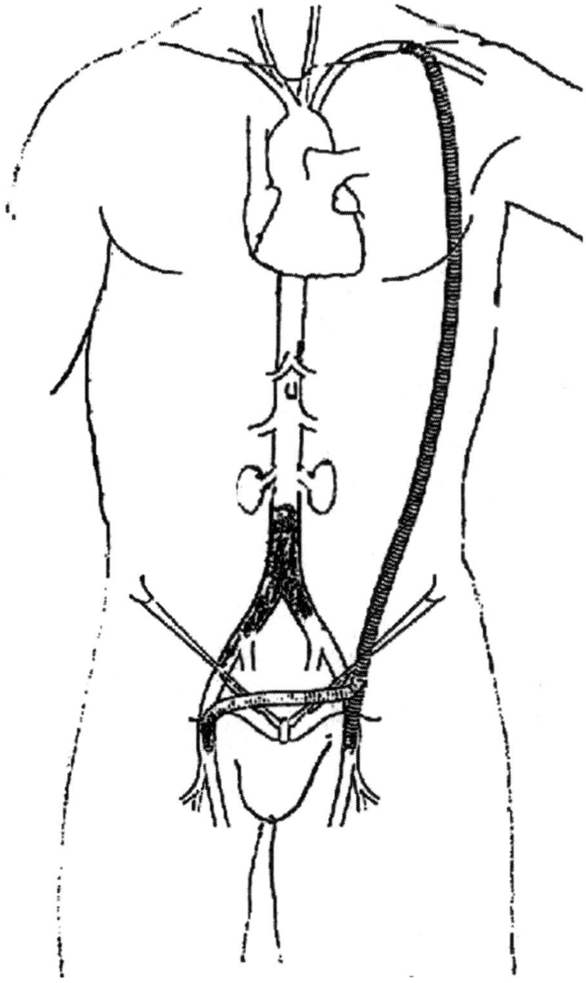

Some patients do not have a good inflow vessel in the aorta or iliacs. In these high-risk patients, when an abdominal procedure is contraindicated because of comorbid conditions or hostile abdomen (eg, multiple prior abdominal operations or an ostomy), the axillary artery can be used as an inflow vessel. Axillofemoral bypasses carry a low overall morbidity and have recently seen improved success with longer patency in both the unifemoral and bifemoral approach. There is much controversy regarding the use of the unifemoral or the bifemoral approach. If patients have bilateral iliac disease they will benefit from the bifemoral approach. If there is unilateral disease, an axillounifemoral or femoral-femoral bypass is an adequate alternative. The 5-year patency for axillofemoral bypasses is associated with the degree of distal disease, but usually approaches 70% at 5 years.[16]

Although the overall mortality in these more limited procedures is lower than in direct aortic repair, they also carry a risk of complication. The occurrence of graft infection and pseudoaneurysm is the same as with the aortic repair and intervention should occur at the time of diagnosis.

Percutaneous angioplasty with or without stenting for aortoiliac occlusive disease is also currently being utilized successfully and has virtually replaced traditional open bypass procedures for certain subsets of patients. Although recanalization of an occluded iliac artery is possible and appropriate in certain situations, percutaneous angioplasty is most appropriate when lesions are short (<5 cm), localized, and not associated with extensive disease proximal or distal to the lesion being treated. Diffuse stenotic or multilevel occlusive disease is still better treated with traditional bypass procedures, provided that the patient does not possess other prohibitive comorbidities that substantially increase the risk of open surgical intervention. Based on currently published reports, guidelines have been put forth in an attempt to define those patients who should undergo percutaneous intervention and those that should proceed directly to open surgery; however, as technology improves and more long-term data is collected, the indications for endovascular versus open surgical intervention will continue to evolve. It is likely that the future trend will continue to favor endovascular techniques when possible.

6. Infrainguinal Bypass

Infrainguinal arterial reconstruction has seen improved success for limb salvage over the past decade. The two major indications for infrainguinal bypass are severe, disabling claudication and limb-threatening ischemia. Claudication is a relative indication, because most of these patients remain stable throughout their lives, with approximately one-half showing improvement on an exercise program, one-third remaining the same, and the remainder progressing to more severe ischemic symptoms or rest pain. These patients have only 1% per year limb loss. The degree of claudication indicating intervention should be individualized to the patient. For young, low-risk patients with moderate claudication, bypass to the suprageniculate popliteal artery is a reasonable approach. For elderly, high-risk patients, or those who would require a bypass to the tibial vessels, a conservative approach should be employed.

Critical ischemia, presenting as rest pain, ischemic ulceration, or tissue loss, inevitably results in limb loss unless a revascularization procedure is performed successfully. In these patients, the overall comorbidities must be evaluated prior to surgical intervention. Patients should also be evaluated for viability prior to embarking on a major revascularization procedure. If the ischemia has progressed to gangrene in a major portion of the leg, any attempt at revascularization is futile. Similarly, if the patient has lost neurologic or motor function, the ischemia is too far progressed and any attempt to salvage the limb should be based on the amount of function that can be restored.

The preoperative evaluation should be undertaken as described earlier in this chapter, depending on the urgency of the situation. In an elective situation with a patient showing symptoms of claudication, a full history and physical examination should be performed, along with vascular lab studies and angiogram prior to revascularization. In the more urgent situation in a patient with an acutely ischemic extremity, urgent angiography either in the radiologic suite or operating room, followed by prompt revascularization, can be performed after a full evaluation showing the need for surgery is done.

Before elective intervention for claudication, the patient should have had at least three months of conservative treatment including a walking program (supervised if possible), tobacco abstinence and treatment with antiplatelet agents, control of hypertension and hyperlipidemia.

Operative Procedures

The ideal operative procedure for each patient depends on the patent arterial anatomy of the patient. The surgeon needs information about the distal patent vessel, and needs to determine if there is adequate runoff from that vessel. The conduit to use for the bypass depends on the level at which the distal anastomosis will be performed. The choices for the conduit include autologous saphenous vein, cephalic vein, prosthetic grafts and cryopreserved vein.

Most patients with claudication will have a patent popliteal vessel either above or below the knee. Above-knee bypasses have patency rates similar to those of prosthetic grafts, expanded polytetrafluoroethylene (PTFE), or the patient's autologous saphenous vein. For the below-knee bypasses, the patency of the grafts is better if vein grafts are used.

Bypasses below the popliteal artery are performed when the popliteal vessel is not suitable for bypass, either because it is occluded, or if occlusion is present in a more distal segment. These small vessel bypasses are performed to the posterior tibial, anterior tibial or peroneal artery. These vessels are considered target vessels when there is runoff into the foot or if major branches are supplied.

Graft Material and Operative Technique

The grafts available today include saphenous vein, cephalic vein, PTFE or cryopreserved vein. Primary 5-year patency rates for autologous saphenous vein grafts range from 63%-75%, with secondary patency rates up to 80%, and limb salvage rates approaching 90%. There is no difference in the overall patency rates between use of *in situ* saphenous vein bypass and reversed vein graft. The overall patency rates for prosthetic bypass grafts have not been as good as those for autologous vein grafts, and rates vary depending on the site of the distal anastomosis. PTFE bypass below the knee is sometimes used to obtain tissue healing, accepting the very limited patency. Upper extremity vein can be used in instances when no other vein is available. These veins are more difficult to work with and require a venous-venous anastomosis to attain the length necessary to bypass the diseased segment. These cephalic and basilic vein grafts may be indicated for limb salvage when an infrapopliteal bypass is to be performed and there is no available leg vein.[18,19,20,25,29] Consideration should be given to future need for upper extremity veins, especially if hemodialysis may become a possible need.

It must be kept in mind that the patencies of all grafts are directly affected by the indication for the bypass, claudication or ischemia, and the disease process distal to the anastomosis. In some situations, the patient who requires infrageniculate bypasses will have no usable vein for bypasses, either because of previous harvest for coronary artery bypass graft, varicose stripping or inadequate size for bypassing. In these situations, to accomplish limb salvage, a combination of prosthetic graft with a vein patch (Taylor) or cuff (Linton) at the distal anastomosis will achieve a better compliance match between the prosthetic graft and artery. This improved compliance match between graft and artery is postulated to decrease the amount of intimal hyperplasia at the distal anastomosis, and may result in longer patencies.[21]

The perioperative mortality rate for lower extremity revascularization ranges from 2%-5%, mostly from concomitant coronary artery disease. The morbidity from myocardial events in the postoperative course can be as high as 10%,[23,24,30] which underscores the association between coronary artery disease and lower extremity peripheral vascular disease. Wound infection also occurs at a significant rate in lower extremity bypasses, up to 15% of cases, because of the large incisions required for vein harvest. Most of these are minor, with just slight erythema and some mild skin breakdown at the skin sutures. Skin flap necrosis secondary to vein harvesting can be avoided by making the incision directly over the saphenous vein. Some are more severe, especially in the diabetic patient, requiring opening of the wound and secondary closure, possibly with split thickness skin grafting. In those patients who received a prosthetic graft, it can become secondarily infected and require removal. Lower extremity edema is common postbypass, secondary to disruption in lymphatics.[26] Unlike with aortoiliac occlusive disease, where percutaneous angioplasty has become the standard of care for many patients (at least initially), the role of angioplasty with or without concomitant stenting in the infrainguinal vessels is more limited. The good initial technical success is often followed by short patency intervals and can lead to reocclusion and further thrombosis requiring reintervention.[27] Again, guidelines have been established to define the appropriateness of percutaneous intervention based on the length and number of stenotic or occlusive lesions as well as the extent of the associated vascular disease. Patient comorbidities and their ability to tolerate open arterial reconstruction must be considered when planning intervention, whether for disabling claudication or limb-threatening ischemia.

7. Conclusion

When evaluating a patient for lower extremity occlusive disease, risk factors should be controlled as much as possible, and conservative treatment should be recommended while a full diagnostic workup is performed to determine the need for possible surgical intervention. The patient's arterial anatomy should then be reviewed, and if the patient is found to be a suitable candidate, surgical intervention should be considered. Based on the extent and location of the disease and the patient's comorbidities, either open surgical bypass or percutaneous intervention can be considered. It is clear that the indications for endovascular intervention versus open surgical bypass have changed over the last several years and will continue to evolve as devices improve, in favor of endovascular techniques. When planning a below-knee surgical bypass, the best long-term patency is still seen with the use of the patient's own vein. Prosthetic grafts, on the other hand, are the conduits of choice when bypassing the aorta and iliac arteries, and can be used infrainguinally in select situations.

8. References

1. Dormandy J, Ludger H, Vig S. Introduction. *Semin Vasc Surg*. 1999;12(2):95.
2. Urdang L. *The Bantam Medical Dictionary*. New York, NY: Random House Bantam; 1992.
3. Depalma R. Atherosclerosis: Pathology, pathogenesis and medical management. In: Moore W, ed. *Vascular Surgery: A Comprehensive Review*. 5th ed. Phildelphia, PA: WB Saunders; 1997:266-304.
4. Starg HC, Chandler AB, Glagou S, et al. American Heart Association. A definition of initial fatty streak and intermediate lesions of atherosclerosis: A report from the committee on vascular lesions. *Atherosclerosis Thrombosis*. 1994;14:840.
5. American Heart Association. A definition of advanced types of atherosclerotic lesions and a histological classification of atherosclerosis. *Atherosclerosis Thrombosis*. 1995;15:1512.
6. Chisolm GM, DiCarleto PE, Erhart LA, et al. Pathogenesis of atherosclerosis. In: Young JR, Graor RA, Olin JW, Bartholomew JR, eds. *Peripheral Vascular Disease Year Book*. St. Louis, MO: Mosby; 1991:137-160.
7. Reisy MA. Biology of disease: A reassessment of endothelial injury and arterial lesion formation. *Lab Invest*. 1985;53:513-520.
8. Yellin A. *The Modern Approach to the Vascular Patient. Vascular Disease: A Multispecialty Approach*. Austin, TX: Landes Bioscience; 1997:1-15.
9. Gomes A. Principles of angiography and interventional radiology. In: Moore W, ed. *Vascular Surgery: A Comprehensive Review*. Philadelphia, PA: WB Saunders; 1997:266-304.
10. Castanada WZ, Knight L, Formanek A, et al. Hemodynamic assessment of obstructive aortoiliac disease. *AJR*. 1976;127:559-561.

11. Haimovich H. Patterns of atherosclerotic lesions of the lower extremities. *Arch Surg*. 1986;95:918-933.

12. Hessel S, Adams D. Complications of angiography. *Radiology*. 1981;138:273.

13. Leriche R, Moral A. The syndrome of thrombotic obliteration of the aortic bifurcation. *Ann Surg*. 1948;127:193.

14. Williams GM, Harrington D, White RI, et al. Mural thrombus of the aorta. *Am Surg*. 1981;194:737.

15. Brewster DC, Perier BA, Robison JG. Aortofemoral graft for multilevel occlusive disease. *Arch Surg*. 1982;117:1593.

16. Brewster DC. Aortoiliac disease. In: Greenfield L, ed. *Surgery: Scientific Principles and Practice*. 1st ed. Philadelphia, PA: Lippincott; 1993:1643-1655.

17. Whitmore AD, Belkin M,. Aortic occlusive disease. In: Moore W, ed. *Vascular Surgery: A Comprehensive Review*. Philadelphia, PA: WB Saunders; 1997:483-496.

18. Bergan JJ, Veith FJ, Bernhardt VM, et al. Randomization of autogenous vein and PTFE grafts in femoral-distal reconstruction. *Surgery*. 1982;92:921-930.

19. Veith FJ, Gupta SK, Ascer E, et al. Six year prospective randomized comparison of autologous saphenous vein and expanded PTFE grafts in infrainguinal arterial reconstructions. *J Vasc Surg*. 1986;3:104-114.

20. Sanchez L, Veith F. Femoral-popliteal-tibial occlusive disease. In: Moore W, ed. *Vascular Surgery: A Comprehensive Review*. Philadelphia, PA: WB Saunders; 1997.

21. Kissen M, Kansel N, Pappas P, et al. Vein interposition cuffs decrease the intimal hyperplastic response of PTFE bypass grafts. *J Vasc Surg*. 2000;31:69-81.

22. Brewster DC, Meir GH, Darling RC, et al Reoperation for aortofemoral graft limb occlusion: optimal methods and long-term results. *J Vasc Surg*. 1987;5:363.

23. Bergamini TM, Town JB, Bandyk DF, et al. Experience with in situ saphenous vein bypasses during 1981-1989: Determinant factors of long term patency. *J Vasc Surg*. 1991;13:137.

24. Donaldson MC, Mannick JA, Wittemore AD. Femoral-distal bypass with greater saphenous vein: Long-term results using the Mills Valvulotome. *Ann Surg*. 1991;213:457.

25. Quinones-Baldrich WJ, Prego AA, Ucelay-Gomez R, et al. Long-term results of infrainguinal revascularization with polytetrafluoroethylene (PTFE). A ten-year experience. *J Vasc Surg*. 1992;16:209-217.

26. Taylor LM, Porter JM, Winek T. Femoropopliteal and infrapopliteal occlusive disease. In: Greenfield L, ed. *Surgery: Scientific Principles and Practice*. 1st ed. Philadelphia, PA: Lippincott; 1993:1656-1667.

27. El-Bayer H, Roberts A, Hye RJ, Davis G, Freischlag JA. Determinants of failure in superficial femoral artery (SFA) angioplasty. *Angiology*. 1992;43:877.

28. Olivera M, Wilson SE, Williams R, Freischlag JA. Is the iliofemoral bypass worthwhile? *J Cardiovasc Surg*. 1993;1:103.

29. Plecha EJ, Seabrook GR, Towne JB, Freischlag JA. Femoropopliteal bypass revisited: An analysis of 138 cases. *J Cardovasc Surg*. 1996;4:195.

30. Mayes BW, Towne JB, Fitzpatrick C, Cambria RA, Seabrook GR, Freischlag JA. Women have increased perioperative myocardial infarction and long term mortality following lower extremity bypass. *J Vasc Surg*. 1999;29:807.

31. Suding PN, McMaster W, Hansen E, Hatfield AW, Gordon IL, Wilson SE. Increased endovascular interventions decrease the rate of lower limb bypass operations without an increase in major amputation rate. *Ann Vasc Surg*. 2008; 22(2):195-19.

9. Questions

1. Which of the following is the *single* risk factor for atherosclerosis?

A. High animal-fat diet

B. Cigarette smoking

C. Male sex

D. Age over 65

2. You are evaluating a patient complaining of pain when walking up and down stairs and he has good pulses on physical exam. Your next step should be:

A. Reassure the patient that he has no vascular disease

B. Assess ankle arm indices

C. Perform exercise noninvasive study

D. Perform angiogram

3. Which two factors are ***not*** associated with Leriche syndrome?

A. Decreased femoral pulses

B. Buttock claudication

C. Rest pain

D. Ulceration

E. Impotence

4. Angiogram is best performed in which two circumstances?

   A. Duplex examination shows evidence of superficial femoral artery occlusion

   B. The patient has one block claudication after conservative treatment

   C. As a preintervention study

   D. Completion study after revascularization

5. Which two of the following statements are true regarding aortoiliac disease?

   A. A late complication of aortofemoral bypass is femoral pseudoaneurysm

   B. A complication of aortofemoral bypass is femoral pseudoaneurysm

   C. The most common early postoperative complication is myocardial infarction

   D. Aortic end-to-end anastomosis has been shown to have better patency than end-to-side

6. The conduit that gives the best long-term patency for infrapopliteal bypass is:

   A. Saphenous vein

   B. PTFE

   C. PTFE with Taylor patch

   D. PTFE with Linton patch

7. Indications for lower extremity bypass include:

   A. Disabling claudication

   B. Rest pain

   C. Ischemic ulceration

   D. Gangrenous change

   E. All of the above

Answers

1. B.
All of the items listed are risk factors for atherosclerotic disease, but a history of cigarette smoking has the greatest association for atherosclerosis.

2. C.
A patient who has exercise-induced claudication with disease at the iliac level often will have peripheral pulses until after exercise. Neither physical examination nor resting AAI will reveal the disease. A treadmill AAI or PVR test will show decreased AAI or waveform.

3. C. and D.
The Leriche syndrome consists of decreased femoral pulses, buttock claudication and impotence. Tissue loss and rest pain are not associated with this syndrome.

4. C and D.
Angiogram should only be performed as a presurgical procedure, and is not indicated for use as a screening study or in patients who are not candidates for surgical intervention. After a revascularization, an intraoperative angiogram should be performed to assure adequacy of the distal anastomosis.

5. B and C.

Axillofemoral bypasses are good alternatives to aortofemoral bypasses, however they cannot achieve the 80% 10-year patency rate of the aortofemoral bypass. The most common late complication after aortofemoral bypass is the formation of femoral pseudoaneurysm, and the early complication seen most commonly is ischemic heart disease. There is no difference in long-term patency between end-to-end and end-to-side anastomoses.

6. A.

Saphenous vein is the best conduit for lower extremity revascularization. PTFE used alone or with vein patches are alternatives in certain situations, but cannot attain the patency rate of vein grafts.

7. E.

All of the above seen in an appropriate situation are indications for revascularization.

Chapter 19: Venous Disease

John J. Bergan, MD, FACS, FRCS (Hon), Eng.
Nisha Bunke, MD

Contents

1. Overview of Venous Disorders

Venous disorders are very common in Western civilization. The precise prevalence is uncertain because, compared to other conditions, relatively little epidemiological research has been conducted in this area. There is a general perception that venous disorders are unimportant because only a few cause death, and it is thought that the visible manifestations of venous disorders are simply a nuisance. However, venous disorders permeate every aspect of medical care, and every specialty and subspecialty must know something about the conditions that are present in their particular patient populations. To organize information about venous disorders, it is helpful to have an overview to address specific conditions. Table 1 shows a broad categorization of venous disorders. The term venous insufficiency as used in the table can cover a wide range of conditions. These can range from as simple a condition as telangiectasias to more severe and disabling entities such as chronic venous leg ulcer.

Table 1

Overview of Venous Disorders

Overview of Venous Disorders
Primary Venous Insufficiency
Telangiectasias
Reticular varicosities
Varicose veins
Chronic Venous Insufficiency
Edema
Lipodermatosclerosis
Venous leg ulcers
Venous Thromboembolic Disease
Superficial phlebitis
Deep venous thrombosis
Pulmonary embolism

Primary Venous Insufficiency

With regard to the category of primary venous insufficiency, it is helpful to know that telangiectasias, reticular varicosities and true varicose veins produce identical symptoms. Therefore, it is appropriate to consider them as a single entity involving vessels that are elongated, dilated, tortuous, pouched and thickened. Each of these entities also involves nonfunctional, incompetent valves; the difference between them is the size of the incompetent valves.[1] The telangiectasias of the skin, the blue-green reticular varicosities under the skin and the large grape-like varicosities that lie even deeper all conform to the same definition, and respond to the same etiologic forces.[2] Their epidemiology, causes, risk factors and other elements will be the subject of further discussion.

Chronic Venous Insufficiency

Chronic venous insufficiency (CVI) is the modern term for what was until recently referred to as the postthrombotic or postphlebitic state.[3] The term encompasses the entities of venous edema, lipodermatosclerosis, and healed or open venous leg ulcer. In the remote past, it was thought that these entities were caused by previous deep venous thrombosis, which in turn had produced venous obstruction and destruction of venous valves. As improved diagnostic methods were applied to limbs with CVI, it was found that a majority of these limbs had never had deep venous thrombosis, and a new term had to be invented. It is useful to refer to this overall condition as CVI because it is chronic and the term "venous insufficiency" implies failure of normal function.

The pathophysiology of primary venous insufficiency and chronic venous insufficiency is dominated by the phenomenon of reflux. The conditions of thromboembolic disease are characterized by obstruction. In general, these are acute conditions in which venous thrombosis forms either in the superficial venous system, the deep venous system, or both, and then portions of the freshly-forming thrombus break off and travel to the heart and lungs, producing all of the manifestations of pulmonary embolization.

2. Venous Anatomy

Anatomy of the venous system as taught in medical school is not useful in everyday practice. Nevertheless, terms used in didactic anatomy are also used clinically. Only the emphasis changes as one views the clinical anatomy of the venous system of the upper and lower extremities.

Lower Extremity Veins

Nomenclature is particularly important since it is difficult to discuss the topic of leg veins without agreement about definitions and meaning. In 2001, an International Interdisciplinary Committee was designated by the Presidents of the International Union of Phlebology (IUP) and the International Federation of Anatomical Associations to update the official Terminologia Anatomica regarding the veins of the lower limbs. Deficiencies in the previous official Terminologia Anatomica had resulted in nonuniform anatomical nomenclature in the clinical literature that complicated international exchange of information and possibly resulted in inappropriate treatment of venous disease. The Committee, with the participation of Members of the Federative International Committee for Anatomical Nomenclature (FICAT), developed a Consensus Document at a meeting held in Rome on the occasion of the 14th World Congress of the IUP. Recommendations of the Committee were published and these new, occasionally unfamiliar terms are shown in Table 2 and are used in the following exposition.

Veins of the lower extremities are subdivided into three systems: the superficial venous system, the deep venous system and the perforating veins that penetrate aponeurotic fascia to connect the superficial to the deep veins. Some texts refer to perforating veins as communicating veins, but it is best to reserve this term for interconnecting veins that do not cross anatomic layers.

It is important to understand that the unique characteristic of veins, the valves, are present in all sizes of veins, including those in the dermis, the subcutaneous tissue and the deep muscular compartment. Valves direct blood flow toward the heart from the superficial and deep veins and prevent the backward flow of blood. In retarding blood flow downward and outward, the valves can be thought of as having a check valve function. The check valve protects

Table 2

Summary of Important Changes in Nomenclature of Lower Extremity Veins

Old Terminology	New Terminology
Femoral vein	Common femoral vein
Superficial femoral vein	Femoral vein
Sural veins	Sural veins Soleal veins Gastrocnemius veins (medial and lateral)
Huntarian perforator	Mid thigh perforator
Cockett's perforators	Paratibial perforator Posterior tibial perforators
May's perforator	
Gastrocnemius point	Intergemellar perforator

Figure 1

Relationship of superficial veins to sensory nerves and medial leg veins

This artist's drawing shows the relationship of the superficial veins to sensory nerves and to the important medial leg perforating veins.

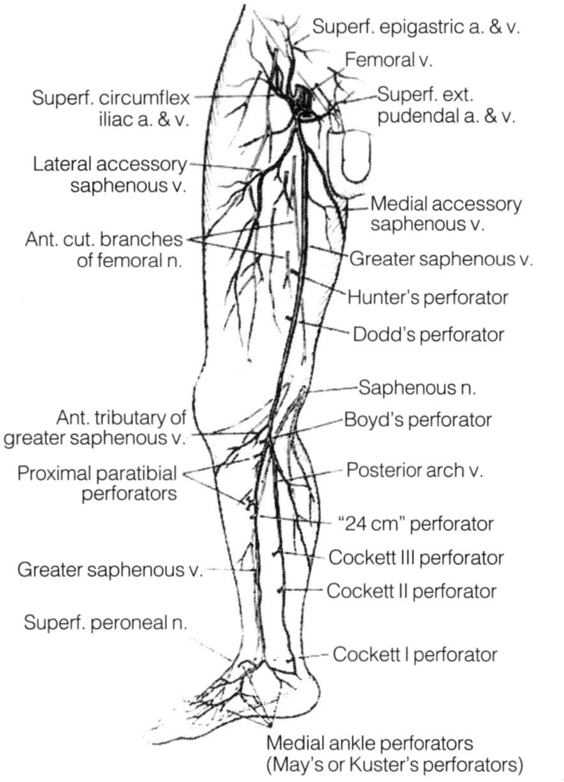

From Ballard JL, Bergan JJ. Chronic Venous Insufficiency: Diagnosis and Treatment. *London, England: Springer-Verlag; 2000.*

distal veins from proximal venous hypertensive forces. Normally, deep veins carry 90% of the lower extremity blood flow. This important fact explains why superficial veins can be removed with no loss of physiologic function.

Superficial Veins

The superficial venous system is different from the deep venous system in that the superficial veins usually do not have accompanying arteries (Figure 1). Instead, the superficial veins are organized into a series of interconnecting subcutaneous channels that drain into 2 major superficial venous systems (Figure 2). These are the great saphenous vein (GSV) and the small saphenous vein (SSV). These 2 systems, the great and small saphenous veins, empty into the deep veins through the saphenofemoral junction (SFJ) in the groin and the saphenopopliteal junction (SPJ) in the popliteal fossa.

The artist's drawing shows the relationship of the superficial veins to sensory nerves and to the important medial leg perforating veins.

Deep Veins

Deep veins in the lower extremities accompany major named arteries. They are frequently doubled, and it is normal for deep veins below the knee to be doubled. In the calf, the paired posterior tibial veins

Figure 2

Relationship of superficial veins of posterolateral calf to perforating veins

This drawing shows the relationships of the superficial veins of the posterolateral calf to perforating veins and to the all-important sural nerve.

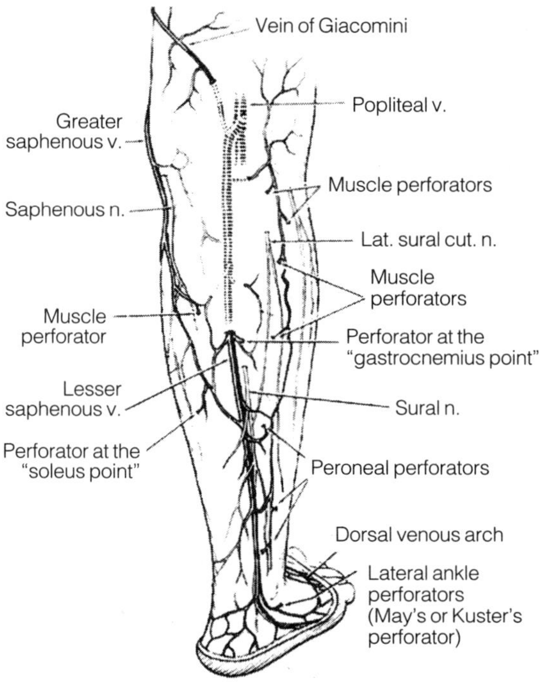

From Ballard JL, Bergan JJ. Chronic Venous Insufficiency Diagnosis and Treatment. *London, England: Springer-Verlag; 2000.*

run under the fascia of the deep posterior compartment between the edges of the flexor digitorum longus and tibialis posterior muscles. These are particularly important because they collect blood through perforating veins from the posterior arch venous circulation as well as the greater saphenous veins. The anterior tibial veins are continuations of the dorsalis pedis veins and ascend between muscles of the anterior compartment of the calf. The paired peroneal veins originate in the distal third of the leg and ascend deep to the flexor hallucis longus muscle. They receive blood through the lateral perforating veins. Large venous sinuses from the soleus muscle also empty into the peroneal veins.

This drawing shows the relationships of the superficial veins of the posterolateral calf to perforating veins and to the all-important sural nerve.

The popliteal and femoral veins are often duplicated in segments of various lengths. Principal tributaries to the popliteal vein are the gastrocnemius veins and the lesser saphenous vein. Proximal to the adductor canal, the femoral vein is the principal deep vein of the thigh. The femoral vein in the thigh receives blood from the perforating veins of the mid and distal thigh. The deep femoral vein drains muscles of the lateral aspect of the thigh and may receive perforators from the lateral accessory saphenous vein. The deep femoral vein unites with the femoral vein to form the common femoral vein. It runs medial to the femoral artery and continues above the level of the inguinal ligament into the external iliac vein.

Generally, the smaller the vein, the more numerous the valves, so the deep veins of the foot, the posterior tibial, anterior tibial and peroneal veins all have many valves, while the popliteal vein has 1 or 2, and there are 3 or more in the femoral vein. Just distal to the saphenofemoral junction is an important valve, the subterminal valve.

The saphenofemoral junction has been of great surgical importance (Figure 3). The great saphenous vein enters the common femoral vein just below the inguinal ligament. It receives proximal tributaries from the superficial circumflex iliac vein, the superficial epigastric vein, the superficial external pudendal vein and the anterolateral vein of the thigh. The most distal tributary is a posteromedial vein that provides a connection to the vein of Giacomini in the posterior thigh. The anatomy of the tributaries may vary considerably as they may be present separately or 2 or more may join to form one common stem. Frequently, it is the tributaries that are incompetent rather than the saphenous vein, and this fact must be determined by duplex scanning before surgical intervention. The external pudendal artery is often posterior to the saphenous vein in the inferior border of the fossa ovalis. Also, it commonly runs in front of the saphenous vein and, in this situation, may be divided.

Figure 3

Anatomy of the saphenofemoral junction

The anatomy of the saphenofemoral junction is of importance to surgeons operating in this area. While the variations in anatomy are numerous, the 4 most common are shown here. The frequency of each variation is: A) 33%, B) 15%, C) 15% and D)13%.

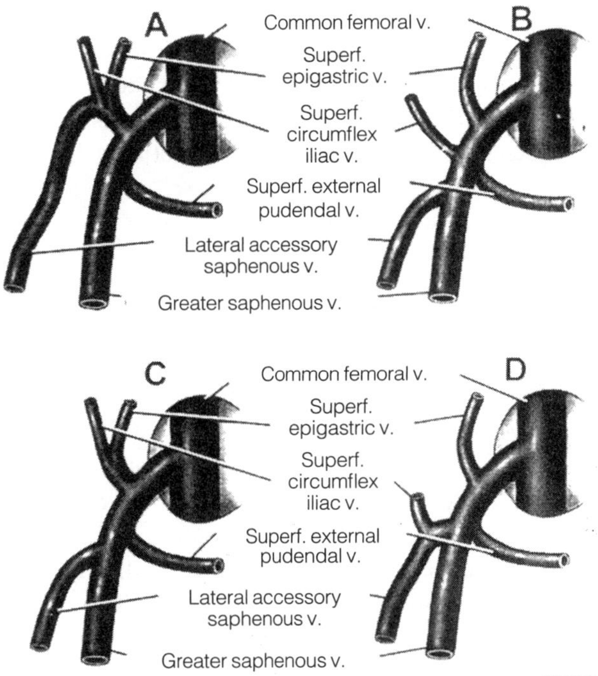

Modified from Gray H. Anatomy of the Human Body. *Goss GM, ed. Philadelphia, PA: Lea & Febiger; 1948.*

Although there are between 120 and 140 perforating veins in the lower extremity, the main ones used to carry the names of important investigators in the field of venous insufficiency. These eponyms will be used in this chapter, although it is expected that their use will fade. On the medial aspect of the leg there is an inframalleolar perforating vein and a retromalleolar perforating vein that is approximately 6 cm from the heel pad. This is called the Cockett I perforating vein. At approximately 6 cm intervals proximally, the Cockett II and Cockett III perforating veins are found. There is also a 24-cm perforating vein and, in the anteromedial leg just below the knee, a perforating vein named for Boyd of Manchester, England. The Dodd perforating veins are in the distal thigh and join the greater saphenous vein to the femoral vein. There is also a midthigh perforating vein named for John Hunter.

For the most part, the perforating veins in the leg (lower extremity, ankle to knee) do not communicate with the greater saphenous vein but instead communicate with the posterior arch circulation. The exception may be the Boyd perforating vein, that may communicate either with the anterior tributary or the posterior tributary to the saphenous vein in the leg, or the saphenous vein itself. Posteriorly, there is a gastrocnemius and a soleus point in the midline of the posterior calf. There is a lateral perforating vein of some importance in venous insufficiency, as well as 5- and 12-cm perforating veins.

Upper Extremity Veins

Unlike the lower extremity where there are 3 major venous systems, in the upper extremity there are only 2 major systems: the superficial and the deep (Figure 4). The superficial system assumes importance because of the need to construct vascular access. The deep circulation is chiefly important at the thoracic outlet or, when referring to the venous system, this might be referred to as the thoracic inlet. There are 2 main superficial veins, the lateral cephalic vein and the medial basilic vein. The basilic vein is a continuation proximally of the median antebrachial vein and the cephalic vein is a continuation of the lateral antebrachial vein.

Figure 4

Veins of the upper extremity

The veins of the upper extremity are diagrammed here. There are 2 main systems with abundant communicating veins connecting them.

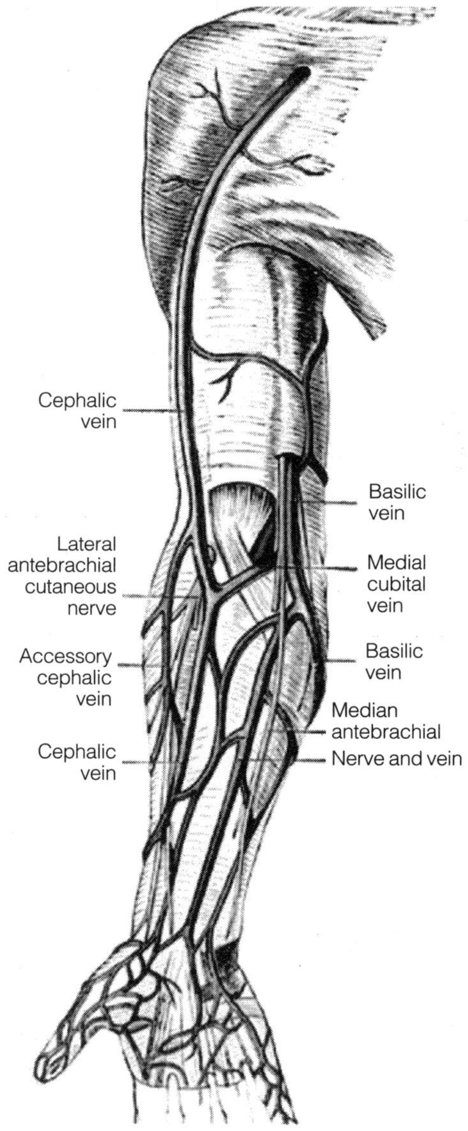

Modified from Gray H. Anatomy of the Human Body. *Goss GM, ed. Philadelphia, PA: Lea & Febiger; 1948.*

3. Physiologic and Anatomic Studies

The clinical examination is of paramount importance in studying patients with venous disorders, but objective evaluation is required to confirm the diagnosis. Furthermore, studies in the vascular laboratory can provide guidelines for subsequent therapy. It is appropriate to consider tests of venous function as providing data regarding either physiology or anatomy. Physiologic testing provides information on the function of the veins and the dysfunction produced by venous disorders. Anatomic studies identify the exact sites of obstruction or reflux flow and may give some indication of venous function as well.

Physiologic Studies

Venous pressure measurements dominated reports of venous physiology and pathophysiology during the 25-year period after 1950 (Table 3). Therefore, much that has been done since then is compared to these studies, so it is necessary to understand these techniques and limitations in assessing venous physiology.

Table 3

Physiologic Studies of Venous Function

Venous pressure measurement
Plethysmography: Impedance plethysmography Mercury strain-gauge plethysmography Photoplethysmography Air plethysmography
Doppler flow

Venous Pressure Measurements

A suitable vein on the dorsum of the foot is cannulated and the needle fixed in place. Superficial veins constitute a single intercommunicating compartment, and it is thought that pressure measured in one vein is representative of the pressure throughout the compartment. The needle is connected to a strain gauge and the transducer fixed level with the tip of the needle. The hydrostatic, or resting pressure is dependent on the height of the patient and is, in essence, the pressure from the right atrium to the tip of the needle on the dorsum of the foot. Systemic abnormalities such as cardiac failure, constrictive pericarditis, ascites and abdominal masses will impede venous return and degrade the accuracy of the venous pressure measurement. After a baseline pressure is taken with the patient standing, the patient exercises by performing tiptoe maneuvers, raising both heels off the ground every second, usually in synchronization with the beats of a metronome. 10 to 20 tiptoe exercises are sufficient to allow the pressure to become stable.

The postexercise pressure and its return to baseline constitute important data relative to venous function. The fall in pressure during exercise indicates efficiency of the calf muscle pump. After the initial fall produced by calf muscle pump emptying of the superficial system, a rise in pressure is produced by arterial inflow, to which is added any venous reflux that might be present. The time taken for 90% refilling, and sometimes the time taken for 50% refilling, are recorded and provide a standard for comparison.

The test is repeated using superficial vein-occluding tourniquets. Placement of these tourniquets may allow detection of major perforating vein outflow vessels (the Trendelenburg test). Thus, reflux can be detected, and the application of tourniquets is done to differentiate deep venous reflux from superficial venous reflux. However, application of the tourniquets is not always accurate, because the tourniquet may be occluding portions of the deep venous circulation as well as the superficial circulation, or the tourniquet may not completely occlude the superficial circulation. Detection of deep venous obstruction by venous pressure measurements is theoretically possible, but in practice is difficult to accomplish except when the occlusion is so gross that the foot vein pressure rises during exercise.

The assumption that the calf muscle pump efficiency is related to symptoms and even findings of venous insufficiency has not proven to be true. Despite this, venous pressure studies have been accepted as the gold standard of calf pump function.[4,5] It is only in recent years that objective clinical findings such as hyperpigmentation and ulceration have been explained by leukocyte activation. Such leukocyte activation is not necessarily dependent on the venous pressure, either hydrostatic pressure or postexercise pressure.[4,5]

Plethysmography

All plethysmographs measure the same thing: volume change. In the extremities, transient changes in volume are attributable to an increase or decrease in blood volume, because the other tissues, bone, muscle, adipose tissue and skin have a constant volume under the conditions of testing. The most common types of plethysmographs used for venous testing are those that use air, mercury strain gauges, or light or electrical impedance.

Impedance plethysmography (IPG) consists of measuring the changes in electrical impedance produced by volume changes detected by electrodes wrapped around the leg below the knee. An increase in volume decreases impedance. This signal is amplified and volume change recorded by a penwriter. In theory, obstruction to venous outflow increases venous outflow resistance, decreases venous compliance, and increases leg volume. These changes can be detected by impedance plethysmography. The method has been used primarily to detect deep venous thrombosis and is dependent on whether the obstructions produced by thrombi are totally or only partially occlusive.[6,7]

In practice, measurement is taken with the patient supine, the leg elevated 20°-30°, and the leg rotated externally at the hip. Flexion of the knee 10°-20° prevents compression of the popliteal vein. The set of 2 electrodes is wrapped around the calf and a pneumatic cuff 20 cm wide is placed around the thigh. The cuff is inflated, pressure is maintained at a steady state and then the cuff is rapidly deflated. The tracing is allowed to return to baseline.[7] The rise of the tracing from the baseline measures the capacity of the venous bed distal to the thigh tourniquet, and the fall of the tracing over a 3-second period is a measurement of venous outflow.[8]

The IPG method of detecting venous thrombosis has been thoroughly studied and validated. However, in patients with previous deep venous thrombosis, the venous collateral circulation may be so well developed that occlusion in major veins is not detected. Similarly, thrombi in tributary veins such as the profunda femoris or internal iliac veins do not impede venous outflow. Also, partially-occluding thrombi, as seen on duplex studies, may not alter flow as measured by impedance plethysmography. Arterial insufficiency will also lead to erroneous readings, as will popliteal cysts or tumors.

An interesting phenomenon occurred as IPG was accepted more and more. Patients were referred to vascular laboratories earlier after onset of symptoms and the prevalence of nonocclusive venous thrombi was higher in this patient group. Thus, the accuracy of IPG appeared to decline.[9]

Strain-Gauge Plethysmography (Mercury Strain-Gauge Plethysmography [MSG])

Although the techniques of using mercury in Silastic tubing or indium-gallium electrodes were highly accurate and sensitive in detecting volume changes in the calf, the fragility of the mercury in Silastic precluded wide acceptance of the techniques. Calf volume expansion, called venous volume or venous capacitance, was determined in a method similar to impedance plethysmography. Measurements of maximum venous outflow improved the sensitivity of the technique. It was possible to devise a graph that plotted venous capacitance against venous outflow and then draw a discriminate line specific for mercury strain-gauge studies. For example, in a group of 45 patients, one group found that the venous outflow:venous capacitance ratio was 100% sensitive and 92% specific in detecting deep venous thrombosis.[10] The sources of error associated with MSG techniques are similar to those using impedance plethysmography.

Photoplethysmography (PPG, also known as Light Reflection Rheography [LRR])

While plethysmographic techniques using electrical impedance were implemented primarily to detect venous obstruction and deep venous thrombosis, the technique of photoplethysmography was applied mostly in detecting reflux. Testing was performed by placing an infrared light source on the skin adjacent to a photoreceptor that received back-scattered light. Continuous recording reflected the volume of the subepidermal venous network. The patient was assessed sitting with the legs unsupported and, after 5 successive plantar flexion/extension maneuvers, the venous refill time was recorded on a strip chart. This venous refill time was similar to that obtained during venous pressure measurements, and was similarly dependent on arterial inflow as well as efficiency of venous outflow as produced by the calf muscle pump. Similarly to venous pressure measurements, when reflux was identified during PPG testing, the placement of tourniquets inflated to 50 mm Hg above and below the knee assisted in localizing the reflux to the deep or superficial venous systems.[11,12]

Accuracy of the PPG, however, depended on physical factors, including the size of the reservoir to be filled and the diameter of the veins that were refluxing. Thus, a long or even normal refill time could be observed when the reflux was occurring in small-diameter vessels. Modifications in the PPG produced the digital PPG in which measurements of venous refill time and muscle pump efficiency had a better quantitative correlation with symptoms than conventional PPG or even LRR.[13,14]

Air Plethysmography (APG)

Clinically, 2 generations of air plethysmographs were developed and used in the noninvasive laboratory. The first to achieve popularity was designed by Raines and was used principally for arterial studies. This was called the pulse-volume recorder.[15] A single pneumatic cuff was placed around the calf, therefore the results were similar to those of strain-gauge plethysmography. Venous capacitance and maximum venous outflow were measured, but this technique was never widely accepted and comparative studies against other noninvasive modalities were not done.

The most recent application of air plethysmography involves measurement of the whole leg, rather than a segment of the leg as was assessed by strain-gauge or small-chamber plethysmographs. The modern air plethysmograph is validated and standardized, and as such has the ability to measure venous reflux, venous obstruction and calf muscle pump function. Studies validating the technique and correlating it with clinical findings have been presented authoritatively.[16,17] Incidence of edema, skin changes and frank ulceration increase with higher values of reflux whether the reflux is superficial or deep.

Venous outflow measurements using the modern air plethysmograph are performed similarly to those using impedance techniques.[18] Of some interest is the ability to measure the ejection capacity of the calf muscle pump. It is felt that the ejection capacity is as important as reflux in the development of the cutaneous changes of CVI. In studies that attempted to correlate physiologic function with clinical findings, a good ejection fraction of greater than 40% was associated with a low incidence of venous ulceration despite marked reflux. A poor ejection fraction of less than 40% was found in limbs with venous ulceration and minimal reflux.[19]

Doppler Flow

Continuous-wave Doppler equipment was the first ultrasound method to be applied to study the venous system. Thus, it was the first to assess the function of each segment of venous anatomy. This precision is the reason the continuous-wave Doppler instrument enjoys such widespread use today. The clinician can perform the continuous-wave Doppler scan immediately, and specific areas of interest indicated by the clinical examination can be examined in detail.

The continuous-wave Doppler instrument emits high-frequency sound waves, which are directed toward the veins under study. The sound waves that are reflected by moving particles in the bloodstream are shifted in frequency by an amount proportional to the velocity of flow. The exact flow velocities are not of interest, but the Doppler equation relates the average flow velocity to 2 times the carrier frequency times the cosine of the Doppler angle. Therefore, it is necessary to preserve the angle to the vein at less than 90°. Otherwise, cosines of this angle approach zero, and there would be little or no detectable signal. Decreasing the Doppler angle to the vein causes an increased distance between the probe and the vein. As this distance is increased, the reflecting ultrasound waves travel the distance twice, and the ultrasound intensity or strength of the signal decreases. Tissue attenuation is proportional to the frequency of the ultrasound waves, and high-frequency probes are more suitable to study superficial veins, and low-frequency probes are more suitable for deep veins. In practice, the 5.4 MHz probe is suitable for venous studies.

The continuous-wave Doppler instrument is used in 2 situations. The first is for detection of deep venous occlusion or thrombosis and the second is for detection of reflux in primary or chronic venous insufficiency. In the former, the patient is supine and relaxed, covered comfortably by a blanket. In the latter, the patient is standing and the nonweight-bearing extremity is examined with the knee slightly flexed. Good acoustic conductivity is promoted by applying ultrasonic gel, and minimal probe pressure should be employed. The Doppler examination should be conducted bilaterally in a systematic fashion so that moderate changes can be noted. An examination of one lower extremity should be followed immediately by examination of the contralateral extremity so that a comparison of parameters can be made.

Spontaneous velocity signals are dependent on respiration. These are cyclic and, as the diaphragm descends, flow is halted. As the diaphragm ascends, flow resumes. Such cyclic variations are mainly present in the thigh veins, and respiratory changes are of less significance in the veins below the knee. Spontaneous flow signals are augmented by pressure maneuvers. For example, in examining the femoral vein, pressure on the abdomen will produce a back pressure which compromises or halts the venous velocity signal. Exhalation against a closed glottis, known as the Valsalva maneuver, will produce increased abdominal pressure and abruptly decrease venous flow. The Valsalva maneuver may detect a competent proximal valve or, conversely, incompetence or absence of a proximal iliac venous valve.

A second maneuver of gentle compression, either proximal or distal to the probe, will lead either to a cessation of flow or an increase in the velocity signal. The distal compression is termed augmentation and proximal pressure may either halt flow or cause a reversal of flow when the venous valve is incompetent. Detection of venous reflux with the patient supine is unfortunately completely inaccurate.

The best method for examining the venous system of the lower extremities for reflux is with the patient standing with the weight supported by the contralateral lower extremity and the knee of the leg under study slightly flexed. A systematic approach from top to bottom includes study of the venous confluence in the groin and the greater saphenous vein in the thigh, including its anterolateral and posteromedial branches. At knee level, the medial aspect is examined for the greater saphenous vein as well as the accessory, or secondary saphenous veins. The greater saphenous vein runs posterior to the femoral condyle and connects to the deep or lesser saphenous system. The preliminary physical examination with the continuous-wave Doppler instrument must be supplemented preoperatively by duplex ultrasonography. In this test the examination is performed during compression and release of distal muscles with reflux defined as reverse flow greater than 0.5 second duration.

Examination of the popliteal fossa is most demanding, and it is possible with the continuous-wave Doppler instrument to mistake crural vessels for the popliteal venous vessels.

Difficulties with the continuous-wave Doppler study occur in patients who are obese and in patients who have had previous superficial venous surgery.

Anatomic Studies

The availability and widespread use of duplex ultrasonography is based on its high level of accuracy and moderate cost. This technology has secured a primary role in the majority of vascular laboratories in the West. Duplex technology has become established as the study of choice for diagnosis of deep venous thrombosis in the ambulatory patient. In practice, it is also used for assessment of venous insufficiency.[20]

For detection of deep venous thrombosis, a 5 MHz to 8 MHz transducer is used. The patient is supine and each of the major veins of the lower extremities is examined with the lower extremity externally rotated. The common femoral, femoral and popliteal veins are scanned in transverse fashion, assessing the patency of each vein throughout its length. Any abnormality that is encountered is verified by longitudinal scanning. Gentle pressure applied to the transducer determines whether easy coaptation of the vein walls occurs. In a normal vein, the anterior and posterior walls should coapt. Interposition of echogenic thrombus will prevent such coaptation. Also, an intraluminal filling defect, a dilated vein, impaired flow or homogeneous echogenicity may be seen. Further, a free-floating thrombus may be encountered. Audible Doppler signals are sampled from each vein and it is these 2 elements of the test which give the term duplex its meaning. As with the continuous-wave Doppler examination, there is spontaneous cyclic flow as well as phasicity with respiration and augmentation with distal or proximal compression. Addition of color can supplement the analysis of audible Doppler signals and is useful for the diagnosis of thrombi below the knee.

In evaluation of a patient for venous reflux, 2 methods are in common use. The first and most accurate is the use of pneumatic tourniquets with rapid deflation to produce a standardized stimulus to venous reflux. The second is the use of augmentation maneuvers of distal compression and release to assess presence or absence of venous reflux. Because the stimulus is not standardized, this is a less accurate method of examination and is not reliably consistent from one patient to another.

In all examinations for reflux, the most accurate method is to have the patient standing with the weight placed upon the contralateral extremity. The standing position allows maximal hydrostatic pressure from the volume of venous blood to be applied to the valves. Standing also amplifies dilation of the venous system, which in turn enhances the detection of venous reflux.[21] Some respected authorities advocate other positions for examination of the patient for reflux, but our experience has been that the standing position is most accurate.[22]

At all times, variations in venous anatomy should be recorded and described. Vein diameter, evidence of obstruction, and evidence of reflux should be noted. The exact protocol varies in each laboratory, but in all cases it should be systematic and thorough. The confluence of veins in the groin will identify the common femoral vein, greater saphenous vein at the saphenofemoral junction and proximal femoral vein. Inflation and deflation of the 24-inch thigh cuff will stimulate reflux flow. Doppler sampling should be done at an angle of insonation of less than 60°. Examination should continue with the 12-inch pneumatic cuff placed on the mid-portion of the calf. The distal one-third of calf veins at the popliteal level should be examined. Then the popliteal vein, the lesser saphenous vein and the gastrocnemius veins should be assessed. The exact confluence of the saphenous vein and popliteal veins should be assessed, and distance from the heel pad recorded, to allow accurate location during surgical intervention.

Perforating veins can be detected using the duplex instrument. The identification of perforating veins is important in chronic venous insufficiency because perforating vein incompetence may lead to transmission of high venous pressure to unsupported subcutaneous veins and intracutaneous post-capillary venules. Identification of perforating veins in the lower extremity can be difficult even for experienced sonographers, and no specific technique has been established as a standard. In the thigh, medial perforating veins are best identified with the use of color Doppler and imaging in a transverse axis. Perforating thigh veins are those that connect the greater saphenous vein to the femoral or popliteal vein.[23]

In the leg, the 5 clusters of medial perforating veins are relatively consistent and connect the posterior arch vein system to the posterior tibial veins. These are identified and distances from the heel pad noted. Lateral calf perforating veins should be sought in situations of stigmata of CVI on the outer aspects of the ankle. After perforating veins are identified on the duplex scan, manual compression can be used to determine directions of flow.[24] Manual compression should be applied both above and below the transducer, and color Doppler will help to determine whether there is superficial to deep venous blood flow or the reverse.

Venography (Phlebography)

Radiographs of the veins after intravenous injection of radio-opaque contrast were first made in the 1920s, but the technique was used little until after the 1950s. The usual contrast media are organic compounds containing iodine. Low-osmolality contrast media are less painful and less thrombogenic than the media used some years ago. Although the correct term for contrast visualization of the venous system is phlebography, in fact the term venography is in common use and therefore will be used throughout this section. All of the commonly-used media give good opacification of the veins but, being heavier than blood, they tend to layer out on the dependent side of the vessels, therefore it is essential to fill the veins with contrast medium.

Ascending Venography

This is a standard technique suitable for well over 90% of the clinical situations in which phlebography is indicated. While the ideal position for the patient is vertical, this is not well tolerated by most patients, and a 20°-60° foot-down position is usually all that is necessary, especially when it is combined with the use of tourniquets to force the contrast media into the deep venous system.

As in assessing venous pressures, cannulation of the vein on the dorsum of the distal half of the forefoot is suitable for puncture. Situations that require venography may cause edema, and this makes intravenous injection difficult. However, prolonged pressure on the area to be cannulated, either with foam rubber or elastic bandage or both will disperse the edema from the forefoot sufficiently to make a distended subcutaneous vein visible. A tourniquet at the ankle will cause the medium to pass directly into the deep venous system through the perforating veins of the dorsum of the foot.

Each lower extremity is examined separately and, in addition to an above-ankle tourniquet, a second tourniquet can be applied above the knee. As indicated, the table is tilted 20°-60° downward and the foot and ankle internally rotated to separate the images of the tibia and fibula. Films are taken of the deep veins of the calf in both the anterolateral and lateral projections. The lateral view is obtained by rotating the foot and ankle outward until the side of the calf lies flat on the tabletop. The upper tourniquet may be removed during the procedure and further exposure is made to show the veins as far as the inferior vena cava. However, inadequate filling of the iliac veins and vena cava may call for direct puncture of the femoral veins. If this is required and there is any suspicion of proximal iliac venous occlusion, a transducer should be attached so that differential pressures can be taken and compared.

Variations of the technique detailed above are in common use. One technique has been popularized by DeWeese.[25] Another which is similar, but is essentially examination of the nonweight-bearing extremity, has been popularized by Rabinov.[26] An alternative technique has been proposed by Nicolaides, in which a bandaged leg is examined so that the images from the soleal veins are less confusing.[27]

Ascending phlebography is used chiefly to detect obstruction of the venous system, either in the search for deep venous thrombosis or for chronic occlusions such as the May-Thurner syndrome. Because the latter can be treated effectively by interventional radiologic techniques, it is important that the iliac veins be well visualized during ascending phlebography. As mentioned above, this may require direct femoral venous puncture.

Descending Phlebography

This procedure can be performed by catheterizing a brachial vein and directing the catheter to the selected femoral vein. However, this technique is flawed by development of upper extremity superficial thrombophlebitis. Jugular cannulation can also be utilized. Direct cannulation of the femoral vein and insertion of guidewire and catheters by the Seldinger technique is preferred by many.

The examination is carried out in a steep, semierect position in which an injection of 10-15 mL aliquots of contrast is given. Fluoroscopic control allows the operator to watch the contrast media descend into the thigh and leg. This descent is recorded on radiographs or by cineradiography. A Valsalva maneuver may be added to assist the retrograde flow of contrast media, but the upright position is usually sufficient. False positives may be obtained because the degree of retrograde flow in normal veins in the upright position depends partly on the specific gravity of the contrast medium. It is always heavier than blood. The force of the injection also influences visualization.

The degree of reflux has been graded using a Kistner classification[28] and standardization of the technique[29] allows comparison of reflux between patients. It is Kistner's contribution to valve repair that makes this technique important. Primary venous valvular insufficiency can be selected for direct surgical repair. Descending phlebography is chosen, particularly when the patient is a candidate for such valve repair.

Perforator Venography

The advent of subfascial perforator vein surgery has increased the utility of perforating vein visualization. Duplex examination is usually sufficient. However, the surgeon may need to know the precise location of incompetent perforating veins in order to plan surgical treatment. The standard technique detailed above is modified by applying the ankle and above-knee tourniquets tightly in order to ensure that the contrast media ascends into the deep veins, rather than remaining in the superficial veins.

With the patient in the semi-upright position, the operator can use fluoroscopy to detect flow outward through perforating veins with incompetent valves.[30] Complications of venography include minor reactions such as nausea, vomiting, a feeling of heat and mild urticaria. Most patients will need no treatment because the symptoms pass rather quickly. Severe reactions, including bronchospasm and glottic edema, may require treatment with oral or intravenous antihistamines or intravenous hydrocortisone.

The term *primary venous insufficiency* implies that no specific cause has been found for the pathologic process. For purposes of this discussion, we will consider telangiectasias, reticular varicosities and varicose veins to have the same causes. This is not a universally-held point of view, since the World Health Organization has defined varicose veins as saccular dilation of the veins which are often tortuous, and this definition specifically excludes dilation of small intradermal subcutaneous veins called telangiectasias.[31] Other studies have separated dilated venules, hyphen-webs or telangiectasias from dilated superficial tributaries, which are reticular veins from dilated saphenous veins or trunk veins. Nevertheless, as our knowledge has increased, we believe that it is best to group telangiectasias, reticular varicosities and varicose veins under a common term, primary venous insufficiency, as aspects of epidemiology and etiology appear to be shared by all of these entities.

In 2002, the president of AVF appointed an ad hoc committee to review classification and make recommendations for change in 2004, 10 years after the CEAP inception. The ad hoc committee has been working together with an international committee in order to reach an international consensus on the suggested changes.

The following is the report on definitions:

Telangiectasia. A confluence of dilated intradermal venules of less than 1 mm in caliber. Synonyms include spider veins, hyphen webs and thread veins.

Reticular veins. Dilated bluish intradermal veins usually from 1 mm in diameter to less than 3 mm in diameter. They are usually tortuous. This excludes normal visible veins in people with transparent skin. Synonyms include blue veins, intradermal varices and venulectasies.

Varicose veins. Subcutaneous dilated veins equal to or more than 3 mm in diameter in the upright position. Varicose veins are usually tortuous, but refluxing tubular veins may be classified as varicose veins. These may involve saphenous veins, saphenous tributaries or nonsaphenous veins. Synonyms include varix, varices and varicosities.

Corona phlebectatica. Fan-shaped pattern of numerous small intradermal veins on the medial or lateral aspects of the ankle and foot. Its significance is unclear, but commonly thought to be an early sign of advanced venous disease. Synonyms include malleolar flare and ankle flare.

Edema. Perceptible increase in volume of fluid in the skin and subcutaneous tissue characterized by indentation with pressure. Venous edema usually occurs in the ankle region, but it may extend to the leg and foot. It can be difficult to differentiate from lymphedema, which usually involves the toes.

Pigmentation. Brownish darkening of the skin initiated by extravasated blood, which usually occurs in the ankle region but may extend to the leg and foot.

Eczema. Erythematous dermatitis, which may progress to a blistering, weeping or scaling eruption of the skin of the leg. It is often located near varicose veins but may be located anywhere in the leg. Eczema is usually caused by chronic venous disease or by sensitization to local therapy. Synonyms include stasis dermatitis.

Lipodermatosclerosis. Localized chronic inflammation and fibrosis of the skin and subcutaneous tissues, sometimes associated with scarring or contracture of the Achilles tendon. LDS is sometimes preceded by diffuse inflammatory edema of the skin, which may be painful and which is often referred to as hypodermitis. The absence of lymphangitis, lymphadenitis and fever differentiates this condition from erysipelas or cellulitis. LDS is a sign of severe chronic venous disease.

Atrophie blanche or ***white atrophy.*** Circumscribed, often circular whitish and atrophic skin areas surrounded by dilated capillary spots and sometimes hyperpigmentation. This is a sign of severe chronic venous disease. Scars of healed ulceration are excluded in this definition.

Venous ulcer. Chronic defect of the skin most frequently around the ankle that fails to heal spontaneously because of chronic venous disease.

The term primary venous insufficiency is also applicable to limbs with ankle hyperpigmentation and even ulceration because it is well known that superficial venous reflux can cause these entities in the absence of any other cause, such as deep venous thrombosis. When hyperpigmentation and ulceration is present, the term chronic venous insufficiency applies. This does not exclude primary venous insufficiency as the cause of this condition.

Epidemiology

Until now, all studies of epidemiology of varicose veins and primary venous insufficiency have been flawed. In the United States, surveys in 1935 and again in 1959 were conducted by lay interviewers, as was the UK Survey of Sickness in England and Wales in 1950. Other studies in Denmark and Canada, and regional surveys have similarly been flawed. However, if we take the findings of all of the studies, we find a remarkably consistent prevalence of varicose veins in approximately 2% of the general population.

The prevalence of a condition is the estimated number of patients in whom the condition exists at a specific time. Some local surveys have shown a greater prevalence, with a variation between 4% and 15%, and this disparity is due to varying diagnostic criteria as well as varying levels of proficiency of the observers. One can accept the prevalence figure of 2% of the population, and should also recognize that the incidence of varicose veins increases with age, so as the average age of the population increases, the incidence of venous insufficiency will also increase.[5]

Causes of Varicose Veins

Historically, a number of theories have been proposed for the development of varicose veins. None of these theories has been totally accepted, so one must be content with observations rather than a unifying theory of origin. In general, the concept that varicose veins are caused by descending valvular incompetence has been accepted for more than 100 years. There is no firm proof that this is actually true, but it is logical. Clinical experience suggests that tributary veins to longitudinal, axial veins may become varicose and incompetent before there is any evidence of greater saphenous incompetence (Figure 5).

We believe that the forces of gravitational hydrostatic pressure and hydrodynamic pressure from muscular contraction can both be transmitted to unsupported superficial veins, causing dilation of reticular veins to produce reticular varicosities, dilation of tributary veins to the saphenous system to produce varicose veins, and dilation of venules in the dermis and epidermis to produce telangiectasias. This is a unified theory that allows all risk factors to act together or separately to produce primary venous insufficiency.[2]

The theory of defective structure of the vein wall has been under study for many years. In general, it is agreed that the number of valves in varicose greater

Figure 5

Causation of varicose veins

The theory of causation of varicose veins by descending valvular incompetence is well known. Less well understood is the fact that tributary varicose veins become elongated, dilated and stretched because of pressure from within the muscular compartments. As shown here, the tributary varicosities may precede the development of incompetence in the greater and lesser saphenous veins.

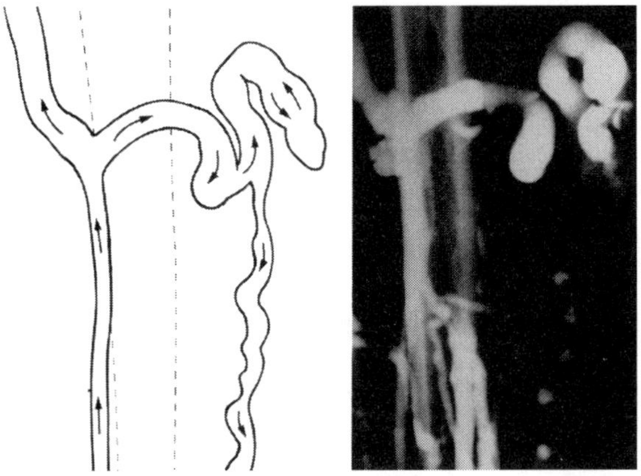

From Browse NL, Burnand KG, Irvine AT, Wilson NM. Diseases of the Veins. *London, England: Edward Arnold & Co; 1999.*

saphenous veins is significantly fewer than the number found in normal greater saphenous veins, and that prominent dilations occur below the cornua of the valve cusps and not proximal to the valve cusps.[32] The fact that tributaries of perforating veins are elongated and tortuous suggests that reversal of flow through the perforating vein dilates the tributaries and, finally, the greater saphenous vein for the most part shows little evidence of lengthening, while varicose tributaries are greatly elongated and tortuous. Defects in the vein wall have been studied, and in general it can be said that the collagen content of varicose veins is lower than that of normal veins, and more muscle fibers are found in varicose than in normal veins.[33]

A number of studies support the theory of vein wall weakness.[34] For example, the normal saphenous vein, when inserted as an arterial conduit, has no difficulty withstanding arterial pressure, but when varicose veins are used as conduits in the arterial system, these segments invariably dilate or develop localized aneurysms. Some have suggested that arteriovenous shunts are the cause of varicose veins.[35] Varices may have an increased oxygen content compared to normal veins. We believe that these observations, though correct, are secondary to chronic venous hypertension that disrupts the normal capillary barrier. It may be that oxygen-free radicals and reduction in antiperoxidase activity may have a role in the development of vein wall weakness.[36]

A number of elements have been described as predisposing causative factors for developing varicose veins and Table 4 lists them. Among all of these, one can generalize that an inherited structural weakness is highly correlated with development of varicose veins. Advanced age, female sex, previous pregnancy, race and occupation may all contribute to the development of varicose veins.

Table 5 lists symptoms and signs that may be caused by primary venous insufficiency.

Natural History of Primary Varicose Veins

It is generally assumed that varicose veins are a naturally progressive condition. However, it is clear that telangiectasias do not progress to varicose veins. Instead, they remain telangiectasias and spread either in an upward or downward direction. The natural history studies of the Bochum children verify that varicosities are progressive and telangiectasias tend to spread.[37]

Although progression is the rule, certain circumstances may cause varicose veins to regress. Chief among these is regression after pregnancy. Multiple pregnancies clearly cause varicose veins to enlarge and progress distally. Palliative treatment such as proximal saphenous vein ligation may also cause temporary regression of superficial varicosities, but it is clear that varicose veins recurring following such surgery are frequently associated with return of saphenous vein reflux. Similarly, palliative treatment with external elastic support seems to relieve some symptoms but does not prevent progression of the varicosities. Now that long-term studies are becoming available, it is clear that patients with large varicose veins will progress within 12-15 years to leg ulcer in 20% of cases. Thus, the statement that the propensity to develop varicose veins is progressive and incurable is generally accepted to be true. This does not mean that treatment should be abandoned, because satisfactory palliation of the condition is quite readily available.[38]

Observations of perforating vein blood flow can be important in defining the natural history of varicose veins.[39] Some perforating veins allow reentry of blood into the deep venous system from reflux down the saphenous vein. Other perforating veins have an opposite direction of blood flow, outward from the deep circulation veins. The first group of limbs does not appear to suffer from skin changes; it is the second group of limbs with venous outflow through perforating veins that seems to be prone to skin changes.

Diagnostic Studies

The history and physical examination are the basis for initial evaluation of patients with varicose veins and telangiectasias. Continuous-wave Doppler can be used at the time of initial clinical evaluation to assist in confirming the clinical diagnosis.[40,41] Reflux can be detected by a Valsalva maneuver or limb compression and release. The Valsalva test will be unreliable if there is proximal valve competence such as in the external iliac or common

Table 4

Potential Causative Factors for Primary Venous Insufficiency

Advanced age
Left lower extremity versus right
Female sex
Bowel habits
Race
Sedentary occupation
Weight
Family history
Alcohol use
Previous pregnancy
Diet
Possible contributing causes:
Obesity
Height
Tight clothing
Erect stance

Table 5

Symptoms and Signs of Primary Venous Insufficiency

Indications for Intervention

Unsightliness
Superficial thrombophlebitis
Aching pain
External hemorrhage
Nocturnal cramps
Hyperpigmentation
Ankle edema
Lipodermatosclerosis
Dermatitis with or without itching
Ulceration

femoral vein. The continuous-wave Doppler examination is a subjective evaluation, and before any intervention is attempted preliminary findings should be followed by objective testing. If the patient presents with large varices or symptoms that are questionably related to venous insufficiency, such as mild edema or aching, duplex scanning should be done.[42,43]

Confirmatory testing with strain gauge plethysmography[40] or air plethysmography may be performed, but the accuracy of photoplethysmography has been challenged recently, and there is some doubt about the reliability of air plethysmography as well. Because all plethysmographic testing gives a global view of the limb, duplex scanning has become the method of choice for testing individual veins of the superficial, deep, and perforating systems.[44,45] Duplex scanning determines whether deep or superficial veins are involved, and gives information about the specific segments of veins which are either incompetent or obstructed. Duplex scanning can detect the presence of incompetent perforating veins and can determine the anatomy of veins in the popliteal fossa. In further investigation of varicose veins, it is usually unnecessary to proceed to phlebography. Similarly, ambulatory venous pressure gives no additional information that will guide therapy.

Treatment of Primary Venous Insufficiency

Recalling that primary venous insufficiency encompasses telangiectasias and reticular varicosities as well as varicose veins, it is logical to assume that the minor conditions without symptoms require no treatment at all. Individuals who tolerate the appearance of telangiectasias and minor varicose veins, and who are without aching pain relieved by leg elevation need not have any treatment whatsoever. However, physicians do see patients who have sought out medical advice due to symptoms, and the options for treatment must be explained to each patient (Table 6).

All practitioners agree that compression is the first line of treatment of all venous insufficiency, and in fact is treatment of choice of the chronically swollen limb. Some general rules apply in this situation. The first is that stockings that cross the popliteal space interfere with return of blood flow from the leg below the knee. Admittedly, some patients need elastic support in the distal and middle thirds of the thigh, and it should be recognized that elastic support in this area would compromise some flow in the popliteal space. The second rule is that varying grades of stockings will produce various results. Over-the-counter and antiembolism stockings have approximately 18 mm Hg pressure at the ankle with a gradient decreasing to virtually zero at the top of the stocking. The lowest grade of therapeutic stockings has 20-30 mm Hg at the ankle, and use of this stocking will reduce symptoms of venous insufficiency. Most cases of CVI with ankle pigmentation, corona phlebectatica and lipodermatosclerosis will require stockings of 30-40 mm Hg compression at the ankle.

The most severe forms of chronic swelling, such as class 6 with open ulcer or class 5 with healed ulcer, as well as lymphedema, will require no-stretch bandaging such as the CircAid® or short-stretch bandaging in multiple layers as is used in Europe. In Europe, the Hohenstein Institute has set certain standards for stockings, and they are classified according to the ankle compression that is delivered. According to this scale, class 1 stockings deliver 18.4-21.05 mm Hg compression at the ankle, class 2 stockings deliver 25.2-32.2 mm Hg, and class 3 stockings deliver 36.5-46.6 mm Hg. There is also a class 4 stocking which delivers 59 mm Hg pressure. The Institute approves stockings and assures the consumer that the compression that is advertised will be delivered by the stocking.

Table 6

Treatment of Primary Venous Insufficiency

None (if symptoms are minor and tolerated by the patient)
External elastic compression
Sclerotherapy
Laser therapy
Surgical intervention

Sclerotherapy is used for telangiectasias and reticular varicosities. Many practitioners also use sclerotherapy for large varicose veins, and this has been in common practice from the 1940s onward. Modern methods of diagnosis have shown that axial reflux defeats attempts at sclerotherapy, and that the overall rule that the smaller the venulectasia, the greater the success with sclerotherapy still holds. Some experts also attempt to obliterate axial reflux by performing sclerotherapy of the greater and the lesser saphenous vein. There are dangers in doing this, just as there are liabilities of performing surgery. The technique is not generally accepted at this time.

Laser and other light therapies have been used extensively to obliterate telangiectasias and venulectasias. However, the margin between success of treatment and production of skin necrosis is very small, and most would agree that the use of laser should be confined to the upper extremities, neck, and face, rather than in treatment of lower extremity blemishes.

Surgical Intervention

Indications for intervention in primary venous insufficiency include unsightly appearance, aching pain, leg heaviness, easy leg fatigue, superficial thrombophlebitis, external bleeding, ankle hyperpigmentation, lipodermatosclerosis, atrophie blanche and venous ulcer. Often, it is the appearance of telangiectatic blemishes or protuberant varicosities that stimulates consultation. Ultimately, this may be the only indication for intervention (Table 7).

Unfortunately, negative physician perception regarding availability and efficacy of treatment of varices may deny the patient the precise care which is sought.[46] Furthermore, symptoms of primary venous insufficiency may be present but not recognized by the patient until sought for during thorough history taking. The characteristic symptoms include aching pain, easy leg fatigue and leg heaviness, all worsening as the day progresses, so that the patient must sit down in the afternoon and elevate the legs for some relief. These symptoms will be most severe on the first day of a menstrual period. The symptoms may not be recognized by the patient as being due to the varicose veins or telangiectasias, and must be inquired about by the examining physician. Neither the patient nor the physician may understand that these symptoms may arise from telangiectatic blemishes just as easily as from venous varicosities, but this is the fact. Some 50% of patients with telangiectasias will have such symptoms, and 85% will be able to find relief with appropriate therapy.[47]

Saphenous Ligation Versus Stripping

Objectives of treatment of severe CVI should be ablation of the hydrostatic forces of axial reflux and removal of the hydrodynamic forces of perforator vein outward flow. Table 7 lists surgical options in such treatment. Saphenectomy should be combined with phlebectomy of vein clusters to achieve ablation of high-pressure conduits and excision or obliteration of their target vessels. Fundamentally, only 2 surgical approaches, ligation alone and ligation plus removal or stripping, have been used in treatment of primary venous insufficiency.

In an old Mayo Clinic study, Lofgren examined limbs of patients for up to 5 years following high saphenous ligation or complete ankle-to-groin stripping. He reported 94% excellent or good results after stripping, compared to 40% after high tie.[48]

Table 7

Surgical Intervention of Primary Venous Insufficiency

Saphenous vein ligation

Greater saphenous vein ligation and stripping
    Stripping ankle to groin
    Stripping groin to ankle

Short stripping of saphenous vein
    Groin to knee
    Lesser saphenous vein ligation
    Gastrocnemius vein ligation
    Stripping of lesser saphenous vein

Radiofrequency ablation of the saphenous vein
Restoration of proximal valve competence (external banding)

This and other old studies were dismissed by some as being too subjective.[49,50]

More recently, saphenous vein stripping and stab avulsion has been compared to saphenous high tie and midthigh perforator interruption.[50] This study found no differences in either patient or physician evaluation of the limbs at 3 years. The report has also been criticized because the evaluation was felt to be subjective, not objective.[51]

Six prospective studies have compared stripping of the saphenous vein to high ligation,[51-54,57,58] and these were the subject of an editorial analysis.[56] The Middlesex group,[51] in their prospective, randomized study, used duplex scanning for postoperative examination of valvular incompetence and PPG as a measure of overall venous physiology, and found that "both objective tests of venous function as well as subjective assessment suggest that the results 21 months after surgery . . . are improved by . . . long saphenous vein stripping from groin to calf."

At Maastricht,[52] stripping and ligation were prospectively randomized. Physician and patient assessment of results at 3 years was supplemented by Doppler ultrasound examination with the conclusion that ". . . the results remained significantly better for the stripping group . . ."

In Copenhagen, Jakobsen's prospective evaluation[53] (confirmed by Carl Arnoldi[1]) concluded that saphenous varices are best treated by radical operation (stripping as compared to high tie), in spite of the fact that the period of disability is significantly longer.[53] In a New Zealand trial, each patient served as their own control, and evaluation was by a single observer at intervals up to 3-5 years after operation.[54,55] Results, judged only by incidence of recurrent varicosities ". . . were significantly better in limbs from which the long saphenous vein had been stripped. However, saphenous nerve paresthesias biased patient evaluation against ankle-to-groin stripping."

At Lund, conventional subjective and objective evaluation was supplemented by foot volumetry before and after treatment.[56,57] The authors concluded "this study clearly supports the conclusion that CST (compression sclerotherapy) alone or in combination with high tie cannot replace radical surgery (saphenous stripping, perforator interruption, and stab avulsion) for varicose vein disease with saphenous incompetence."

Only Hammarstein's study concluded ". . . that the removal of the long saphenous vein per se is of no therapeutic value if all perforators have been ligated."[58] However, as he emphasized in a later letter, only "by means of a thorough (ascending and descending) phlebographic mapping of the insufficient perforators . . . was precise perforator ligation possible."[59] In commenting on this, Darke suggested that with regard to elimination of perforator-induced saphenous recurrences, ". . . the simplest and least costly and uncomplicated way of eradicating the problem is to remove the saphenous trunk along with the existing and potentially incompetent perforators."[60]

Saphenous Preservation

Despite objective verification of lasting benefit of groin-to-knee stripping, ligation of the saphenous vein at the saphenofemoral junction has been practiced widely. This is being done in the belief that it will control gravitational reflux and preserve the vein for subsequent arterial bypass. It is true that the saphenous vein is largely preserved after proximal ligation.[61] However, its reflux continues and hydrostatic forces are not controlled.[62] As stated above: 1.) recurrent varicose veins are more frequent after saphenous ligation than after stripping of the saphenous vein in the thigh; 2.) recurrent varicose veins are more frequent after saphenous ligation and sclerotherapy than after stripping and sclerotherapy; and 3.) prospective, randomized trials comparing proximal saphenous ligation and stab avulsion of varices to stripping of the thigh portion of the saphenous vein and stab avulsion of varices has shown superior results of the latter procedure.

In summary, careful duplex evaluation of proximal saphenous vein ligation 2 years following intervention has shown that, "a large group of patients (33%) had developed significant collateral veins at the level of the operative site." 95% of the saphenous veins were patent to within 10 cm of ligation and 88% were incompetent.[63]

Finally, in studying recurrent varicose veins, preservation of patency of the saphenous vein and continued reflux in the saphenous vein have been found to be the most frequent elements in varicose recurrence. In patients presenting for surgical relief of recurrent varicosities, it has been found that two-thirds required removal of the saphenous vein as part of the repeat procedure.

Ankle-to-Groin Stripping

Before accurate delineation of site of origin of varicosities was made possible by duplex scan, ankle-to-groin stripping of the saphenous vein was considered to be the standard operation to be performed in every operated case. Turn-of-the-century publications conveyed the belief that reflux was uniformly distributed over the entire length of the saphenous vein.

Now the object of excision of the saphenous vein is to remove its gravitational reflux and detach its perforator vein tributaries in the thigh. It has been found to be unnecessary to remove the portion below the knee. Removing the thigh portion detaches perforating veins and communicating veins that enter the saphenous vein.[64] In the leg below the knee, perforating veins enter the posterior arch vein circulation for the most part. There are many venous variations on this general theme of perforator attachments and these variations may be the cause of postoperative recurrent varicosities and persistent perforating veins. However, in legs with severe CVI, the perforating veins of the posterior arch system can only be approached subfascially.

Excision of Varicose Clusters

Table 8 shows the location of common patterns of clusters of varicosities and indicates which perforating veins will be detached from the superficial venous circulation by local phlebectomy. In a significant number of patients, the saphenofemoral junction will be found to be competent and therefore can be left intact. When this is true, thigh varicosities often arise from a refluxing anterolateral tributary to the saphenofemoral junction. Judgment will determine whether the saphenous vein should be removed, left in place intact or ligated. Stab avulsion of clusters of varicosities derived from reflux from Hunterian or Dodd perforating veins may also remove segments of the greater saphenous vein. Those patients who are found to have lesser saphenous venous incompetence will need to have careful removal or ligation of some or all of that structure.

Saphenous Vein Ablation

Removal of the great saphenous vein (GSV) from the circulation is one of two essential steps in treating lower limb varicose veins. Incompetent valves along the GSV allow blood to reflux down the vein and into its tributaries, transmitting high pressure into smaller tributaries, which become varicose as a result. Much emphasis has been placed on the correct technique of high sapheno-femoral ligation, in which meticulous attention is paid to identifying, ligating and dividing all the tributaries of the GSV as they join the vein in the groin. It has always been a matter of surgical dogma that overlooking any of these allows continued reflux into the residual tributary and subsequent development of recurrent varicose veins.

A number of studies have confirmed that patients in whom the GSV is stripped tend to have fewer recurrences than those undergoing simple high ligation of the sapheno-femoral junction (SFJ). Sarin et al studied 89 limbs in 69 patients with LSV incompetence. Legs were randomized to SFJ ligation with or without stripping, and evaluated by photoplethys-

Table 8

Targets of Phlebectomy of Varicose Clusters

Location of varices	Perforator
Medial thigh, mid third	Hunterian
Medial thigh, distal third	Dodd
Medial leg, upper third	Boyd
Ankle, posteromedial	Cockett
Ankle, anteromedial	Sherman
Posterolateral knee crease	Unnamed

mography (PPG), Duplex scanning, clinical examination and patient satisfaction. The follow-up period was 18 months. Significant differences in favor of the stripped group were found in all 4 parameters at final evaluation.

A similar study of 78 patients (110 limbs) was reported by Dwerryhouse et al in 1999, with a longer follow-up period of 5 years. This demonstrated a significantly lower reoperation rate among patients undergoing GSV stripping (6%), as opposed to 20% in those undergoing high SFJ ligation alone. Duplex scanning showed a much lower incidence of residual reflux in the remaining GSV when the proximal vein had been stripped to the knee than when it had not. However, the patient satisfaction rate was not significantly different between the two groups. 90% of the stripped group were satisfied, as opposed to 77% in the non-stripped group (*P* = NS).

A further study from Jones et al came to similar conclusions 100 patients (133 limbs) were randomized as before. After 2 years, 43% of those who had not had GSV stripping demonstrated recurrent varicose veins, as opposed to 25% who had. There was a statistically significant difference.

Of great importance was the fact that Duplex scanning showed that neovascularisation in the groin was the commonest cause of recurrence. It is often seen that reflux through the neovascularization enters the residual saphenous vein and perpetuates the old varices while new ones develop. The authors concluded that by stripping the GSV one was removing the run-off into which the new vessels could drain. Again, however, the satisfaction was broadly similar between the 2 groups: 91% in the stripped group and 87% in the unstripped.

All of these authors concluded that stripping the long GSV gave better long-term results than simple high saphenous ligation. This appears to be true in terms of objective assessment of recurrence rates and in objective measurement of postoperative venous function, but is not generally reflected in patient satisfaction rates, which tend to be similar whichever procedure is performed. This led Woodyer and Dormandy to reach a contrary conclusion—that stripping the LSV was a procedure based on surgical dogma, and one that did not confer subjective benefit to the patients so treated.

RF and Laser Ablation

In recent years, endovenous ablation has been found to be safe and effective in eliminating the proximal portion of the GSV from the venous circulation, with even faster recovery and better cosmetic results than stripping. The currently available methods used to achieve ablation of the GSV are: the early Closure© procedure using a radiofrequency (RF) catheter and generator (VNUS Medical Technologies, Inc., Sunnyvale, California); and the newer Closure© procedure using a Closure-FAST TM radiofrequency catheter that utilizes segmental ablation instead of the old pull-back approach, resulting in a shorter treatment time; and the endovenous laser ablation (EVLA) procedure using a laser fiber and generator (various manufacturers). Both systems use electromagnetic energy to destroy the GSV *in situ*.

The endovenous techniques appear to be as effective as surgery in treating varicose veins. In a meta-analysis comparing varicose vein treatments of 12,320 limbs, radiofrequency ablation (RFA) and EVLA were reported to be more effective than surgery or ultrasound guided sclerotherapy (UGS).[65] At 3 months, the success rates of surgery, UGFS, RFA and EVLA were 80.4%, 82.1%, 88.8% and 92.9%, correspondingly. EVLA was reported to be the most effective long-term treatment modality. At 5 years, the success rates of surgery, UGFS and RFA fell under 80% whereas the success rate of EVLA was 95.4%. Outcome measures were based on ultrasound evidence of obliteration/closure of the insufficient veins. Large, comparative randomized clinical trials do not yet exist, and standardized outcome measures have not been established.

One of the difficulties in evaluating reports of successful ablation of the great saphenous vein lies in the definition of "success." Some, especially in the RF ablation reports, define success as "no reflux in any segment longer than 5 cm." Some laser reports refer to success as "stable occlusion" or "reduction in reflux," while Min has applied the much clearer standard of success as "no flow by color flow Doppler." Those who report results have not used the life table method, which takes into consideration dropouts and early and mid term failures. Thus, the favorable reported 4- and 5-year rates of elimination of reflux may be exaggerated.

The major difficulty with defining success as reduction or absence of reflux is that attempts to establish whether reflux is present in a portion of a previously closed GSV may be inaccurate. Also, most recurrent patency is seen in the proximal portion of the treated GSV; therefore, distal compression of the closed portion of the GSV to identify reflux in a proximal segment is futile. Likewise, using the Valsalva maneuver is unreliable and lacks reproducibility. Finally, the importance of distinguishing a partially patent channel with flow from one with reflux is academic, since the valves are just as thoroughly destroyed as the rest of the vein wall.

Initially, reports of successful ablation of the GSV using either radiofrequency or laser energy without ligation or stripping were treated with great skepticism. However, the absence of neovascularization is striking and many skeptics have begun to believe that former emphasis on a clean groin dissection may have been in error. Patient acceptance of these minimally invasive procedures is overwhelmingly better than with stripping.

Choosing which procedure to adopt, according to Morrison, is influenced by a variety of factors, including reported results (and especially reporting methods); economic factors, such as equipment and disposables costs, reimbursement, procedure time; availability of and experience with ultrasound equipment and trained personnel; individual support by industry before, during and after acquisition of the generator; and the practitioner's own level of expertise and comfort with ultrasound guided techniques and minimally invasive surgery.

Chemical Venous Closure

Some phlebologists have advocated liquid sclerotherapy of the saphenous vein, but the results of such treatment have been disappointing and published long-term results are absent. Comparisons between liquid and foam sclerotherapy have been done and the results strongly favor foam. Ultrasound-guided sclerotherapy (USGS) with foam must be considered as a completely new treatment of varicose veins. Although it needs proper training and some skill, it is simple, affordable and extremely efficient.

Sclerosing agents produce a lesion of the venous wall, predominantly of the endothelium and, to a minor extent, of the media. The reaction that follows depends on the concentration of the agent and on the duration of the contact. If the venous diameter is greater than 3 mm, injections of liquid do not achieve this aim and dilution with blood quickly decreases their efficacy at short distances from the point of injection. Injections of foam have the advantage of a total filling of the vein, at least under 12 mm diameter. A further reduction in venous diameter can be obtained by reverse Trendelenberg position, compression with the hand, Duplex probe or bandage, and by venous spasm. In very large veins, foam will float over blood and induce a lesion of the upper venous wall, despite an apparent correct filling of the vein observed on duplex, thus the importance of massaging and compression.

Making the foam is easy and quick. Based on the technique initially described by Tessari, it can be prepared with two 5 cc syringes and a three-way stopcock. Only detergent sclerosing agents can be used: Sotradecol® and polidocanol at any desired concentration from 0.25% to 3%. Microbubbles of foam sclerosing agents are hyperechogenic and represent an excellent contrast medium for ultrasound techniques. They appear as a shadow within the lumen early, and like a hyperechogenic mass later with an acoustic shadow. Massaging the sclerosing agent to the desired part of the varicose network with the duplex probe or the hand is also very easily carried out. Progression from the varicose clusters to the GSV and then to the SFJ is always visible, provided a sufficient volume has been injected. Venous spasm is usually observed within minutes. The importance of the initial spasm has been emphasized in several studies and protocols.

Postsclerotherapy compression is mandatory: on the varicose clusters for 48 hours, and then whole limb compression with 20-30 mmHg thigh-high medical elastic stockings. They must be worn during the day for at least 15 days. Patients must be examined both clinically and with Duplex at 7 to 15 days.

In a European review of 67 studies evaluating over 9000 limbs treated with foam sclerotherapy, it was concluded that UGS is safe and effective for treating varicose veins.[66] Serious adverse events, such as deep venous thrombosis and pulmonary embolism, and arterial events such as stroke were statistically rare. The absolute risk of deep venous thrombosis is not confirmed. A few cases have been reported, most of them are gastrocnemius veins thrombosis, typically after telangiectasias and reticular veins sclerotherapy. Systemic adverse events such as visual disturbance, transient confusion, or cough were reported in rates that ranged from 0%-5.9%. Headaches ranged from 0%-23%. Visual disturbances have been observed also with liquid sclerosing agents, but their incidence is much higher with foam, and can be estimated at 0.5-1 per 100 foam sessions. They are observed more frequently in patients suffering from migraine with visual aura. They usually reproduce this aura. The pathophysiology of this phenomenon has been questioned but there is no given answer at this point. The existence of a patent foramen oval is the most likely explanation, as well as the liberation of toxic component associated with endothelial cells destruction (endothelin). Local adverse events such as thrombophlebitis, skin matting and pain at the injection site were variable, but more common. Overall, the risk of adverse events was not significantly different from that of liquid sclerotherapy or open surgery.

All published results demonstrate an immediate efficacy better than 80% in terms of immediate/primary venous occlusion. Repetition of injections in case of initial failure allows closure to approach 95% of efficacy with 2-3 sessions. Early and mid-term results demonstrate a recurrence rate about 20%. The re-do injections remain as simple as primary injections and are at least as efficient.

If saphenopopliteal incompetence is found, attention must be paid to the small aphenous vein. As most lesser saphenous vein reflux is segmental, many surgeons practice ligation and division of the lesser saphenous vein and ligation and division of gastrocnemius veins, rather than performing stripping of the lesser saphenous vein. It is the specter of sural nerve injury that validates this approach.

Imaging of the saphenopopliteal junction must be carried out preoperatively. Varicography allowed this in the past, but now duplex examination is perfectly adequate, and the ultrasonographer must document the exact level of the saphenopopliteal junction prior to surgery.

5. Chronic Venous Insufficiency

Epidemiology

Although there are no universally accepted definitions of chronic venous insufficiency, gradually the CEAP classes 4, 5 and 6 are delineating the criteria of this entity and classifications used in the past can be translated into this classification. This gives consistent meaning to the terms when one refers to hyperpigmentation at the ankle or depigmentation in chronic scars, as well as open venous leg ulcers or previously healed leg ulcers.

Risk Factors

Although no epidemiologic studies have been done using the CEAP classification, one can glean from a perusal of past epidemiologic studies that the age of the population under consideration is the most important factor. There is a progressive rise in prevalence with age for all grades of chronic venous insufficiency and leg ulceration. The prevalence of all CVI is less certain, and there is a great deal of variation between study methodologies and results. However, using the best available data, we can estimate that for the whole adult population, the overall prevalence of CVI is 1%-3%, with open leg ulcer having a prevalence of 1%.[67] Many more women than men present for treatment, but that may be in part due to their longer lifespan, and perhaps the sex difference in prevalence has been overstated in the past.

Theories of Etiology of Venous Ulceration

It is generally agreed that venous ulceration occurs when the muscle pump is impaired due to disordered function, either in the superficial or deep venous system.[68] As indicated earlier, this may be due entirely to varicose veins or primary venous insufficiency,[69] or may develop as a result of failure of valve function in the deep veins. That condition may be due to a previous deep venous thrombosis or primary valve failure in a manner similar to valve failure in superficial venous incompetence.[70] Venous hypertension is linked to development of CVI, but is not the only factor involved. Others may include minor trauma, edema, obesity, arthritis and neuropathies.

Venous Stasis Theory

The prevalent theory of etiology of venous ulceration was proposed by Homans in 1917,[71] and was predominant for nearly 60 years.[72] The theory was that static blood in varices became totally deoxygenated and tissue breakdown was caused by ischemia. We now understand that when the patient stands, there is no difference in venous oxygenation between normal subjects and patients with varicose veins and in fact, the raised blood oxygen content in veins of patients with venous disease leads to the suggestion that arteriovenous fistulae are present. Some have suggested that this deprives the skin of oxygen,[73] but that theory has been thoroughly discredited.[74]

The most prevalent theory of etiology of venous ulceration in the last 25 years of the 20 century has been that oxygen diffusion into the tissues of the skin was restricted by a pericapillary fibrin cuff.[75] This theory posits that venous ulceration occurs when the tissues are deprived of oxygen, much like Homans' original suggestion in 1917. There is no published evidence to prove that fibrin provides a barrier to oxygen diffusion, and there is no reliable evidence that skin and subcutaneous tissues are hypoxic in lipodermatosclerotic skin. Although there is disagreement about this point, methodological differences in measurements can account for most of the data that support the theory of hypoxia. This theory is also now discredited.

White Cell Trapping Hypothesis

White blood cells have been implicated as mediators of ischemia in many tissues, including myocardium, brain, lung and kidneys.[76-79] Activation of leukocytes allows proteolytic enzymes to be released and in addition, a nonmitochondrial respiratory burst which permits these cells to release free radicals including the superoxide radical. These in turn have destructive effects on lipid membranes, proteins and many connective tissue elements.[80] While actual white cell trapping may occur in the lower extremities, it is clear that this does not cause capillary occlusion sufficient to impair oxygenation of the skin.

Histology and capillary microscopy show apparent capillary proliferation in skin affected by severe CVI. Careful recent studies suggest that this is more apparent than real, and that the vessels appear more like a glomerulus than a proliferation of capillaries. Nevertheless, the increased endothelial area allows leukocyte adhesion, especially in areas where adhesion molecules ICAM-1 and ELAM-1 are upregulated. A profound leukocyte infiltration has been seen in patients with CVI79 and both macrophages and T lymphocytes are seen.[81] Cytokines have been identified in such an infiltrate, including interleukins IL-1α and IL-1β, however TNF-α has not been detected. Such an infiltrate is seen in other chronic inflammatory conditions, therefore it is difficult to ascertain which comes first, the inflammation or the leukocyte infiltration.

In studying patients with varicose veins and comparing them to patients with skin changes of lipodermatosclerosis, it has been found that leukocytes initially roll along the endothelium, binding in a loose manner. As binding occurs, soluble L-selectin is released and can be detected by ELISA. In plasma, soluble L-selectin levels rise during venous hypertension, confirming that endothelial leukocyte interaction has occurred. Firm binding of neutrophils and monocytes occurs later and these are linked to endothelial ICAM (Figure 6).[82,83]

Exactly what these events lead to is uncertain and questions remain regarding why ulcers form and why they fail to heal. Nevertheless, the present theories are most attractive and lead to implications for pharmacologic treatment of venous disease. When the fibrin cuff theory was popular, enhancing fibri nolysis was attempted to promote removal of the fibrin cuff, but this treatment did not improve ulcer healing. Clinical trials using pentoxifylline to decrease leukocyte adhesion and activation have yielded conflicting results, but in general the ulcer healing rate seems to be improved, especially when levels of external compression are increased.

There are 2 elements that interact to cause all of the manifestations of lower extremity venous insufficiency. These are failure of the vein valves and vein walls and skin changes at the ankles, both of which are related to venous hypertension.

Figure 6

Surface ligands of neutrophils and monocytes and the endothelial adhesion molecules with which they interact

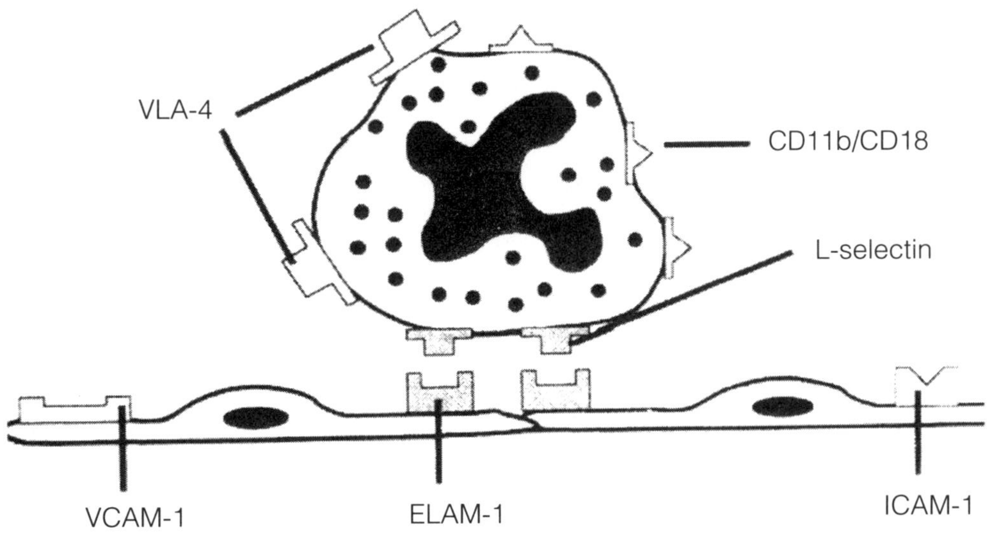

From Ruckley CV, Fowkes FGR, Bradbury A, eds. Venous Disease. *London, England: Springer-Verlag; 1999.*

Our work suggests that venous hypertension causes a sheer stress-dependent leukocyte-endothelial interaction, which has all of the manifestations of chronic inflammation. These are leukocyte rolling, firm adhesion to endothelium and subsequent migration of the cells through the endothelial barrier into parenchyma of valves and vein walls. There, macrophages elaborate matrix metalloproteases, which destroy elastin and possibly collagen as well. Vein walls become stretched and elongated. Vein valves become perforated, torn and even scarred to the point of near total absence. These changes are seen both macroscopically and angioscopically.[15] These changes have been produced in the experimental animal by constructing an arteriovenous fistula.

The second manifestation of chronic venous insufficiency is expressed in the skin where leukocytes are also responsible for the changes which are observed. Skin biopsies have shown that lipodermatosclerotic eczematous skin showed that macrophages and lymphocytes were predominant in such diseased skin. Infiltration of leukocytes into the extracellular space has been documented by observing the localization of these leukocytes around capillaries and postcapillary venules. Accompanying the leukocytes is a disorganized collagen deposition. Clearly, chronic venous insufficiency of the skin and its subcutaneous tissues is a disease of chronic inflammation, again dependent upon venous hypertension.

The primary injury is extravasation of macromolecules and red blood cells into the dermal interstitium. Red blood cell degradation products and intersitial protein extravasations are potent chemoattractants and represent the initial chronic inflammatory signal responsible for leukocyte recruitment.

Diagnostic Studies

As in the assessment of primary venous insufficiency, tests of lower extremity function in CVI may be divided into those that provide anatomic information and those that provide hemodynamic information.

Ascending phlebography has been used to detect obstruction and it remains the most reliable test for obstruction, especially in the iliofemoral system. Because the prevalence of iliofemoral venous thrombosis and resultant impaired blood flow is important in CVI, ascending phlebography must still be considered as part of the diagnostic armamentarium.

Descending phlebography demonstrates reflux in either the superficial or deep veins and determines the exact points of leakage. It is essential that descending phlebography be performed whenever surgical intervention to correct venous valve insufficiency is contemplated. Duplex technology has replaced descending phlebography to a great extent in situations where venous valve repair is not contemplated.

Continuous-wave Doppler ultrasound remains a useful diagnostic test at the time of initial physical examination and is routine in outpatient clinics. It is extremely accurate at detecting popliteal venous reflux. However, the limitation of continuous-wave Doppler ultrasound is that it cannot insonate an individual vessel. It detects flow in any vessel in the path of the ultrasound beam. It is generally agreed that preliminary Doppler ultrasound examination should be confirmed with duplex scanning if surgical intervention is contemplated.

Duplex scanning remains the cornerstone of objective evaluation in limbs with CVI.[84] Multisegmental reflux is usually found in legs with venous ulceration, and patterns of the reflux involve at least 2 of 3 venous systems in about 65% of patients in CEAP classes 4 to 6.[85,86]

Physiologic Testing

Ambulatory venous pressure measurements are always referred to as tests of venous function in CVI. However, the technique is invasive, not easily repeated, and not useful for screening, and therefore has been replaced by plethysmographic techniques. The single exception is the arm/foot differential test of Raju.[87] It provides hemodynamic information on severity of obstruction and the adequacy of recanalization of the collateral circulation. The technique is not used universally and remains a global measure of hemodynamic obstruction due to outflow blockage. In the past, it was used most in selection of patients for venous bypass. The advent of endoluminal therapy to relieve obstruction has caused a reconsideration of use of this test in selection of patients for interventional radiologic treatment.

Plethysmographic techniques have been discussed earlier and are in general use. However, a study of air plethysmography has provided disappointing findings.[88] This report concluded: "Out of the 68 patients, nine were not able to perform the total investigative protocol (13%). Reflux measurement and ejection capacity of the calf muscle pump correlated well with severe venous disease but correlated poorly with mild or absent signs of venous insufficiency. Abnormal refill time measured with the photo techniques was in accordance in 82% with increased reflux with APG but a normal refill time was only correlated with normal-reflux APG in 60% of limbs. It was not possible to distinguish between deep and superficial venous insufficiency. In conclusion, the APG did not turn out to be either a quick or a handy method for quick and accurate screening of venous insufficiency. Its place in the clinical evaluation of venous patients is not yet clear."

In summary, in testing in CVI for simple varicose veins and telangiectasias, a history, physical examination, and hand-held Doppler study is sufficient. When edema is present, these tests may be adequate. However, duplex scanning will often be added depending on its availability. In all cases of CVI with skin changes, with or without ulceration, the simple clinical examination must be supplemented with duplex evaluation, and in cases suspected to need venous reconstruction, ascending and descending phlebography are probably indicated.

Treatment of Chronic Venous Insufficiency

Best medical care of CVI remains nonoperative. This consists of intermittent extremity elevation, strong external elastic support, good wound care, and patient education. Experience teaches that ulcers heal over time in 92%-100% of cases. Nevertheless, the treatment requires prolonged disability and extraordinarily high rates of ulcer recurrence despite persistent utilization of highly skilled care. It is this factor that is of major concern.[89,90]

Ulcer recurrence rates following medical treatment range from 29%-41% in patients who are most compliant and range as high as 70%-100% in noncompliant patients. Unfortunately, when nonoperative treatment fails, surgery is frequently not recommended. Surgical treatment for venous ulcers in those patients with superficial venous incompetence alone consists of total ablation of superficial reflux by saphenofemoral and saphenopopliteal ligation with or without saphenous vein stripping, as well as removal of all varicosities. A cumulative ulcer healing rate of 82%-100% at 18 months has been reported in this subset of patients with only superficial venous insufficiency.[91,92]

While patients with only superficial incompetence may comprise as many as 50% of those with CVI, a significant portion of patients remains who have concomitant perforator vein insufficiency and/or deep venous insufficiency. Interest in correcting these abnormalities goes back to the 1930s and the time of Robert Linton, who suggested ligation of incompetent perforating veins to decrease ulcer recurrence rates. Those direct procedures, often involving a knee-to-ankle incision, did decrease the rate of recurrent ulcerations.[93,94] However, some studies failed to show benefit from perforator interruption alone.[95,96] This controversy has never been settled, but the high rates of wound complications and the prolonged hospitalization required caused the Linton procedure to fall into disuse.[97,98]

Availability of minimally invasive surgical techniques has caused resurgent interest in subfascial endoscopic perforator surgery (SEPS). Experience with this technique has been generally positive and it has been shown that SEPS is effective, safe and promotes more rapid ulcer healing. It has been shown that in limbs with severe CVI, venous hypertension is transmitted to the microcirculation, where it is closely correlated with trophic skin changes. It is the refluxing superficial veins and the incompetent perforating veins that ultimately transmit venous hypertension to the microcirculation. The objective of surgical treatment as described above has been to reduce that microcirculatory hypertension. This is achieved indirectly by superficial vein stripping and perforating vein interruption.

Sclerosant foam reaches the microcirculation just as it does the macrocirculation. The mixture of air with liquid sclerosant displaces the blood from the affected vessel so that there is virtually no dilution of the active agent. Air with its contained nitrogen allows prolonged contact of the agent with the venous endothelium so that fibrosis and obliteration of the lumen occur without damage to surrounding tissue. Thus the effect of the foamed sclerosant is exerted at the end point of venous hypertension—the microcirculation which is inaccessible to all surgical techniques.

Lessons learned from early experience with sclerosant foam in treating venous leg ulcers include the fact that there is no reason to delay treatment if active, invasive infection is absent. Because of this experience, the treatment algorithm for CVI has changed. The simplicity of the treatment, its evident success and the relative freedom from serious complications makes this the first line treatment for venous ulcer and for painful lipodermatosclerosis as well. Ulcer healing is not required before definitive treatment is begun because the effect of foam is to obliterate the abnormal tangle of vessels in the ulcer bed and in the area of lipodermatosclerosis. These vessels are seen by ultrasound to be occluded by the foam ultrasound examination after treatment. Currently, effective compression is applied at the initial patient visit and the ultrasound scan is scheduled. Treatment is given after completion of the venous mapping. The treatment has evolved and is now variable depending on the size of the veins. Specific perforating vein injection is not done at the first treatment. Cannulation is performed in larger veins that are tributary to refluxing saphenous veins. Perforating veins are targeted if the first treatment seems inadequate. In patients who are edema-free when first seen because of effective compression, a preliminary ultrasound scan is done and treatment initiated at the time of the first visit.

Adjunctive Therapy in Chronic Venous Insufficiency

An international task force made up of a panel of 16 experts was assembled to review and objectively evaluate all aspects of CVI. All publications issued from 1983 to 1997 were reviewed by these experts and opinions expressed.[99] The results can be summarized as follows:

Compression remains a mainstay of treatment of CVI, and elastic and stretched bandages have been shown to be effective. Compression stockings may be used, but compression needs to be in excess of 35 mm Hg to be effective. Preliminary results with medications have shown beneficial effects of several vasodilators and oral micronized purified flavonoid fractions, but the evidence for the effectiveness of medications on venous ulcer healing is still limited and further studies are required. There is no evidence that favors the routine administration of antibiotics, and local therapy has as yet unproven adjunctive roles. Sclerotherapy is unlikely to be effective unless there is superficial venous insufficiency, and even so its role is unproven. Patients with active venous ulcer and saphenofemoral or saphenopopliteal junction incompetence do benefit from surgical treatment. Superficial vein surgery has been shown to significantly reduce the rate of ulcer recurrence, with a sustained effect to 4 years. The reduction in ulcer recurrence following superficial vein surgery is irrespective of the presence of deep vein incompetence.[100]

Compression therapy has been taken a step further into nonelastic, nonstretch therapy, and a recent study has shown that this nonstretch therapy is significantly less costly and that it favors faster healing.[101]

6. Venous Thromboembolism

A vast number of clinical studies have been done due to the serious nature of venous thromboembolic disease. It is in this area that evidence-based medicine has had its primary impact. Recent estimates place the mortality from pulmonary embolization at 50,000 per year, and somewhere between 300,000 and 600,000 hospitalizations per year are associated with venous thromboembolic disease.[102] Although it is generally thought that pulmonary embolism is a significant contributor to hospital deaths, and a figure of 10%-15% has been agreed on, a recent autopsy review in a large teaching hospital documented massive fatal pulmonary embolism in only 6% of patients that died there.[103] A major stimulus to investigation of the causes of deep venous thrombosis and pulmonary embolism was the occurrence of pulmonary embolization after major surgical procedures. It is this phenomenon that continues to involve interested surgeons in research on this topic.

The strongest association between surgery and deep venous thrombosis is in cases of orthopedic surgery. The incidence of venous thrombosis in tibial fractures or knee surgery ranges from 50%-65%.[104] Fatal pulmonary embolism appears to have a case frequency of 2%-3%.[105] The incidence of venous thrombosis in patients undergoing general thoracic and abdominal surgery varies widely, ranging from close to zero in young patients undergoing minor elective surgery to 33% or more in elderly patients undergoing major surgery for malignancy.

Multivariate analysis of large groups of surgical patients has identified the risk factors that are associated with venous thromboembolic disease. These include age, magnitude of the surgical procedure, presence of malignancy, duration and type of anesthesia, and use of hormonal preparations, as well as previous thromboembolic events.[106] A consistent feature of venous thromboembolic disease has been the positive association of thrombosis with increasing age. As indicated above, the incidence varies from near zero in younger patients to an incidence of 800 per 100,000 operations by the ninth decade.[107] The association between thromboembolic disease and malignancy has been known since the early reports of Trousseau, and there have been many more recent studies verifying this observation.[108] Several constituents of tumors are highly thrombogenic. The best characterized is the cysteine protease that directly activates factor X.[109]

Obesity has been recognized as one of the traditional risk factors for postoperative venous thrombosis, however, accurate studies on this subject present conflicting data. There are many reasons for this, but one is the association of obesity with more severe operations.[106] Previous deep venous thrombosis may identify individuals with coagulopathy, and a history of DVT is associated with a 2- to 3-fold increase in postoperative thrombosis.[106,108]

Pathophysiology of Venous Thromboembolism

No discussion on this subject would be complete without a mention of Rudolph Virchow. At a very young age, he recognized the association of venous wall damage with low flow or venous stasis. He proposed that a third factor of hypercoagulability contributed to venous thrombosis. Analysis of the coagulation cascade has added a new dimension to the original concepts proposed by Virchow.

Vein wall injury has been highly suspect in the triad of Virchow, however, scanning electron microscopy has revealed this to be only somewhat important. Experimentally, jugular venous stasis and femoral venous stasis have been produced by gentle finger occlusion of the veins and coincidental trauma has been applied to another distant part of the experimental animal.[110,111] Neither the distant trauma nor venous stasis alone consistently produced thrombosis, but a combination of the 2 factors caused early changes of thrombosis to develop. White blood cells began to adhere to the endothelial surface of the occluded vein[112] and patchy endothelial desquamation followed. This exposed large areas of subendothelial collagen. Endothelium, when stimulated by cytokines such as interleukin-1 and tumor necrosis factor, undergoes metabolic changes and participates in an inflammatory process.

5 major changes occur: loss of vascular integrity, expression of adhesion molecules, secretion of cytokines, prothrombotic changes and upregulation of leukocyte antigen molecules. This prothrombotic activity of the endothelium is balanced by

antiplatelet, anticoagulant and fibrinolytic activity of the endothelium. A fundamental prevention of thrombosis by endothelium is produced by synthesizing and releasing antiplatelet and vasodilator factors such as prostacyclin, nitric oxide and other substances that reduce platelet activity. While endothelial cells can inhibit platelet aggregation, platelet-activator factor is produced by many of the agonists that induce prostacyclin synthesis. Activated platelets release adenosine triphosphate and diphosphate from their dense granules. This latter agent is a potent stimulus to platelet thrombosis.

A number of substances participate in the anticoagulant pathways. Among the most important of these is heparan sulfate. It potentiates antithrombin, a powerful inhibitor of intrinsic coagulation proteases. Another glycoprotein expressed on the endothelial surface is thrombomodulin, an important receptor in the protein C anticoagulant system. Thrombin bound to thrombomodulin on the surface of endothelial cells activates protein C and this, together with its cofactor protein S, acts as an anticoagulant by inactivating coagulation factors Va and VIIIa. Tissue factor inhibitor is also produced by endothelium and inhibits the first steps of the extrinsic coagulation pathway. It is thought that this factor is essential for maintaining a normal hemostatic balance.

There are procoagulant factors as well. Among these is von Willebrand factor. It is present free in plasma and anchored in the subendothelium. It acts as a ligand for platelet adhesion when platelets are activated. As indicated above, tissue factor is an important membrane component that serves to stimulate coagulation through factors VII, X and IX.

Diagnosis of Deep Venous Thrombosis

Clinical assessment remains very valuable in diagnosis of DVT even though it is considered generally unreliable. Symptomatic DVT is characterized by unilateral leg swelling, pain and tenderness to palpation of the site of thrombus. These findings can be assessed in relationship to age over 40, immobilization, recent surgery, trauma or presence of malignancy.

The clinical evaluation cannot be used as the sole method of diagnosis; it must be confirmed by objective findings. Venography was felt to be the best of the objective tests for many years, but it has been replaced by real-time B-mode ultrasonography and duplex ultrasonography. Plethysmography has fallen into disuse because of the advent of duplex scanning, and scintigraphic studies using radiolabeled compounds are of limited help in identifying pulmonary embolization. Both computed tomography and magnetic resonance imaging allow visualization of intravenous thrombi and can be used to evaluate pelvic and abdominal veins that are usually inaccessible to ultrasound diagnosis.[113]

Both CT and MRI can visualize slowed venous blood flow, and these techniques are particularly valuable in detecting proximal vein thrombosis where duplex ultrasound is more or less unreliable.[114,115] Blood tests generally have proven disappointing in diagnosis of deep venous thrombosis, but one has shown the potential to be of clinical utility, the D-dimer test.[116] The test is very sensitive but produces an unacceptably high percentage of false-positive results. Nevertheless, the whole blood agglutination assay performed at the patient's bedside on a blood sample obtained by fingerstick gives results within 5 minutes. A negative result obtained with this test has a negative predictive value of 95% for deep venous thrombosis.

Clinically, use of ultrasound as the initial diagnostic modality is practical. If the test is negative, further testing will probably not be necessary. On the other hand, if the ultrasound testing is negative and the patient has had a pulmonary embolism, then imaging studies to visualize central veins must be done. Difficulties occur when the patient has had a previous deep venous thrombosis. In this situation, an ultrasound test may not be able to differentiate between previous DVT and a new event. Venography or serial ultrasonography may need to be done in this situation. A D-dimer assay in conjunction with serial testing may provide supportive data.

Treatment of Deep Venous Thrombosis

Since low molecular weight heparins (LMWH) can be given in a once- or twice-daily subcutaneous injection and do not require monitoring, they have challenged the position of unfractionated heparin (UFH) as the treatment of choice in deep venous thrombosis. A meta-analysis of 13 randomized trials has shown that use of subcutaneous low-molecular weight heparin is associated with lower rates of recurrence, bleeding and mortality than intravenous unfractionated heparin.[117] Certainly, home treatment is associated with an improved quality of life and may save as much as $6000 per patient compared to inpatient therapy. The LMWHs approved by the FDA for the treatment of thromboembolism include enoxaparin, dalteparin, tinzaparin and fondaparinux.

The diagnosis of deep venous thrombosis must be confirmed, and treatment should begin when the diagnosis is suspected if there is a high probability of DVT uncovered by physical examination. The 2008 guidelines published by the American College of Chest Physicians recommend that initial DVT treatment include LMWH or UFH for at least 5 days.[118] Warfarin should be started on the first day of treatment and discontinued when the INR exceeds 2.0 for 24 hours.

In selecting patients for home therapy, outpatients not at high risk for bleeding and without any comorbid conditions can be treated at home. Patient education is necessary and home health services must be arranged. Patients with multilevel severe venous thrombosis with massive edema should be admitted and considered for thrombolysis. While 1.5 mg/kg of enoxaparin has been given in a once-daily injection, that dose is only approved for patients with concomitant pulmonary embolization treated as inpatients. The twice-daily administration may be better in cancer patients. Warfarin may be prescribed concomitantly. A good starting dose of warfarin is 5 mg/day with the patient being supplied with 7 days of enoxaparin. Platelet counts should be obtained on days 3 and 7 of heparin therapy and daily prothrombin time/INR ratios should be done beginning on day 3 of warfarin therapy.

Chronic venous insufficiency occurs in 25%-50% of patients with proximal DVT receiving standard anticoagulant therapy. To reduce the risk of such sequelae, catheter-directed thrombolysis is recommended in select patients with acute iliofemoral DVT.[118] The use of catheter-directed thrombolysis in patients with acute iliofemoral DVT has been shown to reduce symptoms and improve quality of life.[119,120]

Thrombophilia

Table 9 lists the more common known abnormalities associated with coagulopathy or thrombophilia. Antithrombins were first described in the late 1930s. They inactivate thrombin in other serine proteases as well as several of the coagulation factors. Hereditary antithrombin deficiency is inherited as an autosomal dominant disorder and produces reduced synthesis of antithrombin or production of dysfunctional antithrombin molecules. Acquired antithrombin deficiency is caused by acute thrombosis and disseminated intravascular coagulation, as well as liver disease, the nephrotic syndrome and oral contraceptive use. Protein C deficiency is also inherited as an autosomal-dominant disorder and it may be a more common cause of thrombosis than antithrombin deficiency. Protein C is a vitamin K-dependent protein that exerts its primary inhibitory activity by inactivating factors V and VIII. Acquired protein C deficiency may occur during disseminated intravascular coagulation, extensive deep venous thrombosis or severe liver disease.

Table 9

Common Abnormalities Associated with Thrombophilia

- Antithrombin (formerly antithrombin III) deficiency
- Protein C deficiency
- Protein S deficiency
- Activated protein C resistance/factor V Leiden
- Hyperhomocysteinemia
- Hereditary dysfibrinogenemia
- Deficiencies of:
  - Thrombomodulin
  - Plasminogen
  - Factor VII
- Antiphospholipid syndrome
- Prothrombin gene mutation

Activated protein C resistance is currently thought to be the most common risk factor for venous thrombosis. It is caused by a single-point mutation in the factor V gene. This change results in impaired inactivation of activated factor V, which produces a hypercoagulable state. This factor V has been termed factor V Leiden, and may be prevalent in as much as 15% of the general population. It is more prevalent in Caucasians than non-Caucasians,and less frequent in Hispanic Americans, African Americans and Asian Americans.

Protein S deficiency serves as a cofactor for inactivation of plasma factor V and platelet factor V. It exists in a congenital form as well as an acquired deficiency. It is seen in patients on warfarin therapy because protein S is a vitamin K-dependent factor.

The prothrombin A20210 allele is independently associated with the occurrence of venous thrombosis, particularly in patients with a history of deep venous thrombosis or pulmonary embolization.[121] It is associated with higher plasma prothrombin levels, and carriers of this allele have a 2- to 3-fold increased risk for venous thrombosis. This is similar to the risk associated with the factor V mutation.

Diagnosis of Thrombophilia

As increased knowledge of hypercoagulability has been gained, it has become important to recognize which patients should be studied and what methods should be used to find the exact cause of the hypercoagulability. Clinically, a thrombophilic state is manifested by thrombosis at an early age, a familial tendency towards thrombosis, thrombosis at unusual sites such as cerebral veins and by recurrent thrombosis. The value in making the diagnosis is that the presence of hypercoagulability may dictate longer duration of anticoagulant therapy and vice versa. Furthermore, patients with antithrombin deficiency might require administration of concentrates during surgery. Patients with anticardiolipin antibodies require increased intensity of anticoagulation, and family screening is obviously of value in providing advice to such families.

Because there are both inherited hypercoagulable states and acquired hypercoagulable states, patients should be screened for both. The inherited states can be diagnosed by activity assays for protein C antithrombin, protein S, factor V Leiden and PCR assay, as well as study of anticardiolipin antibodies. The conditions that should be screened for are seen in Table 10.[122]

Table 10

Conditions Requiring Family Screening

Antiphospholipid antibodies
Antihyperhomocysteinemia
Malignancy
Nephrotic syndrome
Crohn's disease
Myeloproliferative syndromes
Paroxysmal nocturnal hemoglobinuria
Behçet's disease

Pulmonary Embolization

Pulmonary embolization remains an important cause of death following surgery. The premortem diagnosis is difficult to establish because the symptoms and signs are relatively nonspecific.[123] As many as 50,000 to 100,000 deaths occur annually from pulmonary embolization.[124] With proper treatment, the mortality of pulmonary embolization can be decreased from a level of 30% to 3%.[125]

Diagnosis of pulmonary embolization is aided by ventilation-perfusion radionuclide lung scanning. Although the sensitivity of such scanning is high, the specificity is low. Pulmonary embolization can be diagnosed accurately with pulmonary arteriography. This test is recognized as the reference standard against which all other testing is compared. It has a sensitivity and specificity greater than 95%, but pulmonary arteriography is invasive, not particularly acceptable to patients and carries its own morbidity.

Contrast-enhanced computed tomography of the pulmonary arteries has been suggested as a technique that would have a high sensitivity and specificity. In fact, helical CT scanning and pulmonary arteriography have been compared,[126] and a sensitivity of 100% and specificity of 96% were found for the helical CT diagnosis of pulmonary embolization. A later report from the same institution reported sensitivity of 91% and specificity of 78%.[127] More recent studies have revealed that helical CT has excellent specificity but suboptimal sensitivity.[128] Helical CT scanning is best used when major pulmonary artery emboli are suspected and it is least useful when it is necessary to identify small, peripherally placed emboli. An effective algorithm including ventilation-perfusion scanning, D-dimer analysis, arteriography, venous ultrasonography and helical CT scanning has yet to be constructed.

Treatment of pulmonary embolization is virtually the same as treatment for deep venous thrombosis, consisting of anticoagulation and support. However, if hemodynamic disturbances are present in patients with pulmonary embolization, survival requires providing a speedy reduction in total pulmonary vascular resistance. Impending hemodynamic instability requires rapid reversal of right-sided heart failure to increase survival and decrease the rate of recurrent pulmonary embolization.[129] If lung scans reveal evidence of obstruction greater than 30% of the pulmonary vascular bed, echocardiography should be performed. Patients with hypotension should be considered for thrombolytic therapy.[130,131] Favorable results using reteplase in treatment of massive pulmonary embolization have shown that this agent, given in two bolus doses 30 minutes apart rapidly improves blood flow through the pulmonary artery, and that a significant reduction in total pulmonary vascular resistance can be expected within 30 minutes after initiation of this form of treatment. Because nearly two-thirds of pulmonary embolism-related deaths occur within the first few hours of onset of symptoms, patients need to be considered for treatment as early as possible. Finally, data from randomized clinical trials have shown that there is evidence that recurrence of pulmonary embolization following thrombolytic therapy and heparin treatment are equivalent.[132]

Prevention of Deep Venous Thromboembolism

As knowledge about the silent nature of deep venous thrombosis has grown, and the awareness of the paucity of heralding symptoms of pulmonary embolization has surfaced, the need for means of prevention of venous thromboembolic disease has become apparent. There is now overwhelming evidence in the literature supporting the effectiveness of prophylactic regimens developed to prevent sudden death from pulmonary embolization.[133,134] Nevertheless, studies published as late as 1991 showed that only one-third of patients with multiple risk factors for thromboembolic disease received prophylactic treatment.[135] Even as late as 1998, an epidemiologic study of Medicare patients undergoing major abdominothoracic surgery documented widespread underutilization of preventive measures.[136]

Risk Factors

Research on causes of venous thromboembolic disease has turned up a number of risk factors for deep venous thrombosis and pulmonary embolization. An additional risk is rarely mentioned, namely risk to the physician. Increasingly, there is evidence that malpractice claims are being filed against physicians who fail to use prophylactic measures in patients who are at moderate or high risk of venous thromboembolism. Risk factors include age over 40 with risk increasing with higher age, prolonged immobility or paralysis, previous thromboembolic disease, malignancy, major surgery involving abdomen, pelvis and lower extremities, obesity, presence of varicose veins or congestive heart failure, myocardial infarction, stroke, pelvic or long-bone fractures, inflammatory bowel disease, nephrotic syndrome and estrogen use.[137-139]

Patients with previous documented deep venous thrombosis or pulmonary embolism may have hemostatic abnormalities. Among the most prevalent is activated protein C resistance (Leiden mutation). Almost as frequent is prothrombin gene20210 abnormality. Others of historical importance include antithrombin (formerly antithrombin III) deficiency, protein C deficiency, protein S deficiency, dysfibrinogenemia, disorders of plasminogen, plasminogen activation, antiphospholipid antibodies and presence of lupus anticoagulant. Other conditions include heparin-induced thrombocytopenia, hyperhomocysteinemia, myeloproliferative disorders and hyperviscosity syndrome.[140-143]

Classification of Level of Risk

It is convenient to classify patients undergoing surgery by level of risk for venous thromboembolic disease. This defines categories of patients who must receive prophylactic treatment.

At low risk would be patients with uncomplicated surgery of less than 1-hour duration, age less than 40 years and none of the risk factors mentioned previously. At moderate risk would be surgical patients 40 to 50 years of age, but without the risk factors mentioned above. An additional subgroup at moderate risk would be candidates for major surgery less than 40 years of age without additional risk factors, or perhaps a small group of patients with lesser surgery having risk factors. An example of high-risk patients would be those requiring major surgery that are greater than 60 years of age without additional risk factors, or major surgery in the 40- to 60-year-old age group with additional risk factors. Certainly, patients with myocardial infarction and medical patients with risk factors are in the high-risk category as well.

The highest risk category is major surgery in patients greater than 40 years of age with a history of previous venous thromboembolic disease or malignant disease or hypercoagulable state. Also in this category are patients with elective major lower extremity orthopedic surgery or hip fracture, or patients with stroke, multiple trauma including pelvic trauma or spinal cord injury.[139]

With regard to application of prophylactic measures, it is generally agreed that low-risk patients need no specific prophylaxis other than early ambulation. Patients with moderate risk may receive prophylaxis with unfractionated or fractionated heparin. Some feel that elastic support or intermittent pneumatic calf compression would be good alternatives to these measures.

Patients at high risk of pulmonary embolization should receive effective prophylaxis. Low-dose unfractionated heparin may be given as 5000 units at 8- to 12-hour intervals. Low molecular weight heparins are also effective. Intermittent pneumatic calf compression can be used, and adding elastic support to any of these measures will give added protection. It is also generally agreed that in very high-risk patients with multiple risk factors not only must prophylaxis be given, but multiple measures can be used effectively. For example, intermittent pneumatic compression can be used with pharmacologic agents.

Venous Thromboembolism in General Surgery Patients

The prophylactic coverage mentioned above is applicable to general surgery patients because the risk of deep venous thrombosis noted in many reports ranges from 19%-25%, and rises to 29% in patients being treated for malignant disease. It is generally agreed that deep venous thrombosis involving the femoral iliac segment occurs in 7% of patients, and that pulmonary emboli develop in 1.6% of all general surgery patients, with fatal pulmonary emboli in 0.9%. Relative risk reduction by various prophylactic regimens is as follows: aspirin 19%, dextran 28%, intermittent pneumatic compression 60%, elastic support 64%, unfractionated low-dose heparin 68% and low molecular weight heparin 72%. As mentioned previously, the effects of multiple means of prophylaxis are additive.[144]

Anticoagulants recommended for DVT prophylaxis for trauma and surgical patients include low-molecular-weight heparins (LMWH), low-dose unfractionated heparin (LDUH) or fondaparinux. Pharmacologic therapy includes LMWH 40 mg subcutaneously (SC) daily, LDUH 5000 units SC 2-3 times daily or fondaparinux 2.5mg SC daily. Patients with renal insufficiency (creatinine clearance [CrCl] <30mL/min) should not receive fondaparinux.[118] All are safe and effective, and a great deal of experience has been gained in the high-risk groups of total hip replacement and total knee replacement. For example, it is generally recognized that after total knee replacement, the total DVT prevalence is 61%. This can be reduced 20% by low-dose warfarin treatment, 31% by low-dose heparin and 49% with low molecular weight heparin prophylaxis. Interestingly, intermittent pneumatic compression of the calves reduces the risk by 82%.

The low-molecular weight heparins do not require laboratory monitoring and, in North America, most experience includes an initial dose given between 12 and 24 hours postoperatively on a twice-daily dosing schedule. In contrast, most European experience includes giving the initial low-molecular-weight heparin 12 hours preoperatively, and subsequently a calculated dose on a once-daily schedule. It should be noted that regional anesthesia should be avoided in patients receiving aspirin, nonsteroidal anti-inflammatory drugs, platelet inhibitors or anticoagulants. Initiation of regional anesthesia should be delayed at least 12 hours after any initiation of prophylaxis. Subsequent prophylactic doses should be delayed at least 2 hours after spinal needle or epidural catheter removal. The optimal duration of postoperative prophylaxis is unsettled, and because the current duration of hospitalization is less than 5 days, it would be helpful to know if 5 days of prophylaxis would provide adequate protection.

This discussion of prophylaxis of venous thromboembolic disease should be considered preliminary, because many issues regarding neurosurgery, spinal cord injury, multiple trauma, burns, ischemic stroke and medical conditions such as myocardial infarction are beyond the scope of the present discussion.

7. References

1. Arnoldi CC. The aetiology of primary varicose veins. *Dan Med Bull*. 1957;4:102-107.

2. Bergan JJ. A unifying concept of primary venous insufficiency. *Dermatol Surg*. 1998;24:425-428.

3. Ballard JL, Bergan JJ, eds. *Chronic Venous Insufficiency: Diagnosis and Treatment*. London, England: Springer-Verlag; 2000.

4. Ludbrook J. *Aspects of Venous Function in the Lower Limbs*. Springfield, IL: Charles C. Thomas; 1966.

5. Browse NL, Burnand KG, Irvine AT, Wilson NM. *Diseases of the Veins*. 2nd ed. London, England: Edward Arnold & Co; 1999.

6. Wheeler HB, Hirsh J, Wells P, Anderson FA. Diagnostic tests for deep vein thrombosis. *Arch Intern Med*. 1994;154:1921-1928.

7. Sumner DS. Diagnosis of deep venous thrombosis. In: Rutherford RB, ed. *Vascular Surgery*. Philadelphia, PA: WB Saunders; 1995:1698-1743.

8. Hull R, van Aken WG, Hirsh J, et al. Impedance plethysmography: Using the occlusive cuff technique in the diagnosis of venous thrombosis. *Circulation*. 1976;53:696.

9. Cogo A, Prandoni P, Villalta S, et al. Changing features of proximal vein thrombosis over time. *Angiology*. 1994;45:377-382.

10. Cramer M, Beach KW, Strandness DE Jr. The detection of proximal deep venous thrombosis by strain-gauge plethysmography through the use of an outflow-capacitance discriminate line. *Bruit*. 1983;7:17.

11. Criado E. Laboratory evaluation of the patient with chronic venous insufficiency. In: Rutherford RB, ed. *Vascular Surgery*. Philadelphia, PA: WB Saunders; 1995: 1771-1785.

12. AbuRahma AF. Methods of noninvasive techniques in the diagnosis of venous disease. In: AbuRahma AF, Diethrich EB, eds. *Current Noninvasive Vascular Diagnosis*. Littleton, MA: PSG; 1988:263-269.

13. Schultz-Ehrenburg U, Blazek V. New possibilities for photoplethysmography. *Phlebol Digest*. 1993;5:5-11.

14. Schultz-Ehrenburg U, Blazek V. Quantitative digital photoplethysmography (D-PPG): First results with online registration and significance of V0 (Venous pump power). In: Schultz-Ehrenburg U, Blazek V, eds. *Advances in Computer-Aided Noninvasive Vascular Diagnostics*. Dusseldorf, Germany: VDI Verlag; 1994.

15. Raines JK, Jaffrin MY, Rao S. A noninvasive pressure-pulse recorder: Development and rationale. *Med Instrum*. 1973;7:245.

16. Christopoulos D, Nicolaides AN, Szendro G. Venous reflux: Quantification and correlation with the clinical severity of chronic venous disease. *Br J Surg*. 1998;75:352-356.

17. Christopoulos D, Nicolaides AN, Duffy P, Georgiou I. Noninvasive diagnosis and quantification of outflow obstruction in venous disease. *J Cardiovasc Surg*. 1989;30:72-73.

18. Nicolaides AN, Sumner DS, eds. *Investigations of Patients with Deep Venous Thrombosis and Chronic Venous Insufficiency*. London, England: Med-Orion Publishing Co; 1991.

19. Christopoulos D, Nicolaides AN, Cook A, Irvine A, Galloway JM, Wilkinson A. Pathogenesis of venous ulceration in relation to the calf muscle pump function. *Surgery*. 1989;106:829-835.

20. Vasdekis SN, Clarke GH, Nicolaides AN. Quantification of venous reflux by means of duplex scanning. *J Vasc Surg*. 1989;10: 670-677.

21. van Bemmelen PS, Bedford G, Beach K, Strandness DE Jr. Quantitative segmental evaluation of venous valvular reflux with ultrasound scanning. *J Vasc Surg*. 1989;10:425-431.

22. Masuda EM, Kistner KL, Eklof B. Prospective study of duplex scanning for venous reflux: Comparison of Valsalva and pneumatic cuff techniques in the reverse Trendelenburg and standing position. *J Vasc Surg*. 1994;20:711-719.

23. O'Donnell TF Jr. Surgical treatment of incompetent communicating veins. In: Bergan JJ, Kistner RL, eds. *Atlas of Venous Surgery*. Philadelphia, PA: WB Saunders; 1992:111-118.

24. Lees TA, Lambert D. Patterns of venous reflux in limbs with skin changes associated with chronic venous insufficiency. *Br J Surg*. 1993;6:725-728.

25. DeWeese JA, Rogoff SM. Clinical uses of functional ascending phlebography of the lower extremity. *Angiology*. 1958;9:268.

26. Rabinov K, Paulin S. Roentgen diagnosis of venous thrombosis in the leg. *Arch Surg*. 1972;104:134.

27. Nicolaides AN, Kakkar VV, Field ES, Renney JTG. The origin of deep vein thrombosis: A venographic study. *Br J Radiol*. 1971;44:653.

28. Kistner RL. Surgical repair of the incompetent femoral vein valve. *Arch Surg*. 1975;110:1936.

29. Herman R, Neiman HL, Yao JST. Descending venography: A method of evaluating lower extremity venous valvular function. *Radiology*. 1980;137:63.

30. Lea Thomas M, McAllister V, Rose DH, Tonge K. A simplified technique for phlebography for the localization of incomplete perforating veins of the legs. *Clin Radiol*. 1972;23:486.

31. Prerovsky I. Diseases of the Veins. World Health Organization: internal communication. MHO-PA 10964.

32. Cotton LT. Varicose veins: gross anatomy and development. *Br J Surg*. 1961;48:589-598.

33. Svejcar J, Prerovsky I, Linhart J, Kruml J. Content of collagen, elastin, and water in walls of the internal saphenous vein in man. *Circ Res*. 1962;11:296.

34. Rose SS, Ahmed A. Some thoughts on the aetiology of varicose veins. *J Cardiovasc Surg*. 1986;27:534-543.

35. Schalin L. Role of arteriovenous shunting in the development of varicose veins. In: Eklof B, Gjores JE, Thulesius O, Bergqvist D, eds. *Controversies in the Management of Venous Disorders*. London, England: Butterworth; 1989:182-192.

36. Bergan JJ. Classification of venous insufficiency. In: Goldman MP, Weiss RA, Bergan JJ. *Varicose Veins & Telangiectasias: Diagnosis and Management*. 2nd ed. St. Louis, MA: Quality Medical Publishing, Inc; 1999:87-93.

37. Schultz-Ehrenberg U, Weindorf N, VonUslar D, Hirche H. Prospective epidemiological investigations in early and preclinical stages of varicosis. In: Davy A, Stemmer R, eds. *Phlebology 1989*. Paris, France: John Libbey, Eurotext; 1989:163-165.

38. Tibbs DJ, Fletcher EWL. Direction of flow in superficial veins as a guide to venous disorders of the lower limbs. *Surgery*. 1983;93:758-767.

39. Watts GT. The treatment of varicose veins. *Lancet*. 1973;1:435.

40. Barnes RW, Ross EA, Strandness DE Jr. Differentiation of primary from secondary varicose veins by Doppler ultrasound and strain-gauge plethysmography. *Surg Gynecol Obstet*. 1975;141:207-211.

41. Shull KC, Nicolaides AN, Fernandes E, Fernandes J, et al. Significance of popliteal reflux in relation to ambulatory venous pressure and ulceration. *Arch Surg*. 1979;114:1304-1306.

42. Labropoulos N, Leon M, Nicolaides AN, et al. Venous reflux in patients with previous deep venous thrombosis: Correlation with ulceration and other systems. *J Vasc Surg*. 1994;20:953-958.

43. Vasdekis SN, Clarke GH, Nicolaides AN. Quantification of venous reflux by means of duplex scanning. *J Vasc Surg*. 1989;10:670-677.

44. Masuda EM, Kistner RL. Prospective comparison of duplex scanning and descending venography in assessment of venous insufficiency. *Am J Surg*. 1992;164:254-259.

45. Valentin LI, Valentin WH, Mercado S, Rosado CJ. Venous reflux localization: Comparative study of venography and duplex scanning. *Phlebology*. 1993;8:124-127.

46. Weiss RA, Weiss MA, Goldman MP. Physicians' negative perception of sclerotherapy for venous disorders: Review of a 7-year experience with modern sclerotherapy. *South Med J*. 1992;85:1101-1106.

47. Weiss RA, Weiss MA. Resolution of pain associated with varicose and telangiectatic leg veins after compression sclerotherapy. *Dermatol Surg*. 1990;16:333-336.

48. Lofgren KA, Ribisi AP, Myers TT. An evaluation of stripping versus ligation for varicose veins. *Arch Surg*. 1958;76:310-316.

49. Larson RH, Lofgren ED, Myers TT, Lofgren KA. Long-term results after vein surgery. Study of 1000 cases after ten years. *Mayo Clin Proc*. 1974;49:114-117.

50. Woodyer AB, Reddy PJ, Dormandy JA. *Should We Strip the Long Saphenous Vein?* London, England: John Libbey & Co; 1986:151-154.

51. Sarin S, Scurr JH, Coleridge-Smith PD. Stripping of the long saphenous vein in the treatment of primary varicose veins. *Br J Surg*. 1994;81:1455-1458.

52. Rutgers PH, Kistlaar PJEHM. Randomized trial of stripping versus high ligation combined with sclerotherapy in the treatment of the incompetent greater saphenous vein. *Am J Surg*. 1994;168:311-315.

53. Jakobsen BH. The value of different forms of treatment for varicose veins. *Br J Surg*. 1979;66:182-184.

54. Munn SR, Morton JB, MacBeth WAAG, McLeish AR. To strip or not to strip the long saphenous vein? A varicose veins trial. *Br J Surg*. 1981;68:426-428.

55. Bergan JJ. Saphenous stripping and quality of outcome. Leading article. *Br J Surg*. 1996;83:1025-1027.

56. Neglen P, Einarsson E, Eklof B. The functional long-term value of different types of treatment for saphenous vein incompetence. *J Cardiovasc Surg (Torino)*. 1993;34:295-301.

57. Neglen P. Treatment of varicosities of saphenous origin: Comparison of ligation, selective excision, and sclerotherapy. In: Bergan JJ, Goldman MP, eds. *Varicose Veins and Telangiectasias: Diagnosis and Treatment*. St. Louis, MO: Quality Medical Publishing, Inc; 1993.

58. Hammarsten J, Pedersen P, Cederlund C-G, Campanello M. Long saphenous saving surgery for varicose veins: A long-term followup. *Eur J Vasc Surg*. 1990;4:361-364.

59. Hammersten J, Campanello M, Pederson P. Long saphenous vein-saving surgery for varicose veins (letter/comment). *Eur J Vasc Surg*. 1993;7:763-764.

60. Darke SG. Fewer recurrences with stripping. (letter). *Eur J Vasc Surg*. 1993;7:764.

61. Fligelston L, Carolan G, Pugh N, Minst P, Shandall A, Lane I. An assessment of the long saphenous vein for potential use as a vascular conduit after varicose vein surgery. *J Vasc Surg*. 1993;18:836-840.

62. McMullin GM, Coleridge Smith PD, Scurr JH. Objective assessment of high ligation without stripping the long saphenous vein. *Br J Surg*. 1991;78:1139-1142.

63. Fitridge RA, Fronek HS, Dilley RB, Bernstein EF, Benveniste GL. Assessment of reflux in the greater saphenous vein (GSV) two years following high ligation. *Cardiovasc Surg*. 1995;3:71.

64. Papadakis K, Christodoulou C, Christopoulos D, et al. Number and anatomical distribution of incompetent thigh perforating veins. *Br J Surg*. 1989;76:581-584.

65. Van den Bos R, Arends L, Kockaert M, Neumann M, Nijsten T. Endovenous therapies of lower extremity varicosities: a meta-analysis. *J Vasc Surg*. 2009 Jan; 49(1):230-239. Epub 2008 Aug 9.

66. Jia X, Mowatt G, Burr JM, Cassar K, Cook J, Fraser C. Systematic review of foam sclerotherapy for varicose veins. *Br J Surg*. 2007;94(8):925-936. Review.

67. Callam MJ. Leg ulcer in chronic venous insufficiency in the community. In: Ruckley CV, Fowkes FGR, Bradbury AW, eds. Venous Disease: Epidemiology, Management, and Delivery of Care. London, England: Springer-Verlag; 1999.

68. Nicolaides AN, Zukowski A, Lewis R, Kyprianou P, Malouf GM. Venous pressure measurements in venous problems. In: Bergan JJ, Yao JST, eds. Surgery of the Veins. Orlando, FL: Grune & Stratton; 1985:111-118.

68. Hoare MC, Nicolaides AN, Miles CR, et al. The role of primary varicose veins in venous ulceration. *Surgery*. 1982;92:450-453.

69. Kistner RL. Primary venous valve incompetence of the leg. *Am J Surg*. 1980;140:218-224.

70. Homans J. The etiology and treatment of varicose ulcer of the leg. *Surg Gynecol Obstet*. 1917;24:300-311.

71. Blumhoff RL, Johnson G. Perforating veins PpO_2 in patients with varicose veins. *J Surg Res*. 1977;23:35-36.

72. Pratt GH. Arterial varices: a syndrome. *Am J Surg*. 1949;77:456-460.

73. Lindmayr W, Lofferer O, Mostbeck A, Partsch H. Arteriovenous shunts in primary varicosis: A critical essay. *Vasc Surg*. 1972;6:9-14.

74. Browse NL, Burnand KG. The cause of venous ulceration. *Lancet*. 19822(8292);243-245.

75. Wilson JW. Leukocyte sequestration and morphologic augmentation in the pulmonary network following hemorrhagic shock and related forms of stress. *Adv Microcirc*. 1972;58:197-232.

76. Linas DL, Shanley PF, Whittenburg D, Berger E, Repine JE. Neutrophils accentuate ischemia-reperfusion injury in isolated perfused rat kidneys. *Am J Physiol*. 1988;255:F728-F735.

77. Yamakawa T, Suguyama I, Niimi H. Behavior of white blood cells in microcirculation of the cat brain cortex during hemorrhagic shock: Intravital microscopic study. *Int J Microcirc Clin Exp*. 1984;3:554.

78. Braide M, Blixt A, Bagge U. Leukocyte effects on the vascular resistance and glomerular filtration of the isolated rat kidney at normal and low flow rates. *Circ Shock*. 1986;20:71-80.

79. Babior BM. Oxidants from phagocytes: Agents of defense and destruction. *Blood*. 1984;64:959-966.

80. Scott HJ, McMullin GM, Coleridge Smith PD, Scurr JH. A histological study into white blood cells and their association with lipodermatosclerosis and ulceration. *Br J Surg*. 1990;78:210-211.

81. Wilkinson LS, Bunker C, Edwards JC, Scurr JH, Coleridge Smith PD. Leukocytes: Their role in the etiopathogenesis of skin damage in venous disease. *J Vasc Surg*. 1993;17: 669-675.

82. Saharay M, Shields DA, Porter JB, Scurr JH, Coleridge Smith PD. Leukocyte activity in the microcirculation of the leg in patients with chronic venous disease. *J Vasc Surg*. 1997;25:265-273.

83. Markel A, Manzo RA, Bergelin RO, Strandness DE. Valvular reflux after deep venous thrombosis: Incidence and time of occurrence. *J Vasc Surg*. 1992;15:377-384.

84. Labropoulos N, Delis K, Nicolaides AN, Leon M, Ramaswami G, Volteas N. The role of the distribution and anatomic extent of reflux in the development of signs and symptoms in chronic venous insufficiency. *J Vasc Surg*. 1996;23:504-510.

85. Weingarten MS, Branas CC, Czeredarczuk BA, Schmidt JD, Wolferth Jr CC. Distribution and quantification of venous reflux in lower extremity chronic venous stasis disease with duplex scanning. *J Vasc Surg*. 1993;18:753-759.

86. Raju S. A pressure-based technique for the detection of acute and chronic venous obstruction. *Phlebology*. 1988;3:207-216.

87. Bossuyt LEG, Neumann HAM. Air plethysmography: A critical evaluation of the technique in patients with chronic venous insufficiency. *Phlebologie*. 1999;28:7-12.

88. Mayberry JC, Moneta GL, Taylor LM Jr, Porter JM. Fifteen-year results of ambulatory compression therapy for chronic venous ulcers. *Surgery*. 1991;109:575-581.

89. Negus D. Prevention and treatment of venous ulceration. *Ann R Coll Surg Engl*. 1985;67:144-148.

90. Bello M, Scriven M, Hartshorne T, Bell PR, Naylor AR, London NJ. Role of superficial venous surgery in the treatment of venous ulceration. *Br J Surg*. 1999;86:755-759.

91. Scriven JM, Hartshorne T, Thrush AJ, Bell PR, Naylor AR, London NJ. Role of saphenous vein surgery in the treatment of venous ulceration. *Br J Surg*. 1998;85:781-784.

92. Zukowski AJ, Nicolaides AN, Szendro G, et al. Haemodynamic significance of incompetent perforating veins. *Br J Surg*. 1991;78:625-629.

93. Labropoulos N, Leon M, Geroulakos G, Volteas N, Chan P, Nicolaides AN. Venous hemodynamic abnormalities in patients with leg ulcerations. *Am J Surg*. 1995;169:572-574.

94. Burnand K, Thomas ML, O'Donnell T, Browse NL. Relation between postphlebitic changes in the deep veins and results of surgical treatment of venous ulcers. *Lancet*. 1976;1:936-938.

95. Burnand KG, O'Donnell TF, Lea Thomas M, Browse NL. The relative importance of incompetent communicating veins in the production of varicose veins and venous ulcers. *Surgery*. 1977;82:9-14.

96. Bowen FH. Subfascial ligation of the perforating leg veins to treat post thrombophlebitic syndrome. *Am Surg*. 1975; 148-151.

97. Pierik EGJM, van Urk H, Hop WCJ, Wittens CHA. Endoscopic versus open subfascial division of incompetent perforating veins in the treatment of venous leg ulceration: A randomized trial. *J Vasc Res*. 1997;26:1049-1054.

98. Gohel MS, Barwell JR, Taylor M, et al. Long term results of compression therapy alone versus compression plus surgery in chronic venous ulceration (ESCHAR): randomised controlled trial. *BMJ*. 2007;335(7610):83. Epub 2007 Jun 1.

99. DePalma RG, Kowallek D, Spence RK, et al. Comparison of costs and healing rates of two forms of compression in treating venous ulcers. *Vasc Surg*. 1999; 33:683-690.

100. Consensus Conference. Prevention of venous thrombosis and pulmonary embolism. *JAMA*. 1986; 256:744-779.

101. Hill RB, Anderson RE. *The Autopsy: Medical Practice and Public Policy*. Boston, MA: Butterworth; 1998:153.

102. Cohen SH, Ehrlich GE, Kaufman MS, Cope C. Thrombophlebitis following knee surgery. *J Bone Joint Surg*. 1973;55(1):106-111.

103. Coventry MB, Nolan DR, Beckenbaugh RD. Delayed prophylactic anticoagulation: a study of results in 2012 total hip arthroplasties. *J Bone Joint Surg*. 1973; 55:1487-1492.

104. Nicolaides AN, Irving D. Clinical factors and the risk of deep venous thrombosis. In: Nicolaises AN, ed. *Thromboembolism: Aetiology, Advances in Prevention, and Management*. Lancaster, England: MTP Pressure; 1975:193-204.

105. Nordstrom M, Lindblad B, Bergqvist D, Kjellstrom T. A prospective study of the incidence of deep vein thrombosis within a defined urban population. *J Int Med*. 1992; 232:155-160.

106. Kakkar VV, Howe CT, Nicolaides AN, Renney JTG, Clarke MB. Deep vein thrombosis of the leg. Is there a "high-risk" group? *Am J Surg*.1970; 120:527-530.

107. Gordon SG, Cross BA. A factor X-activating cysteine protease from malignant tissue. *J Clin Invest*. 1981; 67:1665-1671.

108. Stewart GJ, Stern HS, Lynch PR, Malmud LS, Schaub RG. Response of the canine jugular veins and carotid arteries to hysterectomy: Increased permeability and leukocyte adhesions and invasion. *Thromb Res*. 1980;20:473.

109. Stewart GJ, Stern HR, Schaub RG. Endothelial alterations, deposition of blood elements and increased accumulation of 131I-albumin in canine jugular veins following abdominal surgery. *Thromb Res*. 1978;12:555.

110. Stewart GJ, Ritchie WGM, Lynch PR. Venous endothelial damage produced by massive sticking and emigration of leukocytes. *Am J Pathol*. 1974; 74:507.

111. Nemcek AA Jr, Vogelzang RL. Imaging of thrombosis. In: Kwaan HC, Samama MM, eds. *Clinical Thrombosis*. Boca Raton, FL: CRC; 1989:407-458.

112. Carpenter JP, Holland GA, Baum RA, et al. Magnetic resonance venography for the detection of deep venous thrombosis: Comparison with contrast venography and duplex Doppler ultrasonography. *J Vasc Surg*. 1993;18:734-741.

113. Evans AJ, Sostman HD, Knelson MH, et al. Detection of deep venous thrombosis: prospective comparison of MR imaging and contrast venography. *AJR*. 1993; 161:131-139.

114. Boneu B, Bes G, Pelzer H, et al. D-dimers, thrombin antithrombin III complexes and prothrombin fragments 1+2: Diagnostic value in clinically suspected deep vein thrombosis. Thromb Haemost. 1991; 65: 28-31.

115. Bick RL. Low-molecular-weight heparins in the outpatient management of venous thromboembolism. *Sem Thrombosis & Hemostasis*. 1999;25(3):97-99.

116. Kearon C, Kahn S, Agnelli G, Goldhaber S, Raskob G, Comerota A. Antithrombotic therapy for venous thromboembolic disease: American college of chest physicians evidence-based clinical practice guidelines (8th ed). *Chest*. 2008;133;454-545.

117. Comerota AJ, Throm RC, Mathias SD, Haughton S, Mewissen M. Catheter-directed thrombolysis for iliofemoral deep vein thrombosis improves health-related quality of life. *J Vasc Surg*. 2000;32:130-137.

118. Aburama Af, Perkins SE, Wulu JT, Ng HK. Iliofemoral deep vein thrombosis: conventional therapy versus lysis and percutaneous transluminal angioplasty and stenting. *Ann Surg*. 2001;233:752-760.

119. Margaglione M, Brancaccio V, Giuliani N. Increased risk for venous thrombosis in carriers of the prothrombin G-A20210 gene variant. *Ann Intern Med*. 1998;129:89-93.

120. DeLoughery TG. Evaluation of hypercoagulable states. *J Thrombosis and Thrombolysis*. 1998;5:43-47.

121. Moser KM. Venous thromboembolism. *Am Rev Respir Dis*.1990;141:235-249.

122. Henschke CI, Mateescu I, Yankelevitz DF. Changing practice patterns in the workup of pulmonary embolism. *Chest*. 1995;107:940-945.

123. Carson JL, Kelley MA, Duff A, et al. The clinical course of pulmonary embolism. *N Engl J Med*. 1992; 326:1240-1245.

124. Remy-Jardin M, Remy J, Wattinne L, Giraud F. Central pulmonary thromboembolic disease: diagnosis with spiral volumetric CT with the single-breath-hold technique. Comparison with pulmonary angiography. *Radiology*. 1992; 185:381-387.

125. Remy-Jardin M, Remy J, Deschildre F, et al. Pulmonary embolism: diagnosis of pulmonary embolism with spiral CT: comparison with pulmonary angiography and scintigraphy. *Radiology*. 1996;200:699-706.

126. Drucker EA, Rivitz SM, Shepard JO, et al. Acute pulmonary embolism: Assessment of helical CT for diagnosis. *Radiology*. 1998;209:235-241.

127. Cannon CP, Goldhaber SZ. Cardiovascular risk stratification of pulmonary embolism. *Am J Cardiol*. 1996;78:1149-1151.

128. Smalling RW, Bode C, Kalbfleisch J, et al. More rapid, complete, and stable coronary thrombolysis with bolus administration of reteplase compared with alteplase infusion in acute myocardial infarction. RAPID Investigators. *Circulation*. 1995;91:2725-2732.

129. Bode C, Smalling RW, Berg G, et al. Randomized comparison of coronary thrombolysis achieved with double-bolus reteplase (recombinant plasminogen activator) in patients with acute myocardial infarction. RAPID II Investigators. *Circulation*. 1996; 94:891-898.

130. Dalen JE, Alpert JS, Hirsh J. Thrombolytic therapy for pulmonary embolism. Is it effective? Is it safe? When is it indicated? *Arch Intern Med*. 1997;157:2550-2556.

131. Caprini JA, Arcelus JI, Hoffman K, et al. Prevention of venous thromboembolism in North America: results of a survey among general surgeons. *J Vasc Surg*.1994;20:751-758.

132. Bergqvist D. Prophylaxis against postoperative venous thromboembolism: a survey of surveys. *Thromb Haemorrh*. 1990;2:69-73.

133. Anderson FA, Wheeler HB, Goldberg RJ, et al. Physician practices in the prevention of venous thromboembolism. *Ann Intern Med*. 1991;115:591-595.

134. Bratzler DW, Raskob GE, Murray CK, et al. Underuse of venous thromboembolism prophylaxis for general surgery patients. *Arch Intern Med*.1998; 158:1909-1912.

135. Lowe GDO, Greer IA, Cooke TG, et al. Risk of and prophylaxis for venous thromboembolism in hospital patients. *Br Med J*. 1992; 305:567-574.

136. Verstraete M. Prophylaxis of venous thromboembolism. *Br Med J*. 1997; 314:123-125.

137. Nicolaides AN, Bergqvist D, Hull R, et al. *Prevention of Thromboembolism: International Consensus Statement (Guidelines According to Scientific Evidence)*. Nicosia, Cyprus: Med-Orion Publishing Co.; 1997.

138. Nachman RL, Silverstein R. Hypercoagulable states. *Ann Intern Med*.1993;119: 819-827.

139. Svensson PJ, Dahlback B. Resistance to activated protein C as a basis for venous thrombosis. *N Engl J Med*. 1994;330:517-522.

140. Ridker PM, Hennekens CH, Lindpaintner K, et al. Mutation in the gene coding for coagulation factor V and the risk of myocardial infarction, stroke, and venous thrombosis in apparently healthy men. *N Engl J Med*. 1995; 332:912-917.

141. Fermo I, Vigano D'Angelo SV, Paroni R, et al. Prevalence of moderate hyperhomocysteinemia in patients with early onset venous and arterial occlusive disease. *Ann Intern Med*. 1995;123:747-753.

142. Clagett GP, Anderson Jr FA, Geerts WH, et al. Prevention of thromboembolism. *Chest*. 1998;114(suppl 5):531S-5601S.

8. Questions

1. Symptoms of varicose veins include aching pain and fatigue. These are greatest in which of the following?

A. Telangiectasias

B. Reticular varicosities

C. Large subcutaneous varicosities

D. Symptoms unrelated to size

E. Symptoms may be equal in all of the above

2. After the complete history and physical examination is done in a patient with symptomatic varicose veins, which of the following needs to be added to the evaluation?

A. Duplex reflux examination

B. Phlebography

C. Hand-held continuous-wave Doppler evaluation

D. Photoplethysmography

3. Treatment of telangiectasias and/or reticular, flat, blue-green varicosities is done to:

A. Improve the cosmetic appearance of the legs

B. Ameliorate the symptoms of aching, heaviness and pain

C. Neither of the above

D. Both A. and B.

4. Nocturnal leg cramps are chiefly associated with:

   A. Arteriosclerotic occlusive disease

   B. Lymphedema

   C. Telangiectasias

   D. Telangiectasias and varicose veins

5. Venous leg ulcer may be due to:

   A. Saphenous reflux and varicose veins

   B. Deep venous reflux without superficial reflux

   C. Incompetent ankle perforating veins

   D. All of the above

6. Severe venous dysfunction is characterized by ankle hyperpigmentation, induration and open leg ulcers. The correct term for this condition is:

   A. Stasis ulcer

   B. Postphlebitic state

   C. Chronic venous insufficiency

   D. Marjolin ulcer

7. The anatomic cause of venous leg ulcer is:

   A. Superficial reflux

   B. Deep venous reflux

   C. Perforator reflux

   D. All of the above, singly or in combination

8. The Linton and Cockett perforator vein operations were disappointing because of:

   A. Recurrent ulceration

   B. Delayed healing of skin grafts

   C. Systemic infection

   D. General morbidity

9. Conservative treatment of severe venous dysfunction includes:

   A. Induced hyperthermia

   B. Intermittent pneumatic compression

   C. Fitted support

   D. All of the above

10. The fundamental objective of perforator vein interruption is:

   A. Improved calf muscle pump function

   B. Decreased ambulatory venous hypertension

   C. Diminished leukocyte trapping and activation

   D. All of the above

Answers

1. D. and **E.**

D. and E. are both correct, but D. is the best answer. Varicose vein symptoms are poorly explained and relate to hormonal status, pressure on somatic nerves, distension of the affected vessel and unknown factors. The fact that telangiectasias do cause symptoms is not generally appreciated by physicians. (See Weiss RA, Weiss MA. Resolution of pain associated with varicose and telangiectatic leg veins after compression sclerotherapy. *J Dermatol Surg*. 1990;16:333-336 for details.)

2. C.

Duplex examination is unnecessary in limbs with telangiectasias, phlebography is necessary before venous reconstruction, and photoplethysmography is an additive test of function but does not aid in selecting therapy. Doppler examination confirms clinical suspicion, defines axial reflux and assists in selecting patients for surgery vs. sclerotherapy. (See Bergan JJ. Surgical management of primary and recurrent varicose veins. In: Gloviczki P, Yao J, eds. *Handbook of Venous Disorders*. London, England: Chapman and Hall; 1996:394-415.)

3. D.

Same justification as Question 1 above.

4. D.

Night cramps are poorly understood but relate to lessening of edema on recumbency in limbs with some degree of venous insufficiency. Presumably the edema prevents transmission of electrical impulses from nerve ends to the motor end plate of muscle fibers. Since the edema is relieved by the supine position, nerve impluses generated by beginning motion of the limb cross to the motor end plate and throw the muscle into tetanic contraction.

5. D.

The point being made here is that venous leg ulcer is not always caused by previous deep venous thrombosis, and in fact may be prevented by simple removal of nonfunctioning veins.

6. C.

Stasis implies stagnation of blood with deoxygenation, the theory of causation of leg ulcer proposed by Homans before 1920. As stated in question 5, the stigmata of chronic venous insufficiency do not depend upon an episode of previous deep venous thrombosis. A Marjolin ulcer is malignant degeneration of an ancient (burn) scar.

7. D.

The point being made by this question is that precise preoperative diagnosis dictates correct intervention, and that all elements of venous pathology need to be corrected in treatment of venous leg ulcer.

8. D.

While recurrence of leg ulcer plagues all treatments of venous ulcer, it was the total morbidity of the early operations that killed the procedure. Delayed skin graft take is a technical problem and systemic infection is simply one of the contributors to the general morbidity of the pioneering perforator operations.

9. C.

Hyperthermia is an experimental procedure used in treatment of lymphedema, intermittent compression has been used by some in treatment of venous ulcer and does contribute to reduction of edema, subsequent improvement in oxygen transport and more rapid ulcer healing. The cornerstone of treatment of venous insufficiency is external elastic support.

10. D.

While each of the answers is correct in and of itself, it is the sum of all of the factors that produces success in managing severe chronic venous insufficiency.

Chapter 20: Endovascular Treatment of Occlusive Arterial Disease

David D. Kidney, MD

Contents

1. Occlusive Arterial Disease

The most commonly detected pathology in peripheral arterial occlusive disease (PAOD) is atherosclerosis, affecting approximately 5% of men in the 50-plus age group, with a growing incidence as the North American population grows older.[1] Even with claudication, in the majority of patients the natural course is to remain stable with approximately one-third showing some deterioration or progression. 1%-5% of patients with PAOD will eventually require amputation.[1]

Other causes of vascular stenosis include vascular trauma, irradiation or the vasculitides. There is a significantly increased relative risk of mortality secondary to cardiovascular problems in patients with severe or symptomatic PAOD.[2] This is critical to keep in mind when clinically evaluating these patients and advising therapeutic interventions.

There has been a dramatic increase in the use of interventional percutaneous radiological procedures for the treatment of both acute and chronic PAOD in recent years. The technical and imaging advancements in interventional procedures has led to increased use of percutaneous transluminal angioplasty (PTA), stent deployment, and intraarterial thrombolysis in the treatment of peripheral arterial stenosis and thrombosis.

Pathology

The current thinking regarding the pathogenesis of atherosclerosis centers on the combination of a tissue response to injury, infiltration with lipid and modification. Initial injury causes the endothelium of the vascular tree to increase the uptake of plasma lipid. Primarily increased plasma lipids and the presence of oxidized forms may exacerbate the injury. Plaque growth is therefore intraluminal and is the cause of arterial stenosis. Most atheromatous plaques contain a large central pool of lipids and cellular debris. More advanced atherosclerotic plaques can have calcification, surface ulceration, thrombosis, intraplaque hemorrhage or aneurysmal dilatation.

2. PTA and Stents

Historical Perspective

The first described PTA was performed in January 1964, and 11 patients were described by November 1964 by Dotter and Judkins.[3] They utilized rigid polytetrafluoroethylene (PTFE) catheters introduced via the ipsilateral common femoral arteries and advanced across iliac artery lesions with sequentially larger catheters to dilate the flow-restricting stenosis.

Porstman published the first study using a balloon-type device for angioplasty in 1973.[4] In 1974 Gruntzig and Hopff made a fundamental improvement by changing the balloon material from the latex of the embolectomy balloon to polyvinyl chloride, which allowed for more forceful radial dilation and more effective disruption of the atherosclerotic plaque.[5] Since Gruntzig and Hopff's initial balloon designs, advances in technology, particularly in materials and size as well as strides made in development of new pharmacological adjuncts, have advanced the science, technique, and performance of angioplasty significantly. These advances, combined with the vast improvements in imaging quality and digital subtraction, help explain the progressive growth in the number of endovascular procedures.

Mechanism of Plaque Disruption

Compression of atherosclerotic plaque was the theory originally suggested as being responsible for transluminal dilatation of atherosclerotic stenoses.[3] Histologic studies by Casteñada-Zúñiga have shown that the expansive forces of the angioplasty balloon have a more complex mechanism of action, that leads to fracture, dissection, and partial separation of the plaque following severance from the underlying media.[6] This plaque disruption then allows the vessel to dilate without the cast-like restraints of the rigid atherosclerotic plaque. Despite histologic evidence of significant and traumatic plaque disruption, angioplasty has been shown to be surprisingly durable, and to be more reliable than endovascular atherectomy or laser angioplasty.[7] The Achilles' heel of the procedure is restenosis secondary to a combination of intimal proliferation and chronic elastic recoil, which limits the long-term efficacy and durability of the procedure.

One method now accepted for the prevention of immediate restenosis is the use of metallic stents. Initially, the stent serves to maintain the luminal cross-sectional area after angioplasty due to its radial expansion and mechanical enlargement of the arterial diameter. Unfortunately, there may also be a tendency to exacerbate smooth muscle cell hypoplasia, leading to accelerated myointimal hyperplasia.

The ideal stent would have the following characteristics: trackability (ie, ease of deployment at the lesion site), radiopacity for ease and accuracy of placement, and flexibility and resistance to elastic recoil and external deforming radial forces. In addition, the stent would not promote thrombosis, and would become endothelialized rapidly without accelerating myointimal hypoplasia. This ideal stent is not presently available, but a number of stents are now on the market.

Currently available intravascular stents are either balloon expandable (eg, the Palmaz® and Strecker stents) or self-expandable (eg, the Wallstent® and Gianturco stents). The Palmaz stent (Johnson & Johnson Interventional Systems, Warren, NJ), is a rigid, slotted stainless steel tube less suitable for tortuous areas or areas subject to external compression due to its rigidity. In 1990 the first large trial evaluating the Palmaz stent showed a 2% stent thrombosis rate at 6 months, with almost 90% of patients experiencing some clinical benefit. The Wallstent is a self-expanding cylindrical wire mesh device that shortens longitudinally as it expands. Since the final length of the endoprosthesis depends on the amount of radial expansion, it can be more technically challenging to precisely position it. When balloon-expandable stents were compared to self-expandable stents, there was little difference in their performance.[8]

Endovascular atherectomy devices have been used in conjunction with angioplasty in an attempt to improve outcomes by debulking the plaque. The Collaborative Rotablator Atherectomy Group found their device to be significantly inferior to simple angioplasty in the superficial femoral artery.[7] Transluminal atherectomy currently has no recognized beneficial role in the treatment of aortoiliac occlusive disease.

Mechanisms of Failure

Failure of an initial technically successful PTA within 1 year is usually attributed to smooth muscle cell proliferation or myointimal hyperplasia.[6,9] These can lead to hemodynamically significant restenosis and even thrombosis, causing the majority of intermediate failures between 1 month and 2 years.

Extensive research has been directed at inhibiting postangioplasty smooth muscle cell reaction. Some drug therapies that have been used but not proven efficacious include aspirin, heparins, antineoplastics, calcium channel blockers, cholesterol-lowering agents, colchicine, ACE-inhibitors and fish oils. Radiation therapy, both external and internal beam, has been used to inhibit postangioplasty myointimal hyperplasia. Currently available data on humans are encouraging but are limited to just a few small studies, mainly of the coronary circulation.[10]

The use of stent endoprostheses paradoxically appears to accelerate subsequent myointimal hyperplasia while maintaining the luminal cross-sectional area when compared to an unstented artery following standard angioplasty. Covered stents or stent endoprostheses may theoretically prevent this by isolating the injured artery from the circulation.

PTA and STENT

Angioplasty is more dependent on anatomic criteria than is bypass surgery with respect to long-term patency and results. Intuitive common sense rules of angioplasty have proven correct in multiple studies.[11-14] Angioplasty is more successful under these conditions: when the vessel diameter is larger; the treated lesion is short as opposed to long; single rather than multiple arteries are treated; when the lesion is concentric instead of eccentric; when the lesion is a stenosis rather than an occlusion; and when it is nonostial rather than ostial.

A resting ankle/brachial pressure index (ABI) and computed tomographic angiography are obtained preoperatively to determine perfusion and confirm location of occlusion.

The mere identification of a treatable lesion on diagnostic angiography is not an indication for proceeding with surgery. Consultation with the vascular surgeon is critical. Once the lesion is deemed suitable for PTA and is found to be the source of significant clinical symptoms, the procedure can be performed.

Preprocedure

Ideally, the diagnostic and therapeutic parts of the examination can be performed at one sitting to reduce overall procedure time as well as complications. Standard preprocedure management should be performed with appropriate review of history, physical examination and diagnostic tests. The patient's renal function and coagulation parameters need to be reviewed and their medications identified (eg, if the patient is diabetic, caution should be used with respect to use of metformin and iodinated contrast). The patient needs to abstain from metformin for 48 hours pre- and post-administration of iodinated contrast to prevent potential nephrotoxicity. Consent for diagnostic angiography should include a discussion of potential therapeutic options-angioplasty, stent deployment and thrombolysis. The patient should be well hydrated and started on daily low-dose aspirin.

A complete study of the involved vasculature is obtained prior to focusing on the offending lesion. This is performed using a right common femoral arterial approach with a flush catheter proximal to the lesion. First, document and characterize the lesion with two-view angiography—determine its location, degree of calcification, concentricity, length, and whether it is diffuse or focal, and identify the distal runoff vasculature. Using digital subtraction angiography (DSA) and roadmapping techniques, procedure time and the volume of nephrotoxic contrast required has decreased significantly. The use of new iso-osmolar nonionic contrast agents and the use of CO_2 and gadolinium for contrast angiography reduce nephrotoxicity.

Following demonstration of a focal stenosis, arterial pressures can be obtained if there is question regarding the hemodynamic significance of the lesion. Any pressure gradient is abnormal; however, to perform PTA, a gradient greater than 15 mm Hg following flow augmentation with an intraarterial vasodilator should be present.

If the patient's symptoms are more acute in nature or have shown an acute deterioration, the potential for embolus must be considered and preangioplasty thrombolytic therapy may be considered.

Procedure

The use of heparin during the procedure and the administration of antiplatelet agents postangioplasty are variable. In our practice, intraarterial heparin is felt to be useful both for its anticoagulant and antispasmodic effects. After administration of a systemic bolus of 3000-5000 units, we monitor the activated clotting time (ACT) at the conclusion of the procedure. Other drugs that are of use at the time of the procedure include nitroglycerine, and sublingual nifedipine or intravenous verapamil as antispasmodic drugs. These drugs are used more liberally in procedures involving the smaller vessels, where a higher risk of spasm exists. All of our patients have continuous physiological monitoring and conscious sedation as needed.

The use of a vascular sheath at the entry site is useful, particularly for periprocedural angiography, administration of intraarterial medications, and smooth exchange of guidewire and catheters.

Crossing the lesion is the most critical part of the angiography procedure, therefore direct visualization with roadmapping is advantageous. Typically, if the lesion is concentric, it can be crossed with a floppy-tipped guidewire. If the lesion is somewhat eccentric, a hydrophilic-coated wire (eg, glidewire; Terumo, Meditech, Watertown, MA) is useful and has increased the initial success rate of angioplasty.[15] In the presence of occlusion, either a small J-tipped guidewire or glidewire is useful.

There have been significant technologic advances in balloon materials and manufacturing techniques, giving us balloons with better physical characteristics. Low-compliance balloons offer more dilating force at the stenosis with a predictable diameter and profile retention, and a safer failure mode. A low balloon profile helps minimize entry site complications and aids in the traversing of severely stenotic lesions. High strength, ultrathin wall polymers have decreased folded diameters, increasing inflation size ratios, and allowing the development of high-pressure balloon systems (20 atm). Improved column strength, shaft lateral flexibility, and low lumen friction with the guidewire are the main elements contributing to good trackability. There are hydrophilic-coated, low-profile angioplasty catheters with excellent trackability available in various sizes and lengths, and these have significantly decreased complication rates.

Once the lesion has been crossed, a diagnostic catheter is advanced and a test injection performed to confirm the intraluminal location. A stiffer wire is placed and balloon size selected. The balloon length chosen is slightly longer than the lesion and the diameter is approximately 10%-20% oversized.[16] A safe rule of thumb is to use the minimum force to do the job, so start with low pressure and increase it incrementally. The bursting pressure of the balloon should not be exceeded and the duration of balloon inflation should range from 30 to 120 seconds, with a mixture of contrast and saline, until the lesion "waist" has been obliterated; then the balloon is deflated rapidly. The patient may experience mild pain, which is normal, but severe pain can be indicative of vessel rupture or other complication. A diagnostic angiogram should be performed with the guidewire remaining across the lesion.

In the setting of multiple lesions, it is optimal to dilate the most distal lesion first. If a significant residual stenosis remains, the anatomic result should be optimized using a balloon 1 mm larger and the lesion re-dilated. An unsatisfactory result may be salvaged with further angioplasty or stent placement.

Recent studies have found that PTA followed by stenting for superficial femoral artery occlusion results in better 2- and 3-year patency rates.

Postprocedure

If the patient has had heparin during the procedure, we typically wait until the ACT drops below 170 seconds before sheath withdrawal. The heparin can be reversed with protamine sulfate. Continued heparinization may be indicated if: one has performed infrapopliteal intervention; there is poor run-off or a low flow state, or; significant dissection extending beyond the angioplasty site is present.

Postprocedure antiplatelet therapy is instituted in the hope of reducing early restenosis and thrombosis.[18] We routinely put our patients on aspirin (325 mg) for at least 6 months, but various combinations of agents including aspirin, dipyridamole and ticlopidine are used.

For follow-up, the patient should have an ankle/brachial index (ABI) within 48 hours for baseline and this should be monitored at visits at 3, 6, and 12 months, and subsequent yearly visits.

Complications of Angioplasty

The principal advantages of percutaneous angioplasty over surgical management are reduced risk and cost. Therefore maximizing success and minimizing complications with precise and efficient technique is critical. With continued improvements in techniques, equipment, and materials, we should expect both the occurrence and number of complications to diminish.

Complications requiring treatment and overall complication rates are 2.0%-2.5% and 9%-10%, respectively.[19-21] In a study of 3784 patients, the most common complications occurred at the puncture site (Table 1).[22]

Careful attention to technique with the use of the smallest possible catheters and sheaths decreases local hematoma and pseudoaneurysm occurrence. The timing and method of sheath removal is critical. If heparin has been administered, it must be reversed or coagulation monitored prior to obtaining hemostasis. Most groin hematomas can be managed nonoperatively or with nonemergent groin exploration. Pseudoaneurysms and arteriovenous fistulas can be managed with ultrasound compression or direct thrombin injection. A number of vascular seal devices, for use at arterial puncture sites, that claim to decrease local complications are now available.

Arterial injuries occurring beyond the puncture site consist mostly of dissections, perforations and embolization. Distal embolization is most likely to occur when one is dealing with an occluded vessel, and it can occur during balloon dilation, wire and sheath passage, or even forceful contrast injection. If there is acute limb-threatening ischemia, then the patient should have surgical embolectomy. If the limb remains viable, treatment options include

Table 1

Complications of Angioplasty

Location	Incidence
Puncture site (total)	**4.0%**
Bleeding	3.4%
False aneurysm	0.5%
Arteriovenous fistula	0.1%
Angioplasty site (total)	**3.5%**
Thrombus	3.2%
Rupture	0.3%
Distal vessel (total)	**2.7%**
Dissection	0.4%
Embolization	2.3%
Systemic (total)	**0.4%**
Renal failure	0.2%
Myocardial infarction (fatal)	0.2%
Cerebrovascular accident (fatal)	0.55%
Consequences	**Incidence**
Surgical repair	2.0%
Limb loss	0.2%
Mortality	0.2%

Source: Reference 22.

thrombolysis if the occlusion is felt to be recent in origin; if the lesion is longstanding, it is likely that the embolus is partially plaque or intima, and therefore it will not respond to thrombolytic therapy.

Acute occlusion at the angioplasty site can be secondary to thrombosis, vasospasm or intimal injury. Immediate intraarterial treatment with heparin and a vasolytic agent should be attempted. If this fails, thrombolytic therapy should be considered. If the occlusion is secondary to an intimal flap, the lesion may be traversed again and a stent placed to salvage the procedure. Acute arterial rupture should be controlled by immediate reinflation of the appropriate balloon and the surgical team consulted. In some cases, reinflation of the balloon will occlude the offending lesion and result in sealing the perforation and restoration of intravascular flow. However, if extravasation persists, placement of a stent (or covered stent if one is available) should be considered. Balloon rupture can occur, but fortunately most are longitudinal and do not prevent balloon withdrawal through a sheath.

Mortality (0.2%) usually occurs as a result of hemorrhage or a primary cardiac event. Wolf and colleagues[23] randomized 263 patients to angioplasty or surgery for lower extremity ischemia and found 30-day mortality to be 0% and 2.4% respectively, with no statistical difference between the two groups with respect to primary success or limb salvage.

The systemic complications are related to contrast with respect to renal failure, and the length and difficulty of the procedure with respect to both cerebrovascular accidents and myocardial infarctions, which are the major sources of mortality.

3. Aortoiliac and Infrainguinal Disease

The atherosclerotic process most commonly affects the superficial femoral and popliteal arteries, with the earliest symptoms usually being intermittent claudication localized to the calf. In the infrainguinal arterial tree, occlusions are 3 times more common than stenoses, and most are long, making them less suitable for angioplasty.[13]

The distal aorta and its bifurcation into the 2 iliac arteries are the next most frequent sites of disease involvement. Narrowing or resultant thrombosis of these arteries may initially produce pain in the buttocks or thighs as well as the legs. It is also not uncommon for men to have associated vasculogenic impotence due to hypogastric (internal iliac) artery involvement.

Currently, the primary indications for an interventional procedure in patients with lower extremity arterial disease include: 1.) incapacitating claudication interfering with work or lifestyle; 2.) limb salvage in patients with limb-threatening ischemia as manifested by rest pain, nonhealing ulcers, and/or infection or gangrene; and rarely, 3.) vasculogenic impotence.

For the diagnostic angiogram, arterial access should be contralateral to the symptomatic side and typically via the common femoral artery. Access for the endovascular intervention, however, is somewhat debatable and dependent on the exact location of the lesion. With modern low-profile balloons with good trackability, a contralateral approach is feasible for common femoral, proximal superficial and proximal deep femoral artery angioplasties, while more distal lesions necessitate ipsilateral antegrade femoral arterial puncture.

For infrainguinal lesions inaccessible from a contralateral approach, antegrade common femoral arterial puncture is the choice. It is critical to ensure puncture of the artery below the inguinal ligament in the antegrade common femoral artery to prevent any hemorrhagic complication.[24] Popliteal artery puncture is a rarely used alternative access if an antegrade approach to a difficult superficial femoral lesion has not been successful.

Special care must be taken when dealing with common femoral arterial lesions because of the risk of occluding the non-target vessel. Surgical approach and access is relatively straightforward and should be considered. If PTA is decided upon, then wire and balloon access to both vessels via a sheath traversing the aortic bifurcation is required to protect the non-target vessel from embolus and occlusion during dilatation.

When dealing with occlusions, depending on the suspected time interval, thrombolytic therapy prior to attempted guidewire traversal can be attempted.[25-27] This lengthens the procedure but reduces the incidence of embolism and the uncovered causative lesion may be surprisingly focal and easily dealt with. Forceful recanalization and PTA and/or stenting can then be undertaken.

Graft PTA

PTA of surgical grafts in the infrainguinal region can be performed to lengthen the graft life and to spare the patient further surgery.[17] With greater graft surveillance, stenoses are now being identified before thrombosis, making PTA for hyperplasia, anastomotic stenoses, or valvular stenoses significantly technically easier to perform.

Infrapopliteal

There is less literature on infrapopliteal PTA and the risks are higher.[28-30] The indication for angioplasty is predominantly limited to ischemia and limb salvage, with lifestyle-limiting claudication a potential indication in individual cases. Ideally, one attempts to restore inline flow to the foot.

Because of the vessel size and the critical reduced flow, liberal use of heparin and antispasmodics in the form of nifedipine (10-20 mg) and nitroglycerin (boluses of 100-200 mcg) are encouraged. Balloon catheters now used for distal lesions have shorter and manageable shaft lengths with diameters in the 2- to 4-mm range. Steerable platinum-tipped and small vessel glidewires, 0.018 to 0.025 inch, are also available. For infrapopliteal lesions, the antegrade approach of the common femoral artery is requisite. In the setting of multiple-level disease, a superficial femoral arterial lesion should be angioplastied first, and multiple infrapopliteal lesions should be attempted commencing distally and progressing proximally. In successful infrapopliteal angioplasty, most angiographers maintain the patient on heparin for at least 48 hours postprocedure and subsequently change the patient to antiplatelet agents.

Results of Balloon Angioplasty

Since the first reports on iliac angioplasty in the 1970s, it has become evident that it is a relatively safe and durable procedure. Iliac artery angioplasty is useful not only for dilatation of primary lesions but also as an adjunct to enhance inflow for infrainguinal operations. The success rate for femoropopliteal or femorofemoral surgery following ipsilateral iliac artery angioplasty is high when the procedure is well-performed technically. On average, the initial technical success of iliac angioplasty is greater than 90% with 3-year patency greater than 70%. To help with comparison and interpretation of studies, objective clinical and radiological criteria for improvement have been established. Tables 2 and 3 summarize categories of chronic limb ischemia and grades of clinical response to therapy as proposed by Rutherford and Becker.[31] Most contemporary studies now report success as maintenance of greater than 1 grade of clinical improvement. Radiologic patency does not always correlate to clinical improvement. Sullivan and colleagues[32] found in a series of 288 patients that despite a 24-month 73% angiographic patency rate, only 57% of the patients maintained their clinical improvement. As with standard surgical bypasses, clinical deterioration may also be secondary to progression of disease in the vessels proximal or distal to the treated lesion.

In the University of Toronto series, 313 common iliac and 209 external iliac angioplasties were reported with an overall 3-year patency of 68% and 51%, respectively.[33] Possible but unproved reasons for the

Table 2

Clinical Categories of Chronic Limb Ischemia

Grade	Category	Clinical description	Objective criteria
I	0	Asymptomatic	Normal treadmill/stress test
I	1	Mild claudication	Complete treadmill, postexercise ankle pressure >25 mm Hg below resting level but still >50 mm Hg
I	2	Moderate claudication	Symptoms between category 1 and 3
I	3	Severe claudication	Incomplete treadmill, postexercise ankle pressure <50 mm Hg
II	4	Ischemic rest pain	Resting ankle pressure <40 or toe pressure <30 mm Hg
II	5	Minor tissue loss, nonhealing ulcer, focal gangrene with diffuse pedal edema	Resting ankle pressure <60 mm Hg or toe pressure <40 mm Hg
II	6	Major tissue loss, extending above transmetatarsal level, functional foot not salvageable	Resting ankle pressure <40 or toe pressure <30 mm Hg

Adapted from Reference 31.

Table 3

Outcome Criteria after Therapeutic Intervention

Clinical grade	Change in symptoms
+3	Markedly improved: Asymptomatic with ABI increased to normal (>0.95)
+2	Moderately improved: 1 clinical category and >0.10 ABI improvement
+1	Minimally improved: <0.10 ABI or 1 clinical category improvement
0	No change: <0.10 ABI change and no clinical category change
–1	Minimally worsened: >0.10 ABI or 1 clinical category deterioration
–2	Moderately worsened: 1 clinical category and >0.10 ABI deterioration
–3	Markedly worsened: >1 clinical category deterioration including amputation

Adapted from Jones DN, Rutherford RB. Evaluation of results, standard reporting practices and the computerized vascular registry. In: Rutherford RB ed. Vascular Surgery. *Philadelphia, PA: Saunders; 1995:456-469.*

external iliac lower patency rate may include a smaller arterial diameter, more diffuse atherosclerotic disease, different plaque morphology, hemodynamic factors, or a more aggressive response to arterial injury such as that seen in the adjacent femoral vessels. If stents are placed in a distal external iliac, one needs to be careful not to have them extend to the common femoral artery where the potential risk for stent fracture exists secondary to repeated hip flexion at the groin.

Placement of stents is particularly useful during PTA to serve as an adjunct to reduce the incidence of dissections and prevention of recoil. They are widely used despite their added significant costs and are a routine part of a standard iliac angioplasty in many centers.[32] In general, immediate technical success is 75%-100% with 2- to 4-year patency rates in the range of 53%-91%. The available reports suggest the use of stents increases immediate and long-term patency without increasing the complication rate. Bosch and Hunink[34] published a meta-analysis comparing 8 iliac stent studies (n = 816) and 6 iliac angioplasty studies (n = 1300), all published after 1989. He found that patients receiving stents in comparison to PTA had an immediate technical success rate of 96% versus 91% (P <0.05), and a higher post-procedure ABI (0.87 versus 0.76, P = 0.03). The 4-year primary patency of a stented artery and an angioplastied artery was 77% and 64%, respectively. Stent placement is an important adjunct to transluminal angioplasty when a dissection occurs or when a lesion is particularly complex. Routine stent placement is now commonly employed in conjunction with transluminal angioplasty in both iliac and superficial femoral arteries.

Use of covered endoprostheses in occlusive disease has its origin in its original use in aneurysmal abdominal aortic disease. Cynamon and colleagues[35] reported placement of stent grafts in the aortoiliac system in 17 patients. All of these grafts were extended beyond the common femoral artery to the superficial femoral artery, popliteal artery or deep femoral artery. These composite custom-made stent grafts were constructed with 6 mm PTFE sutured onto 29 mm Palmaz stents at one end with the PTFE serving as a prosthetic conduit distally. The distal end of the PTFE graft was usually hand-sewn at the outflow target artery. Comparison of PTFE nitinol self-expanding stent grafts gave the same results as above knee prosthetic femopopliteal bypass.[70] Covered endoprostheses theoretically may preserve luminal integrity in the event of a major dissection and also reduce the incidence of embolization and myointimal hyperplasia ingrowth through the stent interstics compared to bare metal stents. Potential disadvantages of the covered endoprostheses include a higher profile compared to noncovered stents and a longer graft-arterial interface.

Iliac artery occlusions were once thought to be unsuitable for transluminal angioplasty because of an anticipated unacceptable risk of embolization, rethrombosis, and dissection. However, this perception has evolved significantly over the past decade as technological and pharmaceutical advancements have been made.[31,36-40] Reported series of angioplasty of occluded iliac arteries are presented in Table 4. The immediate success rate ranges from 76%-92% and the 3-year patency ranges from 58%-86%. As shown in Table 4, many authors have achieved good results without using thrombolytic therapy routinely.

Aortic angioplasty, when utilized in the properly selected patient, can be very effective. In general, the reported patency of aortic angioplasty does not significantly differ from that of iliac angioplasty. Technical considerations include the need for a larger balloon, a larger stent and lower inflation pressure.

Table 4

Summary of Some of the Data Available on Angioplasty, with or without Stenting, of Occluded Iliac Arteries

	Inclusive	No.		Success[b]			E	
Author	**years of review[a]**	**patients**	**Immediate**	**1 year**	**3 year**	**5 year**	**Embolization**	**Thrombolytics**
Johnston[31] (1987)	1978-86	82	76	73	58			
Vorwerk[36] (1995)	1987-93	127	77	87	81	51	5%	None
Blum[37] (1993)	1988-92	47	85		86		6%	All
Gupta[38] (1993)	1993	50	79	76		76	8%	None
Reyes[39] (1997)	1990-93	59	92	—	73 (24 months)	—	7%	No
Motarjeme[40] (1995)	Prior to 1995	99	86	—	—	80		All

[a] *Refers to inclusive time interval of study*

[b] *Success refers to radiologically determined or clinically determined primary patency after exclusion of immediate failures. If both were reported, the lower primary patency rate was used*

4. Renal Artery Stenosis

The objective in the treatment of renal artery stenosis (RAS), either surgical or percutaneous intervention, is to decrease the blood pressure to normal or to reduce the pharmacotherapy necessary, and to maintain or restore renal function as the natural history of RAS progresses.[41-42] Prospective studies of patients with RAS have shown that complete occlusions develop in 9%-14% of affected arteries and up to 40% of patients experience contralateral stenosis over a 2- or 3-year period.[13 11] Approximately two-thirds of cases are atherosclerotic in nature, with fibromuscular dysplasia (FMD) representing most of the remaining one-third. Atherosclerotic RAS predominantly affects males with a mean age at presentation of 55 years and it has a slight left-sided dominance, whereas patients with FMD are predominantly younger and female and the disease tends to be right-sided.

Captopril renography at present is widely used as a screening examination, but with false-negative rates of 10%-25%, the search for the ideal diagnostic test continues.[45] At present magnetic resonance angiography (MRA), computed tomography angiography (CTA), and Doppler ultrasound are under investigation and these may be the gold standard of angiography for final diagnosis of RAS. Angiography has the advantage of providing therapeutic options at the time of the diagnostic evaluation.

Only 4% of hypertension patients have nonessential hypertension, with the majority of these related to renal causes. The criteria used for patient selection are new onset hypertension in children and adults younger than 40 years old, accelerated hypertension, hypertension difficult to control, rapidly deteriorating renal function or rapidly worsening hypertension, or hypertension or renal function that deteriorates following administration of angiotensin-converting enzyme (ACE) inhibitors. The presence of an abdominal bruit, neurofibromatosis, or Takayasu disease with hypertension also merits further evaluation.

The incidence of renal failure caused by renovascular disease, with or without accompanying hypertension, is increasing partly because of the growing population of elderly patients. The use of revascularization procedures to halt the progression of renal failure and hopefully improve renal function is now accepted, but still not firmly established. Accordingly, until an ideal noninvasive method of assessing those patients who will actually benefit from renovascular intervention becomes a reality, the final proof in most situations is the posttreatment evaluation, ie, the cure or improved control of hypertension or the improvement of renal function after surgery or percutaneous intervention.

Numerous studies have now been published[46-52] with respect to technique, benefits and results of percutaneous transluminal renal angioplasty (PTRA) (Table 5). Although most reports have reasonably similar definitions for cure, improvement, benefit, and technical success, there are sufficient variations between these reports to make comparisons at times difficult. Cure is defined in most reports as a diastolic pressure less than or equal to 90 mm Hg without the need for hypertensive medication. Improvement is usually defined as either a 15% decrease in diastolic pressure or a diastolic pressure less than 90 mm Hg accompanied by a decrease in the level of antihypertensive medication required to maintain this blood pressure. Benefit is defined as either a cure or improvement.

Patients with atherosclerotic RAS are older than those with FMD and tend to have widespread atheromatous lesions. In addition, atherosclerotic lesions tend to be more complex (eccentric, calcified, longer), may involve branch vessels, and may have a greater propensity for immediate recurrence and local complications. Cure is unusual in renovascular hypertension (RVH) secondary to atherosclerosis and occurs in only approximately 14% of patients, but up to 77% of patients do show clinical improvement. Ostial lesions are more difficult to dilate than lesions along the course of the renal arteries. Most reports also indicate that patients with unilateral disease tend to experience better long-term results than those with bilateral disease or with a solitary kidney. In the only prospective randomized trial of surgery vs. PTRA in patients with atheromatous disease, Weibull and colleagues[51] stated they "recommend PTRA as a first choice of therapy for atherosclerotic renal artery stenosis causing renovascular hypertension." In their report, the primary patency rate was 75% with a secondary patency rate of 90% for PTRA as documented in their 2-year angiographic follow-up.

Table 5

Primary Success Rate and Clinical Results of PTRA in Atherosclerotic RAS

Author(s), year	No. of patients	Primary success (%)	Cure (%)	Improved (%)	Benefit (%)
Tegtmeyer et al[46] (1984)	65	94	23	71	94
Miller et al[47] (1985)	34	87	15	49	64
Klinge et al[48] (1989)	134	77	10	68	78
Martin et al[49] (1992)	94	78	22	46	68
Losinno et al[50] (1993)	153	95	12	51	63
Weibull et al[51] (1993)	29	83	12	71	83
Rodriguez-Perez et al[52] (1994)	37	78	0	81	81
Pooled results	546	85	14	63	77

RAS poses a difficult clinical problem in the setting of RVH in the transplantation patient. A number of studies have shown transplantation PTRA to have significant success, and it has therefore become the first-line therapy.[53]

Patients with renal impairment are the most difficult group to treat. One-third of elderly hypertensive patients with diminished renal function have RAS, and approximately 15% of those who are older than 50 years of age with chronic renal failure have RAS. A number of studies have now established a role for PTRA in patients with both established renal failure and impaired renal function.[50,54] It may be useful to view atherosclerotic renal arterial disease as a potentially correctable cause of renal failure and our goal should be to prevent progression of the disease to renal failure with all of its attendant morbidity. Losinno and associates[50] in their review of 195 patients, 60 of whom had renal impairment, showed improvement or stabilization of renal function in 56 patients.

Although the complication rate for PTRA is not high, the complications can be serious, occasionally leading to death, significant worsening of renal function, or emergency surgery as a result of uncontrollable hemorrhage. However, PTRA has a success rate similar to surgical intervention, as well as a slightly lower mortality and morbidity rate, including a lower nephrectomy rate.[55,56]

Table 6 documents a number of reports and experiences with combined PTRA and renal artery stent placement.[57-62] Dorros and associates[61] have published a multicenter study that involved the placement of the Palmaz-Schatz stent in 92 atherosclerotic RAS patients as the primary method of treatment. Technical success was 100% with a restenosis rate of 25% on 6-month follow-up angiography in 45 patients, which is less than the incidence of restenosis occurring after PTRA without stent placement in a similar group of patients. They conclude that stent placement "appears to be a reasonably durable and beneficial preferential therapeutic alternative to balloon angioplasty or surgical revascularization."

Table 6

Primary Success and Restenosis Rates in Stent Placement in the Renal Artery

Author(s), year	Stent	No. of patients	Success (%)	Restenosis	Follow-up angioplasty (mos)	Ostial lesion
Kuhn[57] (1991)	Strecker	10	75	18	—	0
Rees[58] (1991)	Palmaz	28	97	25	5	28
Hennequin[59] (1994)	Wallstent	21	90	20	29	7
Raynaud[60] (1994)	Wallstent	18	100	12	11	4
Dorros[61] (1995)	Palmaz	76	100	25	6	—
Van De Ven[62] (1995)	Palmaz	24	100	16	6	24
Pooled results		177	94	19	11	63

Until further multicenter prospective trials appear comparing combined PTRA and stent placement with simple PTRA and other therapeutic options, it is likely that stent placement for RAS will remain a secondary level option to be used in the setting of restenosis or technically difficult cases and poor immediate results. However, initial data do suggest that primary stent placement (without prior PTRA) may eventually become the standard method for treating many renal artery lesions in the future.

5. Visceral

The superior and inferior mesenteric arteries supply the vast majority of the gastrointestinal tract while the celiac artery supplies a number of branches to the pylorus and first portion of the duodenum and several branches to the greater curvature of the stomach.

With respect to occlusive disease, there are two distinct clinical entities to be aware of: chronic mesenteric ischemia and acute mesenteric ischemia (CMI, AMI). The classic symptoms of CMI are postprandial abdominal pain and eventual weight loss, with a specific history of "fear of food" occasionally noted. AMI typically presents with abdominal pain that is out of proportion to the physical findings. CMI is an uncommon manifestation of atherosclerotic occlusive disease as there is an abundant collateral circulation that exists among the visceral vessels. Typically, a gradual progressive stenosis of more than one vessel is needed for the patient to have significant symptoms. The classic angiographic finding is of significant stenosis of 2 of the 3 vessels (celiac, superior mesenteric artery [SMA], inferior mesenteric artery [IMA]). In CMI, once the diagnosis has been made, the therapeutic options are operative arterial bypass graft, PTA and stenting. The mean technical success rate and immediate pain relief for PTA are 83% and 75%, respectively, which is comparable to the surgical results of 100% and 84%, respectively. The operative procedure has more durability, with primary and secondary success rates of 80% and 90% vs. 50% and 30% for surgery and PTA, respectively, but it is associated with a higher complication rate.[63] It may be appropriate for those patients with acceptable operative risks to undergo the operative procedures whereas PTA is more appropriate in those patients who carry prohibitive operative risks.

6. Supraaortic

Fear of cerebral embolization has delayed aggressive endovascular therapy in the supraaortic arteries. However, starting in 1980 subclavian arterial angioplasty began and since then there has been a steady increase in the level of intervention. Published incidences of complications associated with PTA in this therapy approach 5% with a 14% restenosis rate.[64-65] As experience has been gained, the feasibility of recanalizing an occlusive lesion in a subclavian vessel, for example, has also been performed more frequently.

Subclavian and Axillary Arteries

Stenotic or occlusive disease of the subclavian and axillary arteries are considered to be uncommon. The typical presenting complaints include arm claudication, upper extremity ischemia or "subclavian steal syndrome," and vertebral basilar symptoms that occur on extremity exertion. A coronary steal syndrome has also been described that refers to blood flow being redirected from an internal mammary to coronary artery graft to the exercising arm. In many ways these problems are more ideally suited to endovascular therapies since the surgical procedures carry significant morbidity and mortality, especially when a transthoracic approach is needed. Extrathoracic and extraanatomic surgical intervention are somewhat more appealing, and include carotid subclavian, axilloaxillary, and femoral axillary bypasses. Most supraaortic arterial stenotic disease is primarily atherosclerosis, but radiation-induced stenosis or aortitis may also be seen. Endovascular therapy is typically used for relief of symptoms only; however, if the internal mammary artery is intended to be used, or indeed if an axillofemoral graft is planned, a proximal asymptotic lesion can be dilated.

Most lesions in the brachiocephalic vessels can be approached from the femoral route, though occasionally an occlusive ostial stenosis is better approached from a brachial route. Left subclavian arterial disease is more common than right. Aggressive anticoagulation is performed with heparinization. As in other locations, a floppy guidewire is initially used in an attempt to cross the occlusive or stenotic area. This is changed to a torque-controlled hydrophilic guidewire when the floppy guidewire fails.

Angioplasty of subclavian artery stenosis has a 92% technical success rate, while stenting and angioplasty for occlusive lesions has a technical success rate approaching 83%.[66-67] The biggest fear with subclavian artery stenosis on the left-hand side is fear of vertebral arterial embolization. PTA of a lesion proximal or distal to the vertebral artery typically does not cause occlusion of the vertebral artery, in spite of the balloon being inflated across the origin of the artery.[68] However, occlusion of the vertebral artery can occur if the plaque is immediately adjacent to the ostial. Interestingly, in recanalization of the subclavian in the presence of a vertebral steal syndrome, vertebral embolization is rare since there is a delay in the redirection of arterial flow during the actual procedure.[69] Balloon angioplasty and stenting of the subclavian and innominate arteries can be accomplished simply, safely, and effectively for both stenotic and occluded vessels.

There is presently significant debate with respect to endovascular therapy of carotid and vertebral artery occlusive disease. It is controversial because of the well-established low morbidity and mortality of surgical carotid endarterectomy. This makes direct comparison with endovascular therapies difficult, and at present a number of trials are underway evaluating these procedures. At present the conventional view is that patients who can undergo conventional surgical endarterectomy should do so, while internal carotid arterial stent placement is an excellent nonsurgical alternative in patients with a prohibitively high surgical risk.

The results of single center studies show a complication rate of approximately 2%-6% and mortality less than 1%. An ongoing prospective trial comparing the safety of percutaneous angioplasty with stenting with those of retrospectively reviewed patients who were treated with carotid endarterectomy is underway. During the same 14-month period, 273 patients underwent treatment of 310 carotid bifurcation stenoses, 107 with stenting following PTA and 166 with carotid endarterectomy (CEA). Nonneurologic complications were evident in 6 stent PTA patients and 2 CEA patients. Combined early stroke and death rates were 3.6% in the CEA group and 3.7% in the stent angioplasty group.

In the vertebral artery territory, the most common site of stenosis is ostial, and treatment is only considered in patients with characteristic clinical signs of vertebral basilar insufficiency. Endovascular treatment is less traumatic and has a lower complication rate than the vascular alternatives and is typically indicated for symptomatic patients with stenosis greater than 70%. Direct clinical correlation of symptoms with the lesion is critical, and in most cases for a vertebral artery lesion to be symptomatic, the contralateral artery is diseased or hypoplastic. The procedure is typically performed with microcatheters and balloons from a femoral approach. Stents are reserved as a salvage procedure for a poor angioplasty result.

With regard to internal carotid artery stenosis, there is ongoing controversy as to the efficacy of stenting (CAS) in comparison to surgical endarterectomy, and the definitive answer will depend on the outcome of a number of trials, including the CREST (Carotid Randomized Endarterectomy Stent Trial) and the CASET (Carotid Arterial Stent Arterectomy Trial). International trials of carotid enarterectomy vs. CAS, conducted in Germany and France without industry support, have shown fewer postoperative neurological events with open operation. The vascular registry of the Society for Vascular Surgery encompassing 6403 procedures recorded a significant difference in outcomes in favor of carotid endartectomy over carotid stenting (death/stroke/myocardial infarction at discharge 6.42% for stenting and 2.62% for open surgery [$P<0.0001$].[71] A conservative approach would reserve endovascular treatment for symptomatic carotid stenosis for which surgical access is hazardous (after neck radiation), symptomatic restenosis following carotid endarterectomy, and in patients who are at high-risk for surgery.

7. References

1. Dormandy J, Mahir M, Ascady G, et al. Fate of a patient with chronic leg ischemia. *J Cardiovasc Surg*. 1989;30:50-57.

2. Criqui MH, Langer, RD, Fronek A, et al. Mortality over a period of 10 years in patients with peripheral arterial disease. *N Engl J Med*. 1992;326:381-386.

3. Dotter CT, Judkins MP. Transluminal treatment of arteriosclerotic obstruction: description of a new technique and a preliminary report of its application. *Circulation* 1964;36:654.

4. Porstman W. Ein neurer Korsett-balloon katheter zur transluminalen rekanalisation nach Dotter unter besondere Berucksichtigung von obliterationen an den Beckenarterien. *Radiol Diagn (Berl)*. 1973;14:239.

5. Gruntzig A, Hopff H. Perkutane Rekanalisation chronischer arterieller Verschlusse mit einem neuen Dilatationskatheter: Modification der Dotter-Technik. *Dtsch Med Wochenschr*. 1974;99:2502-2505.

6. Casteñada-Zúñiga WR, Formanek A, Tradavarthy M, et al. The mechanism of balloon angioplasty. *Radiology* 1980;135:565.

7. The Collaborative Rotablator Atherectomy Group (CRAG). *J Vasc Surg*. 994;19(3):509-515.

8. Rutherford RB, Becker GJ. Standards for evaluating and reporting the results of surgical and percutaneous therapy for peripheral arterial disease. *J Vasc Intervent Radiol*. 1991;2:169-174.

9. Faneli C, Aronoff R. Restenosis following coronary angioplasty. *Am Heart J*. 1990:119:357.

10. Condado JA, Waksman R, Gurdiel O, et al. Long-term angiographic and clinical outcome after percutaneous transluminal coronary angioplasty and intracoronary radiation therapy in humans. *Circulation*. 1997;96:727-732.

11. Krepel VM, van Andel GJ, van Erp WF, Breslau PF. Percutaneous transluminal angioplasty of the femoropopliteal artery: initial and long-term results. *Radiology*. 1985;156:325-328.

12. Hedeman Joosten PP, Ho GH, Breuking FA Jr, et al. Percutaneous transluminal angioplasty of the infrarenal aorta: initial outcome and long-term clinical and angiographic results. *Eur J Vasc Endovasc Surg*. 1996;12(2):201-206.

13. Hewes RC, White Jr RI, Murray RR, et al. Long-term results of superficial femoral artery angioplasty. *AJR*. 1986;146:1025-1029.

14. Stanley B, Teague B, Raptis S, Taylor DJ, Berce M. Efficacy of balloon angioplasty of the superficial femoral artery and popliteal artery in the relief of leg ischemia. *J Vasc Surg*. 1996;23(4):679-685.

15. Hartnell GG, Jones AM, Murphy P. Do hydrophilic guidewires affect the technical success rates of percutaneous angioplasty? *Angiology*. 1995;46(3):229-234.

16. Probst P, Cerny P, Owen A, Mahler F. Patency after femoral angioplasty: correlation of angiographic appearance with clinical findings. *AJR*. 1983;140:1227.

17. Whittemore AD, Donaldson MC, Polak JF, Mannick JA. Limitations of balloon angioplasty for vein graft stenosis. *J Vasc Surg*. 1991;14:340-345.

18. Leon MB, Baim DS, Popma JJ, et al. A clinical trial comparing three antithrombotic drug regimens after coronary-artery stenting. *N Engl J Med*. 1998;339(23):1665-1671.

19. Schwarten DE. Transluminal angioplasty: overview of complications and long-term results. *AJR*. 1985;144:53-57.

20. Weibull H, Bergqvist D, Jonsson K, Karlsson S, Takolander R. Complications after percutaneous transluminal angioplasty in the iliac, femoral and popliteal arteries. *J Vasc Surg*. 1987;5:681-686.

21. Bergqvist D, Jonsson K, Weibull H. Complications after percutaneous transluminal angioplasty of peripheral and renal arteries. *Acta Radiol*. 1987;28:3-12.

22. Pentecost MJ, Criqui MH, Dorros G, et al. Guidelines for peripheral percutaneous transluminal angioplasty of the abdominal aorta and lower extremity vessels. *Circulation*. 1994;89(1).511-531.

23. Wolf GL, Wilson SE, Cross AP, Deupree RH, Stason WB. Surgery or balloon angioplasty for peripheral vascular disease: a randomized clinical trial. *J Vasc Intervent Radiol*. 1993;4(5):639-648.

24. Lechner G, Jantsch H, Waneck R, Kretschmer G. The relationship between the common femoral artery, the inguinal crease, and the inguinal ligament: a guide to accurate angiographic puncture. *Cardiovasc Intervent Radiol*. 1998;11:165-169.

25. Meyerovitz MF, Didier D, Vogel JJ, Soulier-Parmeggiani L, Bounameaux H. Thrombolytic therapy compared with mechanical recanalization in non-acute peripheral arterial occlusions: a randomized trial. *J Vasc Intervent Radiol*. 1995;6(5):775-781.

26. Chalmers RT, Hoballah JJ, Kresowik TF, et al. Late results of a prospective study of direct intra-arterial urokinase infusion for peripheral arterial and bypass graft occlusions. *Cardiovasc Surg*. 1995;3(3):293-297.

27. Motarjeme A, Gordon GI, Bodenhagen K. Thrombolysis and angioplasty of chronic iliac artery occlusions. *J Vasc Intervent Radiol*. 1995;6(6:2 suppl):66S-72S.

28. Brown KT, Schoenberg NY, Moore ED, Saddekni S. Percutaneous transluminal angioplasty of infrapopliteal vessels: preliminary results and technical considerations. *Radiology*. 1988;169:75-78.

29. Bakal CW, Sprayregen S, Scheinbaum K, Cynamon J, Veith FJ. Percutaneous transluminal angioplasty of the infrapopliteal arteries: results in 53 patients. *AJR*. 1990;154:171-174.

30. Leofberg AM, Leorelius LE, Karacgil S, Westman B, Almgren B, Berqgvist D. The use of below-knee percutaneous transluminal angioplasty in arterial occlusive disease causing chronic critical limb ischemia. *Cardiovasc Intervent Radiol*. 1996;19(5):317-322.

31. Rutherford RB, Becker GJ. Standards for evaluating and reporting the results of surgical and percutaneous therapy for peripheral arterial disease. *J Vasc Intervent Radiol*. 1991;2:169-174.

32. Sullivan TM, Childs MB, Bacharach JM, et al. Percutaneous transluminal angioplasty and primary stenting of the iliac arteries in 228 patients. *J Vasc Surg*. 1997;25:829-839.

33. Johnston KW, Rae M, Hogg-Johnston SA, et al. Five year results of a prospective study of percutaneous transluminal angioplasty. *Ann Surg*. 1987;206(4):403-413.

34. Bosch JL, Hunink MGM. Meta-analysis of the results of percutaneous transluminal angioplasty and stent placement for aortoiliac occlusive disease. *Radiology*. 1997;204:87-96.

35. Cynamon J, Marin ML, Veith FJ, et al. Stent-graft repair of aortic-iliac occlusive disease coexisting with common femoral artery disease. *J Vasc Intervent Radiol*. 1997;8(1:1):19-26.

36. Vorverk D, Günther RW, Schürmann K, et al. Primary stent placement for chronic iliac occlusions: Follow-up results in 103 patients. *Radiology*. 1995;194:745-749.

37. Blum U, Gabelmann A, Redecker M, et al. Percutaneous recanalization of iliac artery occlusions: Results of a prospective study. *Radiology*. 1993;189:536-540.

38. Gupta AK, Ravimandalam K, Rao VRK, et al. Total occlusion of iliac arteries: Results of balloon angioplasty. *Cardiovasc Intervent Radiol*. 1993;16:165-177.

39. Reyes R, Maynar M, Lopera J, et al. Treatment of chronic iliac artery occlusions with guide wire recanalization and primary stent placement. *J Vasc Intervent Radiol*. 1997;8(6):1049-1055.

40. Motarjeme A, Gordon GI, Bodenhagen K. Thrombolysis and angioplasty of chronic iliac artery occlusions. *J Vasc Intervent Radiol*. 1995;6(6:2 supp):66S-72S.

41. Mailloux LU. Atherosclerotic renovascular disease causing end-stage renal disease: The case for earlier diagnosis and therapy. *J Vasc Med Biol*. 1993;4:277-284.

42. Schreiber MJ, Pohl A, Novick AC. The natural history of atherosclerotic and fibrous renal artery disease. *Urol Clin North Am*. 1984;11:383-392.

43. Standsby G, Hamilton G, Scoble J. Atherosclerotic renal artery stenosis. *Br J Hosp Med*. 1993;49:388-398.

44. Tollefson DFJ, Ernst CB. Natural history of atherosclerotic renal artery stenosis associated with aortic disease. *J Vasc Surg*. 1991;14:327-331.

45. Mann SJ, Pickering TG, Sos TA, et al. Captopril renography in the diagnosis and treatment of renal artery stenosis: accuracy and limitations. *Am J Med*. 1991;18:289-298.

46. Tegtmeyer CJ, Kellum CD, Ayers C. Percutaneous transluminal angioplasty of the renal artery: Results and long-term followup. *Radiology*. 1984;153:77-84.

47. Miller GA, Ford KK, Braun SD, et al. Percutaneous transluminal angioplasty vs. surgery for renovascular hypertension. *AJR*. 1985;144:447-450.

48. Klinge J, Mali WPTM, Puijlaert CBA, et al. Percutaneous transluminal renal angioplasty: Initial and long-term results. *Radiology*. 1989;171:501-506.

49. Martin LG, Cor RD, Kaufman SL. Long-term results of angioplasty in 110 patients with renal artery stenosis. *J Vasc Intervent Radiol*. 1992;3:619-626.

50. Losinno F, Zuccala A, Busato F, et al. Renal artery angioplasty for renovascular hypertension and preservation of renal function: Long-term angiographic and clinical follow-up. *AJR*. 1994;162:853-857.

51. Weibull H, Bergqvist D, Bergentz S-E, et al. Percutaneous transluminal renal angioplasty versus surgical reconstruction of atherosclerotic renal artery stenosis: A prospective randomized study. *J Vasc Surg*. 1993;18:841-852.

52. Rodriguez Perez JC, Plaza C, Reyes R, et al. Treatment of renovascular hypertension with percutaneous transluminal angioplasty: Experience in Spain. *J Vasc Intervent Radiol*. 1994;5:101-109.

53. Sagalowsky AI, McQuitty DM. The assessment and management of renal vascular hypertension after kidney transplantation. *Semin Urol*. 1994;12(3):211-223.

54. Scoble J, Maher ER, Hamilton G, et al. Atherosclerotic renovascular disease causing renal impairment: A case for treatment. *Clin Nephrol*. 1989;31:119-122.

55. Foster JIL, Maxwell MH, Franklin SS, et al. Renovascular occlusive disease: Results of operative treatment. *JAMA*. 1975;231:1043-1048.

56. Dean RH. Comparison of medical and surgical treatment of renovascular hypertension. *Nephron*. 1986;44(suppl 1):101-104.

57. Kuhn FP, Kutkuhn B, Torsello G, et al. Renal artery stenosis: Preliminary results of treatment with the Strecker stent. *Radiology*. 1991;180:367-372.

58. Rees CR. Palmaz stent in atherosclerotic stenoses involving the ostia of the renal arteries: Preliminary report of a multicenter study. *Radiology*. 1991;181:507-514.

59. Hennequin LM, Joffre FG, Rousseau HP, et al. Renal artery stent placement: Long-term results with the Wallstent endoprosthesis. *Radiology*. 1994;191:713-719.

60. Raynaud AC, Beyssen BM, Turmel-Rodrigues LE, et al. Renal artery stent placement: Immediate and midterm technical and clinical results. *J Vasc Intervent Radiol*. 1994;5:849-858.

61. Dorros G, Jaffe M, Jain A, et al. Follow-up of primary Palmaz-Schatz stent placement for atherosclerotic renal artery stenosis. *Am J Cardiol*. 1995;75:1051-1055.

62. Van de Ven PJG, Beutler JJ, Kaatee R, et al. Transluminal vascular stent for ostial atherosclerotic renal artery stenosis. *Lancet*. 1995;346:672-674.

63. Rose CS, Quigley TM, Raker EJ. Revascularization for chronic mesenteric ischemia: comparison of operative arterial bypass grafting and percutaneous transluminal angioplasty. *J Vasc Intervent Radiol*. 1995;6:339-349.

64. Miilaire A, Trinca M, Marache P, et al. Subclavian angioplasty: Immediate and late results in 50 patients. *Cath Cardiovasc Diagn*. 1993;29:8-17.

65. Queral LA, Criado FJ. The treatment of local aortic arch branch lesions with Palmaz stents. *J Vasc Surg*. 1996;23:368-375.

66. Becker GJ. Noncoronary angioplasty. *Radiology*. 1989;170:921-940.

67. Mathias KD, Lath I, Haarmann P. Percutaneous transluminal angioplasty of proximal subclavian artery occlusions. *Cardiovasc Intervent Radiol*. 1993;16:214-218.

68. Vitek JJ, Keller FS, Duvall ER, Gupta KI, Chandra-Seker B. Brachycephalic artery dilation by percutaneous transluminal angioplasty. *Radiology*. 1986;158:779-785.

69. Ringelstein EB, Zuemer H. Delayed reversal of vertebral artery blood flow following percutaneous transluminal angioplasty for subclavian steal syndrome. *Neuroradiology*. 1984;26:189-198.

70. McQuade K, Gable D, Hohman S, et al. Randomized comparison of ePTFE/nitinol self-expanding stent graft vs. prosthetic femoral-popliteal bypass in the treatment of superficial femoral artery occlusive disease. *J Vasc Surg*. 2009;49:109-116.

71. Sidawy AN, Zwolak RM, White RA, et al. Risk-adjusted 30-day outcomes of carotid stenting and endarterectomy: Results from the SVS Vascular Registry. *J Vasc Surg*. 2009;49:71-79.

8. Questions

1. The initial procedure for percutaneous transluminal angioplasty as described by Dotter in 1964, used a dilating device made of:

   A. PTFE

   B. PVC

   C. Latex

   D. Stainless steel

2. The Palmaz® stent is:

   A. A self-expandable steel stent

   B. A balloon-expandable nitinol stent

   C. A balloon-expandable steel stent

   D. A self-expandable nitinol stent

3. Percutaneous transluminal angioplasty causes the following pathological changes in the vessel wall:

   A. Dissection

   B. Plaque fracture

   C. Plaque separation

   D. All of the above

4. The following therapies have ***not*** been investigated to retard post-angioplasty restenosis:

   A. Smoking

   B. Radiation

   C. Gene therapy

   D. Aspirin

5. With respect to angioplasty complications:

   A. Percutaneous transluminal angioplasty has a higher morbidity and mortality rate than similar surgical procedures

   B. Most angioplasty complications necessitate urgent vascular surgery

   C. Stents can be used to salvage a number of lesion site complications

   D. Complications requiring treatment occur at a rate of 5%

6. With respect to renal artery stenosis:

   A. FMD responds better to angioplasty than atheromatous lesions

   B. FMD is more common in males

   C. One should always primarily stent FMD

   D. FMD is typically bilateral

7. Aortoiliac occlusive disease:

   A. Occlusive iliac lesions respond better than stenosis to angioplasty

   B. One should always attempt percutaneous transluminal angioplasty prior to stent deployment in aortoiliac lesions

   C. Stents are only to be used for salvage of a poor angioplasty result in the iliac arterial territory

   D. Primary stenting of common iliac lesions has better results than angioplasty

8. Infrapopliteal angioplasty:

A. Is only used for patients with claudication

B. Thrombolysis has no benefit

C. One's aim is to achieve in-line flow to the foot

D. Periprocedural anticoagulation is optional

9. With respect to mesenteric ischemia:

A. Chronic mesenteric ischemia typically presents with abdominal pain that is out of proportion to the physical findings

B. Acute mesenteric ischemia typically presents with a history of "fear of food"

C. Single vessel stenosis is the typical finding in chronic mesenteric ischemia

D. In acute mesenteric ischemia secondary to embolism, the origin is most commonly cardiac

10. With respect to supraaortic endovascular intervention:

A. Carotid endarterectomy is no longer a reasonable option for stenotic carotid disease

B. In subclavian steal syndrome, PTA carries a very real risk of vertebral embolism

C. Brachial arterial approach for arch ostial lesions is an option

D. Vertebral artery PTA is indicated in stenotic lesions greater than 90%

Answers

1. A.
Dotter and Judkins[3] advanced sequentially larger PTFE catheters to dilate the flow-restricting stenosis.

2. C.
The Palmaz® stent is the original balloon-expandable steel stent.

3. D.

4. A.
All the other described modalities have been investigated with varied success.

5. C.
Stents can be used to salvage most lesion site complications including immediate restenosis dissection.

6. A.
FMD responds superbly to simple angioplasty with an 80% success rate.

7. D.

8. C.

9. D.
In acute mesenteric arterial embolism, most patients have an underlying cardiac disease such as atrial fibrillation or cardiomyotomy.

10. C.
Ostial lesions are difficult to catheterize from the arch, and the brachial route can significantly increase technical success rates.

Chapter 21: Thyroid and Parathyroid Surgery

David Hsiang, MD

Contents

1. Embryology

The thyroid gland is comprised of endodermal cells that originate from the primitive alimentary tract. During the third week of gestation, it arises as a midline diverticulum from the floor of the pharynx in the region of the foramen cecum.[1] From this point, the main body of the thyroid descends into the neck, where the hollow cylinder of epithelial cells develop into a solid bilobed organ. The original attachment at the foramen cecum then becomes the thyroglossal duct. This structure ruptures and is reabsorbed during the sixth week of gestation. In some cases, the distal end of the duct is retained and develops into the pyramidal lobe of the mature thyroid. The median thyroid anlage develops into the lateral thyroid lobes and isthmus. During the formation of the lateral lobes, calcitonin-producing C cells from the neural crest migrate and concentrate in the upper and middle portions of the thyroid gland.

2. Anatomy

The normal adult thyroid gland weighs approximately 15-20 grams. It is anteriorly bound by the strap muscles (ie, the sternohyoid and sternothyroid), posteriorly bound by the trachea and larynx, and laterally bound by the carotid sheath and sternocleidomastoid muscles. The deep cervical fascia divides into anterior and posterior layers that create a false capsule encompassing the entire thyroid. The posterior layer, more dense and adherent to the trachea, forms the ligament of Berry.

4 major arteries provide the thyroid gland with an abundant blood supply. These arteries include the superior thyroid arteries, which arise bilaterally as the first branch of the external carotid artery and the inferior thyroid arteries, which arise bilaterally from the thyrocervical trunks. Occasionally, there is a fifth artery, the thyroidea ima. It originates from the aortic arch and enters the gland inferiorly in the midline.

The venous blood supply is composed of 3 pairs of vessels. The superior and middle thyroid veins drain into the internal jugular vein; the inferior thyroid vein drains into the innominate vein.

Lymphatic drainage is primarily into the internal jugular nodes. The superior poles and medial isthmus drain into the superior groups of nodes. The inferior groups drain the inferior poles and empty into pretracheal (Delphian) and paratracheal nodes.

There are usually 4 parathyroid glands, each weighing 35 mg. The superior glands are embryologically derived from the fourth brachial pouch. They migrate with the thyroid and lie close to the superior portion of the lateral thyroid lobes. The inferior parathyroid glands and the thymus arise from the third branchial pouch. The inferior parathyroid glands descend with the thyroid but can stop anywhere in between the upper neck and mediastinum. They are most commonly located on the lateral or posterior surface of the inferior pole of the thyroid, but can be located in the top portion of the thymus. A general rule is that the superior parathyroid glands lie laterally to the recurrent laryngeal nerve and the inferior parathyroid glands lie medial to it. Anomalous locations do occur, eg, parathyroid glands can be found in both the anterior and posterior mediastinum, carotid sheath, or behind the esophagus.

Occasionally patients may have more than 4 parathyroid glands. The blood supply to all 4 parathyroid glands usually arises from the inferior thyroid artery.

The recurrent laryngeal nerve is a branch of the vagus nerve that loops around the aortic arch at the ductus arteriosus on the left and around the subclavian artery on the right. The nerve lies in the tracheoesophageal groove, enters the larynx through the cricothyroid membrane, and innervates all of the muscle of the larynx except the cricothyroid muscle. In about 1% of individuals, the right recurrent laryngeal nerve does not loop around the subclavian artery but directly enters the larynx[2] (nonrecurrent laryngeal nerve). On the left side this is extremely rare and is only reported in patients with situs inversus.

There are 3 important anatomic relationships to be aware of when performing a thyroidectomy[3]: the locations of the recurrent laryngeal nerve, the location of the superior laryngeal nerve and the location of parathyroid glands in respect to the thyroid gland itself.

Injury to the recurrent laryngeal nerve results in paralysis of the vocal cord on the ipsilateral side. The cord may remain in a paramedial or abducted position. If the paralyzed cord remains in the paramedial position and the airway is decreased in size, the patient may have a normal but weakened voice with some shortness of breath. If the paralyzed cord remains in an abducted position, its closure is prevented, the voice will be severely impaired, and the patient will have an ineffective cough. Bilateral cord palsies can result in a complete loss of voice or an airway obstruction, both of which require emergency intubation or tracheostomy.

The superior laryngeal nerve arises from the vagus nerve at the base of the skull and divides into 2 branches at the level of the hyoid cornu. The internal branch supplies sensation to the mucosa of the larynx and hypopharynx. The external branch innervates the cricothyroid muscle. The superior laryngeal nerve lies near the upper pole of the thyroid, is closely associated with the superior thyroid vessels, and can easily be damaged during a lobectomy. Injury to this nerve results in vocal fatigue and changes in the strength and pitch of the voice.

The principal blood supply to the parathyroid glands is the inferior thyroid artery. Parathyroid glands invariably have a single end artery supplying them. For this reason, it is preferable to divide only the branches of the inferior thyroid artery medial to those that supply the parathyroid glands. In this way, there will be less chance of disrupting the blood supply to the glands. It is advisable to avoid ligating the main trunk of the inferior thyroid artery.

Thyroglossal Duct Cysts

Thyroglossal duct cysts are midline structures found between the base of the tongue and the suprasternal notch.[4] Up to 75% are found inferior to the hyoid bone. They are most commonly discovered in infancy, but can be found at any age in either sex. Diagnosis is made by asking the patient to protrude their tongue and watching the thyroglossal cyst elevate in the neck. Other symptoms such as choking and dysphagia can occur. Frequently, the cyst becomes infected and surgical excision is required.

Treatment consists of excising the entire cyst and the thyroglossal tract up to its origin at the foramen cecum. Since the tract frequently passes through the center of the hyoid bone, resection of the central portion of the bone is crucial. Failure to entirely excise the tract to the base of the tongue often results in recurrence.

Approximately 1% of thyroglossal duct cysts contain thyroid cancer (usually papillary). If the cancer is limited to the cyst, total excision of cyst and duct may be sufficient; however, in the presence of lymph node metastases, a total thyroidectomy with regional excision of all involved nodes should be considered.

Lingual Thyroid

When the median anlage fails to develop or to descend, the result is a lingual thyroid.[5] In such cases, the lingual thyroid is often the only functioning tissue. When there is airway obstruction, dysphagia or hemorrhage, surgical excision may be required. Most lingual thyroid glands can be treated by exogenous thyroid hormone administration. Since thyroid replacement therapy is well accepted by patients, excision and transplantation of lingual thyroid tissue is rarely performed.

Lateral Aberrant Thyroid

The theory that an embryologic accident can cause normal thyroid tissue to appear in the lateral neck has been abandoned. Such occurrences are almost always due to a follicular variant of papillary carcinoma that has metastasized to the cervical lymph node chain and replaced the nodes with tumor.[6] The diagnosis of lateral aberrant thyroid tissue should always direct the clinician to search for a thyroid cancer in the ipsilateral lobe of the thyroid.

Physiology

The principal function of the thyroid gland is to synthesize and secrete the thyroid hormones necessary for normal metabolic processes. The thyroid gland is also a source of calcitonin, whose role in human physiology is unclear.

Absorption of iodine occurs in the gastrointestinal tract. The necessary dietary iodine intake is between 150-500 mcg/d.[7] The absorbed iodine is distributed in the plasma and extracted by the thyroid or kidney. Approximately two-thirds is excreted in the urine. The iodine is trapped by the thyroid follicular cells and oxidized to a free radical. These activated forms of iodine attach to tyrosine amino acids and form either monoiodotyrosine or diiodotyrosine, which link to form triiodotyrosine (T_3) and thyroxine (T_4). These newly formed molecules are stored on the thyroglobulin molecules located in the colloid center of the thyroid follicle. The thyroid hormones remain stored until their release is initiated by thyroid stimulating hormone.

Thyroid-stimulating hormone (TSH) is a glycoprotein secreted by the anterior pituitary gland. It regulates the synthesis and release of thyroid hormone (T_4/T_3) and iodine trapping by the thyroid cells. The release of TSH from the anterior pituitary gland is controlled by thyrotropin-releasing hormone (TRH). TRH, a peptide produced in the hypothalamus, is transferred to the pituitary by way of the portovenous system.

There are several feedback mechanisms involved in thyroid hormone metabolism. High levels of T^3 and T_4 inhibit the action of TRH on the anterior pituitary by decreasing the secretion of TSH. Also, large amounts of ingested iodine decrease iodine trapping and hormone synthesis.

The thyroid gland is the only endogenous source of T_4, whereas most T_3 is produced by the peripheral conversion of T_4. Once the thyroid hormones are released into the circulation, they are bound to thyronine-binding protein TBG (85%), albumin (10%)

and prealbumin (15%). These binding proteins allow the thyroid hormones to remain soluble in plasma and to be distributed systemically. Both hormones are conjugated in the liver and excreted in bile. T_3 has a half-life of 2-3 days; the half-life of T_4 is 7-10 days.

Hyperthyroidism

The clinical presentation of hyperthyroidism (thyrotoxicosis) consists of tachycardia, fever, weight loss, palpitations, heat intolerance and emotional instability. The cause is due to an elevated circulating level of free T_3, T_4 or both. The 3 most common causes of hyperthyroidism are Graves disease (diffuse toxic goiter), toxic multinodular goiter and a solitary toxic nodule.

Graves Disease (Diffuse Toxic Goiter)

Graves disease is the most common cause of hyperthyroidism. It is 6 times more common in women than men and usually occurs in persons between the ages of 20 and 40. The syndrome is characterized by thyrotoxicosis, diffuse goiter, exophthalmus and pretibial myxedema.

In Graves disease, hyperthyroidism results from the binding of autoantibodies to the TSH receptors on the follicular cells.[8] In about 3% of patients, the thyroid is of normal size, ie, most are diffusely enlarged, symmetric and smooth. ^{131}I uptake is increased symmetrically, a characteristic that helps differentiate Graves disease from other forms of hypothyroidism such as Hashimoto's thyroiditis or toxic multinodular goiter.

The treatment of Graves disease must be individualized for each patient. The three approaches are thionamide drugs, radioactive iodine and thyroidectomy. All are safe and most have good success rates.

Antithyroid drugs, the initial therapy in most patients with Graves disease, may be considered as definitive therapy or as treatment in preparation for ^{131}I or surgical ablation. Long-term thionamide drug use has a high failure rate and its use as a definitive therapy has decreased over the last few years. In addition, there is a small, 0.5% incidence of agranulocytosis risk associated with prolonged thionamide therapy. Success rates are much higher in patients with small or normal sized glands than those with large goiters.

^{131}I has been used for the last 45 years to treat patients with Graves disease. It is a definitive treatment with hypothyroidism as an inevitable result. Most adult patients with Graves disease in the United States are treated with ^{131}I. Exceptions are women during childbearing years, patients with concomitant thyroid nodules, patients with extremely large glands and patients opposed to radiation.

Thyroidectomy for Graves disease is the third option. This is a definitive treatment, but there is controversy about the extent of the operation.[9] The traditional approach is a bilateral subtotal thyroidectomy, which leaves a remnant of 2-4 grams of viable thyroid tissue on either side. A second approach is to perform a total lobectomy on one side, leaving a larger remnant on the contralateral side. Approximately 70% of patients are euthyroid after the procedure, 3%-4% remain hyperthyroid and 25%-30% become hypothyroid. Hypothyroidism is an acceptable end result of the operation, but recurrent hyperthyroidism is not. To correct the recurrent hyperthyroidism involves re-operating or using ^{131}I to ablate the remaining tissue, which negates the reason for choosing surgery in the first place. Consequently, a third approach is to perform a total thyroidectomy as the initial procedure.[10] This has the lowest risk rate but increases two other risks, ie, hypoparathyroidism and recurrent laryngeal nerve injury. Determining the extent of the thyroidectomy requires weighing the risks and benefits. 3 guiding principles should be followed. First, permanent hypoparathyroidism is a serious and lifelong complication that can be avoided by modifying the operation according to the anatomic factors present. Second, since recurrent hyperthyroidism represents an operative failure, the amount of thyroid tissue spared to ensure preservation of the parathyroid glands must be as small as possible. Third, hypothyroidism is not a complication; it is an easily treated consequence of the operation.

Toxic Multinodular Goiter

Toxic multinodular goiter occurs when 1 or more thyroid nodules secrete thyroid hormones independent of TSH. It occurs most often in areas of endemic goiter. This type of hyperthyroidism is milder than hyperthyroidism caused by Graves disease and the patients are usually older. In addition, usually the gland has 1 or more palpable nodules.

The standard treatment is a bilateral subtotal thyroidectomy.[11] ^{131}I is not as effective in treating these nodules; they have lower iodine uptake and require larger doses of radiation for treatment. ^{131}I use should be reserved for poor surgical candidates with no airway obstruction symptoms.

Solitary Toxic Nodule

The solitary toxic nodule represents 5%-10 % of all solitary nodules.[12] There is a female predominance of 13:1 and males are seen in older age groups. Treatment is based on the size of the nodule. For solitary nodules greater than 3 cm, the patients are encouraged to undergo a surgical resection or ^{131}I ablation. There has been a low success rate using antithyroid medication suppression with large nodules.

Thyroiditis

Thyroiditis is an inflammatory condition that may be acute or chronic.

Acute suppurative thyroiditis is an uncommon condition featuring neck pain, a fluctuant gland, fever and chills. Surgical drainage may be required.

Hashimoto's Disease

Hashimoto's disease or chronic lymphocytic thyroiditis, the most common form of thyroiditis, mainly occurs in middle-age women. It is characterized by diffuse indurations of both lobes of the gland. The gland is described as firm and rubbery; it may be asymmetric and nodular in texture. Hashimoto's disease and Graves disease tend to occur in the members of the same family, which suggests a genetic predisposition.

Hashimoto's disease is due to a defect in thyroid hormone synthesis caused by the lack of organification of trapped iodine.[13] This reduced hormone production increases TSH secretion, which results in goiter formation. Most patients eventually become hypothyroid, but in the initial period, mild thyrotoxicosis may occur. The diagnosis is made upon finding lymphocytes and Hurthle cells on biopsy. Additionally, most patients demonstrating elevated levels of antimicrosomal and antithyroglobulin antibodies.

Usually, treatment is with exogenous thyroid hormone. If the goiter continues to grow despite this treatment, a partial thyroidectomy may be required.

De Quervain's Thyroiditis

De Quervain's thyroiditis is a subacute thyroiditis that often follows a viral upper respiratory infection.[14] It usually presents with pain, swelling, fever, fatigue and weight loss. The disease is usually self-limited and symptoms occur for a few weeks. Initially, patients may be hyperthyroid, then hypothyroid and, finally, euthyroid. Symptomatic relief can be achieved with salicylates or steroids.

Riedel Struma

Riedel struma, a rare form of goiter, features a "woody" or fibrous component in the adjacent strap muscles and carotid sheath. Its cause is unknown, but the condition is associated with other types of fibrotic processes, eg, retroperitoneal fibrosis.[15] Clinically, Riedel struma resembles an infiltrative undifferentiated thyroid cancer or lymphoma. Although self-limited, it can cause localized pain and compression of adjacent tissue. Occasionally, a tracheostomy may be required to protect the airway.

Solitary Thyroid Nodule

The prevalence of thyroid nodules in the population ranges from 4%-8 %.[16] Most nodules are colloid nodules or follicular adenomas. In the past, all solitary thyroid nodules that failed to respond to TSH suppression were removed. Presently, selective management is emphasized because of the relatively high frequency of benign nodules.

The history and physical examination are still the most important considerations for patients with thyroid nodules. Often patients are unaware of any thyroid enlargement or symptoms even after the nodule has been identified. The relationship between radiation exposure during infancy or childhood and thyroid cancer is well established. This relationship should always be explored when taking the history. A history of low-dose radiation exposure is a strong factor favoring a more aggressive approach to a thyroid nodule. Other important factors are the use of thyroid hormones in the past and any change in nodule size during treatment. If a nodule is growing or not responding to suppressive doses of thyroid hormone, it would suggest that the nodule is autonomous and may be malignant.

Upon physical exam, certain findings are more likely to point toward thyroid malignancy. Large, firm lymph nodes in the lower third of the neck are often present, particularly in children and in young adults with papillary carcinoma. Lymphadenopathy in association with an ipsilateral thyroid nodule should always be considered to be malignant until proven otherwise. Fixation of a nodule to surrounding tissue also tends to imply malignancy. The palpable consistency of the nodule is more variable. Some malignancies are soft and cystic in nature. The presence of hoarseness without recurrent laryngeal nerve palsy may occur with either benign or malignant nodules. Paralysis of the recurrent laryngeal nerve is more suggestive of a carcinoma.

The most common imaging study is the thyroid scintiscan.[17] The scintiscan should supplement the physical exam. The results are not decisive in choosing the treatment modality. A nodule has to be at least 1 cm or larger to be picked up by the scan. Most patients are referred for surgical treatment for a cold nodule. A scintiscan may be of value when the thyroid gland cannot be completely palpated because of it substernal extension or because the patient's neck is too thick and muscular.

Fine needle aspiration biopsy has been used extensively for 30 years in Scandinavia. Over the last 10 years this technique has gained wide acceptance in the United States.[18] The technique is applicable to any palpable thyroid nodule. The false-negative rate is 10% and the false-positive rate is less than 2%. Because the false-negative rate is 10% this technique has to be used with careful clinical judgment when selecting operative candidates. The cytology studies can identify papillary, medullary and anaplastic carcinoma, but they cannot differentiate malignant from benign follicular or Hurthle cell carcinoma. Follicular and Hurthle cell neoplasia require the excision of the entire tumor to determine if there is any capsule invasion of the gland.

The surgical procedure of choice is a total extracapsular thyroid lobectomy and isthmectomy for removal of the solitary nodule. When the nodule is located in the isthmus, it may be excised with a clear margins on both sides. After a delayed diagnosis of malignancy, an initial total lobectomy is safer than a partial lobectomy followed by a subsequent resection of the residual lobe. Re-operation to complete a lobectomy is associated with greater risk to both recurrent laryngeal nerve and parathyroid glands.

Thyroid Carcinoma

Thyroid carcinomas are classified as papillary, follicular, Hurthle cell, medullary and anaplastic. Their virulence ranges from indolent to highly lethal. Lymphomas can occur as primary neoplasms arising from the thyroid gland or the thyroid gland can be the site of metastatic carcinoma.

Papillary Carcinoma

Papillary carcinoma is divided into 3 groups based on size and local extent of the tumor: minimal, intrathyroidal and extrathyroidal with invasion through the capsule.[19]

Minimal thyroid carcinoma are less than 1 cm in diameter and are not associated with any clinically apparent lymph node metastases. For tumors between 0.5 to 1 cm, a total lobectomy and isthmectomy is adequate.

Intrathyroid carcinomas, the most common, range from 1-4 cm in diameter and are contained within the gland. There is a high rate of multicentricity accounting for 20%-30% of all cases. Cervical lymph node metastasis in the central compartment, anterior mediastinum or lateral cervical nodes are found in 30% of patients with papillary carcinoma.

The presence of lymph nodes metastases correlates more with the age of the patient than the size of the tumor. Nearly all patients younger than 15 years of age have metastases to the regional lymph nodes. The presence or absence of lymph node metastases does not appear to have an appreciable effect on long-term survival of the patient if distant metastases are not present at the time of initial treatment.[20]

Extrathyroidal carcinomas have the worse prognosis. These are not dependent on size. Tumors as small as 1 cm invading through the capsule into the recurrent laryngeal nerve or surrounding structures have been reported. This is a reflection of the biological aggressiveness of the tumor.

There are 2 clinical scoring systems presently used to classify high- and low-risk patients. From the Lahey clinic, there is the AMES system which examines Age, distant Metastasis, Extent of the primary tumor and Size of the tumor.[21,22] The other system, from the Mayo Clinic, is called the AGES system: Age, Grade of tumor, Extent of the primary tumor and Size.[23] Both show age to be most important. Men younger than age 40 and women younger than age 50 have a low risk if no distant metastases are present at the time of initial treatment. Also, patients with tumor sizes greater than 4 cm and capsule extensions have increased risk.

Surgical resection is the treatment for papillary carcinoma. The extent of resection remains controversial.[24] The general agreement is a total lobectomy and isthmectomy. If there is a history of irradiation, a total or near-total thyroidectomy is performed to address the high incidence of multifocal neoplasms. For children, most surgeons perform a total thyroidectomy with a regional or modified neck dissection.

Follicular Carcinoma

The classification of follicular carcinomas is based on macroinvasion or microinvasion of either the capsule or tumor vessels.[25] Another form of classification is based on high-grade angioinvasive or low-grade encapsulated follicular carcinomas.

High-grade angioinvasive follicular carcinomas are usually large, have bone metastases, and show invasion of peri-thyroidal and lateral neck veins at the time of diagnosis. The tumor thrombus may extend into the jugular vein and into the right atrium. There is often extension into surrounding structure and nerve involvement. Patients younger than 40 usually do well; patients over 50 have a poor prognosis.

More commonly, the thyroid resection is for the low-grade encapsulated follicular carcinoma. During the operation, these are seldom diagnosed definitively by either fine needle aspiration cytology or frozen-section. Most often the diagnosis is made from analysis of permanent sections after the operation.

Follicular carcinomas are treated by a total thyroidectomy. Lymphatic dissection is not required since only 5% have lymphatic spread.[26] If there is bone or pulmonary metastases, the use of radioactive iodide is indicated. There is some controversy as to whether it is prudent to perform a total thyroidectomy when low-grade encapsulated follicular carcinoma is identified after a total lobectomy. Usually if there are no distant metastases at the time of presentation, the rate of recurrence in the contralateral lobe and elsewhere is extremely low and no further treatment is needed. If the size is greater than 4 cm, there is high incidence of multicentricity and a total thyroidectomy may be indicated.

Medullary Carcinoma

Medullary carcinoma is a relatively rare tumor. It accounts for only 7% of all thyroid cancers. It is unique in that there is a hereditary component in some individuals and the cells of origin are the parafollicular cells (C cells) . The C cells are derived from the neural crest and can produce peptide and hormones. Medullary carcinoma secretes a biological marker, calcitonin, which can be used for detection and surveillance.[27]

Medullary carcinoma can occur in 3 settings. It can present as a sporadic tumor or as a component of either multiple endocrine neoplasia (MEN IIa) syndrome or MEN IIb syndrome. The sporadic form is usually an isolated nodule in 1 lobe of the gland. The familial types are always bilateral, multicentric and arise from C cell hyperplasia.

The minimal treatment of medullary carcinoma is a total thyroidectomy.[28] Most of the patients with sporadic disease have lymph node metastases and also require a central compartment dissection. If lateral lymph nodes are involved, a modified neck dissection is needed. Patients with MEN II syndromes must be evaluated for possible pheochromocytoma before treatment of the thyroid. Operations for pheochromocytoma should always take precedence over the thyroid operation.

Hurthle Cell Carcinoma

Hurthle cell carcinoma accounts for only 3%-5% of all thyroid cancers. This tumor, previously classified as a variant of follicular carcinoma, is now considered a separate entity because of its unique biological behavior.[29] Derived from follicular cells, the Hurthle cell carcinoma have no ability to take up iodine or to make thyroid hormones. The lesions can spread via the lymphatic or hematogenous route. It is impossible to differentiate benign from malignant Hurthle cell neoplasm based on cytology alone. The capsule must be examined to rule out angioinvasion.

Hurthle cell carcinomas are treated with a total thyroidectomy; the benign Hurthle cell adenomas may be treated with a lobectomy. There is no satisfactory adjunctive therapy because the Hurthle cells do not readily take up radioactive iodine and are unresponsive to chemotherapy. Local and regional recurrences are common after inadequate surgical resection. If the lymphatics are involved, a central compartment is indicated. If lateral lymph nodes are involved, a modified radical neck dissection is indicated.

Anaplastic Carcinoma

Undifferentiated or anaplastic thyroid carcinoma of the spindle or giant cell type usually arise from previous long-standing differentiated thyroid cancers. Most occur in follicular carcinoma but can be seen in papillary, Hurthle and medullary carcinoma. The spindle and giant cell type are among the most rapidly lethal malignancies known. Most patients are too far advanced when the carcinoma is initially discovered. If found early, a total thyroidectomy offers the only possibility of cure.

4. Parathyroid Glands

Embryology

Due to differences in patterns of embryogenesis, the location of the parathyroid glands can vary in individuals. The superior parathyroid arises from the fourth pharyngeal pouch in conjunction with the lateral thyroid during the fourth and fifth week of fetal development. The inferior glands arise from the third pouch with the thymus. The glands tend to migrate with their corresponding pouches. Hence, the superior thyroid remains in close association with the upper pole of the thyroid and the inferior gland descends with the thymus. The migration stop point of the inferior parathyroid is extremely variable and location can be anywhere from the pharynx to the mediastinum.

Anatomy

There are usually 4 parathyroid glands: 2 superior and 2 inferior. They measure approximately 4 mm x 6 mm and weigh between 25-45 mg each.[30] The superior glands are usually located on the backside of the upper thyroid where the recurrent laryngeal nerve enters the larynx. The inferior glands are more variable but are usually found on the posterior side of the inferior pole of the thyroid.

The inferior thyroid arteries provide the principle arterial supply to both the superior and inferior parathyroid glands. There can be arterial variations that originate from the superior thyroid and thyroid ima arteries as well as collaterals from the vessels supplying the larynx, trachea and esophagus.

Physiology

The principle function of the parathyroid gland is to regulate calcium and phosphate metabolism.

Calcium

Calcium is a cation that comprises approximately 2% of the average body weight. Most of it is contained in the skeleton.[31] It is absorbed in the duodenum and proximal jejunum. Calcium is necessary in enzymatic reactions and hormone metabolism. The total serum calcium concentration is a function of serum albumin and pH.

Phosphate

Phosphate is an anion critical in the glycolysis pathway and is the functional group of a number of high-energy compounds such as ATP.[32] The serum phosphate level varies inversely with the serum level of calcium. Its absorption from the diet is relatively constant and renal excretion is the major mechanism for regulating the phosphate levels.

Regulation

The regulation of calcium and phosphate homeostasis is dependent on 3 organ systems: the digestive tract, the skeleton and the kidneys. The hormones involved are parathyroid hormone, vitamin D and calcitonin.

Parathyroid Hormone

Parathyroid hormone (PTH) is synthesized as a precursor (preproparathyroid hormone), which is cleaved in the parathyroid gland to propararthyroid hormone, and finally to parathyroid hormone. PTH is composed of 84-amino acid molecules.[32] Its release into the circulation is controlled by a negative feedback loop dependent on the level of extracellular calcium. In the liver, the parathyroid hormone is cleaved into a biologically active N-terminal fragment and a C-terminal fragment.

The physiological action of PTH is mediated through stimulation of adenylate cyclase to form cyclic AMP in the target tissues. PTH stimulates renal tubular resorption of calcium and the excretion of phosphate. In the intestine, it stimulates calcium absorption indirectly via increase hydroxylation of vitamin D. In bone, the effects are more complex, ie, it stimulates both resorption and new bone formation.

Vitamin D

Vitamin D_3 or cholecalciferol is produced from the action of sunlight on 7-dehydrocholesterol in skin. This is further hydroxylated in the liver (position 25) and kidney (position 1) to its active form 1,25-dihydroxyvitamin D_3 (calcitriol).

Vitamin D has two major sites of action. It increases intestinal absorption of calcium and phosphate, promotes mineralization, and enhances PTH-mediated mobilization of calcium and phosphate in bone. It has no direct effect on the kidney.

Calcitonin

Calcitonin is produced from the parafollicular C cells in the thyroid. It is a 32 amino-acid protein. It is not essential for the normal control of calcium metabolism in humans. It does inhibit bone resorption and can increase urinary calcium and phosphate excretion.

Hypercalcemia

Hypercalcemia is a relatively common problem. The incidence ranges between 0.1%-0.5% of the population. Many of the clinical signs are subtle in presentation:

- Lethargy
- Coma
- Headache
- Depression
- Hearing loss
- Hyporeflexia
- Ataxia
- Constipation
- Anorexia
- Polydipsia
- Weight loss
- Hypertension
- Renal colic
- Polyuria

There are many causes of hypercalcemia. Hyperparathyroidism is a major cause, but all causes of hypercalcemia must be considered and excluded.

5. Hyperparathyroidism

Common causes of hypercalcemia:

- Malignancy
- Vitamin A or D intoxication
- Thiazide use
- Milk-Alkali syndrome
- Sarcoidosis
- Familial hypocalciuric hypercalcemia
- Pagets disease
- Lithium
- Addisonian Crisis
- Hyperthyroidism
- Immobilization

There are 3 states of hyperparathyroidism.

Primary hyperparathyroidism is defined as an elevated PTH level in the presence of hypercalcemia that is often characterized by single or multiple gland enlargements.

Secondary hyperparathyroidism occurs when there is a defect in mineral homeostasis that leads to a compensatory increase in parathyroid function. An example is renal disease with a chronic state of hypocalcemia.

Tertiary hyperparathyroidism can occur with long-standing secondary hyperthyroidism. In this condition, the glands become nonresponsive to the increased serum calcium level. One example is the hyperparathyroidism that occurs after renal transplantation, even after the defect in calcium homeostasis has been corrected.

Pathology

The cell most commonly involved in primary hyperparathyroidism is the chief cell. Affected glands typically have an increase in the proportion of stromal cells and a reduction in the proportion of stromal fat.[33] Adenomas have been classically described as a single enlarged gland in the presence of three normal or small remaining glands with the histological finding of a center of hyperplastic tissue surrounded by a rim of normal-appearing parathyroid tissue. In parathyroid hyperplasia, there is diffuse proliferation in multiple glands with little remaining tissue. Note that these criteria are not always reliable and that all four glands need to be evaluated during the time of surgery. A decision of adenoma or hyperplasia needs to be made on the gross characteristics of the glands identified during the exploration.

Diagnosis

The initial workup is often started after a patient is discovered to have an elevated serum calcium level. Unfortunately, the physical exam is seldom helpful because the parathyroid glands are rarely palpable. Palpable parathyroid glands are usually indicative of malignancy. Consequently, PTH measurement has become an important method of diagnosing hyperparathyroidism. The current assays are sufficiently sensitive and specific that in the setting of an inappropriately elevated serum calcium level and elevated PTH, one can make the diagnosis of hyperparathyroidism. Another helpful index is a serum chloride/phosphate ratio greater than 30. Parathyroid hormones increase bicarbonate excretion and the patients have a hyperchloremic metabolic acidosis. Hypomagnesemia is seen in 5%-10 % of the patients. This is more evident after the parathyroidectomy, when both hypocalcemia and hypomagnesemia can occur.

Localization Studies

Because of the ectopic location of some glands, locating all 4 can be difficult. In the hands of an experienced surgeon, the cure rate for hyperparathyroidism at the initial operation approaches 95%. There is no evidence that preoperative localization reduces the duration or complication of the operation. A recent National Institutes of Health Consensus Development Conference concluded that preoperative localization in patients without prior neck operation is rarely indicated and has not proven to be cost effective.[34]

Treatment

Asymptomatic Hyperparathyroidism

A proportion of patients with the diagnosis of hyperparathyroidism are asymptomatic. In 1990, an NIH Consensus Development Conference suggested that all patients who are symptomatic will need to undergo surgery, but there is a subgroup that can be followed closely every 6 months.[35] This remains an area of controversy because a large percentage (40%) of the patients followed for 10 years eventually require surgery or were lost to follow-up efforts. The following indications mandate surgical intervention:

- Markedly elevated serum calcium
- History of an episode of life-threatening hypercalcemia
- Reduce creatinine clearance
- 1 or more kidney stones
- Elevate 24-hour urinary calcium excretion
- Substantially reduced bone mass

Symptomatic Hyperparathyroidism

The surgical approach to the parathyroid glands is similar to that of the thyroid. The thyroid gland is mobilized anteriorly and medially to expose the glands. All 4 parathyroid glands should be identified. Since the location of the inferior glands can be variable, the operation can be arduous and requires considerable patience. It must be noted that the necessity for re-exploration can usually be avoided by a meticulous initial dissection. Re-operation is predictably more difficult than the initial operation and the risk of recurrent laryngeal nerve injury and hypoparathyroidism is much higher.

Single gland disease (adenoma) is treated by simple excision of the affected gland. 4-gland disease (hyperplasia) is treated by subtotal parathyroidectomy, ie, removing 3 and a half glands or total parathyroidectomy with auto-transplantation into the forearm.

Recurrent Hyperparathyroidism

Recurrent hyperparathyroidism occurs in less than 5% of patients undergoing parathyroid surgery.[36] When evaluating these patients, the diagnosis of hyperparathyroidism must be reconfirmed by excluding all other causes. Next, it is generally agreed that localization studies should be considered. Noninvasive imaging methods are used first, and if not successful, they are followed by selective angiography or venous sampling. Surgical re-exploration can be difficult. The neck should always be re-explored first. If there is a thymic remnant it should be removed. Only 1%-2% of patients need to undergo median sternotomy and exploration.

Parathyroid Carcinoma

Parathyroid carcinoma is very rare and accounts for less than 1% of all cases of hyperparathyroidism. The gland is often palpable on initial physical exam. The patients tend to be younger and the male to female ratio is equal. Initial treatment includes radical resection of the involved gland, the ipsilateral thyroid lobe, and the regional lymph nodes. Chemotherapy and radiation has not proven to be beneficial. The long-term prognosis is poor and survival depends on complete initial resection.[37]

6. References

1. Organ GM, Organ CH Jr. Thyroid gland and surgery of the thyroglossal duct: exercise in applied embryology. *World J Surg*. 2000;24(8):886-90.

2. Hollinshead WH. Anatomy for surgeons, vol 1. *The Head and Neck*. New York, NY: Hoeber-Harper;1968.

3. Thompson NW, Olsen WR, Hoffman GI. The continuing development of the technique of thyroidectomy. *Surgery*.1973;73:913.

4. Athow AC, Fagg NL, Drake DP. Management of Thyroglossal cysts in children. *Br J Surg*. 1989;76(8):811-814.

5. Abdallah-Matta MP, Dubarry PH, Pessey JJ, Caron P. Lingual thyroid and hyperthyroidism: a new case and review of the literature. *J Endocrinol Invest*. 2002;25(3):264-267.

6. Rabinov CR, Ward PH, Pusheck T. Evolution and evaluation of lateral cystic neck masses containing thyroid tissue: "lateral aberrant thyroid" revisited. *Am J Otolarygol*.1996;17(1):12-15.

7. Tong W. Thyroid hormone synthesis and releasing. In: Werner SC, Ingbar SH, eds. *The Thyroid: A Fundamental and Clinical Text*. 3rd ed. New York, NY: Harper & Row;1971:24.

8. Wartofsky L, Glinoer D, Solomon B, et al. Differences and similarities in the diagnosis and treatment of Graves disease in Europe, Japan and the United States. *Thyroid*. 1991;1:129.

9. Falk SA. The management of hyperthyroidism, a surgeon's perspective. *Otolaryngol Clin North Am*. 1990;23:361.

10. Perzik SL. Total thyroidectomy in the management of Graves disease: a review of 282 cases. *Am J Surg*. 1976;132:480.

11. Miller JM, Hamburger JI, Sini S. Diagnosis of thyroid nodules. *JAMA*. 1979;241:481.

12. Thomas CG Jr, Croom RD. Current management of the patient with autonomously functioning nodular goiter. *Surg Clin North Am*. 987;67(2):315-328.

13. Slatosky J, Shipton B, Wahba H. Thyroiditis: differential diagnosis and management. *Am Fam Physician*. 2000;61(4):1047-1052,1054.

14. Thompson LD, Heffess CS. Subacute (deQuervain's) thyroiditis. *Ear Nose Throat J*. 2002;81(9):623.

15. Lloyd RV. The thyroid. In: Lloyd R, ed. *Endocrine pathology*. New York, New York: Springer-Verlag;1990:37.

16. Hoffman GL, Thompson NW, Heffron C. The solitary thyroid nodule: a reassessment. *Arch Surg*.1972;105:379.

17. Oppenheimer J. Thyroid action at the nuclear level. *Ann Intern Med*. 1985;102:374.

18. Lowhagen T, Granberg PO, Lundell G. Aspiration biopsy cytology (ABC) in nodules of the thyroid gland suspected to be malignant. *Surg Clin North Am*. 1979;59:3.

19. Thompson NW, Nishiyama RH, Harness JK. Thyroid carcinoma: current controversies. *Curr Probl Surg*. 1978;15:1.

20. Rossi RL, Cady B, Silverman ML, et al. Current results of conservative surgery for differentiated thyroid carcinoma. *World J Surg*.1986;10:612.

21. Cady B, Rossi R. An expanded view of risk-group definition in undifferentiated thyroid carcinoma. *Surgery*. 1988;104:947.

22. Cady B, Sedgwick CE, Meissner WA, et al. Risk factor analysis in differentiated thyroid cancer. *Cancer*. 1979;43:811.

23. Hay ID. Prognostic factors in thyroid carcinoma. *Thyroid Today*.1989;12:1.

24. Chen H, Udelsman R. Papillary thyroid carcinoma: justification for total thyroidectomy and management of lymph node metastases. *Surg Oncol Clin N Am*. 1988;7(4):645-643.

25. Harness JK, Thompson NW, McLeod MK, Eckhause FE, Lloyd RV. Follicular carcinoma of the thyroid gland: trends and treatment. *Surgery*. 1984;96:972.

26. Yamashita T, Fujimoto Y, Kodama T, et al. When is total thyroidectomy indicated as a treatment of follicular carcinoma? *World J Surg*. 1988;12:539.

27. Giuffrida D, Gharib H. Current diagnosis and management of medullary thyroid carcinoma. *Ann Oncol*. 1998;9(7):695-701.

28. Thompson NW. Surgery for medullary thyroid carcinoma. In: Fee WE Jr, Goepfert H, Johns ME, Strong EW, Ward PH, eds. *Head and Neck Cancer.* Philadelphia, PA: BC Decker;1990:2.

29. Boone RT, Fan CY, Hanna EY. Well-differentiated carcinoma of the thyroid. Otolaryngol *Clin North Am*. 2003;36(1):73-90.

30. Akerstrom G, Malmaeus J, Bergstrom R. Surgical anatomy of human parathyroid glands. *Surgery*. 1984;95:14.

31. Guyton AC. *Basic Human Physiology: Normal Function and Mechanism of Disease*. Philadelphia, PA: Saunders; 1977.

32. Wells SA, Leight GF, Ross A. Primary hyperparathyroidism. *Curr Probl Surg*. 1980;17:398.

33. Roth SI. Recent advances in parathyroid gland pathology. *Am J Med*. 1994;50:612.

34. Potts JT Jr, Ackerman IP, Barker CF, et al. Diagnosis and management of asymptomatic primary hyperparathyroidism: consensus development conference statement. *Ann Intern Med*. 1991;114:593.

35. Scholz DA, Purnell DC. Asymptomatic primary hyperparathyroidism: 10 year prospective study. *Mayo Clin Proc*. 1981;56:473.

36. Moley JF, Wells SA, Dilley WG, et al. Reoperation for recurrent or persistent medullary thyroid cancer. *Surgery*. 1993;114:1090.

37. Wang C, Gaz RD. Natural history of parathyroid carcinoma. Diagnosis, treatment, and results. *Am J Surg*. 1985;149:522.

7. Questions

1. With regard to the embryology of the thyroid gland, which of the following is/are true?

A. The thyroid gland is comprised of ectodermal cells that originate from the primitive alimentary tract.

B. During the fifth week of gestation it arises from a midline diverticulum from the foramen cecum.

C. The thyroglossal duct is the original attachment of the thyroid at the foramen cecum.

D. C cells migrate into and concentrate in the upper and middle portions of the thyroid gland.

2. The vascular supply of the thyroid gland is abundant and is supplied by the:

A. Superior thyroid artery

B. Middle thyroid artery

C. Inferior thyroid artery

D. Thyoidea ima artery

3. Which of the following comments on the nerves and their innervations is/are true?

A. The recurrent laryngeal nerve is a branch of the vagus nerve that loops around the subclavian artery on both the right and left sides.

B. Injury to the recurrent laryngeal nerve will result in paralysis of the vocal cord on the contralateral side.

C. The superior laryngeal nerve arises from the vagus nerve and divides into two branches. The internal branch supplies sensation to the mucosa of the larynx and hypopharynx; the external branch innervates the cricothyroid muscle.

D. Injury to the superior laryngeal nerve has no effect on the voice.

4. With regard to anomalous variations in thyroid embryological development, which of the following statements are true?

   A. The thyroglossal duct frequently passes through the center of the hyoid bone.

   B. The lingual thyroid may be the only functional thyroid tissue present in an individual.

   C. Lateral aberrant thyroid is normal thyroid tissue appearing on the lateral neck as an embryological accident.

   D. Thyroglossal ducts can contain thyroid cancer which is usually papillary in nature.

5. Which of the following statements is/are true?

   A. Thyroid stimulating hormone (TSH) is a glycoprotein secreted by the hypothalamus to stimulate the thyroid.

   B. Graves disease is more likely to occur in men and demonstrates elevated levels of antimicrosomal and antithyroglobulin antibodies.

   C. DeQuervain's thyroiditis is a subacute thyroiditis that usually occurs after a viral upper respiratory infection and is self-limited.

   D. Riedel struma is a high lethal malignancy of the thyroid gland.

6. When working up a solitary thyroid nodule, which of the following statements is/are true?

   A. A history of low-dose radiation exposure is a strong factor favoring a more aggressive workup of a thyroid nodule.

   B. A nodule must be at least 1 cm to be picked up by the scintiscan.

   C. Needle biopsies have a high false positive rate.

   D. Cytological studies can identify papillary, follicular, and anaplastic thyroid carcinoma.

7. With regard to thyroid carcinoma, which of the following statements is/are true?

   A. Papillary thyroid carcinoma spreads via a hematogenous route.

   B. Follicular thyroid carcinoma spreads via a lymphatic route.

   C. In medullary thyroid carcinoma, parafollicular cells (C cells) are the cells of origin.

   D. Hurthle cell carcinoma has the ability to incorporate iodine.

8. With regard to the blood supply to the superior and inferior parathyroid glands, they are usually supplied by the:

   A. Superior thyroid artery

   B. Middle thyroid artery

   C. Inferior thyroid artery

   D. Thyoidea ima artery

9. With regard to hyperparathyroidism, which statements is/are true?

   A. The type of cell most commonly involved in primary hyperparathyroidism is the chief cell.

   B. Because the parathyroid glands are hard to locate, one should always use localization studies such as MRI, sestamibi, and ultrasound.

C. Both the parathyroid hormone and calcium level are usually elevated in primary hyperparathyroidism.

D. A serum chloride/phosphate ratio of less than 30 is highly suggestive of hyperparathyroidism.

10. Which of the following statements is/are true?

A. Single gland disease (adenoma) is treated by simple excision of the affected gland.

B. 4-gland disease (hyperplasia) is treated by subtotal parathyroidectomy or total parathyroidectomy with auto-transplantation.

C. In the initial operation for hyperparathyroidism, one should always perform a median sternotomy to look for occult parathyroid glands.

D. Parathyroid carcinoma is a common condition and has a male predominance.

Answers

1. C., D.
The thyroid gland is comprised of endodermal cells that originate from the primitive alimentary tract. It arises during the third week of gestation from the floor of the pharynx in the region of the foramen cecum.

2. A., C., D.
There are usually 2 sets of arteries that supply the thyroid. There is no middle thyroid artery. There is a middle thyroid vein. Occasionally, a fifth artery, the thyroidea ima, originating from the aortic arch or innominate artery, can enter the thyroid in the midline inferiorly.

3. C.
The recurrent laryngeal nerve loops around the aortic arch at the ductus arteriosus on the left and the subclavian artery on the right. There is about a 1% incidence of nonrecurrent laryngeal nerve on the right. Injury to the recurrent laryngeal nerve results in paralysis of the vocal cords on the ipsilateral side. Bilateral cord palsies can cause complete loss of airway. Injury to the superior laryngeal nerve results in vocal fatigue and loss of strength and pitch of voice.

4. A., B., D.
The theory that normal thyroid tissue appears in the lateral neck as an embryologic accident has been abandoned. There is almost always metastatic well-differentiated thyroid cancer that has replaced the local lymph node.

5. C.
Thyroid-stimulating hormone (TSH) is a glycoprotein secreted by the pituitary to stimulate the thyroid. Thyrotropin-releasing factor (TRH) is released from the hypothalamus to stimulate the pituitary. Graves disease is more likely to occur in women and has autoantibodies that bind to TSH receptors. Hashimoto's disease features elevated levels of antimicrosomal and antithyroglobulin antibodies. Riedel struma is not a malignancy of the thyroid. It is a nonspecific fibrosis of the thyroid gland.

6. A., B.
In the United States, needle biopsy has gained wide acceptance as an essential part of the workup of a solitary thyroid nodule. The false-positive rate is very low, ie, less than 2%. Cytological studies by themselves cannot diagnosis follicular carcinoma. The pathologist needs to evaluate the thyroid tissue specimen for the presence or absence of capsule invasion.

7. C.
Papillary carcinoma has a tendency to spread via a lymphatic route, whereas follicular carcinoma tends to spread via a hematogenous route. The Hurthle cell carcinoma is unique in that it does not have the ability to take up iodine and does not make thyroid hormones.

8. C.
Usually, the superior and inferior parathyroid glands are supplied by the inferior thyroid artery; however, there can be some variations and collateralization with other arteries.

9. A., C.
In a 1990 NIH Consensus Development Conference, it was concluded that preoperative localization in patients without prior neck operation is rarely indicated and not proven to be cost effective. In the hands of an experienced surgeon, the cure rate from hyperparathyroidism at the initial operation approached 95%. Parathyroid hormones increase bicarbonate excretion and patients have a hyperchloremic metabolic acidosis. The serum chloride/phosphate ratio is usually higher than 30 in cases of hyperparathyroidism.

10. A., B.
During the initial operation and after a meticulous exploration of all areas, most surgeons terminate the operation and order localization studies before performing a median sternotomy and exploring the mediastinum. Parathyroid carcinoma is a very rare condition that accounts for less than 1% of all cases of hyperparathyroidism. Male and female ratio is equal for parathyroid carcinoma.

Chapter 22: General Urology and Trauma

Thomas E. Ahlering, MD
Franklin I. Margolis, MD
Leland A. Ronningen, MD
Douglas W. Skarecky, BS

Contents

1. Anatomy and Physiology

Kidneys

Anatomy

The kidneys are paired retroperitoneal organs, protected by perinephric fat within and paranephric fat outside Gerota's fascia. They lie between the T12 and L3 vertebrae, anterior to the 11th and 12th ribs. Their blood supply is from paired renal arteries arising from the aorta at the first lumbar vertebra, just inferior to the superior mesenteric artery. The renal artery is bounded posteriorly by the renal pelvis and anteriorly by the renal vein. The collecting system and renal vessels emanate from the renal sinus centrally through a medial depression in the kidney called the renal hilum. The kidney is structurally and functionally divided into an outer cortex and an inner medulla that is composed of approximately one million nephrons. The nephron consists of a glomerulus, convoluted tubules, a loop of Henle, and a collecting duct ending at the tip of the papilla of a medullary pyramid. Urine is excreted from the papillae into the minor calyces, which join to form major calyces, which in turn join to form the renal pelvis.

Physiology

The kidneys maintain fluid and electrolyte balance as well as excrete nitrogenous wastes. They receive 20% of the cardiac output. Renal blood flow as well as the glomerular filtration rate (GFR) are precisely regulated by hormonal, adrenergic, and vasoactive substances. Normally about 130 mL of plasma is filtered every minute. The proximal tubule absorbs 60% of the glomerular filtrate, along with glucose, amino acids, bicarbonate, and 60% of the filtered sodium. The loop of Henle, relatively impermeable to water, absorbs the remaining 25%-40% of sodium via a cotransport mechanism, setting up a gradient for excretion of maximally dilute urine. The amount of sodium passing through the distal loop determines the activity of the renin-angiotensin-aldosterone system. Low sodium concentration and low blood volume, among other mechanisms, stimulate this system, causing vasoconstriction, sodium reabsorption and increased blood volume. 70% of potassium is reabsorbed by the proximal tubules, another 20% is absorbed in the loop, and the fine tuning for absorption or secretion is accomplished in the distal tubule and collecting duct via the influence of aldosterone. Fluid balance is ultimately managed at the level of the distal collecting duct by antidiuretic hormone (ADH, vasopressin). Loop diuretics work in the loop of Henle to inhibit reabsorption of sodium and potassium, producing a natriuresis and kaliuresis. Thiazides perform a similar function, but at the distal convoluted tubule. Potassium sparing diuretics block sodium reabsorption in the collecting ducts, leading to natriuresis and potassium retention.

Ureters

Anatomy

The renal pelvis narrows inferiorly to become the proximal ureter. The ureter, with the ipsilateral gonadal vessel, courses in the retroperitoneum anterior to the psoas muscle, loosely adherent to the posterior peritoneum and mesentery of the colon. It passes anterior to the iliac vessels at the bifurcation of the external and internal iliac arteries. In females, it is closely associated with the cervix, coursing posterior to the uterine arteries and running along the anterior vaginal wall, putting the ureter at risk during hysterectomy. Separating from the gonadal vessels, it courses posteriorly to enter the trigone near the apex of the bladder. The ureter has many layers of muscle which contract in a coordinated fashion from the renal pelvis to the trigone. The blood supply is segmental, arising from the renal, gonadal, and vesical arteries, forming a rich adventitial network.

Physiology

A layer of smooth muscle covers the renal calyces, pelves and ureters. It is divided into inner longitudinal and outer circular layers. These layers work in concert to propel the urine from the renal calyces through the ureterovesical junction. The peristaltic waves occur at a rate of 5-8 per min and proceed in an organized fashion at 3 cm/sec. They do not secrete nor reabsorb water or electrolytes. During micturition, the trigone of the bladder contracts to prevent reflux of urine into the kidneys.

Bladder

Anatomy

The bladder is a storage organ composed of several layers of intricately interrelated muscle fibers. The distal ureter and bladder trigone are intimately connected to prevent efflux of urine back up the ureter. Like the renal calyces, renal pelves and ureters, the bladder is lined by transitional cell epithelium. The urachus anchors the bladder to the anterior abdominal wall. Vesical branches entering laterally and posteromedially from the internal iliac artery supply the bladder. The venous drainage is through the internal iliac veins while lymphatic drainage is to the external iliac lymph nodes.

Physiology

As a urinary reservoir, the bladder is designed to maintain low pressures during its filling phase. The detrusor remains quiet and the bladder neck is tonically closed. During micturition, the detrusor contracts uniformly and the bladder neck (internal urinary sphincter) relaxes, allowing urine to flow until the bladder is empty.

Prostate

Anatomy and Physiology

The prostate is a ovoid-shaped gland, weighing about 20 grams, located inferior to the bladder. Its function is primarily reproductive, as it secretes the bulk of the ejaculate, and it contains the ejaculatory duct from each vas deferens. It is also traversed in its length by the urethra, which ends distally at the urogenital diaphragm as the voluntary external urethral sphincter. The prostate is almost completely surrounded by a capsule of collagen, elastin, and smooth muscle. It has several distinct anatomic zones, defined based on their structure and anatomic origin. The transition zone, which surrounds the urethra, is the site of benign prostatic hyperplasia (BPH), and is where 20% of all prostate cancers are found. The peripheral zone makes up 70% of the normal-sized prostate, is the site of 70% of all prostate cancers, and is the zone most commonly affected by chronic prostatitis. The vascular supply is from the inferior vesical artery, which divides to form the prostatic, capsular and urethral arteries. Venous drainage is via a periprostatic plexus. Lymphatic drainage is via the obturator, hypogastric and external iliac nodes. Prostate specific antigen (PSA), a serine protease secreted from prostatic glandular epithelial cells, acts to liquefy the ejaculate. In cases of cancer, infection, and BPH, the PSA may be elevated. Determinations of free versus protein-bound forms of PSA (percentage of free PSA) in the serum have aided in differentiating the cause of elevation of the PSA, limiting the number of unnecessary prostate biopsies. Nerve supply is both sympathetic and parasympathetic via the pelvic plexus and cavernous nerves. Parasympathetic nerves cause secretion from the glands, while sympathetic nerves act at the preprostatic sphincter via alpha-1 receptors to maintain tone. Treatments of BPH target blockade of these receptors, improving urinary flow.

Penis and Urethra

Anatomy

The penis is composed of dorsally-located paired copora cavernosa. They are composed of endothelium-lined channels of erectile tissue surrounded by a tough layer called the tunica albuginea. Ventrally located is the corpus spongiosum, which in addition to containing erectile tissue, contains the urethra from the urogenital diaphragm to the tip of the glans penis. Buck's fascia surround both cavernosa and splits to surround the corpus spongiosum. The penis receives its blood supply from the internal pudendal artery, via the cavernosal, bulbar and dorsal arteries of the penis. The overlying skin receives blood supply from the external pudendal artery, running in the dartos layer. It is a richly anastomotic network, thus penile skin is easily mobilized for urethral reconstruction. The male urethra is divided into an anterior and posterior component. The posterior urethra is composed of the membranous and prostatic portions of the urethra, surrounded by the external urethral sphincter and the prostate, respectively. The anterior urethra is composed of the bulbous, pendulous, and glanular portions of the urethra and is covered by the corpus spongiosum throughout its course. Stricture disease is usually the result of trauma or infection and commonly affects the bulbous urethra. The female urethra is about 4 cm long and its lining gradually changes from transitional to squamous epithelium. Estrogen-dependent layers of mucosa and submucosa coapt to provide continence. Additionally, there is a voluntary striated sphincter around the middle third of the urethra.

Testis, Epididymis and Vas

Anatomy

The testes are paired organs of retroperitoneal origin located in the male scrotum. They are composed of several hundred seminiferous (sperm-forming) tubules, each separated by septa. At the apex of the septae, the tubules come together in the mediastinum of the testis to form 12 to 20 efferent ductules. These subsequently pierce the upper pole of the testis to form the head of the epididymis. As they pass to the body and tail of the epididymis, they coalesce and thicken into a single tube, the vas deferens. A parietal layer, the tunica albuginea, and a visceral layer, the tunica vaginalis, cover the testis. Its blood supply is primarily the testicular artery, but there is a rich network of anastomoses from the cremasteric, vasal, and epididymal branches. The venous drainage is via the pampiniform plexus.

Physiology

The main functions of the testes are production of sperm and testosterone. Luteinizing hormone (LH) released from the pituitary gland stimulates testosterone production from Leydig cells in the testicular interstitium. Testosterone in turn supports growth of Sertoli cells within the seminiferous tubules. Spermatogonia lining the tubules are stimulated into mitotic and meiotic division by follicle-stimulating hormone (FSH) released from the pituitary gland. The spermatocytes and spermatids are nurtured by the Sertoli cells as well as the epithelial cells of the epididymis and vas to produce motile sperm capable of fertilization.

2. Developmental Anomalies

Renal

Renal Agenesis

Unilateral agenesis is generally a sporadic phenomenon, seen in 1 in 1000 live births. Bilateral agenesis results in fetal loss due to oligohydramnios. Related ipsilateral loss of ovary, fallopian tube, vas deferens or testicle may be seen. Because adrenal glands develop separately from the kidneys, both are usually present.

Cystic Diseases

There is a spectrum of renal cystic disease ranging from simple cysts to multicystic dysplastic kidneys. Causes may be genetic, as in the case of infantile and adult polycystic kidney disease or tuberous sclerosis-associated cysts. They can also occur without genetic predisposition, as in simple cysts, multicystic dysplastic kidneys, medullary sponge kidney, or acquired renal cystic disease. Simple cysts are lined with epithelium, arising from but no longer connected to the nephron. They become more common with age, with 33% of cases occurring after age 60. Rarely they can cause hypertension, for which needle aspiration has been used successfully. Evaluation is with sonography. Benign cysts are spherical, without internal echoes, have a thin wall and through transmission. CT evaluation is needed for septations, calcifications, or irregular margins. Benign cysts on CT show smooth walls, are spherical and homogeneous, and have a density similar to that of water. The density within the cyst or its wall should not change with contrast administration. Bosniak criteria are used to stratify risk of malignancy based upon sonographic and CT findings.

Horseshoe Kidney

The most common of fusion abnormalities, it usually involves the lower poles of the kidneys joined across the midline anterior to the great vessels. Associated abnormalities are not rare. Trisomy 18 and Turner syndrome have the highest rate of horseshoes. Most remain asymptomatic, while infection, stones, and pain are most likely to belie the presence of the horseshoe kidney.

Medullary Sponge Kidney

Collecting tube ectasia is the primary pathology in medullary sponge kidney. Clinically it is manifested as pain, infection and gross hematuria. Treatment is directed at prevention of stones with thiazides and with culture-directed antibiotics or chronic suppression.

Ureteral

Megaureter

By strict definition, this is a ureter enlarged for any reason. They are categorized as refluxing, obstructed, and nonrefluxing-nonobstructed megaureters. Abnormal muscle development and collagen deposition seems the most likely cause in primary obstructed and refluxing megaureters, but even this is debated. Treatment, indicated for children symptomatic with infection or pain, involves division of the ureter above the obstruction and reimplantation into the bladder.

Duplication

Due to bifurcation of the ureteral bud, duplication is seen in one of 400 individuals. The kidney's upper pole ureter enters the bladder nearest the bladder neck, and is the one more likely to be ectopic and obstructed. The lower pole ureter often has a short tunnel through the bladder and is prone to reflux. Clinically significant anomalies present with pyelonephritis from obstruction or reflux. Treatment involves surgical reimplantation of the ureters. If the upper pole of the kidney is nonfunctional, it is removed with its ureter at the time of reimplantation.

Ureterocele

Ureterocele is a cystic dilation of the distal ureter. Diagnosis is often *in utero* with detection of fetal hydronephrosis. It is more common in Caucasian girls and is usually associated with the upper pole ureter in a duplicated system. Some are clinically diagnosed in infants with urinary tract infections (UTI) or urosepsis. Large ureteroceles can obstruct the bladder neck and contralateral ureter and cause bilateral hydronephrosis. Confirmation is with voiding cystourethrogram and intravenous pyelogram (IVP). Treatment is variable and depends on the size of the ureterocele, its location, and the function of the upper pole kidney it serves. The goal in each case is preserving renal function and eliminating infection and obstruction, while minimizing surgical morbidity.

UPJ Obstruction

Ureteropelvic junction (UPJ) obstruction is one of the more common causes of fetal hydronephrosis and the most common cause of abdominal masses in the newborn. It is most often left-sided, bilateral in up to 40% of cases, and is more common in males. Debate rages about whether crossing renal vessels or intrinsic stenosis is the cause. Diagnosis is almost exclusively by fetal ultrasound. The rest are detected in childhood or later due to UTI, episodic vomiting, and flank pain (Dietl's crisis), or from gross hematuria after minor trauma. IVP or renal scan confirms the diagnosis. Treatment is surgical, however timing is controversial. Some insist on early repair while others advocate observation until some deterioration in function is noted.

Vesicoureteral Reflux

The normal distal ureter is intricately involved with the trigone of the bladder acting to prevent reflux back into the kidney. Classic reflux is due to a deficiency of longitudinal muscle in the distal ureter(s). There is also secondary reflux, which occurs as a result of elevated intravesical pressures from either an anatomic or a functional obstruction. Reflux is suspected in neonates with antenatally diagnosed hydronephrosis. If missed, presentation is later in infancy or childhood with fever, abdominal pain, and failure to thrive. Once a UTI or pyelonephritis is diagnosed, reflux is suspected and a renal ultrasound and a voiding cystourethrogram (VCUG) are performed to determine the presence and grade of reflux (on a scale of 1 to 5, with 5 being most severe). Technetium-99m dimercaptosuccinic acid (DMSA) renal scintigraphy is used to detect renal scarring from reflux and pyelonephritis. Cystoscopy is not indicated unless there is concern for an ectopic ureter or ureterocele, or if there is nonvisualization of the entire urethra on cystourethrography. Urodynamic evaluation is reserved for children with secondary forms of reflux. All these studies can be done without general anesthesia. Management depends on age at diagnosis and the severity of the reflux. Resolution of reflux does occur with growth of the child. Higher grades (4 and 5) are less likely to resolve before further renal scarring occurs. Children with lower grades of reflux are less at risk and are more likely to be managed nonoperatively, with suppressive antibiotics. Follow-up of these children is with nuclear cystography and ultrasonography. Antibiotics are stopped when reflux has resolved. Children with infections while on antibiotics or persistence more than a few years are considered at risk for progressive nephropathy and undergo reimplantation of the ureter(s). Open surgery is directed at lengthening the intravesical portion of the ureter via a transvesical or extravesical approach. Endoscopic approaches attempt to partially obstruct the orifice by submucosal injection of natural or synthetic bulking agents. The task remains to find the best agent that is safe and effective in the long term. Sequela involve renal insufficiency and hypertension.

Vesical

Exstrophy

This is a severe anomaly with complete absence of the anterior bladder and abdominal wall. It is associated with epispadias in boys. Hydronephrosis is common. Squamous cell carcinoma occurs as a late sequela. Single stage bladder closure and phallic reconstruction as a newborn is now recommended.

Penile and Urethral

Hypospadias

Failure of fusion of the urethral folds leads to a midline meatus somewhere proximal to the glans tip. Disproportionate growth of the corpora cavernosa often leads to associated chordee or penile bending in proximal hypospadias. Cryptorchidism (nonpalpable testes) is common, and a midscrotal meatus raises suspicion of a female with masculinized genitalia, as in congenital adrenal hyperplasia. Infants with such ambiguous genitalia must quickly be studied by hormonal and chromosomal analysis to determine their sex of rearing. Most hypospadias is distal and is associated with a ventral hood of foreskin. These infants should not be circumcised, as this skin may be used in future reconstructive surgery.

Cloacal Malformations

Development of the lower gut is intimately associated with the lower genitourinary tract. Anomalies of the rectum and genitals are due to faulty division of the cloaca into the urogenital sinus and rectum. There is a spectrum of disease giving rise to a classification system based upon the position of the rectum with respect to the urogenital sinus. In lower anomalies, the anus may be narrowed, anteriorly ectopic, or imperforate, with insertion into the scrotum or penis in males and the lower vagina of females. In higher anomalies, the rectum may end blindly but usually finds an insertion into the prostatic urethra or bladder in males and upper vagina in females. Evaluation should include MRI of the lumbosacral spine to rule out spinal cord tethering, IVP or ultrasound of the upper tracts, and injection of contrast into the urogenital sinus to visualize the bladder, vagina, and rectal fistula. The most common urologic problems found in association with the fistula are vesicoureteral reflux, cryptorchidism, renal agenesis, ureteral ectopia, UPJ obstruction and horseshoe kidney.

Urethral Strictures

Congenital urethral strictures are rare and usually respond to endoscopic management.

Urethral Diverticula

These congenital lesions arise in the bulbous and pendulous urethra of males. In females, they develop later in life and present with irritative voiding and recurrent UTIs. They can form stone and carcinoma (transitional-cell carcinoma and adenocarcinoma). Treatment in women is by excision and placement of a bladder neck sling for maintenance of continence.

Posterior Urethral Valves

In newborn males, this is the most common cause of urethral obstruction. Valves arise from the verumontanum in the prostatic urethra. Prolonged urinary obstruction results in severe hydronephrosis, renal dysplasia, and abnormal development of the bladder and bladder neck. Boys are seen to have a weak stream with a persistent abdominal mass. Elevated creatinine is noted on laboratory evaluation, as well as UTI. The diagnosis is confirmed with demonstration of a trabeculated, thickened bladder, vesicoureteral reflux, and a dilated posterior urethra on VCUG. Endoscopic fulguration or laser ablation is the immediate treatment of choice following 2 to 3 days of decompressive catheter drainage.

Testicular and Scrotal

Perinatal Torsion

Perinatal torsion presents at birth as a dusky, edematous scrotum that does not transilluminate. Neonatal torsion occurs in an infant who had a normal scrotum documented at birth who subsequently develops scrotal swelling, ecchymosis or a mass. Exploration is warranted to document viability of the testis and perform an orchiopexy of the opposite testis. Because the differential includes hernia, infection, meconium peritonitis, or tumor, an inguinal approach is recommended.

Hernia and Hydrocele

Formation of childhood hernia and hydrocele is due to failure of fusion of the processus vaginalis. Incarceration of bowel may occur and requires immediate exploration to avoid perforation. Infarction of the testis may also occur due to pressure on the spermatic vessels. Hydroceles present clinically as a scrotal mass in which the testis is not palpable and transilluminates. These are usually watched in infancy with surgery reserved for persistence after 6 to 12 months of age. In both entities, the processus vaginalis is divided and ligated high in the inguinal canal at the time of surgery to prevent recurrence.

Cryptorchidism

The normal testis descends at 12 to 17 weeks of gestation from the upper abdomen to a location just within the internal ring. At 7 months, the testis is guided by the gubernaculum through the processus vaginalis into the scrotum. Failure to complete this migration is referred to as cryptorchidism. The causes of cryptorchidism are myriad, including end-organ failure, inadequate gonadotropin stimulus, and mechanical obstruction. Testes may be undescended or ectopic. They may be palpable or nonpalpable. Cryptorchid testes exhibit progressive loss of germinal cells if left untreated. Treatment involves identification of the testis by careful physical examination or laparoscopy and surgical placement in its normal anatomic position.

3. Acquired Lesions

Renal

UPJ Obstruction

This lesion is usually congenital but may be acquired as a result of vesicoureteral reflux, urothelial malignancy, stone disease, benign polyps, or postoperatively from scar or ischemia. Presentation is with abrupt onset of flank pain, usually associated with ingestion of large amounts of fluid or alcohol. Management is based on the nature and degree of the obstruction. Many cases previously managed with open pyeloplasty are now managed with endoscopic incision.

Acquired Renal Cystic Disease

Patients with end-stage kidneys, regardless of whether they receive dialysis, commonly develop acquired renal cystic disease. The etiology is presumed to be a uremic toxin which is more pronounced in men. Symptoms include flank pain, hematuria, and occasionally fever if infected. Infected cysts must be drained either percutaneously or surgically. The incidence of renal cell carcinoma is increased three- to six-fold over that of the general population. One therefore must not ignore the native kidneys in renal transplant patients. Regular CT or ultrasound have been advocated.

Ureteral Obstruction

Intrinsic

Acquired lesions are less common than congenital ones. They are due to injury (trauma, surgery, radiation) and cancer.

Extrinsic

The ureter may be impinged upon by cancerous lymph nodes, an anomalous blood vessel, retroperitoneal fibrosis, aortic aneurysm, cancer of the bladder or cervix, or due to trigone hypertrophy secondary to BPH.

Vesical

Diverticulae

Bladder outlet obstruction from BPH or neurogenic pathology is the usual cause for bladder diverticulae. Transitional-cell carcinoma and stones may be found within a diverticulum. If large enough, they may prevent bladder emptying and lead to frequent bladder infection. Treatment involves intermittent catheterizations or surgical excision.

Penile and Urethral

Peyronie's Disease

Presumed due to a subclinical or incidental trauma to the penis, it results in fibrosis of the tunica albuginea surrounding the corpora cavernosa. This produces a calcified plaque, which causes penile curvature and pain during erection. This is a benign and usually self-limiting condition. However, if intercourse is not possible due to the curvature, plication and/or dermal or venous grafting of the penis may be necessary. No intervention should be attempted until the plaque has matured and the patient is pain-free for at least 6 months.

Phimosis and Paraphimosis

Inability to retract the foreskin over the glans penis is not uncommon before 5 years of age. It is not usually painful or dangerous, but it can cause urinary obstruction and may lead to chronic infection or carcinoma. Paraphimosis is the inability to reduce a previously retracted foreskin. It usually occurs iatrogenically when a health professional fails to replace the foreskin over the glans after examination or catheter placement. It soon develops impaired lymphatic drainage and extensive edema. It is usually possible to manually reduce the paraphimosis by gently squeezing out the edema fluid from the prepuce and gently pulling the foreskin while pushing the glans inward. A dorsal slit (a longitudinal incision of the underlying fibrotic tissues) may be required to reduce the foreskin. Failure to reduce the foreskin can lead to necrosis of the glans penis.

Condyloma Acuminata

Human papillomavirus (HPV) is the cause of these warty growths of the penis, scrotum, urethra, perineum, vagina and cervix. HPV infection of the cervix can cause dysplasia and is considered the precursor lesion to cervical cancer. Condyloma is usually sexually transmitted. Presentation is with pain and bleeding. Treatment is with podophyllin, liquid nitrogen, or laser therapy, depending on the location of the warts.

Priapism

Deriving its name from the Greek god of fertility, Priapus, priapism refers to erections lasting more than several hours not related to intercourse or relieved by orgasm. They are usually very painful and a sign of underlying pathology. It occurs most commonly in young sickle cell patients, but is also seen in older individuals with malignancy, coagulation disorders and pulmonary disease. Treatment should be instituted quickly to prevent penile ischemia and subsequent fibrosis and impotence. When medical management fails, surgery is performed to create a shunt to drain the blood from the penis.

Female Urethral Diverticulum

Previously underdiagnosed, this lesion is found in up to 5% of women. Classically, women with these complain of recurrent urinary tract infections, stress urinary incontinence, postvoid dribbling and dyspareunia. Compression of the urethra, which is often tender, may express purulent or bloody material from the urethral meatus. Urethrography may confirm the diagnosis. Management is by surgical excision and meticulous layered closure. A concomitant procedure for stress incontinence may be necessary.

Urethral Strictures

Strictures of the urethra are commonly due to infection and trauma. They can affect any part of the urethra (bulbous, pendulous, or fossa navicularis). The onset of symptoms leading to diagnosis is often insidious. Typical complaints are of decreased urinary stream, spraying of urine, and need to Valsalva to empty the bladder. Cystoscopy identifies the stricture, but retrograde urethrography is essential to determine its length and position. Patients who are poor surgical candidates are treated with direct visualization internal urethrotomy or balloon dilation. The remainder are treated with open urethroplasty.

Prostatic

Benign Prostatic Hyperplasia (BPH)

In the strictest sense, BPH is a pathologic diagnosis reflecting the overgrowth of the glandular and stromal components of the prostate gland. The term has been used over the years to describe the symptoms associated with prostatic enlargement. The symptoms are more properly termed lower urinary tract symptoms or LUTS. These include incomplete emptying, frequency, intermittency, urgency, weak stream, straining and nocturia. Enlarged prostates do not uniformly cause these symptoms, nor are these symptoms found exclusively with BPH. BPH becomes evident in the fourth decade of life. The prevalence of BPH increases with each decade until it approaches 100% in the ninth decade of life. Treatment is directed at management of symptoms. Alpha-adrenergic blocking agents are the first line treatment in standard medical management of BPH. 5-alpha-reductase inhibitors are often used to shrink larger glands or prevent troublesome prostatic variceal bleeding. Recent studies have shown that combination medical therapy with the use of an alpha-blocker, plus a 5-alpha-reductase inhibitor is more effective than either medication alone. Combination medical therapy is frequently used in these patients. Surgeries, such as transurethral resection of the prostate or TURP, are reserved for severely affected individuals, those who cannot tolerate medical therapy, and those in urinary retention. Laser procedures are becoming much more common, and include laser vaporization of the prostate and laser enucleation of the prostate.

Bladder Neck Contracture

Radical prostatectomy for prostate cancer results in bladder neck contracture in 2%-3% of cases. It is usually apparent within 2 months postoperatively. Management is with dilation or endoscopic incision (cold knife or laser). Recurrence is common.

Testicular

Torsion

Torsion is twisting of the testicle on the spermatic cord, causing strangulation and infarction of the testicle. Presentation is a sudden onset of pain and swelling of the testicle in males aged 12 to 20. On examination, it is difficult to distinguish the testicle from the epididymis, frequently leading to missed diagnosis. In postpuberty sexually active males, torsion is less likely than epididymitis. Ultrasound is a negative confirmatory test reserved for those individuals in whom you have a low clinical suspicion for torsion. Treatment is emergent scrotal exploration, detorsion if possible, and bilateral fixation of the testes. Occasionally torsion of the testicular appendage will present with pain localized to the upper pole of the testicle. Physical examination may identify a "blue dot sign" representing a thrombosed, torsed appendix testis. These can be observed if the ultrasound shows good flow to the testicle.

4. Stones

Epidemiology

Nephrolithiasis has plagued man for centuries, as attested to by the stone found in an Egyptian mummy from 4800 BC. Presently the prevalence is about 5%, with a lifetime risk of stone disease up to 15%. Higher prevalence of stone disease is found in hot, arid, or dry climates. Men are affected more than women, 2 to 3:1 and whites are affected more than other races. Stone disease is not common before the age of 20 and peak incidence occurs in the fourth to sixth decades of life. High fluid intake and low protein intake can have a beneficial effect on stone formation. The risk of stone disease seems to correlate with weight and body mass index with obesity being an independent risk factor for stones.

Calcium-Containing Stones

Stones containing calcium represent 75%-80% of urinary stones. The most common are calcium oxalate (monohydrate and dihydrate forms), calcium phosphate (apatite), and calcium hydrogen phosphate (brushite). Common causes of calcium stone formation are absorptive hypercalciuria, renal hypercalciuria, resorptive hypercalciuria, and idiopathic hypercalciuria. Hypercalcemia as a cause is related to hyperparathyroidism, sarcoidosis, malignancy, hyperthyroidism, chronic steroid or thiazide use, and prolonged bedrest. Oxalate-containing stones are caused by primary hyperoxaluria, enteric hyperoxaluria, metabolic hyperoxaluria, hyperuricosuria, hypocitraturia and hypomagnesemia. Calcium phosphate (apatite and brushite) stones are found in approximately 70% of distal renal tubular acidosis (type I RTA) patients. Stones do not occur in other forms of RTA.

Non-Calcium-Containing Stones

Uric Acid (5%-7%)

These stones are lucent on plain radiograph, but bright on CT scan. The three main determinants of uric acid stone formation are low urine pH, low urine volume and hyperuricosuria. These can result from many causes to include primary gout, high animal protein intake, obesity, diarrheal states, myeloproliferate disorders and uricosuric medications. Low urinary volume can also be related to living in warmer climates.

Struvite (5%-15%)

These stones, composed of magnesium ammonium phosphate, are also referred to as infection stones. They are formed by urea-splitting organisms in basic urine. Struvite stones account for the majority of staghorn calculi. The treatment of choice is percutaneous nephrolithotripsy, with extracorporeal shock wave lithotripsy (ESWL) for any residual stones.

Cystine (1%-2%)

Cystine stones result from cystinuria. Cystinuria is an autosomal recessive disorder that results in excessive urinary excretion of cystine. Cystine stones are rare, but are the cause of up to 10% of all stones in children. The stones are faintly radiopaque, and are often large and multiple. Occurrence peaks in the second to third decade of life. Diagnosis is made with a 24-hour urinalysis for cystine. Treatment is directed at stone dissolution with diet (low methionine and high fluid intake), alkalinization of the urine and oral cystine-binding agents. Surgery may be needed initially to remove large stones. Renal transplant corrects the defect in patients with renal failure.

Indinavir Stones

This is an increasingly common occurrence with the development of protease inhibitors used in the treatment of HIV infection. The stones are crystals of the medication, which form in concentrated urine and lead to obstruction of the ureter. Suspicion is the key to diagnosis since the stones are radiolucent on KUB as well as CT. Treatment is with analgesics, hydration and cessation of the medication for several days.

Physical Findings

Nonobstructing stones are painless, however stones acutely obstructing the ureteropelvic junction or a calyx may cause renal pain, nausea and vomiting. Migration of the stone down the ureter is experienced as loin pain that eventually radiates to the bladder and genitalia as the stone approaches the ureterovesical junction. Feelings of urgency and dysuria are common as the stone traverses the intravesical ureter. Costovertebral angle tenderness in association with fever is a sign of secondary infection.

Laboratory Findings

Urinalysis may reveal hematuria, pyuria and crystals. High pH suggests urea-splitting organisms, while low pH may indicate uric acid or cystine stones. If the pH is between 6 and 7, consideration should be given to renal tubular acidosis, especially as a cause of nephrocalcinosis. Acutely, 24-hour urine collections are inaccurate.

Differential Diagnosis

Pyelonephritis can present with flank pain and fever suggestive of an obstructing stone. Intravenous urogram or CT urogram fails to reveal a stone. Cancer of the kidney or ureter can cause flank pain or lead to infection from obstruction. Tumors of the renal pelvis may mimic radiolucent stones on an excretory urogram. CT scan or ultrasound will easily demonstrate the stone. Papillary sloughing can present with pain and hematuria, but is easily diagnosed with excretory urography. Appendicitis should still be considered in right lower quadrant pain, even with pyuria or hematuria.

Imaging Studies

An abdominal radiograph is an excellent first test since up to 70% of stones will be radiopaque. If a stone is suspected, an intravenous pyelogram or noncontrast CT scan should be done. CT scan or renal ultrasound are anatomic studies and cannot establish the degree of obstruction caused by the stone. Patients with iodine allergy and suspicion of a stone on CT may require retrograde pyelography.

Management

Hospital admission is required for high-grade unilateral obstruction, any obstruction of a solitary kidney, bilateral obstruction, obstruction with fever or azotemia, severe pain not controlled by oral narcotics, severe nausea and vomiting, or obstruction with a stone too large to be expected to pass. A rule of thumb is that 50% of 5-mm stones will pass. If possible, patients should be given several weeks to try to pass their stone. Instruction is given to increase fluid intake to 3 L/day, strain the urine, take oral narcotics for pain, and return for worsening pain, fevers, gross hematuria, or nausea and vomiting. Alpha-blocker medication can be given as they have been shown to increase the rate of stone passage from the ureter.

An obstructing ureteral stone associated with signs of significant infection is a medical emergency. This situation can lead to bacteremia, sepsis and death. The kidney needs to be decompressed with either a ureteral stent or a nephrostomy tube.

There are multiple minimally invasive treatment options for renal and ureteral stones. ESWL can be performed for renal and ureteral stones smaller than 2.0 cm, but success can depend on the size of the patient and the hardness of the stone. Ureteroscope technology has improved to the point where stones throughout the entire collecting system and ureter are treated with this approach. Percutaneous nephrolithotripsy (PCNL) is usually reserved for staghorn calculi, ESWL failures and stones in a calyceal diverticulum. Open stone surgery is rarely required with present day technology.

Prevention

Patients should be advised of the 50% recurrence rate at 10 years, unless sufficient attention is paid to measures for prevention of stone formation. Fluid intake should be increased to 3 to 4 L/day. Diets that reduce animal protein intake and sodium intake have shown to reduce stone formation as well. Specific diet and medical therapy is recommended on the basis of stone analysis, serum chemistry analysis, and evaluation of a 24-hour urine collection for specific electrolytes.

5. Trauma

Kidneys

Though well protected in the retroperitoneum, the kidneys are vulnerable to both blunt and penetrating trauma. Blunt trauma can cause hematoma, laceration, avulsion of the renal parenchyma (grades I to V), or injury to the collecting system. Penetrating trauma causes similar injury. Gunshot wounds produce ischemia in an area larger than the projectile's path might indicate. Higher-velocity rounds do the most damage, with delayed necrosis causing urine leak, bleeding, and infection. Patients present with flank pain, nausea and vomiting, gross hematuria, and occasionally a flank mass or ecchymosis. When stable, patients should have a plain abdominal film to look for fractures of ribs or transverse processes. Abdominopelvic contrast CT scan is the study of choice to evaluate the extent of injury. Unstable patients should undergo laparotomy and repair of associated injuries. Renal exploration is indicated for uncontrolled bleeding, urinary extravasation or devitalized parenchyma. Shattered kidneys from blunt trauma should be managed nonoperatively in stable patients. Partial nephrectomy, renorrhaphy and vascular reconstruction are only occasionally successful.

Ureters

Injury is iatrogenic from gynecologic, urologic and general surgical procedures. Inadvertent ureteral ligation leads to hydronephrosis and loss of renal function. Laceration leads to urinoma and fistula formation. Patients with delayed diagnoses often present with flank pain and ileus. Intravenous urography or retrograde pyelography will demonstrate the injury. Repair depends on the mechanism and level of injury, with early recognition of injury providing better outcomes.

Bladder

Blunt trauma with or without pelvic fracture is the most common cause of injury. Suprapubic pain and hematuria are common. Meatal bleeding may indicate urethral injury, so a retrograde urethrogram should precede catheterization. Cystography with a drainage film or CT cystogram confirms the diagnosis. Extraperitoneal bladder rupture presents as a pelvic mass with contrast confined to the pelvis on cystography. Treatment is with antibiotics and catheter drainage. Operative repair is for massive perforation or if coincident with other surgical procedures. Abscess formation is a delayed complication. Intraperitoneal perforations cause ileus, oliguria and azotemia. Operative repair of these is via laparotomy, bladder closure and catheter drainage.

Urethra

Posterior Urethra

This involves the prostatic and membranous urethra up to the urogenital diaphragm. History is of blunt pelvic trauma with pelvic fracture present in over 90% of cases. Digital rectal examination is performed to identify prostate and bladder elevation and presence of hematoma. Gross blood at the urethral meatus is almost invariable with urethral injury. Patients suspected of injury should be told not to void until a retrograde urethrogram (RUG) is completed. The RUG identifies the degree and position of the injury. Stretch injury and partial tears of the urethra can be managed with temporary catheter drainage. More severe injuries are initially managed with placement of a suprapubic tube. Primary repair has been associated with lower rates of urethral stricture, but higher rates of incontinence and impotence, as well as pelvic infection and bleeding. Delayed repair allows several months for strictures to mature and for appropriate imaging to be obtained. Repair is usually endoscopic, but open repair is preferred. Disruption in children is initially managed with vesicostomy, but stricture forms in approximately 95% of cases.

Anterior Urethra

Injuries to the bulbous and pendulous urethra are usually due to direct blows to the perineum or by penetrating injury. Tears of the urethra can occur with sex, masturbation or self-mutilation. Inflation of a Foley balloon in the urethra or its accidental removal while inflated can also cause injury. Bleeding is contained within Buck's or Colles' fascia. RUG should be performed if blood is seen at the meatus. Exploration, debridement, and repair are indicated if rupture is present. Proctoscopy is essential for bullet wounds of the perineum or suprapubic region.

Table 1

2002 AJCC TNM Staging for Renal Cell Carcinoma

Tumor (T)	
T0	No evidence of tumor
T1a	Tumor 4 cm or less in greatest dimension, confined to the kidney
T1b	Tumor >4 cm but not more than 7 cm in greatest dimension, confined to the kidney
T2	Tumor greater than 7 cm in greatest dimension, confined to the kidney
T3	Tumor extends into the major veins, the adrenal vein, or perinephric tissues but not beyond Gerota's fascia
T4	Tumor invades beyond Gerota's fascia
Regional lymph nodes (N)	
N0	No regional lymph node metastasis
N1	Metastasis in a single regional lymph node
N2	Metastasis in more than one regional lymph node
Distant metastasis (M)	
M0	No distant metastasis
M1	Distant metastasis

Female Urethra

Trauma in women is the result of pelvic fracture and often involves the bladder neck and vagina.

6. Tumors

Renal Cell Carcinoma

Renal cell carcinoma (RCC) represents 3% of all adult malignancies. It is associated with von Hippel-Lindau disease, adult polycystic kidney disease, acquired renal cystic disease and smoking. The disease is twice as common in men as in women.

Clinical Findings

Hematuria is the most common presenting symp tom. Though a classic triad of hematuria, flank pain, and palpable abdominal mass suggest RCC, it is present in fewer than 10% of cases. Metastatic lesions may present with bone pain, weight loss or dyspnea. There are no laboratory tests specific for RCC, however paraneoplastic syndromes are common (30%). These patients may have elevated liver function tests and fever, suggestive of metastases (Stauffer's syndrome), but have normalization of labs after the nephrectomy. Failure to normalize results in poor prognosis. Anemia, polycythemia, hypercalcemia and hypertension are also seen in association with RCC. Lesions are often detected incidentally on ultrasound or CT scan. Intravenous urography (IVU) done as part of the hematuria workup may also demonstrate a mass lesion, prompting follow-up with a CT scan. Ultrasound is also helpful in evaluating lesions seen on IVU, differentiating solid from cystic lesions. It has the benefit of identifying caval tumor thrombus. Magnetic resonance angiography (MRA) is the most sensitive noninvasive test for detecting renal vein or vena caval thrombi.

Staging

The most recent staging is from the American Joint Committee on Cancer, 2002, and is depicted in Table 1. Metastatic workup should include chest radiograph, bone scan if indicated, lymph node examination, neurologic examination, and comprehensive chemistry panel.

Treatment

Treatment of RCC is dependent upon the extent of disease at diagnosis and on the patient's overall performance status. Historically, one-third of patients have presented with metastatic disease. Radical nephrectomy (en bloc removal of the kidney, perirenal fat, ipsilateral adrenal and proximal ureter) and regional lymphadenectomy are indicated for any patient without multiple metastases. Solitary metastases can be resected at the time of the nephrectomy, sometimes for cure. This is more likely with pulmonary metastases. RCC with multiple metastases can be treated with high-dose IL-2 therapy, with or without nephrectomy. The recent introduction of tyrokinase inhibitors, such as sunitinib, for advanced RCC has lengthened the survival of patients with advanced disease. Temsirolimus provided a 2-3 month prolongation in patients who were considered poor risk and to have an advanced stage RCC. Radiation is for palliation of brain or bone metastases. Partial nephrectomy (nephron-sparing surgery) is reserved for individuals with peripheral lesions less than 4 cm in diameter, solitary kidneys, bilateral tumors, obviously benign lesions, poor renal function or an at-risk contralateral kidney. Warm ischemia time should be kept under 30 minutes, or the kidney should be chilled to 15°C after the artery is clamped.

Prognosis

The overall prognosis depends upon the TNM stage and the nuclear grade of the tumor. Survival at 5 years is: T1, 83%; T2, 57%; T3, 42%; and T4, 28%. Higher-grade lesions have worse prognosis within each stage.

Wilms' Tumor

Wilms' tumor is the most common malignancy of the urinary tract in children. There are 350 new cases diagnosed each year, with peak incidence at ages 3 to 4. The tumor results from abnormal metanephric blastemal proliferation. Chromosome 11, containing the gene for a tumor suppressor, is implicated in pathogenesis. Associated anomalies are common. Wilms' tumors may exhibit different microscopic features. Diffuse anaplasia in the specimen confers a poorer prognosis. Rhabdoid and clear cell sarcoma variants are now considered separate from Wilms' tumor.

Angiomyolipoma

These are hamartomas of the kidney that contain fat and blood vessels. They are found in association with tuberous sclerosis, a neurological disorder. They have a propensity to grow and present with pain from retroperitoneal bleeding, gastrointestinal

Table 2

2002 AJCC TNM Staging for Bladder Cancer

Tumor (T)	
T0	No evidence of tumor
Ta	Papillary noninvasive carcinoma
Tis	Carcinoma *in situ*
T1	Tumor invades subepithelial connective tissue
T2	Tumor invades muscularis propria
T2a	Tumor invades superficial muscle
T2b	Tumor invades deep muscle
T3	Tumor invades perivesical tissue:
T3a	Microscopically
T3b	Macroscopically
T4	Tumor invades prostate, uterus, vagina, pelvic wall, abdominal wall
Regional lymph nodes (N)	
N0	No regional lymph node metastasis
N1	Metastasis in a single lymph node, 2 cm or less in diameter
N2	Metastasis in a single lymph node, more than 2 cm but not more than 5 cm in diameter; or multiple lymph nodes, none more than 5 cm in diameter
N3	Metastasis in a lymph node greater than 5 cm in diameter
Distant metastasis (M)	
M0	No distant metastasis
M1	Distant metastasis

obstruction, or are found incidentally on CT scan. Initial management of lesions over 4 cm involves angioembolization, with surgery reserved for failures or for those lesions with calcifications or areas suspicious for cancer.

Oncocytoma

Hard to distinguish from renal cell carcinoma, these usually benign tumors are discovered incidentally. Some have a characteristic central scar on CT scan, however management is still partial or radical nephrectomy, depending on the age of the patient and the size and location of the lesion.

Transitional-Cell Carcinoma of the Bladder

These account for 2% of all cancers. The male to female ratio is 2:1. Most are related to smoking (70%) or industrial chemical exposure. The lesions are usually superficial. Recurrences are not uncommon and are usually also superficial.

Clinical Findings

The most common presentation is painless gross or microscopic hematuria. Those with carcinoma *in situ* may present with irritative voiding symptoms. Obstructive symptoms can develop due to bladder neck obstruction. Flank pain can develop if the tumor obstructs a ureter. Physical examination is not usually helpful, but bimanual examination may demonstrate a mass. IVP may demonstrate a filling defect in the bladder or hydronephrosis if the ureteral orifice is involved. CT scan may show extension outside the bladder along with pelvic or retroperitoneal adenopathy. Urinary cytologic evaluation may demonstrate atypia (higher-grade lesions are most likely to slough into the urine). Cystoscopy is essential in any patient with gross hematuria or greater than 3 red blood cells per HPF on 2 separate occasions.

Staging

Treatment depends heavily upon the stage of the tumor. The most recent American Joint Committee on Cancer staging is listed in Table 2. Metastatic workup should include lymph node examination, bimanual examination, chest radiograph, and comprehensive chemistry panel. CT scan is indicated for

Table 3

2002 AJCC TNM Staging for Cancer of the Renal Pelvis and Ureter

Tumor (T)	
T0	No evidence of tumor
Ta	Papillary noninvasive carcinoma
Tis	Carcinoma in situ
T1	Tumor invades subepithelial connective tissue
T2	Tumor invades muscularis
T3	For renal pelvis only: Tumor invades beyond the muscularis, into peripelvic fat or renal parenchyma
T3	For ureter only: Tumor invades beyond muscularis into periureteric fat
T4	Tumor invades adjacent organs or through the kidney into perinephric fat
Regional lymph nodes (N)	
N0	No regional lymph node metastasis
N1	Metastasis in a single lymph node, 2 cm or less in diameter
N2	Metastasis in a single lymph node, more than 2 cm but not more than 5 cm in diameter; or multiple lymph nodes, none more than 5 cm in diameter
N3	Metastasis in a lymph node greater than 5 cm in diameter
Distant metastasis (M)	
M0	No distant metastasis
M1	Distant metastasis

invasive (T1 or above) lesions. Bone scanning is done if clinically indicated.

Treatment

Treatment is based upon the stage and grade of the tumor. Superficial lesions can be cured with transurethral resection. Occasionally, adjunctive treatment is necessary for those with recurrent superficial lesions, multiple lesions at diagnosis, minimally invasive lesions (T1) or for carcinoma *in situ*. Standard therapies include intravesical bacille Calmette-Guérin (BCG), mitomycin or thiotepa. Refractory bladder cancer has been treated with intravesical interferon and valrubicin with some success. Surveillance after definitive treatment involves cystoscopy quarterly for 1 year, twice a year for 1 year, and annually thereafter. Urine cytology should be done annually as well as an IVP every 2 years. In cases of lesions that invade muscle, radical cystectomy and pelvic lymphadenectomy with urinary diversion are required. Diversion can be achieved via an ileal conduit to the skin, a continent cutaneous diversion such as an Indiana or Mainz pouch, or by an orthotopic neobladder to the native urethra. Positive urethra margins or urethral recurrences require urethrectomy. Chemotherapy is reserved for node-positive or metastatic disease.

Prognosis

Most superficial lesions will not recur. Higher-grade lesions are more likely to recur and progress to invasive disease. Intravesical agents have been shown to prolong the time to tumor recurrence. Submucosal invasion results in a 92% 5-year survival rate. Organ-confined muscle-invasive tumors result in 76% 5-year survival, while non-organ confined lesions produce about a 40% 5-year survival. Nodal metastases portend a very poor prognosis (30% 5-year survival in N1, 22% in N2, and 0% in N3 disease). Chemotherapy with MVAC (methotrexate, vinblastine, adriamycin, and cisplatin) has provided substantial prolongation of time to progression (36 vs. 63 months).

Transitional-Cell Carcinoma—Renal Pelvis and Ureter

Clinical Findings

Painless gross or microscopic hematuria with or without abnormal urine cytology is common. Diagnosis is suggested by IVU and confirmed by retrograde pyelography. Tissue for diagnosis is obtained ureteroscopically with brush or biopsy.

Staging

The most recent American Joint Committee on Cancer staging is listed in Table 3. Metastatic workup should include lymph node examination, chest radiograph and comprehensive chemistry panel. CT scan is useful in ruling out stones or metastases. Bone scanning is done if clinically indicated.

Treatment

Lesions in the renal pelvis are not usually metastatic so nephroureterectomy with excision of a cuff of bladder is curative. If they are low-grade, lesions in the ureter can be managed with segmental resection of the ureter. Endoscopic management is preferred when the lesions are low-grade and there is a solitary kidney or renal insufficiency. Follow-up requires periodic cystoscopy and annual IVP.

Prognosis

Grade of tumor and stage of disease dictate prognosis. Low-grade lesions are rarely fatal. High-grade or invasive lesions have a worse prognosis, while metastases portend a less than 10% 5-year survival rate.

Prostate Cancer

This is the most common non-skin tumor in US men and the second leading cause of cancer death in the United States. Adenocarcinoma is the most common type, but others include neuroendocrine, transitional-cell, sarcoma, and squamous cell carcinoma. Tumors arise in the peripheral zone (70%) and transition zone (20%) most commonly. Risk factors include first-degree relative with prostate cancer, African American race and age over 65. Benign hyperplasia is not a precursor of cancer. Prostate cancer is usually slow growing.

Clinical Findings

Presenting symptoms are absent in early stages of disease. Advanced disease may present with urinary difficulty or infection. Metastatic disease may present with bone pain, weight loss, anemia or neurologic deficit if the spine is involved with tumor. Digital rectal examination (DRE) may confirm the pres-

Table 4

2002 AJCC TNM Staging for Prostate Cancer

Tumor (T)	
T0	No evidence of tumor
T1	Clinically inapparent tumor not palpable or visible by imaging
T1a	Incidental histologic finding of tumor in 5% or less of tissue resected
T1b	Incidental histologic finding of tumor in more than 5% of tissue resected
T1c	Tumor identified by needle biopsy (eg, because of elevated PSA)
T2	Palpable tumor confined within the prostate (into capsule, not through)
T2a	Tumor involves ½ of one lobe or less
T2b	Tumor involves >½ of one lobe, but not both lobes
T2c	Tumor involves both lobes
T3	Tumor extends through the prostatic capsule
T3a	Extracapsular extension (unilateral or bilateral)
T3b	Tumor invades seminal vesicle(s)
T4	Tumor is fixed or invades adjacent structures other than seminal vesicles
Regional lymph nodes (N)	
N0	No regional lymph node metastasis
N1	Metastasis in one or more regional lymph nodes
Distant metastasis (M)	
M0	No distant metastasis
M1	Distant metastasis

ence of induration or a nodule on the prostate. Fixation to the pelvic side wall may be detected. Laboratory evaluation may reveal elevated PSA (prostate specific antigen), elevated creatinine due to urinary obstruction, or anemia due to marrow replacement by tumor. The American Urological Association (AUA) and American Cancer Society recommend annual PSA testing and DRE for men beginning at age 50, if a life expectancy of >10 years. African Americans and men with first-degree relatives represent higher risk, and screening should be offered at an earlier age, 40-45 years old. Transrectal ultrasound may reveal hypoechoic areas of the prostate. Its prime function is as a guide to needle biopsy. CT and MRI have not proved helpful to stage prostate cancer. Chest radiograph is rarely positive for lung lesions, however it may show lytic rib lesions. Bone scan is performed for high-grade lesions (Gleason's 8 and above), for PSA 20 ng/mL and above, and if there is suspicion of metastatic disease.

Staging

The most recent staging is from the American Joint Committee on Cancer, 2002, and is depicted in Table 4. Metastatic workup should include chest radiograph, bone scan if indicated, lymph node examination, PSA, CBC and comprehensive chemistry panel.

Treatment

Low-grade disease in older patients may be observed. Moderate-grade disease requires some form of therapy. Choices today include radical prostatectomy (removal of the prostate and seminal vesicles), external beam radiation therapy, interstitial seed implantation (radioactive iodide or palladium) or total androgen ablation (orchiectomy or medical castration). Pelvic lymph node dissection accompanies prostatectomy for staging purposes only. Prostatectomy offers the best chance of cure, but is complicated by risks of impotence, incontinence, transfusion, deep venous thrombosis (DVT) and bladder neck contracture. It is usually only offered to those with a life expectancy of 10 or more years. Neither chemotherapy nor immunotherapy has been helpful in treatment.

Prognosis

Gleason's score is the primary determinant of successful treatment. High-grade tumors grow and spread more quickly and act independently of

Table 5

2002 AJCC TNM Staging for Testis Cancer

Tumor (T)	
pT0	No evidence of tumor
pTis	Intratubular germ cell neoplasia (carcinoma *in situ*)
pT1	Tumor limited to the testis and epididymis without vascular/lymphatic invasion (Tumor may invade into the tunica albuginea but not the tunica vaginalis)
pT2	Tumor limited to the testis and epididymis with vascular/lymphatic invasion, or tumor extending through the tunica albuginea with involvement of the tunica vaginalis
pT3	Tumor invades the spermatic cord with or without vascular/lymphatic invasion
pT4	Tumor involves the scrotum with or without vascular/lymphatic invasion
Regional lymph nodes (N)	
N0	No regional lymph node metastasis
N1	Metastasis in one or more lymph nodes, all 2 cm or less in diameter
N2	Metastasis in one or more lymph nodes, more than 2 cm but not more than 5 cm in diameter
N3	Metastasis with a lymph node mass greater than 5 cm in diameter
Distant metastasis (M)	
M0	No distant metastasis
M1	Distant metastasis
M1a	Nonregional nodal or pulmonary metastasis
M1b	Distant metastasis other than to nonregional lymph nodes and lungs
Serum markers (S)	
S0	Normal markers
S1	LDH <1.5 times upper normal limit (unl) and HCG (mIu/ml) <5000 and AFP (ng/ml) <1000
S2	LDH 1.5 to 10 times unl and HCG (mIu/ml) 5000 to 50,000 and AFP (ng/ml) 1000 to 10,000
S3	LDH >10 times unl and HCG (mIu/ml) >50,000 and AFP (ng/ml) >10,000

testosterone. Men with low cancers confined to the prostate achieve near 85%-90% progression-free survival, with moderate, 75% and with high-grade cancers 35%-50% rates, respectively. Radiation is almost as effective in those with localized low-grade disease. Follow-up with annual digital rectal examination and frequent PSA monitoring is essential to detect recurrence or progression of disease.

Testis Cancer

Testis cancer is relatively rare, but it receives a great deal of attention because it is the most common malignancy in males aged 15 to 35. It is incredibly chemosensitive and is one of the few cancers with accurate tumor markers. Testicular tumors are usually of germ cell origin. Exceptions are Sertoli and Leydig cell tumors, which occur infrequently and are usually benign. Germ cell tumors are further divided into seminomatous (40%) and nonseminomatous (teratocarcinoma, 40%; embryonal, 20%; teratoma, 5%; and choriocarcinoma, 2%) varieties. Cryptorchidism increases the risk of cancer 5- to 15-fold. Yolk sac tumors and pure teratomas are usually seen in children. Seminoma is seen in men aged 35 to 39 and rarely over age 60. Lesions after age 50 are likely lymphoma.

Clinical Findings

Presentation is a history of a painless, hard mass in the testis, which may have grown rapidly in size over several months. Delay in evaluation may cause back pain, weight loss and anorexia from metastases. Examination confirms the mass. A hydrocele may obscure the lesion, so a testicular ultrasound is indicated; otherwise ultrasound is unnecessary. Serum testing for lactate dehydrogenase (LDH), beta-human chorionic gonadotropin (β-hCG), and alpha-fetoprotein (AFP) are done prior to treatment. β-hCG is found in the majority of nonseminomas and 10% of seminomas. AFP is elevated in 70% of nonseminomas. Pure seminomas in patients with elevated AFP indicate other elements missed by the pathologist. Abdominopelvic CT scan should always be done to rule out retroperitoneal adenopathy that may require neoadjuvant chemotherapy. CT scan fails to diagnose 20%-25% of micrometastatic disease.

Staging

The most recent American Joint Committee on Cancer staging is listed in Table 5. Metastatic workup should include lymph node examination, chest radiograph, abdominopelvic CT scan, LDH, AFP, β-hCG and a comprehensive chemistry panel.

Treatment

Inguinal orchiectomy with high ligation of the cord structures is required. Tumor markers, if elevated, should be checked in 4 to 6 weeks. The half-life of β-hCG is 1 day, and for AFP it is 5 to 7 days. Failure to normalize markers is a sign of residual metastatic disease and chemotherapy with 3 cycles of PEB (cisplatin, etoposide, and bleomycin) is indicated. If markers are normal, the patient chooses between lifelong surveillance with tumor markers and CT scans, or prophylactic retroperitoneal lymphadenectomy (RPLAD). RPLAD involves removal of lymphatic tissue from around the vena cava and aorta in a template fashion and removal of the remaining cord structures. Prospectively identifying the sympathetic nerves and limiting the dissection to above the inferior mesenteric artery (IMA) results in maintenance of seminal emission and ejaculation. Bulky retroperitoneal disease is treated with chemotherapy (bleomycin, vinblastine and cisplatin) and subsequent postchemotherapy RPLAD if residual disease remains. Seminoma is exquisitely radiosensitive so treatment after orchiectomy is irradiation (2500 cGy) of the abdomen. Bulky seminoma is also treated with multiagent chemotherapy.

Prognosis

Overall, prognosis is excellent. Low-stage disease is cured with orchiectomy and RPLAD or irradiation for seminoma 95% of the time. Low-volume retroperitoneal disease patients can expect an 85% to 90% chance of cure. Bulky retroperitoneal adenopathy, with the most aggressive treatment, yields success in about 70% of individuals. An exception to this is choriocarcinoma, which metastasizes hematogenously. RPLAD is not helpful, nor is chemotherapy. Survival in these cases is 35% at 5 years.

Penile Cancer

Cancer of the penis is rare in circumcised men. The cause is uncertain; however, HPV has been implicated. It usually occurs in men aged 50 and older. It may present as a painless erythematous patch or fungating lesion. Incisional biopsy confirms the presence of squamous cell carcinoma. Superficial lesions may be treated with fluorouracil (5-FU), radiation, or laser therapy. Larger or more invasive lesions require partial or total penectomy, depending upon its location. Ilioinguinal lymphadenectomy is performed for palpable inguinal nodes, invasion of tumor into the corporal bodies, or in moderate- to poorly-differentiated lesions. Note that palpable inguinal nodes may be a sign of metastasis or simply secondary infection or reaction. A six week course of antibiotics should be given before considering ilioinguinal lymphadenectomy. Dissection should be bilateral. Radiation therapy and chemotherapy have no place in the management of penile cancer. Five-year survival is 80% in low-grade noninvasive lesions, 50% in node-positive cases and 0% for distant metastatic disease.

7. Infections

Kidney

Acute Pyelonephritis

These are infections of the renal parenchyma due to ascending bacterial pathogens. The clinical picture includes fevers, chills, flank pain, malaise, dysuria, urgency and frequency. Physical examination often reveals unilateral costovertebral angle tenderness. Laboratory studies reveal leukocytosis, pyuria, bacteriuria and bacterial growth of cultured urine. Intravenous urography may demonstrate delay in excretion or hydronephrosis if a stone is present. CT scan may reveal perinephric stranding, gas in the tissues or obstructing ureteral stone. Differential diagnosis includes pancreatitis, diverticulitis and intestinal angina. Failure to document obstruction can be fatal.

Xanthogranulomatous Pyelonephritis

Patients harboring infectious stones related to urea-splitting organisms can develop a large, nonfunctional kidney which is hard to distinguish from renal cell carcinoma. Microscopic examination reveals macrophages laden with lipid (foam cells). Treatment is with radical nephrectomy via a transperitoneal approach. There is extensive desmoplastic reaction and early control of the vessels is essential.

Emphysematous Pyelonephritis

This is an acute necrotizing pyelonephritis involving facultative anaerobic organisms (*Escherichia coli*, *Proteus mirabilis*, and *Klebsiella pneumoniae*) that produce carbon dioxide from glucose in the renal parenchyma of diabetics. Patients present with fever, flank pain, and vomiting. The diagnosis is made based upon the presence of gas seen within the parenchyma on plain radiograph as well as CT scan. Focal pockets of gas belie the full extent of renal destruction. Management involves broad-spectrum antibiotics and immediate nephrectomy. Mortality approaches 50% even with aggressive treatment. Percutaneous drainage is not an option in this situation.

Abscess

Renal abscess forms within the parenchyma of the kidney in response to lower or upper tract infection, calculi, or vesicoureteral reflux disease. Higher incidence is seen in diabetics, the immunocompromised, and drug users. Treatment includes 1 to 2 weeks of broad-spectrum antibiotics and early percutaneous drainage. Perirenal abscess is an occasional complication of renal abscess due to rupture into the perinephric space (within Gerota's fascia) and is often treated by open drainage or nephrectomy.

Bladder and Urethra

Cystitis

Acute cystitis involves symptoms of frequency, urgency, dysuria, hematuria, and occasionally suprapubic or low back pain. There is rarely fever or leukocytosis unless the upper tracts are involved. Treatment is usually empirical. Culture of the urine is reserved for cases of persistence or recurrence of symptoms. Chronic cystitis is due to urethral or prostatic obstruction, prostatitis, or presence of foreign bodies, tumors or stones. Women with chronic infections may be treated with several months of suppressive oral antibiotics or postcoitally if infections are so related.

Prostate

There are 2 million diagnoses of prostatitis each year with a cumulative incidence approaching 50% by 80 years of age. NIH classification includes acute and chronic bacterial prostatitis, chronic nonbacterial prostatitis (no demonstrable infection) with and without inflammatory cells, and asymptomatic inflammatory prostatitis. Only 5% are bacterial. Symptoms include fever, chills, and low back and perineal pain. Enteric pathogens are causative and severe cases require broad-spectrum parenteral antibiotics. Mild cases are managed with a quinolone or trimethoprim-sulfamethoxazole for at least 4 weeks. Repeat courses are given for non or partial responders. Nonbacterial cases are managed with hot baths, increased fluid intake, exercise, and well-balanced meals without soda, alcohol or caffeine.

Testis and Epididymis

Orchitis/Epididymitis

Acute orchitis/epididymitis usually occurs in young, sexually active men due to ascending infection from the prostate and urethra. There is often fever, pain in the scrotum and tenderness of the spermatic cord, epididymis and testis. Pyuria, bacteriuria and leukocytosis are common. Treatment includes urine culture, antibiotics (ceftriaxone, 125 mg IM once and doxycycline for 10 days), bedrest and scrotal elevation. Severe infections require hospitalization and intravenous antibiotics. Complications include abscess formation, testis infarction, chronic pain and infertility.

Penis and Scrotum

Balanoposthitis

Inflammation of the foreskin and glans penis is most commonly seen in young men with phimosis. The cause is usually bacterial or fungal and biopsy is rarely required. Treatment is with antibiotics, antifungal agents or topical steroid cream. If it is recurrent, circumcision is required.

Fournier's Gangrene

Fournier's gangrene, described in the 1880s, is a necrotizing fasciitis of the male genitalia, perineum, and abdominal wall. Predisposition is from diabetes, perirectal or perineal infection, paraphimosis, local trauma and recent pelvic surgery. Infecting organisms are usually anaerobic and multiple. Presentation is with fever and pain. Examination may reveal cellulitis, purpura of gangrene and crepitus of the skin. Prompt diagnosis, based on the toxic appearance of the patient, is essential. Treatment includes broad-spectrum antibiotics, fluid resuscitation and aggressive surgical debridement. Mortality averages 20%, but is higher in diabetics and alcoholics.

Genital Warts

These are most often caused by HPV types 6 and 11. Transmission is via sexual contact. Women with HPV are more likely to have cervical dysplasia leading to cancer. Lesions are usually painless but unsightly. The goal of treatment is to remove the lesions, not to rid the body of the virus. Common methods include topical podophyllin, cryotherapy, 5-FU, and surgical and laser removal. Patients should be made aware that they are always infectious, so use of condoms is recommended.

8. Neurogenic Bladder

Clinical Evaluation

History

A thorough history and physical examination is essential in patients with voiding dysfunction. Symptoms present since childhood suggest a congenital lesion. Past medical history should include questions about neurologic conditions, spinal cord injury, or spinal surgery. Patients should be asked about a history of strokes, Parkinson's or multiple sclerosis. Medications affecting urination such as cold medicines, antidepressants and anticholinergics should be inquired about. Prior pelvic, genital or prostatic surgery is also extremely important. Voiding diaries, which record intake and output for 3 days, are very helpful. Frequency, timing and bladder capacity can be determined. Issues of urgency, urge incontinence, frequency, nocturia, urinary tract infections, stone formation and bladder emptying form a basis for a working diagnosis.

Physical Examination

This should include a general neurologic examination, including mental status, motor and sensory examinations. General reflexes as well as the bulbocavernosus reflex (S2-S4) should be tested. Urologic examination should concentrate on palpation for a distended abdomen, and pelvic examination in women to identify perineal skin excoriation, pelvic prolapse and urethra hypermobility. Rectal examination in both sexes is done to check for a bulbocavernosus reflex. Women are also evaluated for rectocele and constipation. Men are evaluated for infection, prostatic enlargement and nodules suggestive of cancer.

Urine Examination

A urinalysis is essential in patients with voiding complaints. Simple reagent strip tests can be misleading. The nitrite test is sensitive only to organisms that convert nitrate to nitrite and thus is only 40%-60% accurate in detecting infection. The leukocyte esterase test is performed to demonstrate presence of leukocytes, indicating inflammation. Bacteriuria is not the only cause of inflammatory cells. These tests should be performed along with microscopic examination of the urine to guide further therapy.

Radiologic Evaluation

Renal ultrasound is used to identify scars, measure kidney size, and to demonstrate signs of obstruction. In patients with neurogenic bladders, ultrasound is useful for following upper tract deterioration. IVU is less commonly used, however it is excellent for evaluating the structure of the upper tracts. Nuclear medicine studies are useful for detecting renal scars, identifying vesicoureteral reflux, and quantifying urinary obstruction. Cystography is important to document reflux, diverticulae, stones and residual urine.

Cystoscopic Examination

Cystoscopy detects stones, urethra and bladder diverticulae, and tumors that may occur as a result of chronic indwelling catheters.

Urodynamic Evaluation

Urodynamics are used to characterize detrusor function, evaluate the bladder outlet and determine activity of the urinary sphincter. The cystometrogram and pressure-flow and sphincter electromyograms are the components of the standard urodynamics study. Occasionally, video examination with contrast and fluoroscopy are added. In general, the studies involve filling the bladder with saline, while simultaneously measuring pressures within the bladder and rectum. Detrusor pressures equal the difference between vesical and rectal pressures. Urinary sphincter activity is measured with skin patches or needle electrodes in the perineal region, and compared to detrusor activity. Bladder capacity, compliance (ability to fill without generating high intravesical pressure) and activity are measured. Pressure-flow studies evaluate how much pressure is required per volume of urine flowing from the bladder during voiding. This helps to differentiate obstruction from a poorly functioning bladder as the cause for weak urination.

Neurologic Disorders

Introduction

Lesions involving different areas of the nervous system produce consistent abnormalities of bladder filling and emptying. Lesions of the brain and brainstem generally result in overactivity of the bladder with normal sensation. Lesions of the spinal cord above S2 usually cause involuntary bladder activity without sensation. Lesions below S2 result in an areflexic, flaccid bladder.

Diseases of the Brain

Cerebrovascular accidents are due to thrombosis, hemorrhage, and occlusion. Incidence is estimated at 6 to 12 per 1000 persons per year. Only 10% exhibit no permanent sequelae. The most common finding is detrusor hyperreflexia. Early incontinence resolves in 75% of cases. Areflexia can also occur. Dementia involves loss of gray and white matter in the frontal lobes, leaving the patient with indifference to voiding and incontinence without any evidence of hyperreflexia. Parkinson's disease is due to a loss of dopamine in the central nervous system. It presents with the typical bradykinesia, but can affect urination in 35%-70% of patients. The clinical picture is one of frequency, urgency, nocturia and incontinence. The bladder is hyperreflexic. TURP should be done with caution.

Diseases of the Spinal Cord

Multiple sclerosis (MS) is a result of demyelination of the neurons, sparing the axons. Of MS patients, at least 50% complain of voiding problems at some time, and for 10% urologic complaints are the first manifestation of the disease. Detrusor hyperreflexia is the most common finding. Treatment involves anticholinergic drugs and clean intermittent catheterization. Still, 10% will require surgery. Spinal cord injury can result in early detrusor flaccidity due to spinal shock. Urinary retention seen with spinal shock can last from days to months. As communication with higher centers returns, the bladder becomes progressively more hyperreflexic, exhibiting involuntary voiding. Damage to the cord above the sacral centers of micturition but below the sympathetic centers results in a bladder that neither stores well nor empties well. The external sphincter is active at the time of voiding, leading to an obstructive picture. Treatment is based on particular factors: bladder distention, bladder storage pressures, leak pressures and presence of reflux. Usually CIC (clean intermittent catheterization) is performed. Injury of the sacral spinal cord usually produces an areflexic bladder; however, decreased compliance may develop. Urethra sphincter tone is fixed and Valsalva voiding is ineffective. CIC and anticholinergic medicine is the usual treatment.

Diseases Below the Spinal Cord

Disc disease causes compression of the spinal roots of L4-L5 or L5-S1. Voiding problems occur up to 18% of the time. These patients complain of difficulty voiding, straining and urinary retention. Laminectomy may not improve bladder function. Urodynamic evaluation should be done pre- and postoperatively. Pelvic surgery results in urinary dysfunction in 10%-60% of patients, with permanent dysfunction in 15%-20%. When dysfunction persists, the pattern is generally a failure of contractility with obstruction from the external striated sphincter. Some develop high bladder pressures and have leakage across an uncontrolled yet weak external sphincter. Patience is mandatory, as dysfunction may be transient. CIC should be performed in the interim. Lastly, diabetes is a common cause of bladder dysfunction. The common picture is of an insensate, compliant, distended bladder, incapable of normal contraction due to prolonged distention. Early on, timed voiding may be helpful to prevent distention.

9. Minimally Invasive Surgery

History

Two decades ago, minimally invasive surgery was pioneered in urology to decrease mortality and morbidity in high-risk patients. Through perseverance, the feasibility and effectiveness of the laparoscopic technique has been shown in many urologic indications such as nephrectomy, adrenalectomy and radical prostatectomy, and is emerging as the standard of care for these procedures, even in low-risk patients, to decrease morbidity. Standard laparoscopy has several inherent limitations. The two-dimensional view of the single lens camera system causes difficulty determining spatial distance and depth, and due to the rigidity of the instrument shaft and the fixed trocar position in the abdominal wall, the degrees of freedom of movement are limited to four. Most significantly, all movements are "counter intuitive" and precise positioning of the endoscope light source remains in the hands of an assistant. Lastly, the tactile feedback from the instrumentation is minimal. Despite initial pessimism due to its difficulty, and longer learning curves, laparoscopic urology has developed into a standardized procedure of choice at many medical centers.

Robotic-assisted Laparoscopic Surgery in Urology

The introduction of the master-slave system of "robotic-assisted" laparoscopic surgery has extended to new and challenging procedures that were difficult due to the drawbacks of standard laparoscopy. Originally developed for performing battlefield open trauma surgery with the surgeon controlling the surgical manipulators from a safe distance, robotic-assisted systems have now been adapted for medical use in the civilian world, initially proven to be effective in cardiac surgery. Robotic laparoscopic surgery offers several advantages over standard laparoscopy for the operator, most notably with "normal" intuitive motion, true 3D high definition color vision, six degrees of freedom, tremor filtering and motion scaling. The master unit allows full range of movement which is transmitted accurately to the surgical arms; indeed, the "wrist" on the robot can rotate beyond human physiologic limits, given its ability to rotate 540 degrees. The robotic system that is FDA-approved for laparoscopic prostatectomy is the da Vinci® system (Intuitive Surgical Inc., Sunnyvale, CA). This system provides the surgeon with a true three-dimensional image providing magnification up to 12x. The entire system is operated from an ergonomic console at which the surgeon sits with his arms and head supported. The stereoscopic viewing system is one of "total immersion" and the control of the camera is by a foot pedal, which is both rapid and accurate. The one major ongoing disadvantage of pure laparoscopic surgery, and even more so with robotic systems, is the lack of tactile feedback for the novice. Through experience, the operating surgeon has to compensate for this by taking visual cues using the endoscopic image. Indeed, for handling tissues and for suturing, it is necessary for the surgeon to "feel" with his eyes; the tension on tissues or sutures is visually estimated rather than felt. Cost is a significant concern as well, as the da Vinci unit runs greater than $1,000,000 plus annual service contract costs.

Laparoscopic Outcomes in Urology

Laparoscopic surgery has significantly decreased patient morbidity in recuperation, blood loss and transfusion rates, in part due to induced pneumoperitoneum during surgery, and reduced lengths of incision. Robotic-assisted radical prostatectomy has shown to be a more easily acquired laparoscopic technique, with shorter learning curves, and now rivals the open procedure as best practice. Less than a decade old, the five year outcomes of robotic prostatectomy are now beginning to emerge, and evidence-based accounting of this and other robotic techniques will have to bear out, if this is a true technical advance in oncologic and quality of life outcomes.

10. References

Ahlering TE, Boyd SD, Skinner DG. Emphysematous pyelonephritis: A 5-year experience with 13 patients. *J Urol*. 1985;134:1086.

Feldman DR, Bosl GJ, Sheinfeld J, Motzer RJ. Medical treatment of advanced testicular cancer. *JAMA*. 2008:299(6):672-684.

Fulgham PF, Ed. Urologic Imaging. *Urol Clin North Am*. 2006;33(3):279-423.

Greene FL, Page DL, Fleming ID, et al, eds. *AJCC Cancer Staging Manual*. 6th Ed. New York, NY:Springer-Velag;2002.

Hohenfellner M, Santucci RA. *Emergencies in Urology*. New York, NY:Springer-Velag;2007.

Kirby RS, Partin AW, Feneley M, Parsons JK. *Prostate Cancer: Principles and Practice*. London, England:Taylor and Francis;2006.

Lapides J. Observations on normal and abnormal bladder physiology. *J Urol*. 1953;70:74.

Loughlin ED, ed. *Complications of Urologic Surgery and Practice*. New York, NY:Informa Healthcare;2007.

McAninch JW, ed. Genitourinary Trauma. *Urol Clin North Am*. 2006;33(1):1-127.

McConnell JD, Roehrborn CG, Bautista OM, et al. The long term effect of Doxazosin, Finasteride and Combination therapy on the clinical progression of Benign Prostatic Hyperplasia. *New Engl J Med*. 2003;349(25):2387-2398.

Mundy AR, Fitzpatrick JM, Neal DE, George NJR. *The Scientific Basis of Urology*, 2nd ed. United Kingdom:Taylor and Francis;2004.

Nickel JC, ed. New Developments in Infection and Inflammation in *Urology. Urol Clin North Am*. 2008;35(1):1-97.

Padzur R, Wagman LD, Camphausen KA, Hoskins WJ. *Cancer Management: A Multidisciplinary Aproach*. 11th ed. Lawrence, KS:CMP Medica; 2008.

Patel VP. *Robotic Urologic Surgery*. London, England:Springer-Verlag;2007.

Pearle MS, ed. Urolithiasis. *Urol Clin North Am*. 2007;34(3):287-453.

Pitts WR, Muecke EC. Horseshoe kidneys: A 40 year experience. *J Urol*. 1975;113:743.

Smith AD, Badlani G, Bagley D, et al. *Smith's Textbook of Endourology*. 2nd ed. Ontario, Canada: BC Decker Inc.;2007.

Stephens FD, Smith ED, Hutson JM. Congenital Anomalies of the Kidney, Urinary and Genital Tracts. 2nd ed., London, England:Martin Dunitz;2002.

Sturgeon CM, Duffy MJ, Stenman UH, et al. National Academy of Clinical Biochemistry laboratory medicine practice guidelines for use of tumor markers in testicular, prostate, colorectal, breast and ovarian cancers. *Clinical Chemistry*. 2008;52 (12):e11-e79.

Tanagho EA, McAnich JW. *Smith's General Urology*. 17th ed. New York, NY:McGraw Medical, New York;2008.

Wein AJ. *Campbell-Walsh Urology*. 9th ed. Philadelphia, PA: Saunders/Elsevier; 2007.

Williams PL, Bannisster LH, Berry MM, et al. *Gray's Anatomy*. 38th ed. New York, NY: Churchill Livingstone; 1995.

Winfield HN. Minimally Invasive Genitourinary Procedures. *Urol Clin North Am*. 2008;35(3):351-533.

11. Questions

1. A 66-year-old man presents with right flank pain. Urinalysis reveals 35 RBC, 25 WBC and moderate bacteria. IVP demonstrates obstruction of the right ureter down to the pelvic brim. His prior surgical history is significant for an aortobifemoral reconstruction. The most likely cause for obstruction is:

   A. Ischemia of the ureter

   B. Pseudoaneurysm formation

   C. Retroperitoneal fibrosis

   D. Ligation of the ureter

   E. Compression by the graft

2. Morbidity following a renal trauma is often due to:

   A. Acute blood loss

   B. Delayed hypertension

   C. Nonurologic injuries

   D. All of the above

3. A 4-year-old boy falls from monkey bars. His physical examination is only significant for pain, tenderness and fullness of his right flank. He has no signs of peritonitis and his urine is absent red cells and white cells. The next step is:

   A. Abdominopelvic CT scan

   B. IVP

   C. Abdominal renal ultrasound

   D. Diagnostic peritoneal lavage (DPL)

   E. Observation

4. A 61-year-old man undergoes an abdominoperineal resection (APR) for colon cancer. Four weeks postoperatively he is complaining of urinary incontinence day and night. He demonstrates a postvoid residual of 410 cc. He has a history of urinary hesitancy and a large prostate on physical examination. The most appropriate next step would be:

   A. TURP

   B. Cystoscopy

   C. IVP

   D. Clean intermittent catheterization

   E. Alpha-blocker and bethanechol

5. A 27-year-old man with Crohn's disease has had recurrent urinary tract infections with multiple organisms for 6 months. The best study to establish a diagnosis is:

   A. Cystoscopy and cystogram

   B. Upper GI with small bowel follow-through

   C. Barium enema

   D. IVP

   E. CT scan

6. A 35-year-old man undergoes an orchiectomy for seminoma. His tumor markers and CT scan are negative. He opts for surveillance. The statement which reflects his outcome over the next 2 years is:

   A. 20% chance of retroperitoneal relapse

   B. 5% chance of pulmonary metastases

   C. Similar relapse rate to patients treated with radiation

D. 50% chance of relapse with nonseminomatous tumor

E. 20% chance of contralateral testicular tumor

7. Approximately what percentage of prostate cancer develops in the peripheral zone?

A. 30%

B. 50%

C. 70%

D. 90%

E. 100%

8. A 54-year-old diabetic woman presents with 2 days of left flank pain and fever. A KUB reveals gas overlying the left kidney. CT scan confirms air in the parenchyma. What is the appropriate management?

A. Emergent nephrectomy

B. Percutaneous drainage of kidney

C. Retrograde ureteral stent placement

D. Broad-spectrum antibiotics and pressors

E. Outpatient therapy with oral antibiotics for 4 weeks

9. The current standard chemotherapeutic regimen for metastatic germ cell tumors is:

A. MOPP (mechlorethamine, oncovin, prednisone and procarbazine)

B. ABVD (doxorubicin, bleomycin, vinblastine and dacarbazine)

C. M-VAC (methotrexate, vinblastine, doxorubicin and cisplatin)

D. PEB (cisplatin, etoposide and bleomycin)

E. CISCA (cisplatin, cytoxan and doxorubicin)

10. Of the five major types of renal calculi, the most common is:

A. Cystine

B. Uric acid

C. Calcium oxalate

D. Calcium phosphate

E. Calcium magnesium ammonium phosphate

Answers

1. C.
Reconstructive vascular procedures have a known risk of ureteral obstruction. Transient obstruction is seen in 12%-30% of procedures and permanent obstruction in 2%-14%. Most develop symptoms within 1 year. Retroperitoneal fibrosis from the surgical procedure is the most common cause of ureteral obstruction. Excessive bleeding and dissection are the most likely reasons for fibrosis.

2. D.
Major renal trauma may be associated with other intrabdominal injuries and post traumatic renal artery obstruction could give rise to hypertension.

3. A.
The most likely injury is avulsion of the renal pelvis at the ureteropelvic junction due to deceleration from the fall. Hematuria is not always present. DPL or renal ultrasound may not identify bleeding from the kidney. Of IVP and CT scan, the CT is more likely to be diagnostic for associated injuries, such as liver or spleen lacerations.

4. D.

Any injury to the pelvic nerves, as in pelvic surgery, results in a flaccid or atonic bladder. Large residual urine volumes are seen. While cystoscopy may demonstrate prostatic obstruction, TURP will not help generate a detrusor contraction. The sphincter and bladder neck are usually less competent so alpha-blockers are not indicated. IVP will only reveal large postvoid residual.

5. E.

Crohn's disease has a 10% incidence of ileovesical fistula. Abdominopelvic CT is an excellent test to demonstrate air in the bladder, thickening of the bladder wall, and a soft tissue mass outside the bladder. Cystoscopy is required, but demonstrates nonspecific erythema and ulceration. IVP is not helpful. While barium enema and cystography may be very helpful, they are often nondiagnostic given the low pressures between the bladder and bowel lumen.

6. A.

With a negative initial CT scan, there is still a 20% chance of having microscopic retroperitoneal disease at the time of orchiectomy that will present later. Pulmonary metastases are uncommon early on. Contralateral tumors are uncommon. Nonseminomatous recurrence is unlikely if there was none in the original specimen and tumor markers are not elevated. Radiation treatment decreases the risk for relapse to 5%.

7. C.

The peripheral zone is the most frequent site of origin of prostate cancer, accounting for about 70% of cases. The central zone is the least common site with approximately 10%, and the transition zone accounts for the remaining 20%.

8. A.

This is the presentation of a patient with emphysematous pyelonephritis. It is common in diabetics. The infection is caused by *E coli*, and *Proteus* and *Klebsiella* spp, which act as facultative anaerobes. Nephrectomy is the standard treatment. Anything less risks the patient's survival, as mortality reaches 50%. Broad-spectrum antibiotics are given in preparation for surgery. Pressors are often necessary to treat sepsis prior to nephrectomy.

9. D.

The original regimen of bleomycin and vinblastine was improved upon in the early 1970s with the addition of cisplatin. Further studies with T3 disease demonstrated that exchange of etoposide for vinblastine further improved survival rates. Three cycles of PEB suffices in most cases. For IgG-GCG classification "good risk" patients can get either 4 cycle EP or 3 cycle BEP. For "intermediate" or "high risk," only BEP x 4 cycles.

10. C.

Calcium oxalate is the most common stone in the developed world (70%). It is radiopaque and easily seen on KUB and CT scan. Calcium phosphate is common in cases of hyperparathyroidism, renal tubular acidosis, and medullary sponge kidney. Magnesium ammonium phosphate stones are also known as struvite or infection stones. They make up 15% of all stones. Uric acid and cystine are rarer at 5% -10% each.